PHARMACEUTICAL PACKAGING
TECHNOLOGY

New and Forthcoming Titles in the Pharmaceutical Sciences

Nuclear Medicine in Pharmaceutical Research, *Perkins & Frier (Eds)* 1999, 0 7484 0688 3 (Hbk)

Electrically Assisted Transdermal and Topical Drug Delivery, *Ajay K. Banga* 1998, 0 7484 0687 5 (Hbk)

Physiological Pharmaceutics Barriers to Drug Absorption (2nd Edition), *Washington & Wilson* 1999, 0 7484 0562 3 (Hbk), 0 7484 0610 7 (Pbk)

Microbial Quality Assurance in Cosmetics, Toiletries and Non-Sterile Pharmaceuticals (2nd Edition), *Baird with Bloomfield (Eds)* 1996, 0 7484 90437 6 (Hbk)

Immunoassay A Practical Guide, *Law (Ed.)* 1996, 0 7484 0560 7 (Hbk)

Cytochromes P450 Structure, Function and Mechanism, *Lewis* 1996, 0 7484 0443 0 (Hbk)

Autonomic Pharmacology, *Broadley* 1996, 0 7484 0556 9 (Hbk)

Pharmaceutical Experimental Design and Interpretation (2nd Edition), *Armstrong & James* 1996, 0 7484 0436 8 (Hbk)

Pharmaceutical Production Facilities (2nd Edition), *Cole* 1998, 0 7484 0438 4 (Hbk)

Pharmaceutical Aspects of Oligonucleotides, *Couvreur & Malvy (Eds)* 2000, 0 7484 0841 X (Hbk)

Pharmaceutical Formulation Development of Peptides and Proteins, *Frokjaer & Hovgaard (Eds)* 2000, 0 7484 0745 6 (Hbk)

Handbook of Microbiological Quality Control in Pharmaceuticals and Medical Devices, *Denyer, Baird & Hodges* 2000, 0 7484 0614 X (Hbk)

full pharmaceutical science catalogue available
or visit our website on: http://www.tandf.co.uk

11 New Fetter Lane
London, EC4P 4EE, UK
Tel: +44 (0)20-7583 9855
Fax: +44 (0)20-7842 2293

29 West 35th Street
New York, NY 10001, USA
Tel: +1 (212) 216 7800
Fax: +1 (212) 564 7854

PHARMACEUTICAL PACKAGING TECHNOLOGY

Edited by

D. A. Dean
Packaging Consultancy, Education and Training, Nottingham, UK

E. R. Evans
Pharmaceutical Quality Assurance Consultant, Wiltshire, UK

I. H. Hall
Packaging Consultant for Pharmaceuticals and Security,
Buckinghamshire, UK

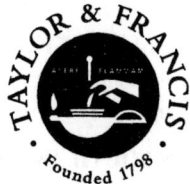

TAYLOR & FRANCIS · Founded 1798 ·

London and New York

SECOND INDIAN REPRINT, 2011

Taylor & Francis is an imprint of the Taylor & Francis Group

© 2000 Taylor & Francis

Printed and bound in India by Nutech Photolithographers

British Library Cataloguing in Publication Data
A catalogue record for this book is available from the British Library

Library of Congress Cataloging in Publication Data
Pharmaceutical packaging technology / edited by D.A. Dean, R. Evans, I. Hall.
p. ; cm.
Includes bibliographical references and index.
ISBN 0-7484-0440-6 (hardback)
1. Drugs – Packaging. I. Dean, D. A. (Dixie A.), 1923- II. Evans, R. (Roy) III. Hall, I. (Ian)
[DNLM: 1. Drug Packaging. 2. Technology, Pharmaceutical. QV 825 P536 2000]
RS159.5 .P495 2000
615'.18--dc21
99-051910

"This book is printed on ECF card and ECF environment-friendly paper manufactured from unconventional and other raw materials sourced from sustainable and identified sources."

FOR SALE IN SOUTH ASIA ONLY.

CONTENTS

CONTRIBUTORS

P. L. Corby
(BA, F.Inst.Pkg.)
Retired

D. A. Dean
(B.Pharm., F.R.Pharm.S., FSS, DBA, F.Inst.Pkg., FIP, SA)
Consultant
Dixie Dean Packaging Consultancy
Education and Training

E. R. Evans
(F.Inst.Pkg., MIQA)
Consultant
Pharmaceutical Quality Assurance

Dr N. Frampton
(Ph.D., C.Chem., MRSC)
Business Development Manager
Ernest Jackson Ltd

Dr J. Glasby
(Ph.D., B.Pharm., BA (Law), M.R.Pharm.S.)
Managing Director
Kendle International Ltd

I. H. Hall
(BA, M.I.Mgt., M.Inst.Pkg.)
Consultant
Packaging Consultants for Pharmaceuticals and Security

PREFACE

For many years, the role of packaging has been low-profile and rarely understood by the general public who, other than at the point of sale, have considered it almost invisible. However, the increasing publicity associated with environmental issues had tended to identify packaging as environmentally unfriendly. This masked the more important and essential roles of the pack, i.e. its influence on product shelf life and the protection it provides against the various hazards which might cause the product to deteriorate.

Although for many years pharmaceutical packaging has been thought to have a rather dull and negative role, it is now being increasingly realised not only that the pack has a very important function, but that pharmaceutical packaging requires an intensity of testing which exceeds that required for all other products. This is necessary to safeguard both the end user, i.e. the professional person or patient, and the company under the general 'product liability' requirements. It is particularly relevant with certain higher risk products, (i.e. IV solutions, injections and implants) and where the pack is increasingly involved in terms of product administration. Often in these circumstances product and pack cannot be segregated.

In trying to provide a broad overview of packaging for pharmaceuticals it will be inevitable, as with any technical or scientific subject, that certain aspects will quickly become out of date. This is especially likely in the area of directives, guidelines, compendial standards, national standards, etc. where attempts to harmonise, standardise and rationalise are constantly ongoing.

The situation is complicated by the fact that the world can be divided according to its purchasing power. This means that the most profitable areas (EU, Japan, USA, etc.) form a significant part of the pharmaceutical market as the more expensive drugs cannot be purchased in developing countries. In terms of packaging, technical weaknesses can be readily highlighted by the fact that problems found and solved in the developed world (even 30–40 years ago) tend to repeat themselves in the less developed territories (e.g. those associated with moving from glass to plastics). This book, therefore, endeavours to span the historical detail of the past as well as giving insight into the trends of tomorrow for the developed world. For example, the problem of environmental stress cracking was experienced in the mid–1950s when detergent solutions moved from metal and glass packaging into plastic. However, the same problem was found 35 years later in a developing country on a very large scale, as people there were unaware of the problem and its solution. Thus while international travel (to the masses) was virtually non-existent before 1960 but is well accepted today, it is suggested that a book on pharmaceutical packaging must involve at least a similar period of history, as learning must start with a certain level of basic knowledge. For example, glass packaging 60 years ago was in an era of long necks, square corners, sunken panels, heavy in weight, to achieve adequate distribution of wall thickness and closed with corks or ground glass stoppers. Today most of these features would be associated with antiquity and poor design. However, some of these designs can still be found in developing countries being manufactured on second- and third-hand equipment which started its life in the developed world. This is common to many industries.

In this book I have drawn from the past 50 years of experience in the packaging industry together with valuable contributions from P. L. Corby, E. R. Evans, N. Frampton, J. Glasby and I. Hall, which in total will provide an in-depth background for the next generations.

One inevitable conclusion is that the subject of pharmaceutical packaging can only become more complex with the passage of time, and hence will need even greater attention to detail.

D. A. Dean

Technical editor's note

Technology is synonymous with change and this is as true of pharmaceutical packaging as it is of electronics.

As this book is finalised for publication, I have seen advisory notices on several new British Standards (e.g. BS EN 12377:1999, Packaging flexible tubes – test methods for the airtightness of closures; and BS EN 14632:1999, Extruded sheets of polyethylene, requirements and test methods). There has been further reference to increased legislation (e.g. regulatory control of suppliers of pharmaceutical starting materials), and I can anticipate that the impending launch of ISO 9000, in its ISO 9000:2000 format, will result in increased customer demands on suppliers.

Compared with the relative price stabilty of oil throughout the 1990s, the year 2000 has been accompanied by continuing price escalation which, if it continues, will eventually filter through to increased plastic costs and the possible decline in some applications where there are alternatives.

A further, possibly even greater change concerns the rationalisation of the pharmaceutical industry where well-known companies apparently disappear and are lost within a new derived company identity. Here it seems too easy to lose the accumulated data, wisdom and experience that went into the creation of a specification, a standard or even a product.

The modern history of packaging is one of change, often but not always leading to improvement, and the readers of this book, particularly those with a career in the supply or use of packaging materials, must above all maintain an awareness of changes to materials, specification, standards and regulatory legislation.

Lastly, a close technical relationship with the supplier(s) is essential, not only for operational efficiency but also to ensure the supplier's/suppliers' appreciation of the implication of uncontrolled change on the stability of the pharmaceutical product.

E. R. Evans

1

AN INTRODUCTION TO PHARMACEUTICAL PACKAGING

D. A. Dean

Introduction

This chapter endeavours to set out the important role of the pack and the need to consider the total packaging operation as part of any drug discovery and development programme. Although demands on the type of pack (material, style, etc.) will vary according to the characteristics of the product; how it is produced and distributed; where, how and to whom it is sold; how it is used/administered; etc., certain factors are shared irrespective of the product classification (i.e. ethical, over the counter (OTC), veterinary, etc.). Pharmaceutical products generally require a standard of packaging which is superior to that of most other products in order to support and comply with their main requirements, i.e. proven efficacy, safety, uniformity, reproducibility, integrity, purity with limited impurities, minimum side-effects coupled to minimum product liability risks, and a good shelf-life stability profile. Since all these terms tend to be well established, but not always fully understood, it may be useful to emphasise the importance of each and its relevance to product pack development. Thus although packaging technology may be a clearly defined discipline, it must have as its basis a thorough understanding of pharmaceutical products generally, the characteristics of formulations and dosage forms, and the general physical and chemical properties of drug substances. Such background detail must include factors associated with medical and marketing input, the methods of manufacture and packaging, warehousing and distribution, sale, the ultimate customer and product use, coupled to adequate profitability. Quality associated with aspects of good manufacturing practice has to be clearly defined at all stages. This chapter therefore starts with some background information.

Uniformity

Uniformity applies within and between batches and usually refers to the quantification of active ingredients, excipients and impurities/degradation. The term applies to the minimum of variation between items, doses, etc., both as active constituents and excipients and any factors which control dissolution, bioavailability, etc. It may be expressed as a percentage of the initial target figure since in this way any relationship with storage time, temperature, etc. can be quantified. However, changes in uniformity or variable uniformity after storage may relate to variations in the product, the pack or the environment.

Purity

Purity today embraces both the percentage of active ingredient and, when possible, the identity and level of impurities present. If one looks back to pharmacopoeias of say 55 years ago it is quite remarkable that in accepting a purity of 99.0%, 98.5%, 95.0%, etc., little attention was paid to the remaining percentage which could consist of impurities or degradation of products related to the process of manufacture and the drug entity itself. Today greater emphasis is placed on the 'other constituents' as by-products of the manufacturing process and/or degradation of the drug or formulation. In the same way that modern analytical methods have made the quantifications of impurities practical, modern chemical techniques have made it more readily possible to separate major impurities. As a result, purer drug substances are being produced today. Impurity levels of 0.1% or more normally have to be identified and safety detail quantified.

Integrity

Integrity covers any assurance that the ingredients are correct in quality and quantity, the formulation is correctly compounded and exhibits the required bioavailability profile, and the pack is to specification and correctly assembled with the quantity of product and the product-pack correctly labelled and identified. Integrity, therefore, covers all aspects related to quality, quantity and security and is thus a function of production and quality control/assurance. Security against counterfeiting has recently increased in importance.

Minimum side-effects

It is perhaps not always recognised that most drugs have some side-effects. Provided these are minor the drug usually will be accepted. This is generally known as a risk–benefit ratio, and therefore varies according to the severity of the disease. A person using a life-extending drug usually accepts side-effects which would be unacceptable for a milder disease. These side-effects may occur from the drug itself or other excipients in the formulation. In this context any move towards simpler formulations, e.g. the removal of colourants, flavours, preservatives, etc., can reduce some of the risks associated with side-effects. Since packaging, by interaction, extraction, or migration may change, add to or even subtract from the product, this can contribute as a side-effect factor.

Good stability with a clearly defined shelf-life profile

Occasionally drugs have a limited shelf life irrespective of the pack used, but at the other extreme, some drug formulations are inherently stable and therefore a pack is needed only to prevent direct contamination, i.e. dirt, dust, bacteria, etc. from the outside atmosphere, and for containment. However, few pharmaceutical products can exist without the supporting role of a pack, as many of the above product factors are not only interdependent with the pack, but ultimately represent a compromise between these and other conflicting needs. Traditionally pharmaceutical products have aimed for a 5 year shelf life where practical, or at least 3 years. General stability is currently supported through the International Conference on Harmonisation (ICH) guidelines.

Some factors that may influence the pharmaceutical pack

Pharmaceutical products and/or their packs can be classified under a number of categories, i.e.

- the type of dosage form
- the route or mode of administration or use
- the type of pack
- the mode of· sale/marketing area
- the mode of dispensing via a combined device/pack
- administration by a device separate to the pack.

Although a brief explanation is given below of these classifications, it can be seen that all are concerned with the broad product–pack interface, hence no method of approach is of necessity better than another.

The type of dosage form is primarily related to the physical state, e.g. solid, liquid or gas, and whether it is sterile, non-sterile, unit dose or multi-dose.

- Solids may be regular, irregular, free-flowing, cohesive, i.e. powders, tablets, capsules, suppositories, etc.
- Liquid or semi-liquid products may be based on water, alcohol, solvents, oils, gels, etc., i.e. emulsions, suspensions, creams, ointments, solutions, etc.
- Gases may be liquefied, pressurised, volatile, inert, i.e. vapours, inhalations, aerosols.

With each group or sub-group, certain basic properties can be identified which lead to specific packaging requirements in terms of both the packaging processes and the materials to be employed.

Route or mode of administration

The route of administration may make certain packaging features desirable or necessary. Possible routes include the following.

- Oral — dispensing, dosing, with absorption/mode of action occurring between mouth and colon.
- Local — topical applications to the skin, hair.
- Parenteral (large and small volume) — sterile products administered intravenously, intramuscularly, intrathecally, subcutaneously, etc., in single or multi-dose packs.
- Orifice introduction — ear, nose, eye, rectal, vaginal, etc.
- Inhalation — via mouth or nose using a face mask, breathing tube or direct inhalation into mouth or lungs.

Type of pack/material

Type of pack can refer to either the basic materials employed, i.e. glass, plastic, metal, etc. or the pack style/type, e.g. bottle, tube, sachet, blister. Packs may provide single (non-reclosable) use, or multi-use (reclosable). Both groups have influences on the product and have to be considered in terms of the material characteristics and the total packaging concept involving such factors as product compatibility, functional and aesthetic design, production performance, material costs, production costs and user convenience.

Mode of sale or market area

The 'sale' of a pharmaceutical product may be by retail (community pharmacy), wholesale, health centre, hospital, dental, health care centres, special homes, home trade or export, etc. These may be further broken down into ethical and over the counter (OTC) sales. Ethical products are normally available only through or via the profession, i.e. pharmacist, doctor, dentist, nurse, veterinarian, etc. They may be supplied either as a bulk pack which is then broken down into a smaller quantity at the patient–dispenser interface or as an original pack whereby a course of treatment is supplied in the pack as produced by the pharmaceutical manufacturer (also called patient pack or unit of use pack).

OTC or proprietary products, as their name suggests, are products designed for direct sale to the general public. How the sale occurs, i.e. through pharmacies, drug stores, etc., largely depends on legal requirements of the country concerned, and how the drug is classified in terms of the prevailing poison enactments, food and drugs legislation, etc.

Pharmaceutical sales may also include bulk quantities of the drug and the compounded drug for further processing, and/or packing in contractors, overseas countries, etc.

The market may involve and be influenced by how an ethical product is paid for, i.e. privately, by national insurance or by some other form of reimbursement through governmental authorities. Markets are also identified by diseases or illnesses which may vary from country to country, continent to continent and be related to age, ethnic origin, sex, etc., i.e. demographic factors.

Packaging may have to be varied to fulfil any of these various needs – for example, tamper resistance or child resistance.

Administration

The mode of dispensing and the use of packs which act as a device are both related to how a product is administered, and the route or mode of administration. To help the administration, the pack may be required to act as a dispensing aid or a device, e.g. an aerosol, or have accessories which can either be made part of the pack or used as a separate unit, e.g. a dropper assembly.

Finally, the pack may either become part of a device, e.g. a cartridge tube which may be used with a reusable or disposable syringe, or have a separate device which administers the product once removed from the pack, e.g. a hand- or power-operated nebuliser.

From this broad introduction it should be recognised that the main objective of most pharmaceutical products is to deliver, introduce or apply a drug of proven stability and safety to a specific site where the most effective activity can be achieved. General investigations to select this dosage form and the dose, by dose ranging studies, must therefore be identified at an early stage in a drug development programme. Prior to formulation of the drug entity, the drug substance should be challenged by a range of factors such as light, temperature range, oxygen, carbon dioxide, water/moisture, so that modes of degradation or physico-chemical change can be established. Formulation then proceeds through a series of stages, such as preformulation studies where any possible interactions between ingredients and the drug entity can be identified, through to formulations which involve feasibility–stability tests and finally to formal stability activities. In the last stage, where the formulation is normally produced on a production scale and packed in the final pack of sale, evaluation is usually carried out on three separately produced batches of the drug, i.e. formal stability. Through all these activities data are gradually accumulated to provide total confidence in terms of the product and the pack, and to satisfy both the company and the regulatory authorities.

Before detailing the broader functions of the pack, the importance of the product–pack relationship cannot be over-emphasised, as it must be considered an essential partnership. Thus any future reference to the pack must ultimately bear some correlation with a product. Most of what follows may appear to be considered in isolation, but in practice this must not occur.

The pack

A pack has a number of functions to perform during its life, including storage, carriage, display, sale, use, etc., all of which require in-depth consideration.

A simple definition of a pack is: a pack is the *economical* means of providing for a *product*

- *presentation*
- *protection*
- *identification/information*
- *convenience/containment/compliance*

until such time as the product is used or administered, paying due attention to any relevant environmental issues.

The term 'pack' in the above covers all the components involved, i.e. the primary or immediate pack which consists of those materials in direct contact with the product. The secondary pack and sometimes tertiary components enable the product to be stored, transported and displayed, and possibly assist use. Tertiary components may include ancillary components, e.g. leaflets or inserts, separate dispensing spoons and measures.

As each of the above contributes to the total function of the pack, the separate factors included in the definition are expanded below.

'Economical'

This term is preferred to that found in some other textbooks – 'minimal (overall) cost' – since a primary function of a pack in certain circumstances (e.g. OTC products) is to maximise both sales and confidence. It can therefore be seen that a pack of minimal cost that limits sales does not meet the prime requirement of all companies – to achieve the highest return on investment (ROI), i.e. profitability. This may be far more effectively achieved by a pack which costs more but shows a significant increase in sales. 'Economical' also covers the total cost, which includes such factors as space used for incoming packaging materials, finished packed stock, handling, labour and distribution. However, as this total costing may vary in the way it is calculated from company to company, material costs, wastage plus production costs, including labour, are widely used for simple initial cost comparisons, i.e. cost as the packed product leaves the production line.

Presentation

Presentation is important in providing confidence and enhancement of the product image. This may be achieved by the aesthetics and/or functional aspects of the pack. The emphasis tends to vary according to the product type, i.e. ethical, semi-ethical, OTC, etc. For instance, an ethical product usually has a high standard of packaging which is relatively simple, elegant, but not over-dressed. On the other hand, an OTC pack which may sell through rigorous advertising may be designed with a view to eye appeal and include a sales gimmick. Pack confidence is often reflected in 'belief' in the medication.

Identification/information

The printed pack or its ancillary printed components (e.g. package inserts) serves the functions of providing both identity and information. Much of this information may have to meet the legal requirements of the country of sale. These are likely to cover some of the following points:

- type of product
- product trade name
- official name, i.e. compendium reference
- strength
- quantity
- mode of usage/administration
- batch number
- expiry date or date of manufacture
- shelf-life declaration
- storage instructions
- contra-indications – precautions
- product licence number/manufacturing licence number
- product category (OTC, ethical, etc.) and GSL, P, POM in the UK
- manufacturer's name and address

- bar code and/or similar security code (UPC, EAN), pharma-code
- warnings (mandatory or voluntary), e.g. 'keep out of the reach of children'
- product formulation, including excipients, preservatives, colourants, etc.

In a pharmaceutical context, information is likely to become a more important aspect, particularly in terms of the pharmacist–patient relationship. Thus although the primary pack may give only the briefest details, more in-depth information will be available both to the professional person, i.e. the pharmacist, nurse or doctor, and the patient. This may be achieved from published literature (which may be collected, for example, by an information service in a hospital), a computer base or the package insert or leaflet. It is therefore envisaged that the final screen for possible incompatibility between prescribed drugs, making the patient aware of possible secondary reactions which arise either directly from the drug or from other combined sources (i.e. drowsiness arising from alcohol and certain antihistamines), will move more towards the responsibility of the pharmacist issuing the product, as a part of counselling. Patient-friendly leaflets are now an EU requirement.

The legality of other information such as storage instructions, how to use the product, how to open/administer the product and reclose the pack may also need additional consideration.

Convenience

Convenience is normally associated with product use or administration. It may be a feature related to the pack, e.g. a metered dose aerosol, or related to the product–pack, e.g. a unit dose eye drop which both eliminates the need for a preservative and reduces risks associated with cross-infection, by administering only a single dose.

A unit dose pack also offers a number of other convenience factors, i.e. no risks associated with opening and reclosing, a few doses can be more readily carried at a time, size of pack, etc. Most pack devices demonstrate convenience advantages over earlier forms of presentation. However, convenience can also be extended to warehousing and production as well as the end user, i.e. in terms of incoming materials, reel-fed packs need less storage space than glass, metal and plastic containers.

Containment

Containment is probably the most basic aspect of any pack. Whereas it was possible in the past to buy certain vegetable drugs, herbs and spices literally unpacked, this is virtually impossible today. Powders, gases and liquids can only be purchased if they are 'contained' in a pack. Remember, a liquid which is not contained is 'a puddle on the floor'.

Compliance

Compliance has recently times become an 'in' word based on the fact that a pack can either detract from or encourage compliance. The advent of the sustained release or delayed release type of product will lead not only to smaller packs, but to a simpler dosage regime that should in theory improve the chances of compliance. This is based on the belief that in taking a product three or four times a day (traditional medication), at least one period could be overlooked. Medication based on delayed or sustained release once or twice daily is currently preferred. This on occasions conflicts with policies which encourage aids aimed at administering the drug to the site where the drug is most effective, giving the fastest response to the symptoms. Thus, rather like packaging, compliance is inevitably a compromise between a selection of factors.

Protection

Protection has been left to last, as it is almost invariably the most important factor and frequently the most complex. Broadly, the pack must afford protection against the following primary hazards:

- *climatic*, i.e. those associated with the surrounding atmosphere
- *biological* – these involve microbiological (bacteria, moulds and yeasts) and biological factors (insects, rodents, human pilferage, etc.)
- *mechanical*, i.e. physical hazards associated with storage, carriage, etc. – general handling
- *chemical* – aspects of interaction and exchange between product and pack, i.e. compatibility, ingress and egress, and combinations of these and the factors above
- *use* – professional and patient, including any possibilities of misuse or abuse.

Many of the individual factors involved tend to be so obvious that there is always a danger that some will be overlooked. The author therefore presents these in a mnemonic form in order to assist memory recall and provide a check list (SCRAP CART MIST MARD).

S – shock
C – compression
R – rattle (vibration) ⎫ Physical hazards associated with storage and carriage, i.e.
A – abrasion ⎬ during loading, unloading, movement, handling, warehousing,
P – puncture ⎭ etc.

C – contamination/compatibility between pack and product
A – ageing (certain combinations involving several sources)
R – rodents or similar animal sources of contamination
T – theft

M – moisture (relative humidity (RH), rain, sea water)
I – insects
S – sunlight or any light sources
T – temperature (extremes)

M – microbiological
A – atmospheric – gases, pressure differentials, dirt, dust, oxygen, carbon dioxide, etc.
R – reuse/recycling/recovery/reduce, i.e. 'the four Rs'
D – disposal – indirect hazards associated with ultimate disposal of pack–product including any pollution risks.

Although the above provides a fairly comprehensive check list, each item requires a fuller explanation.

Physical or mechanical hazards

A product–pack system can either be static (during storage) or in a state of motion (during carriage, handling or use). Physical hazards arising from both can occur at any time to the packaging material, the product and/or the packed product. Any material delivered to the site of a pharmaceutical operation also needs to have attention paid to the way it is packed, handled and delivered. This equally applies to in-house intermediate and bulk products stored prior to packing into smaller quantities. Damage is not therefore solely related to journey hazards, although these are likely to be a prime cause.

Physical or mechanical hazards can be identified as follows.

Shock–impact

Shock or impact arises from a change in velocity. The more rapid the change in terms of acceleration or deceleration, the greater will be the shock or impact applied to the object in question. Normally this deceleration is expressed as the number of times greater than the deceleration due to gravity (g). When the article is broken, the number of g thereby derived is called the G factor, or impact load factor. The aim of the pack, particularly where it acts as a cushion, is to limit the shock conveyed to the product–pack to an acceptable level. Knowledge of how, when and where shock can occur is essential for any packaging study, irrespective of the type of product involved. The severity of damage which may occur varies very much according to the handling facilities and the type of distribution media used in each country. The fragility factor is the maximum force an item (and pack) will withstand before it is damaged to a point where it becomes unusable or non-saleable.

Loads which are distributed in their entirety, e.g. lorries or trucks with fully palletised loads, containerised loads, etc., where movement is minimal during transportation, providing stacking strength is adequate, invariably incur the least risk. Mixed or part loads, items despatched individually or where transhipment occurs, are likely to suffer more damage and hence require a higher standard of protective packaging.

Examples of where shock or impact can occur are as follows:

- drops from tops of pallets, back of trucks, during stacking, loading or unloading, etc.
- impact from slings, hooks, shunting, rapid braking, forks of lifting trucks, etc.

Drops and impacts can usually be visualised from a study of warehousing and the main modes of sophisticated transportation, i.e.

- inland – road, rail, inland waterways
- sea – cargo, tramp, container ships, etc.
- air – cargo, passenger.

However, other forms of transport such as mules, donkeys, camels, horsedrawn cart or bullock cart with solid wheels may be all that is available in less developed countries, and these are less easy to visualise and quantify.

An assessment of drop-impact damage risks can be made by direct observation, self-contained instruments (within packs), and special recording instruments to identify how simulated laboratory tests can ultimately be substituted for travel tests. Data loggers are now capable of recording temperatures, RH, impacts and vibrations.

Compression

Compression is usually associated with stacking. Compression, as with shock, can be approached on a scientific basis by hydraulic compression tests equated with stacking loads. However, other factors may influence what happens in practice, i.e. the evenness of the floor, the type and style of pallet or stillage and, where paper-based outers are used, the temperature and RH of the surrounding atmosphere. In some instances, shock and compression may both be involved.

The height to which items can be stacked will depend on both the outer packaging and whether the item contained therein is rigid or collapsible. Articles such as sachets or plastic containers may require higher strength outer packaging than those containing glass or metal products which will accept high stacking stresses. However, certain points should be borne in mind:

- a pallet of glass containers may be significantly heavier than plastic
- for the same volume of pallet, the plastic container is likely to be 25–30% smaller, hence a greater weight of product can be stacked on the same pallet volume.

Whether a pack suffers from compression depends on both the design of the primary pack and the way it is positioned in the final pack. For instance, blister and strip packs afford little protection to the product if they are placed in a horizontal position, as all the top weight tends to be taken by the product. However, on-edge positioning not only maximises the strength of the packaging material, but also eliminates direct compression of the product.

Top weight or compression which is transmitted through the pack to a primary pack may cause changes and subsequent failure in function of some closuring systems. In turn such compression may provide the necessary stress to cause environmental stress cracking (ESC) should the product contain a stress cracking agent and the packaging material used be prone to ESC. Cracking or damage due to pure physical stress can also occur.

Although compression is obviously a serious hazard, there is a tendency for most pharmaceutical companies to over-pack on the outer packaging. Subsequent reappraisal of the outer packaging may therefore offer substantial cost savings. This is not taken advantage of by many companies.

Vibration

Vibration is defined by frequency and amplitude. At the extremes it can be a 'bump' or a high-frequency vibration. A bump may be a rise and fall of say 1–3 cm, such as may occur when a vehicle travels along a rutted or bumpy road.

Under certain circumstances vibration may cause direct problems with the product, independent of the pack, i.e. segregation of powders, separation of emulsions, surface dulling of tablets, settling down of product, etc. Vibration will also act in combination with compression forces and thereby possibly accelerate the weakening or distortion of board outers, cartons, etc. It can also lead to the distortion of flexible packs such as strips or sachets.

One significant vibratory effect is associated with abrasion or rub, particularly where printed or decorated surfaces are involved. This effect is likely to be more severe on round containers which will revolve (clockwise and anti-clockwise), and move side to side and up and down in either a carton or a divisioned outer. Rectangular or square containers under the same circumstances will usually show less movement. Thus unless the label is recessed, superior rub resistance is usually required for a label on a cylindrical pack.

Vibration, in conjunction with compression, may also cause loosening or leakage from closures. Distortion of flexible materials, i.e. plastic bottles, cartons, etc., which can produce 'high spot' areas where the item bulges, may lead to excessive lateral rub.

Puncture

Puncture, where a pack is penetrated by an internal or external object, is a fairly rare occurrence in the pharmaceutical industry. Although the problem is ever-present from such objects as fork trucks, sharp corners of pallets, slings and hooks, mixed loads inevitably present the more serious risk. The resistance of a pack to penetration can be measured by burst and puncture (swinging pendulum) tests.

Damage caused by the primary pack or a component of the pack on its outer packaging should not be overlooked (i.e. penetration from within the pack).

Climatic hazards

Before proceeding to how the product–pack may have to stand up to certain hazards, it is reasonable to assume that the drug entity, the ingredients associated with the formulation, and the final formulation have been challenged to a range of conditions prior to full packaging investigations being started. It can therefore be expected that the susceptibility to temperature, pressure, oxygen, carbon dioxide, heavy metals, bacteria, mould, pH, etc. has provided guidelines on the sensitivity of the product and its ingredients. This information provides a broad indication of what 'protection' is required. It is essential that the packaging technologist has access to such reports.

Temperature

Let it immediately be said that temperatures cannot strictly be broken into such simple categories as were once envisaged, i.e. 'home' and 'export' markets. The fact that many pharmaceuticals will finish up in the kitchen or bathroom invariably means that extremes of temperature and humidity may be worse in the home than in export-type conditions. Companies should also note that goods transported in the boot or trunk of a representative's car may occasionally reach temperatures in excess of 60°C. If outdoor arctic or antarctic conditions are included, then products may be exposed from −60°C to +60°C depending on the circumstances. As temperature scales used for test conditions frequently bear some relationship with the past, those selected for testing may tend to be related to a rather arbitrary selection or even what manufacturers of cabinets have available. The pharmaceutical industry therefore, until recently, tended to operate to no particular standard and selected from the following conditions for testing purposes:

- $-18\,^\circ$C to $-22\,^\circ$C   deep freeze conditions (arctic, antarctic conditions)
- freeze–thaw   recommended for drug substance
- $4\,^\circ$C   i.e. refrigeration 0–$8\,^\circ$C
- $10\,^\circ$C
- $15\,^\circ$C   (lower temperate)
- $20\,^\circ$C
- $25\,^\circ$C   (upper temperate/lower tropical)
- $30\,^\circ$C
- $37\,^\circ$C or $38\,^\circ$C   (tropical, body temperature)
- $40\,^\circ$C   a preferred condition for certain Japanese tests
- $45\,^\circ$C or $50\,^\circ$C   upper maximums for medium-term storage, i.e. 3–6 months
- $55\,^\circ$C, $60\,^\circ$C, and $80\,^\circ$C   usually short-term upper challenge conditions

The phrases in parentheses, other than body temperature, have evolved by tradition rather than on any scientific basis and should be interpreted accordingly.

Recent investigations based on kinetic mean (km) temperatures have divided the world into four zones:

zone I   km temperature $21\,^\circ$C mean RH 45% (lower temperate Europe)
zone II   km temperature $26\,^\circ$C mean RH 60% (upper temperate Europe)
zone III   km temperature $31\,^\circ$C mean RH 40% (tropical dry)
zone IV   km temperature $31\,^\circ$C mean RH 70% (tropical humid)

These temperatures are usually 'rounded' to $25\,^\circ$C (zones I and II) and $30\,^\circ$C (zones III and IV) for stability-type programmes.

$40\,^\circ$C 75% RH is now being widely adopted as an accelerated condition where practical. It has been used in Japan for many years. The above forms the basis of harmonisation (ICH) investigation carried out by Europe, Japan and the USA.

The use of a series of conditions at $10\,^\circ$C intervals has some advantage, in that chemical changes which follow Arrhenius plots can clearly be identified. However, with the ever-increasing cost of tests there is a tendency either to reduce the range of storage temperatures or, if product–packs are stored over a range of conditions, to limit full analysis to, say, one or two conditions until such time as a change is identified or suspected. Accelerated tests may not proceed to the expected rules, especially where certain plastics are under strain. In these circumstances the strain may be increased by lowering the temperature and reduced (by cold flow) by raising the temperature. In addition, quite a few packaging materials will weaken, break down, or not function properly if consistently stored at temperatures of $45\,^\circ$C and above. Thus certain higher temperature testing may accelerate product degradation through pack breakdown, hence even short-term storage at higher temperatures cannot always provide a scientific means of predicting a shelf life. It should also be noted that testing at an accurately controlled temperature condition does not compare with any actual climate where temperature fluctuations can lead to dimensional and pressure changes which may encourage exchange between the product and the outside atmosphere. Long-term formal stability which uses controlled conditions can therefore be fully justified only if the true effects of temperature, RH and pressure differentials are evaluated in the investigational or feasibility stage of a pack–product assessment. Most formal stability work also involves static conditions, i.e. it does not include effects due to handling, warehousing and distribution.

A few cases where variable conditions may cause changes other than arise from storage at a controlled temperature are:

1   the pack 'breathes' – exchange may be in or out, or both
2   the closure loosens or tightens
3   laminates separate or delaminate, usually starting at the edges.
4   materials 'age' faster.

Declared storage conditions (temperature)

Serious attempts have recently been made to clarify the storage statements used for pharmaceutical products, with a view to eliminating such vague phrases as 'store in a cool dry place'.

Single label statement (no storage temperature statement) is acceptable if product has the ability to withstand temperatures to 30°C (based on support data). Below 30°C, storage statements are necessary, e.g.:

- up to 25°C
- 2–8°C – refrigerate, do not freeze
- below 8°C – refrigerate
- below −5°C – freeze
- below −18°C – deep freeze
- protect from light
- store in a dry place.

These statements formed part of ICH harmonisation discussions, hence there are currently variants on these, i.e.:

- 8–15°C (USA) – a cool place
- 30–40°C (USA) – warm
- above 40°C (USA) – excessive heat.

Controlled room temperature (USA) refers to an expected control between 20 and 25°C with excursions which allow a total range of 15–30°C.

Moisture

There is perhaps a tendency to challenge packs, particularly during storage tests, to higher conditions of controlled RH which may be difficult to equate with a lower 'norm'. Suffice it to say that if the product and pack pass a stringent test, then any subsequent risk may be small. However, failure may make decisions difficult, particularly where a combination of conditions is involved. For instance, the author has experienced a number of occasions where deterioration at 25 °C 75% RH has been greater than at 37 °C 90% RH storage. It might be suggested that higher vapour pressures in the pack at the higher temperatures are playing a different role.

Moisture can exist as either a vapour or a liquid. The latter can be associated with rain, sea water, flooding, etc., or occasions where a reduction in temperature causes dew point to be reached and, literally, a 'shower' within the pack or the surrounding packaging materials. Although water vapour ingress and egress may occur from a variety of causes, the product changes which may result can be extremely diverse, e.g.:

- hydrolysis
- weight gain, e.g. stickiness with sugar-based products
- weight loss – note the increased concentration effect when water or solvent is lost; loss of more volatile constituents can also occur (flavours, alcohol, etc.)
- chemical interaction (e.g. effervescence)
- drying out, caking, hardening, softening
- changes in dissolution, disintegration times
- changes in microbial growth or microbial effectiveness
- dimensional changes, swelling, contraction (packaging and product)
- change in appearance – dulling, loss of gloss
- organoleptic change in flavour or odour
- changes in electrostatic effects – under dry conditions many plastics become more highly charged, and collect dust and dirt.

Exchange of moisture between a pack–product and the surrounding atmosphere may occur for a number of reasons.

1 The closuring system is not fully effective (some moisture exchange is likely to occur with most closure systems, even heat seal systems involving foil laminates may allow low permeation via the edge seals).
2 The materials used are permeable – this occurs to some degree with all plastics.
3 The pack may 'breathe' – not a truly scientific form of terminology but a means of indicating that loss or gain will be increased or reduced by external influences such as changes in temperature and pressure (i.e. where capillary channels may exist in creased heat or cold seals – see (6) below).
4 Increasing or reducing the pressure within a pack, e.g. a reduction of pressure within a pack can occur if a warm or hot fill is employed or if a flexible container is compressed during capping.
5 Changing the atmosphere surrounding the product by absorbing the moisture (e.g. a desiccant or substance which is hygroscopic in nature) or the emission of moisture whereby an equilibrium moisture level between the product and air space is set up. Both absorption and emission may be temperature-dependent.
6 Capillaries and capillary attraction: if folds occur in areas where seals are made, exchange may occur by capillary channels. Similar surface effects can occur with bottles employing an internal plug system. Sinkage or furrows in bottle bores,

which may arise from shrinkage at the thicker thread section, crizzles or hair lines, etc. may all act as an encouragement to capillary-type leakage or seepage.

7 Wicking: this is an expression originally applied to strands of cotton wool which straddle the sealing surface of the bottle. As a result moisture enters (or leaves) via the raw ends of the strands, which literally act as a wick. However, the term has now been extended to any material which will transport moisture via an exposed end. For instance, reels of regenerated cellulose may expand or shrink due to moisture uptake or loss via the raw cut edges (this in turn can change the tension of the reels, whereby machine running performance is drastically impaired).

Whether a product gains or loses moisture depends on its affinity to water, the nature of the pack and the seal, and the RH (or water) in the area which surrounds it. Packs which are basically impermeable, i.e. metal, glass and most types of foil, largely rely on the effectiveness of the seal or closure. The torque of screw closures, for example, may vary according to the temperature and the relative expansion and contraction of differing materials. Increasing the RH differential gradient between the inside and outside of the pack will increase the rate of loss or gain.

The above should further indicate why moisture must be considered as a serious hazard. It should also clearly establish that moisture constitutes a far more critical hazard than the simple effects associated with loss or gain.

Moisture both in the product and in the environment in which the product is produced, processed, packed or used may also be relevant. Thus in some circumstances the apparently simple action of opening and reclosing a pack under an adverse atmosphere may lead to product deterioration.

The atmosphere and atmospheric gases

Although a simple analysis of the atmosphere identifies the main gases as oxygen, carbon dioxide, nitrogen, etc., traces of localised gases cannot be ignored. Oxygen invariably gives the most problems due to oxidative type interactions. In the case of oils and fats, oxidation will lead to rancidity and unpleasant off odours or flavours. Volatile oils are also subject to oxidation to a point where resinification may occur with the production of light brown to black, viscous, possibly odorous, residues. Oxygen can also be absorbed by certain types of product with the result that a headspace may be reduced into a partial vacuum, and materials which are flexible will partially collapse (for example, panelling in low-density polyethylene bottles). Chemical degradation by oxygen may be sometimes avoided or reduced by minimising the headspace (e.g. vacuum packaging), gas flushing with an inert gas such as nitrogen, plus an effective closuring system and correct barrier materials. Oxidative effects may be accelerated by the presence of light, higher temperatures or the presence of catalytic substances. The degradation of Vitamin B_1 is a typical example of an oxidation process that can be accelerated by the presence of copper.

Carbon dioxide, although less of a hazard than oxygen, can act as a weak acid and cause either a pH shift or a reaction with alkaline substances (possible precipitation as carbonates). A pH shift is most likely to occur with non-buffered aqueous solutions stored in materials (e.g. low-density polyethylene bottles) which are highly permeable to carbon dioxide.

Nitrogen, by its inert nature, is not likely to cause any problems. However, it should be recorded that the simple act of nitrogen flushing does not overcome all problems, particularly if the material used is permeable to oxygen and carbon dioxide.

Under this general heading of the atmosphere, it should be noted that a pack has two atmospheres which need consideration, i.e. those internal and external to the pack. Exchange both within the pack and between product and the external atmosphere is usually related to a 'gradient' based on concentration, and pressure differentials between the two.

Changes of internal pressure within a pack, irrespective of whether they are created by the processing (accidental or devised), the product or the environment, therefore need to be carefully monitored. The following are examples.

1   Hot-filling leading to product and airspace contraction/condensation causing a partial vacuum, assuming that significant exchange does not occur via the closure. Flexible containers may show a state of partial collapse, especially if hot-fill is followed by storage under colder conditions.

2   Terminal autoclaving.

   •   Changes in closure efficiency during autoclave cycle whereby the closure may seal less or more effectively at some stage.
   •   Dimensional changes which, due to differential cooling, may lead to pack distortion, i.e. in cooling of pack, hot contents extend pack. Can contribute to the 'dimpling' of plastics.
   •   Pressure in pack (liquid and air space expansion) which is not sufficiently counteracted by over-pressure so that the pack distends and distorts (due to content pressures – airspace and product). Can contribute to the 'dimpling' of plastics.

3   External changes in atmospheric pressure.

   •   Packs filled at sea level then transported to higher altitudes (negative pressure). Can apply to both non-pressurised and pressurised aircraft.
   •   Packs filled at high altitudes then transported to lower altitudes (positive pressure). Can apply to both non-pressurised and pressurised aircraft.

4   Capping a flexible container whereby the container is compressed, flexed or distorted (i.e. squats) to an extent that the content momentarily occupies more volume in the container. Thus if a good seal is then obtained, a partial vacuum can then be created in the pack. This type of operation may be extremely sensitive for plastic containers which show changes in wall thickness and compress (e.g. concertina) easily.

5   Inadequate ullage in the container. This is especially relevant where ingredients either exert high vapour pressures or have high thermal coefficients of expansion (e.g. alcohol).

6   Vacuum packaging – degree and efficiency of vacuum retention.

7   Product change leading to pressure changes (acid/alkali interaction, metal acid/alkali reaction, leading to release of hydrogen or the absorption of oxygen or CO_2 from container headspace etc.).

8   Efficiency of nitrogen flushing – frequently an operation which is difficult to monitor and control. Flushing an empty container then filling tends to be more effective than trying to nitrogen-flush the headspace once filled.

9 Extremes of temperature, particularly when unexpected, e.g. non-insulated vehicle caught in subzero temperatures, warehouses where goods are stacked near heat sources, may cause pressure changes.

10 Filling to incorrect weight, volume, number, whereby product to ullage ratio is adversely altered.

Sunlight/light

Sunlight covers a range of wavelengths from infrared (IR) through the visible spectrum to ultraviolet (UV). While certain packaging materials, e.g. metals and foil, will reflect the IR rays, some colours will absorb IR (e.g. amber glass bottles) and show a corresponding temperature rise. UV offers the most serious risk as it can cause photochemical changes to both the product and the pack. These changes can be visible (discoloration) or invisible. Whereas the effects of light can be accelerated by the use of light sources which intensify all or certain wavelengths (e.g. UV) it is somewhat difficult to divorce such effects from higher temperatures, particularly if IR wavelengths are also involved. Tests using certain accelerated light apparatus (e.g. xenon test), although providing excellent comparative data, are frequently difficult to interpret in the degree of protection from light actually required. It should, however, be noted that most products spend a significant part of their shelf life in a carton surrounded by secondary packaging. Adequate protection from light may therefore be necessary only in the latter or final exposed stages of storage or use. For total exclusion of light it is not sufficient to use opaque materials since thinner papers and board, most plastics except those pigmented with carbon black, and coloured glasses (even amber and actinitic green) do allow the passage of some light waves. Metal-based materials, aluminium, tinplate and aluminium foil provide an absolute barrier.

Selected amber and actinitic green glasses provide substantial protection against the short UV wavelengths provided the glass is of adequate thickness (usually 2 mm or more).

The Japanese recommend that a light test use 1.2×10^6 lux hours as a drug substance–product challenge (now part of the ICH Guidelines).

Ageing

Ageing is used as a general term when either the cause cannot be clearly identified or a combination of climatic effects is involved. Natural rubber materials suffer from ageing, which can be accelerated by the combined effects of light, higher temperatures, oxygen, ozone and moisture in that the elastic properties are lost and the rubber can ultimately become tacky or surface-crazed to a point where it splits or disintegrates when stretched. Many companies now put re-examine dates on packaging materials so that any long-term ageing can be established.

Contamination

Contamination may arise from chemical interaction, organoleptic effects, exchange of ingredients between product and pack, or from particulates or biological–microbiological causes. Further details of some of these are given below.

Particulate contamination

Under the broad terminology of atmospheric contamination, both microbiological and particulate airborne contamination can be considered. These two aspects should partly be considered together, especially as microbial contamination will frequently increase or reduce according to the 'cleanliness' of both the product and the pack, i.e. particulates can be a bioburden carrier.

Particulate contamination, although mainly airborne, can also arise when materials are cut, torn, rubbed, fractured, punctured or penetrated. In these cases any airborne phase may be either short or non-existent, i.e. direct contamination can occur. However, for the purpose of this preview, particulate contamination will be related to how it may arise.

Airborne environmental sources

Dirt, dust, fibres, grit and hairs are ever-present in a non-filtered atmosphere and vary from submicrometre, invisible particles to visible, clearly definable units. Particles of below 50 μm are not easily seen by persons with normal eyes. Contamination from the environment is also dependent on the prevailing atmospheric conditions and any electrical charges carried by the particles and the materials which may become contaminated. Such charges are usually increased by dry, low-RH conditions and lessen as humidity rises.

Environmental sources – not airborne

As above but with the inclusion of larger particles or agglomerates which contaminate by direct contact, i.e. placing a product or component onto a precontaminated surface. Particles may adhere initially by gravity, electrical charges, or due to the adhesive nature of the surface or particle.

Contamination arising from physical actions

Examples are as follows.

- Fracturing, breaking, e.g. glass fragments arising from the opening of a glass ampoule.
- Sawing, cutting, tearing, e.g. paper fibres from paper (cellulosic) based products.
- Abrasion/vibration – between the same or different surfaces; aluminium, for example, is particularly prone to abrasion from both a raw edge and a flat surface.
- Rubber also suffers from a form of abrasion when a needle passes through it, i.e. fragmentation.
- Removal of surface acting substances from plastics, e.g. lubricants, slip additives, such as stearamide, stearates, anti-static agents.

Contamination arising from the fabrication processes

Although fabrication processes may involve some of the examples in the above list, certain processes may further encourage contamination, e.g. trimming metal, paper, board, etc.; flash from trimmed and untrimmed plastic components, flash from residues from tumbling or freeze tumbling operations; friction-generating processes, shaping, swaging, seaming, extruding, cutting dies, grinding, polishing, excessive handling.

Contamination arising from in-house production and processing (including packaging) operations

For example, excessive rubbing of plastic materials may induce high static charges, thereby increasing the attraction of particles. Unscrambling and printing can also be a source of particulates.

Chemical contamination

For example, a partially corroded metal surface from which particles of corroded metal can become detached.

Avoidance or elimination of particulate contamination

Minimising particulate contamination is obviously related to the product–pack form, the type and source of contamination, and the environment. Although adequate control of these will produce a relatively particle-free situation (i.e. prevention), either the introduction of processes to eliminate contamination or a combination of relatively clean materials plus limited processing may be equally acceptable. The latter may therefore involve a number of cleaning type activities, i.e. dry oil-free air blowing of components plus vacuum extraction. Alternatively, washing with water or water plus detergents with an adequate rinsing procedure followed by drying may be used. Drying may vary between air drying, hot air drying with or without filtered air, etc. As hot air drying tends to produce high levels of static, recontamination at the drying stage represents a high risk unless the area and atmosphere are reasonably particle-free. This risk is particularly significant with plastics. Producing sealed preformed containers which are opened immediately prior to filling and resealing, e.g. closed ampoules, is a further option that is becoming increasingly available.

Solvent washing

Provided materials are compatible with solvents, solvent washing is a useful alternative to water, especially where surface residues (oils, greases, lubricants, release agents) may either act as an adhesive bond for particles or give rise to a form of chemical contamination.

Ultrasonic washing

An effective cleaning process can, under certain conditions, create particles. Ultrasonic energy usually detaches particles into a liquid, thus diluting the particle population.

Fixing particles

This can be done by annealing or firing (i.e. fixing glass particles on to glass), burning off organic matter (glass), lacquering or coating.

Avoidance of electrostatic build-up

This can be achieved by neutralising charges, i.e. use of ionised air, raising the humidity or using material incorporating anti-static additives (plastics).

As indicated previously, the alternative to cleaning is producing a material/product and/or pack under clean conditions. To achieve this in totality means that all operations must match those of a sterile or aseptic type of process in terms of cleanliness. However, as this is not totally practical, attention to special detail, such as filtered air to feed plastic moulding equipment, production under laminar flow and positive air pressure, avoidance of draughts, minimum of handling by operators and good housekeeping goes a long way towards cleaner manufacture.

Before any efforts are made to reduce contamination, knowledge of the materials, the processes by which they are made, the packaging materials in which they may be packed, how such packs may be opened, removed/unscrambled, etc., are an essential part of total control. Basically these are all part of good manufacturing practice (GMP). However, before this can be done some agreement must be reached on what constitutes contamination and how it may be detected.

Detection options

1. Visual observation – largely dependent on the eye sight of the operator; tends to be very subjective.
2. Visual under low magnification, i.e. 2–10 times magnification, including use of hand lenses with and without graticules.
3. Polarised light – with and without magnification.
4. Microscope – low- to high-power magnification.
5. Counters, which operate on a number of principles:

   - electrical resistivity, e.g. Coulter counter
   - light scattering, Royco
   - light blockage, Royco, HIAC
   - lasers, e.g. Malvern.

These may require the particles to be suspended in a solution, hence in terms of containers and components results are dependent on how the particles are removed from the surfaces to the solutions.

There is no obvious standardisation on levels of particulate matter permitted in a product.

EXAMPLE 1. EYE OINTMENT – TEST ON PRODUCT

British Pharmacopoeia (BP): this takes an approximate 10 mg smear on a microscope slide with the following acceptance limits. Number of particles:

- not greater than 25 μm – 20
- not greater than 50 μm – 2
- not greater than 90 μm – none.

BS 4237 applies limits to metal fragments in collapsible tubes.

United States Pharmacopoeia (USP): This takes the contents of ten tubes which are melted in separate Petri dishes, cooled and inverted. Examined under 30× magnification, and particles of 50 μm and more measured. The test is passed if particles do not exceed 50 for ten tubes and not more than one tube has eight particles. If test fails, twenty further tubes are taken. The test passes if the particles do not exceed 150 for thirty tubes and not more than three tubes have eight or more particles.

EXAMPLE 2. IV SOLUTIONS

The USP uses a filtration technique whereby the particles are retained by a membrane filter and then measured under 100× magnification. Particles are gauged by their effective linear dimension. Limits are:

- not more than fifty particles equal to or greater than 10 μm
- not more than fifty particles equal to or greater than 25 μm.

The BP 1980 test permits the use of an instrument based on either:

1 electrical zone – sensing principle, i.e. Coulter counter, or
2 the light blockage principle.

Different limits are specified for each method. These limits are:

1 not more than 1,000 greater than 2 μm and not more than 100 greater than 5 μm
2 not more than 500 greater than 2 μm and not more than eighty greater than 5 μm.

Both estimated per ml of undiluted solution.

Finally it should be noted that whatever the methods of particulate detection employed, each remains a somewhat subjective judgement and is constantly being updated.

Biological contamination

Under this heading the following will be considered:

1 insects, including termites
2 animals, including rodents
3 human pilferage, adulteration, etc.
4 moulds, bacteria and yeasts, i.e. microbiological aspects (bioburden).

Insects

While drugs are still obtained from vegetable and animal origins, some contamination risks from insects etc. will remain. The frequent gassing of stores and warehouses has done much to reduce the general level of infestation.

The types of insect that create the most damage are moths and small beetles. Moths and flying insects in general can be minimised by control of doors, windows, etc., or through use of 'Insectocuters' etc. Termites are of minute size and usually exist in very large colonies, in total darkness, attacking paper, board and wood-based materials, and require specialist attention. Traps for crawling insects are also available.

Animals

Damage caused by animals in general and rodents in particular may relate to penetration (leading to possible product spillage) or general fouling leading to an unhygienic situation.

Bulk stored and transported items tend to be more prone to infestation by insects and animals. Attention to properly maintained storage conditions is essential if infestation and general fouling is to be prevented.

Pilferage

As the pilferage of pharmaceutical products can be a profitable business, particularly with highly priced items in countries of either high unemployment or low wages, the use of tamper-resistant (a preferred term to pilfer-proof) closures or packs may be advised. Such systems may also be used and are indeed a mandatory requirement with certain sterile products to indicate that the container seal has not been disturbed and the product has not been subjected to contamination from external sources.

Tamper resistance and adulteration

The Tylenol incidents of 1982 caused serious concern to governments and the pharmaceutical industry in particular. The USA immediately brought in legislation (5 November 1982) to ensure that OTC products had some form of tamper evidence, with 1984 as a deadline for virtually all OTC and certain cosmetic and toiletry products. Tamper-evident seals at that time included glued or taped cartons (provided a fibre tearing seal was achieved), carton (film) overwraps (clear material had to be printed with a recognised design), diaphragm seals, various closure break systems, shrink seals or bands, sealed tubes (i.e. collapsible metal tube with a blind end), pouches, blisters, bubbles or strips, etc. All had to show some distinct form of evidence of having been tampered with or opened. Each pack also has to indicate (in print) the primary means by which tamper evidence had been achieved. Although as part of a pharmaceutical image the legislation may appear ethically sound, virtually all systems can be circumnavigated by a skilful and dedicated person via an alternative route to the main closure system. The customer opening the pack may not always observe the state of the tamper-evident seal, particularly if it is carefully and cunningly replaced.

Microbiological aspects

Microbiological aspects of pharmaceuticals are of importance not only to sterile products but to all products, in that gross contamination should be avoided irrespective of how the product is used or administered. Although bacteria, moulds and yeasts constitute the major sources of contamination, pyrogens are also included under this heading.

Bacteria are widely distributed in all surroundings unless special precautions are taken to eliminate or partially exclude them. Bacteria can be pathogenic (disease-producing organisms), non-pathogenic or commensals (i.e. bacteria which occur naturally on or in the body without doing any obvious harm). Some bacteria may produce dormant forms of spores which are very resistant to heat and disinfectants, hence are more difficult to destroy.

METABOLISM OF BACTERIA

Bacterial cells are nuclear structures bounded by a cell wall. Although as with other cellular structures the moisture content is high (75–90%) other constituents may include sulphate, silica, sodium, phosphorus, potassium, magnesium, calcium, chloride, carbohydrates, fats and lipids.

In order to survive, bacteria require water (free liquid water), food (usually in the form of organic substates with a supply of nitrogen and carbon), particular temperature conditions and certain atmospheric gases.

Some bacteria will only grow in the presence of oxygen and are known as obligatory aerobes. Those which will grow in either the presence or absence of oxygen are called facultative anaerobes; those which will only grow in the absence of oxygen are obligatory anaerobes. A few bacteria will only grow in the presence of relatively large amounts of carbon dioxide. pH is also critical for the survival and growth of most bacteria with the optimum range being pH 7.0–7.8 for many and pH 5.0–8.0 covering most pathogenic types. However, some bacteria will flourish at abnormally low or high pHs. As with human beings, bacteria have a definitive life cycle.

TEMPERATURE

The normal growth temperature for most bacteria is 15–40°C, with pathogenic organisms growing best at 37°C. A few bacteria, called thermophilic, can live at temperatures of 45–70°C. Bacteria can, however, generally withstand low temperatures and remain viable. Bacteria can be killed by exposure to high temperatures which can be quantified as a time–temperature reaction: the higher the temperature, the shorter the kill time (see 'Sterilisation' below).

LIGHT

Light frequently inhibits the growth of bacteria, although there are species which readily survive in the light (UV light has surface sterilising properties).

MOULDS AND FUNGI

Moulds and fungi consist of filaments or masses of filaments of one cell in width which initially extend as hyphae, branch and grow and form a readily visible colony mass known as mycelium. This in turn produces spores on the surface either by sporangium or conidiospores, or by a process of reproduction. Moulds can produce enzymes which break down surrounding substances, which can be then adsorbed as a food. Some acids can be made by fungal fermentation. Such acidic excretions can lead to corrosion of metal-based materials. Moulds require similar conditions of growth to bacteria, except that high RH is necessary rather than liquid water. Properties of moulds are as follows.

1   Best growth condition is around 25°C; moulds are less resistant to low and high temperatures.
2   Moulds do not need liquid water but will use atmospheric moisture. An RH of 75% and above is usually necessary.
3   A source of organic food which includes fairly simple chemical substances is required.
4   All moulds require oxygen, although some will grow under relatively low concentrations.
5   Some moulds will grow under both light and dark conditions. Others will be either inhibited or stimulated by one of these conditions.
6   Moulds will tolerate wide ranges of pH, with a preference towards acid medium. Some not only produce acidic substances but will survive in a relatively low pH (e.g. in vinegar).

YEASTS

Although yeasts are basically closely aligned to moulds and fungi, they frequently exist in an unicellular form. Yeasts ferment sugars forming alcohols, and will grow in high CO_2 concentrations.

The above outline on the characteristics of bacteria, moulds, fungi and yeasts is necessary to understand:

1   the requirements of sterile products and aseptic packaging
2   the need to minimise microbiological contamination and the involvement of GMP and good laboratory practice (GLP)
3   how these organisms can survive and hence be controlled
4   the special pack characteristics associated with the above.

An obvious way of controlling organisms relates to aspects of cleanliness, good hygiene and the removal or control of those factors which are necessary to the survival of viable organisms, i.e.:

•   removal of moisture

- removal of oxygen (note that certain organisms can still survive)
- removal of nutrients (unless product itself provides a nutrient base).

It should be immediately seen that the pack must be an effective barrier to moisture and gases so that entry does not support growth or, if the product is made sterile, re-entry of bioburden is prevented. Control can also be exerted by the use of preservative systems. These may involve disinfectants, germicides, bactericides (kill bacteria), fungicides (kill fungi, mould or yeasts) and bacteriostatics (inhibit growth but do not necessarily have a significant rate of kill). The activity of any preservative system is influenced by concentration, temperature, time in contact, the test organisms (or the contaminating organisms), the pH, presence or absence of organic matter, and surface tension (wetting power) of the solution. Other factors may be involved, e.g. effects related to the drug entity, the presence of other ingredients such as EDTA, which can increase the effectiveness of certain preservative systems, etc. (e.g. benzalkonium chloride). Typical preservatives include:

- mercurial compounds – inorganic and organic
- medicinal dyes
- phenols and chlorophenols, i.e. phenols, cresols, chlorocresol, chloroxylenol
- anionic and cationic detergents.

Product changes which may be related to the pack characteristics can reduce (or increase) the microbial effectiveness of a product. Examples include adsorption and absorption of preservatives with plastics, and the change of pH due to the passage of carbon dioxide through certain plastics.

Sterilisation

Sterilisation is the finite method for microbial control and can be achieved either by sterilising each component (product and packaging materials) followed by assembly, i.e. aseptic processing, or by a terminal sterilising process which involves both product and pack. The latter is the preferred method as it entails less risk of a non-sterile product being produced.
    These processes of sterilization are used in pharmaceutical production:

1   dry heat (160–180°C) for 1 h or more
2   moist heat (autoclaving) 115–118°C for 30 min or 121–123°C for 15 min or an appropriate temperature/time cycle; high-pressure steam is also employed
3   filtration (of liquids) by use of a 0.2 μm filter
4   irradiation, either gamma irradiation or accelerated electrons (beta irradiation)
5   gas treatment (ethylene oxide)
6   heating with a bactericide
7   UV (non-official).

Heat and irradiation

Each of these processes imposes different demands on the packaging materials. Dry heat (temperatures of 160–180°) can only be withstood by glass, metals and a few selected plastics. Glass often uses 320°C or slightly higher for 3–4 min.

Autoclaving by moist heat involves the effects of temperature, expansion and contraction, pressure differentials and moisture. Gamma irradiation of 2.5 Mrad (25 kGy) can be used to sterilise materials and filled packs. Packaging materials sterilised by this process are normally double-sealed in a polythene bag, in a second sealed polythene bag within a fibre board outer. This enables the outer bag to be removed in a non-sterile area; the inner bag and contents may then be passed through a hatch to a sterile area where the inner bag is removed. Gamma irradiation normally uses a cobalt 60 source of 2.5 Mrad. The rays will penetrate most materials. Caution is, however, required as many of the possible effects have not been fully identified or quantified. Glass, for example, is darkened to the extent that white flint glass becomes a smoky grey-brown and amber changes to almost black. Although this discoloration tends to fade with time, the appearance remains unsightly and variable from container to container. Paper-based materials are reported as not being affected, but as these are usually only used for the secondary packaging operation, any change is less critical. Rubber, other than certain synthetic grades, is generally listed as suitable for gamma irradiation. With the increase in the use of plastics, many of which are aseptically processed, the question as to whether irradiation can be employed is very important. For example, certain polymers pronounced as suitable have been found to have some grades which are either unsuitable or suitable only for certain products. Thermosets, thermoplastics and their suitability for each process of sterilisation are more fully covered in Chapter 7. Suffice it to say, at this stage, that as the use of gamma irradiation is extended, further detail as to possible packaging material changes will be identified. To approve the irradiation of a filled pack requires additional attention to safety and the identification of any possible degradation compounds associated with the product.

An alternative method of irradiation sterilisation is the use of accelerated electrons, i.e. beta irradiation. This generally has a milder effect on both the product and the packaging material than gamma irradiation. Although it has less penetrating power than the latter, it is equally effective in terms of sterilisation. The cycle time is short (seconds) whereas gamma irradiation takes hours. UV rays have been used to control microbial growth in liquids flowing through narrow tubes, e.g. water.

Gaseous sterilisation

Although several gases will kill bacteria (ethylene oxide, formaldehyde, propylene oxide), ethylene oxide is the one which has been most widely adopted for pharmaceuticals, instruments, and dressings. Sterilisation by ethylene oxide involves either a gas concentration of 10–20% with an inert gas such as carbon dioxide or nitrogen, or the gas in a pure state. The dilution method is usually preferred, particularly as ethylene oxide can form an explosive mixture with air.

For the lower concentrations of ethylene oxide a temperature of 50–60°C is employed, together with a degree of humidification, as moisture assists the penetration of the gas. The exposure time for the above is normally around 16 h. Degassing can be achieved by forced aeration, vacuum cycles or storage for a period (7–14 days) in a well-ventilated area to allow natural degassing. However, the material being sterilised must be permeable to the gas.

Virtually all sterilisation processes impose some hazard or risk of adverse effects on the packaging material, and they all need study before they can be pronounced as completely satisfactory. Those processes which may be critical to a particular material will be reviewed in great detail in the respective material section.

Pyrogens

Pyrogens are mainly liposaccharide components of dead gram negative bacterial cell walls which can cause disease and temperature increase. They are difficult to destroy (dry heat temperatures of 250°C and above are required) and are detected by either the rabbit injection test or the LAL test (Limulus amoebocyte lysate), the latter now being the preferred test. Keeping microbiological contamination low is an essential part of reducing pyrogens to a minimum. Preventing such contamination (microbial entry or re-entry) therefore partly relies on the type of pack employed.

Chemical hazards and compatibility

Compatibility basically covers any exchange which will occur either between product and pack or between pack and product. Incompatibility may be associated with inter-action, migration, leaching, adsorption, absorption, extraction, whereby ingredients may be lost, gained, or chemically or physically altered. Such exchanges may be identi-fied as organoleptic changes, increase in toxicity/irritancy, loss or gain of microbial effectiveness, precipitation, haze, turbidity, colour change, pH shift, degradation, etc. Again other external influences may catalyse, induce or even nullify chemical changes. Chemical changes may also be followed by further chemical reactions.

Chemical interaction or contamination can also arise from impurities in the ingredi-ents, accidental ingredients arising from the production processes, or abrasion between contact surfaces. Examples of these are, respectively, as follows.

1   An oxidative reaction accelerated by the presence of low levels of copper.
2   Contamination arising from the extraction of plasticisers from PVC pipelines.
3   A bulk product involving a clarity of solution test was packed in a low-density polyethy-lene bag inside a metal drum. On reaching its destination the product failed the clarity of solution test. This was traced to a lubricant in the polyethylene which achieved its effect by being present at the surface of the film. During transportation the lubricant was physically removed from the film surface, by vibration with the solid product.

Other examples of incompatibility or partial incompatibility are as follows.

- Adsorption of chemical entities onto component surfaces which are frequently related to the surface areas involved – losses of EDTA and certain preservatives have been known to occur due to surface adsorption.
- Absorption and surface evaporation. The more volatile preservatives, e.g. chlorbu-tol, phenol, 2-phenylethanol, show fairly rapid loss through low-density polythene. If an external overwrap which is not permeable to the preservative is used, the loss can be restricted to relatively low levels, i.e. less than 10%.
- Other surface active ingredients which may be found in plastic materials and suffer loss into product by solution, surface abrasion, etc. include anti-static additives, slip additives, mould release agents, etc.

- Detachment of glass spicules may occur when alkaline solutions of citrates, tartrates, chlorides or salicylates are stored in soda glass containers. It may occasionally occur when treated glass is autoclaved in the presence of similar alkaline salts.
- Organoleptic changes – permeation of volatile or odorous substances through plastic materials (conversely to loss of perfume through plastic containers).

Environmental issues

To complete this introductory chapter, attention must be drawn to certain environmental issues. These are receiving increasing publicity, and include:

- conservation of the earth's natural resources (renewable and non-renewable)
- conservation of energy and minimum use of energy
- minimising pollution, from raw material production to pack disposal
- disposal of packaging materials following fulfilment of purpose
- modes of material disposal and recovery, including recycling, reuse, and chemical recovery
- packaging as a prime cause of litter.

These have recently been emphasised under the 'four Rs' of recovery, recycling, reuse and reduce (the materials involved).

As the packaging technologist of the future will certainly be required to have a basic understanding of these and life cycle analysis (LCA), some explanations are offered. All processes involve the use of energy irrespective of whether the energy can be related to a mechanical, chemical, biological, electrical or environmental activity. Thus any packaging material can be quantified in terms of total energy arising from the processes associated with obtaining the raw material, conversion into a finished container and the auxiliary activities related to storage, transportation, etc. One early estimate on the energy involved for a range of material/containers is given later. However, figures will vary considerably for individual containers depending on size to weight ratio, the conversion process employed, the distance materials are transported, etc., and therefore figures may have to be continually updated as new data become available, usually as part of life cycle analysis. They do provide a broad guide and readily reveal the more energy-intensive activities in the life span of a packaging material.

Once a packaging material has completed its function, i.e. the product has been removed or administered, the next critical question is the disposal or recovery of the material(s). This may appear to be the simple act of placing the materials in the dustbin or garbage can. However, consideration must be given to whether the material is best recycled, reused, used in part or whole to generate some form of energy, or broken down into a reusable chemical form. Until recently, disposal in a dustbin subsequently led to one of the following means of disposal. In Europe this is covered by The Packaging and Packaging Waste Directive 94/62/EC.

Open dumping – a rather primitive method for solid waste disposal whereby the material is left to break down naturally or deliberately fired to reduce volume. Since both constitute health hazards (rats, mice, etc. and noxious fumes), open dumping is not encouraged.

Sanitary landfill – this mainly uses large holes in the ground and prepared areas where the top soil has been set aside for reclamation. Once the holes are filled, the surface can be covered with the top soil and eventually reused. However landfill can still generate undesirable gases, e.g. methane.

Incineration – this is a process of controlled combustion (contrast with direct burning) whereby any release of atmospheric pollutants (carbon, noxious gases, etc.) is kept to a minimum. The heat generated in the burning process can be used as an energy source. Modern sophisticated incinerators are, however, very costly to install and maintain. Experiments continue to establish how energy released in the process can be maximised and costs of running incineration plants minimised. Segregation of certain low-energy materials is now preferred.

Composting – this normally consists of a grinding or breaking down process to give a fairly fine–coarse mixture of compost involving most of the materials found in the dustbin. Although the resulting compost has good agricultural/horticultural applications, the process is again relatively energy-intensive for what is achieved.

In the UK, landfill, incineration and composting are the normal disposal processes (ratio approximately 86 : 13 : 1). However, segregation of waste to encourage recycling and reuse (returnable containers) now has more emphasis, with landfill and incineration being seen as poor substitutes (a general but not finally approved opinion).

Reuse – this describes a practice whereby a container is returned, cleaned and used for the same or a similar product over a number of trips, as has been used for such products as milk and beer for many years. Initially this may appear the route to use for many other containers, and attempts have been made within the EU and in Oregon to bring in legislation to introduce deposit systems to encourage the return of the more widely used packs (particularly glass). However, when the proposition is studied in greater detail it becomes less clear how the advantages and disadvantages can be further quantified. For example, the UK milk bottle only remains economical if the trip-page is above fifteen and the bottles are collected on a regular basis. Once the milk bottle reaches the dairy, energy is involved in the cleaning process (hot water) and significant quantities of detergents, alkalis, water, etc. are necessary to guarantee a clean, hygienic container. These chemicals can be considered as industrial pollutants if they reach the normal effluent systems in quantity, unless they are subjected to further treatment processes. However, it must be recognised that milk bottles (and beer bottles for that matter) are specific products where reuse has been calculated and built into all stages, from sale to return. Return of many food-type containers would mean that retail outlets would not only have to build special storage extensions or reduce selling space, but also allocate staff to the segregation of containers and keeping the areas clean and sanitary, otherwise vermin, moulds and bacteria could produce a most unhygienic situation. One can immediately see that legislation would ultimately be required to control such areas which otherwise could create a hygiene risk to the main selling area. There would be a need not only for capital investment but also for labour resources to return deposits, segregate various types of containers, take stock of types and quantities, arrange returns with invoices, etc., plus other transportation and handling costs etc. No doubt retail pharmacists who have been involved with the simpler return of glass dispensing containers will appreciate the complexities of larger scale reuse.

The above should serve two purposes: establish that the reuse of containers is not as simple as first envisaged, and indicate that the recycling of materials may become a

Table 1.1 Recycling prospects and requirements of basic materials

Material	Requirements	Comments on recovery
Soda glass	Segregation into colour. Removal of closures (metal). Removal of labels. Removal of more toxic contents! Options: wash cullet; add scrubbing towers to melters.	High temperatures, process burns off virtually all impurities (into the atmosphere). Hygienic process. No known deterioration of properties. Recovery value £40–50 per tonne.
Neutral glass	Has a higher melt temperature than soda glass. Not readily distinguishable from soda glass. Could change properties if contaminated with soda glass or vice versa.	As soda glass, but would need guarantee on material in order to be further used for pharmaceuticals.
Paper board	Can readily be repulped. Requires segregation from plastic, foil, etc. Total removal of contaminants including inks present some difficulties.	Difficult to maintain high-quality, high-purity material, but suitable for slightly downgraded usage. Constant recycling reduces fibre length, hence reduces strength. Recovery value varies from £25 to £100 per tonne depending on quality.
Aluminium	Non-magnetic. Various alloys of aluminium not easily distinguished. Highly energy-intensive, basic material.	High melt temperature, removes virtually all impurities, but possible pollutant source. Recovery value £600–700 per tonne.
Tin plate	Magnetic separation possible. Separation of tin from steel required, otherwise basic characteristics will change.	Recovery of tin from basic steel plate economical provided cost of tin remains high. High temperatures as for aluminium.
Plastics	Suitable for virgin machine scrap where regrind is permitted. Used plastics highly likely to be contaminated. Individual plastic types difficult to identify, unless adequately coded.	Regrind only used when permission is given (pharmaceutically). Increasing use as a middle layer. Certain plastics may be mixed for downgraded usages. Unsuitable for pharmaceutical primary packs. Difficult to remove contaminants. Recovery value varies – mixed £40–60 per tonne.
Composites	May consist of mixtures of paper, board, plastic and metal. Multiple coextrusions present obvious difficulties.	Unless components are easily segregated or separation can be done mechanically, recovery generally is not economically favourable – may be economic if metal component is aluminium.

more logical way of limiting the depletion of the earth's natural resources. Recycling can be defined as the recovery of a basic material which can be reprocessed into a further usage. The ability of a material to be recycled varies considerably. Glass, which is most readily recyclable, is the least energy-intensive of the packaging materials. Aluminium is the most energy-intensive material, therefore may more readily justify recovery. Table 1.1 provides a summary of the recycling prospects of the major materials.

The future packaging technologist may therefore have to consider disposal as part of the brief and even design the pack from materials with the most effective disposal or recovery in mind. To this end, the material factors which have to be considered may include the following:

- energy used to obtain the basic raw material
- waste value
- weight/density
- volume
- crushability
- separability
- combustibility
- risks relative to material contamination (from product)
- material changes (physical and chemical) which may result from reuse or recycling, i.e. whether the material will be downgraded by reprocessing, impurities, contaminants, etc.

These factors are relatively complex, and as yet no simple approach is obvious nor have the factors been fully evaluated and quantified.

Energy used in container production is given in the Table 1.2 by the kind permission of the Metal Box Co plc (now Carnaud plc). Although this data is 'old', it does indicate some of the factors which need considering on an ongoing basis.

The above has provided a broad introduction to the environmental issues associated with packaging. These issues although more obviously applicable to the higher volume users in food, beverages, etc., may in the longer term influence material usage in other industries. It is important to have a broad understanding, particularly as most information which reaches the general public via the media treats packaging as a villain rather than a necessity. It must therefore be recognised that few of the public understand the role of packaging and that packaging technologists in industry should be well versed to challenge some of these adverse comments. Table 1.3 quantifies what was found in the average London dustbin in (1935–36, 1968 and 1980) and is often quoted

Table 1.2 Energy used in container production (tonnes of oil equivalent, TOE)

	Aluminium	Plastics	Paper	Tinplate	Glass
Raw material production	6.00	2.30	1.45	1.00	–
Conversion to containers	0.20	0.40	0.05	0.10	0.35
Heating and lighting factors	0.08	0.16	0.07	0.04	0.02
Transport to user	0.06	0.06	0.02	0.02	0.01
Total	6.34	2.92	1.59	1.16	0.38

Table 1.3 Contents of London dustbins

Item	Year 1935–36	1968	1980
Dust and cinders	57.0	22.0	12.0
Vegetables	14.0	17.5	17.0
Paper	14.0	37.0	43.0
Metal	4.0	9.0	9.0
Rags	2.0	2.0	3.0
Glassware	3.0	9.0	9.0
Unclassified	6.0	2.0	2.0
Plastics	–	1.1	5.0

to show how growth in packaging has occurred, with suggestions that packaging must be greater than the actual need (i.e. that a large number of products are overpacked). This has not significantly changed since 1980, when domestic waste still represented only about 4% of the total 'solid waste' in the UK.

However, Table 1.3 also gives other social information, such as the swing from coal fires to central heating. It is not surprising that ash has considerably reduced and other materials have as a result changed in proportion. The reduction in coal fires has also meant that the dustbin is filled with materials which had been previously burnt on household fires.

By the early 1990s plastic had increased to around 7% with a marginal reduction in metal and glass. Since then actual amounts have reduced due to the use of various 'recycling banks'. The average dustbin content weight per week in the 1980s was as follows: towns, 16 kg; rural, 13.5 kg; London, 18 kg.

Conclusions

To conclude, it should be emphasised that packaging does go hand in hand with higher standards of living. Maintaining the balance whereby any pack meets an acceptable compromise between all the factors involved is always a matter of judgement. In the case of pharmaceuticals this judgement requires not only a greater in-depth knowledge as identified in this chapter, but a far more critical appraisal than for virtually any other product. This approach to packaging, from the initiation of a new product to ultimate withdrawal from the market after a successful sales period, varies considerably between companies. Even so, the total packaging organisation does not always receive either the overall co-ordination or emphasis required for the most effective and economical operation, even though many pharmaceutical companies spend more money on packaging materials and the storage of packaging materials than on raw drugs or chemicals. The next chapter therefore covers the broader issues of packaging management and the organisation of a packaging function.

Having explored the broad role of the pack, it is now necessary to consider the information required prior to the development of a pack. This needs to be supported by the many disciplines identified in detail in Chapter 2, where one of the first stages may be the creation of a broad 'packaging brief'. This normally includes certain key information in an initial outline form such as the following:

- name of product
- broad purpose of product and likely route of administration
- dosage form and likely dosage regime
- pack size or sizes
- type of pack preference(s)
- territories of launch outline
- predicted quantities per territory for launch and follow-up sales
- competitive products with list of main features including costs
- any relevant cost restraints
- any quality factors
- legal aspects and implications
- distribution factors
- any environment-related issues.

The above will subsequently be expanded under such headings as facts on the:

- product
- market (and medical)
- warehousing and distribution
- manufacture and pack assembly.

How the above information is handled will very much depend on the type of product. For example, detail will be more readily available on an OTC product than on a new ethical product based on a new chemical entity. The more detail is available, the easier it will be to develop the pack rapidly.

To summarise, this chapter has attempted to identify the following.

1   The role of the pack in its broadest context.
2   The fact that most packs are a *compromise* derived from many considerations.
3   The many, sometimes obvious, factors that have to be considered to obtain a satisfactory marriage between the product and the pack (some of which may conflict with each other).
4   The fact that packaging requires a searching mind and a disciplined approach to ensure that these many and often simple factors produce a logical and acceptable answer for both the company and the end user (patient).
5   The fact that the pack helps to optimise sales and increase profits by being economically viable.
6   A realisation that not only must the product and pack be considered as one entity, but good knowledge of the product characteristics is essential to any effective packaging option.

Each factor taken in isolation could be seen as simple, but the possible reactions between the many hundreds of factors involved turn this into a complex function. Unfortunately, most of the older packaging technologists have learnt only from experience (the way much learning starts), hence it is hoped that this book will be seen to start with a wealth of experience from which a more logical and predictable approach can be derived.

2

THE PACKAGING FUNCTION: MANAGEMENT, DEVELOPMENT AND PRODUCT SHELF LIFE

D. A. Dean

Packaging management

It must first be stressed that the packaging function cannot and should not be separated from the product, particularly as the pack primarily serves as a means of selling and protecting the product. The functions within a company which are either directly or indirectly associated with packaging become more diverse in terms of individual job responsibilities as a company increases in size. Whereas in a small company one person may cover every activity and probably not realise that one is involved in packaging, many specific jobs can be identified with larger companies. Although the job titles may vary, the list below covers most of the major activities. These are not listed in any particular order of importance, and a study of various companies will establish that the authority endowed in a specific function varies significantly, depending on whether the overall activities are marketing, purchasing, development, engineering-oriented, etc. Any one of a number of areas could therefore have the responsibility of leading a packaging co-ordination function. The following job titles or activities are frequently found in the pharmaceutical industry:

- marketing and sales
- packaging supplies buying, packaging buyer or package purchasing
- supplies manager, warehouse supplies, warehouse manager, finished stock manager
- package development, packaging technology, pack or package research or engineering
- production, product manufacture and packaging
- production engineering, machinery purchasing, spare-part supplies and maintenance
- analytical method development for product and 'pack'
- pack design, packaging design – graphical and functional; design purchasing
- legal aspects of packaging; legal department
- works technical, technical support – usually based as a support function to production
- quality control (QC), packaging
- quality assurance (QA), packaging

- specifications, pack assembly details, general documentation associated with packaging (may be seen as an administration/clerical function)
- transportation manager
- project management and packaging co-ordination management
- market research – user opinions/attitudes
- clinical trials – particularly relevant where pack is administration-oriented
- costing, package costing
- regulatory affairs (product–pack registration)
- medical – advising on dosage regime, method and site of administration
- formal stability testing and ongoing product stability testing.

The functions which these disciplines broadly cover can be expanded as follows.

Marketing and sales

This area is usually involved in defining the product and pack marketing requirements; identifying competition; stressing the importance of the dosage regime; maximising compliance, optimising the mode of administration; considering marketing strategies in conjunction with medical support and clinical evidence; assisting with instructions for leaflets and publicity for both OTC and ethical products; establishing prices and profit levels; calculating initial launch quantities and predicting future sales for all the markets in which the product will be sold; deciding a target date for launch; and dealing with initial launch strategy, sample packs for the profession, prelaunch publicity, training of representatives and, in particular, how to introduce and 'pitch' a new product image. Instruction on product administration may also be advised, in conjunction with medical opinions.

Packaging supplies buying, package buyer, package purchasing

Responsibilities are likely to cover purchasing of packaging supplies; identifying possible suppliers; evaluating suppliers commercially and technically; inspecting suppliers' premises and noting documentation; evaluating ability of suppliers to meet delivery dates in terms of quantity and quality (auditing of suppliers or contractors is usually a joint function with QA/QC, sometimes with assistance from development staff); keeping abreast of new packaging developments and obtaining samples/supplies; co-ordinating technical liaison between internal and external expertise as it affects commercial activities; and advising on suitable contract packers.

Supplies manager, warehouse supplies, warehouse manager

This usually involves the planning of deliveries, the warehousing of both raw materials and finished stock, covering possibly ordering (supplies management), storage and movement from and to the warehouse and all closely related functions; defining how materials must be handled to prevent damage, stacked in a suitable manner and under suitable conditions, held in quarantine until cleared by QC; organising proper and effective identification with consideration being given to re-examination should materials be stored for prolonged periods or subjected to adverse conditions; stock keeping, correct rotation of stock, cleanliness and environmental control of premises, maximising use of space, controlling revenue and capital budgets related to warehousing and the movement of stock; knowledge of handling methods, stacking systems (automated or otherwise), types of pallets, stillages, etc. and their maintenance, etc.; introducing and operating computerised systems where these are cost-effective and relevant to stock control.

Packaging development

This may be called packaging engineering, packaging research, packaging technology, etc. in some companies. Package development is normally closely related with product development. The function covers knowledge of packaging materials; investigations into basic materials, packs and packaging systems; carrying out feasibility/investigational programmes on primary (immediate) and secondary packs with the product, devising test procedures for product and pack; establishing packaging procedures for formal stability tests; creating provisional and completed (verified) specifications in liaison with QC, engineering, etc.; providing, proving and updating test methods for materials and finished packs; recommending pack assembly methods; assisting in the selection of packaging equipment; considering cost saving exercises. It may have its own analytical support activity and an internal QC type unit.

Production function

Production covers the manufacturing of the pharmaceutical formulation, the holding of the product under bulk storage until cleared, and the carrying out of the packing of the product. The last of these involves the organisation, training, safety, maintenance and control of packaging lines covering the primary and secondary packaging operations. Since line efficiency and output depends not only on the machinery but on maintenance and the quality of the materials, close liaison is essential with those involved in specifications, QC, development, machinery, safety, engineering, etc.

Production engineering, maintenance and machinery purchasing

Production engineering is likely to be associated with the purchase of packaging machinery, the life expectancy of machinery, the care and maintenance of equipment, the training of maintenance fitters and basic production line training of management, supervisors and line operators. To achieve these functions effectively, good knowledge is required on materials, pack components and pack specifications. As a result, engineering is usually involved in the pack specification clearance to indicate that the specification is compatible with the machinery requirements.

Works technical, production support

Production support and works technical type functions are frequently operated as a support activity to production and may cover chemical and formulation processes, packaging, etc. concentrating on product–pack introductions, including scale-up operations and cost savings which are broadly related to any part of the 'production' process. Many of these activities require a technical and scientific support group covering, in the case of pack changes, packaging operation changes, further evaluation of both the primary and secondary packaging and related equipment technical 'qualification' (i.e. validation) and efficiency. Such a unit may operate a similar packaging operation to the initial packaging development area, covering production line assessment, feasibility testing of new and changed packs, including packaging materials, which is supported where necessary with full stability testing. Some companies may limit such tests to, say, a year or six months until equivalence is established with the previously cleared pack. Although this approach may be quite suitable for minor changes, it is essential to generate actual long-term stability data where significant product or pack changes are involved. Placing the first production batches (usually three) on stability test following a proposed change is one way of confirming that the change was acceptable, assuming initial judgement recommended this from earlier evaluation investigations.

Production support activities may also fall under packaging development (related to initial drug discovery of new products), engineering or production.

Pack design

Pack design can be divided into graphics/aesthetics and function. The latter cannot usually be divorced from development and therefore is part of the initial product–pack activities prior to the launch of a new product. Graphics is closely linked with the market, sales, publicity and legal requirements of the product and pack. It is therefore possible to have a separate graphics department or a graphics buyer whereby designs are carried out by external agencies. Alternatively it may be found as an internal activity under one of the other main disciplines (i.e. marketing, general purchasing, packaging development, etc.). Both functional and aesthetic design may involve market research so that external (or internal) opinion is sought on how best the product can be presented and administered. In total, pack design must provide a suitable marriage between graphics and pack performance and consultation with production on where and how variable detail such as batch coding and expiry dating is added. DAR (digital artwork and reproduction) or DTP (desk top publishing) can be used to assist graphic design.

Legal aspects (see also Chapter 3)

The legal aspects of packaging are always broadening. They cover a wide range of legislation which may include product (and pack) liability – general function including accuracy of dosage administered (where relevant) and risks associated with the product, any hazards associated with pack usage, etc.; and correct description and wording as per labelling legislation. In the UK up to fourteen pieces of information are required on most packs. Fewer are required on smaller packs where the area limits what can be legibly achieved. Legal aspects also include type of sales category (e.g. prescription only), permitted phrases (e.g. 'keep out of the reach of children') and general medicines and poisons regulations.

Quality control and quality assurance, and specifications

These two 'quality' titles are not synonymous, although they are occasionally used indiscriminately. QC can be defined as the function responsible for the maintenance of quality to an agreed standard. QA covers the activities and functions concerned with the attainment of quality, i.e. building quality into processes by broad association with GMP, GLP, etc.

The control of quality may be covered as a central function where incoming raw materials, intermediate and manufactured chemical entities, intermediate and bulk formulations, packaging materials, the packaging line, the packed end product, complaints, etc. all undergo some form of check or analysis. The same function may also be responsible for the analysis of development work (on new products or modifications to product–pack of an established product), the checking and validation of new methodology/equipment, supplier audits and the formal stability programme. Close liaison between packaging QC and packaging development has distinct advantages and these two functions may sometimes be under the same management. Specifications are always a common link to both, as these activities tend to be the basis of any project. A provisional specification is essential for any material before it is subjected to a test procedure, irrespective of whether it is related to feasibility, stability studies or subsequent ongoing production. Specifications are also built up over a period of time (tentative, provisional, agreed or verified). As a result of this, specifications are likely to be initially established via a development operation and then handed over to a QC function. This transfer is the most important part of any liaison link and it should be likened to baton change-over in a relay event, and not one where responsibility ends when the other receives the specification. Best motivation is frequently achieved where the QC operation is involved in the stages of development, and 'development' has a responsibility with a new product–pack until it has been 'successfully launched'. This latter phrase has been deliberately selected since the time scale to define when a product is successful may vary with each launch, i.e. usually the first x batches or 3, 6 months of a new production operation.

'Specification' must be looked on as a word which can be used to describe a number of activities whereby a process, an assembly or a material is defined and agreed between a number of parties. The ultimate success of any product is therefore related to having:

1 a specified product including the processes by which it is manufactured, with individually specified ingredients
2 a specified pack including the materials and components from which it is assembled
3 a specified method of assembly of product–pack and the processes involved, e.g. standard operation procedures derived via a product manual.

Where relevant, process detail should include environmental conditions (humidity, temperature, time, duration, etc.); documentation of procedures, tests, etc.; details of records to be kept (GMP); written instructions for operators; reference to machinery to be employed; etc. It can therefore be concluded that an effective level of specification is required for any pharmaceutical product and the appropriate detail must be similarly treated for the packaging function. As specification detail and tests associated with specifications frequently show a tendency to expand with time, it is important that these are constantly reviewed in terms of both the quality level necessary and the procedures by which materials are judged as satisfactory. Although the setting-up of a specification system is relatively simple, maintenance and updating frequently cause problems. It is therefore recommended that any specification distribution system have the absolute minimum of recipients.

The tendency to have a pack component specification which is all-embracing is also changing. A simpler procedure utilises a series of information documents which lay out the procedures that a supplier has to follow for selective package forms, i.e. glass bottles, plastic bottles, laminates, labels, collapsible tubes, etc. It is then possible to have an abbreviated specification document which covers critical, major and minor defect classifications, advice on delivery and identification, and basic information on the material to be employed, etc. The specification therefore cross-references to its respective information (component manual) document and becomes considerably simplified in terms of both layout and detail. This is particularly important now that specifications are being computerised in conjunction with stock control and purchasing.

The main areas of packaging/pack specification are as follows.

1   Basic packaging materials and components (possibly divided into purchasing and performance specifications).
2   Finished pack specification:

- normally requires an agreement between user and supplier, i.e. acts as a purchasing specification; occasionally there may be a separate 'performance' document
- an in-house standard which will be acceptable to marketing, sales, medical, development, production, QC, etc.

QA/QC plays an important link role in the above. However, there are no hard and fast rules on the area that should create, issue and control any specification system. With the advent of computerisation, the 'control' may arise from those who are most competent to initiate and maintain computer programs.

Transportation – direction and control

This involves the safe movement of goods to agreed time schedules supported by adequate documentation. Since no pack can be expected to meet every rigour of transportation, packs are normally produced to withstand certain handling conditions plus a safety factor. Studies are therefore required of transit conditions irrespective of whether own transport, contractor's transport or nationalised transport is used. Actual conditions will vary between air, road, rail, sea and inland waterways. Knowledge is equally essential of intermediate storage/transhipment points which may be encountered on a journey. As products move from home trade to export the supportive documentation becomes increasingly important. Since the cost of transportation may relate to either size or weight, the economies of transportation may vary significantly according to the materials of the primary pack, the size/weight of contents and the secondary protective materials. For some export markets the use of containerised loads is likely to be more economical.

A study of warehousing arrangements external to the producing company, the handling facilities, types of pallet and stacking systems is also required as part of the total evaluation. Due attention must be given to hazardous goods, in terms of safety and adequate labelling.

Project management and package co-ordination

Project management operating across the hierarchical systems by a matrix approach is being increasingly used within the pharmaceutical industry, particularly where new products are involved. This usually brings together all the major company packaging disciplines previously identified. However, as the role of the pack becomes increasingly important, a separate packaging co-ordination role may be required to bring together all those who can contribute to the successful launch of a product.

The costing of projects both before they commence and during progress is an essential part of project management. There is also the costing of the product–pack so that the sale price can be worked out at an early stage, covering the various stages of profitability, i.e. pharmaceutical company, wholesaler, retailer, etc. Methods of costing covering production, materials, direct and indirect costs, etc. tend to vary between companies, hence the most important feature is to compare like with like. Fully effective cost comparisons are sometimes difficult to achieve as, depending on how a product is packed, significant costs (or cost savings) may be incurred in warehousing and transportation. How materials are warehoused and whether transportation relates to weight or volume, partial or full loads, etc. is frequently a neglected aspect of the total packaging operation. The difference between the production cost (into the company's warehouse) and the cost sold on is normally referred to as the 'contribution'. Profit is the part of the contribution remaining after various other costs such as warehousing, distribution, etc. are deducted. Since warehousing has become a costly operation, long-term storage reduces profitability, hence the justification of 'just in time' philosophies (JIT) which improve cash flow.

Final thoughts on packaging management

A company's reputation depends largely on how it is seen by the outside world. Part of this outside world includes those who supply to the company. Too much diversification of job responsibilities may make it difficult and confusing for such supplying companies, especially when they are contacted by a large number of persons, i.e. works technical, engineering, project management, production, design management, development, purchasing, etc. Although two levels of contact between users and suppliers are obviously desirable, i.e. commercial and technical, some central co-ordination is required to monitor all levels of information exchange. The initial choice of supplier for a new product concept tends to be particularly difficult, as a number of functions within a company may consider it their responsibility. There are dangers if the QC–GMP type operation of an external company is judged too critically at this early development stage, as quite a number of projects are not likely to reach fruition. Choosing a company because it operates an excellent QC system may therefore be fruitless if the expertise within the supplying company is insufficient to meet the design demands of a new concept. The author argues that it is easier to teach quality managcment than innovation, since experience has shown that entrepreneurial innovative companies have been condemned because of a lack of initial investment into quality standards.

Packaging management ideally should involve the total co-ordination of all direct and indirect packaging activities. Once a company has recognised that packaging is an essential activity, then any of a number of systems will undoubtedly satisfactorily control this function. In fact many companies simply leave these contributory factors to reach their own level, relying on individuals to compensate for any over- or under-emphasis of specific areas. However, the most effective system must be where there is some centralised control, probably through a packaging co-ordinator.

A check on the total cost of all incoming materials may frequently reveal that incoming packaging materials cost more than those ingredients which are 'product'-oriented. Although this may be overlooked, added value ultimately becomes the main yardstick by which cost-effectiveness is measured.

Finally, no management system can be considered without the support of a planning operation with various types of bar charts, PERT (Program Evaluation and Review Technique) charts and full critical path analysis. Although these systems are a useful tool for management, occasionally there is a risk that the system takes over management.

Product and pack development

Following the above introduction to total packaging management it is necessary to revert to the main aspect of the pharmaceutical industry, i.e. the development of new products and packs. For this part of the exercise the technical detail will be defined, rather than the management system by which the end-point, i.e. the successful launch of a product, is achieved.

The first requirement for any development programme is to identify the type of development involved, i.e.

1   new product–new pack (note that a new pack may be a modified existing pack since all new pharmaceutical products must pass through a full development programme)
2   existing or established product in a new pack, i.e. a major pack change
3   major product change (reformulation of a product) associated with a major pack change or no pack change; could be a product extension e.g. a new disease treatment
4   minor product change–no pack change (possibly limited testing required)
5   existing product–minor pack change (possibly limited testing required)
6   special pack with existing product or new product for promotional purposes, usually distributed to professional people or used by representatives for demonstration purposes
7   pack either acting as an administrative aid or being used in a device (note that this can apply to any of the above).

The next and probably the most important stage is the defining of *objectives*. This includes what is generally known as a packaging brief, covering the more important packaging aspects listed below.

1   Product name/identity, i.e. project title.
2   Route of administration, likely dose, dosage frequency, etc.
3   Detail of product characteristics, i.e. physical, chemical and biological properties.
4   General pack requirements:

- type of pack suggested
- pack sizes, primary and secondary; warehouse versus distribution number for transit pack
- product strengths
- any special requirements, e.g. tamper-evidence, child resistance, administration aids.

5   Estimated sales, against initial launch and follow-up quantities; territorial sales, initial and follow-up.
6   Suggested launch date; initial launch (which territories?); other territories – priorities.
7   Tentative cost schedule for product–pack.
8   Any special legal requirements, e.g. product category, poison schedule, weights and measures, labelling.
9   Customer requirements – may be unknown initially, but simulated usage is essential as pack is probably more likely to fail during use than when it remains unopened.
10 Similar products on market, i.e. competitors' products and costs.
11 Safety hazards if relevant, i.e. internally and externally, including pack–product liability.
12 Any environmental issues, restraints.

If it is assumed that most pharmaceutical companies will have some form of pharmaceutical/packaging development operation, then the activities which stem from the above brief are likely to involve the following.

Keeping up to date on materials, components and innovative packs in terms of physical and chemical properties – note that pharmaceuticals use virtually all materials offered and therefore this field is not only as wide as in any other industry (food, confectionery, etc.) but requires greater in-depth knowledge and background investigation. Most companies will therefore need to do some type of research investigation on components, materials, packs and test procedures on an ongoing basis. The above serves to strengthen the information base line within any company. Note that certain pack innovations can be patented, hence extending the patent life of product.

Assisting in or actually specifying the packs to be used for any R&D investigation, i.e. covering safety, animal and human studies (clinical pharmacology), clinical trials, as well as formulation development and package development. These activities also provide a useful source of early information on product-pack compatibility which can be supported by pack observations and general stability-type studies (see Chapter 3).

Feasibility or investigational tests

This phrase normally covers any tests carried out between the areas of formulation, drug substance, and packaging to establish the suitability of possible packs and materials. It is important that any material used is covered by a provisional specification and then cleared through a formal QC process prior to being used for a test. The indiscriminate use of unidentifiable materials (e.g. testing in 100 ml plastic bottles where grade and type of material cannot be identified and/or bottles which have not been cleared by a closure test) serves virtually no purpose. It should be noted that challenge tests carried out on chemical entities, preformulation studies and formulation studies should provide excellent knowledge of how a product is likely to deteriorate, i.e. through moisture, oxygen, carbon dioxide, losses due to migration, etc. Packs with the required protection characteristics can be readily selected once compatibility studies (part of the feasibility programme) have been covered. Developing test procedures to evaluate materials and packs is also part of the development programme. Where suitable, such tests may ultimately become part of a more formal QC clearance procedure. This stage needs the services of an analytical unit, certainly for the full identification of plastics.

Formal stability tests

The final stage of any product–pack clearance is usually a formal stability test. Although this is basically an analytical programme, packaging examination and pack analysis should also form an important part of the procedures. The final assessment of shelf life should therefore be agreed by a number of interested parties, i.e. analysts, microbiologists, formulators, packaging technologists, etc. Any use of accelerated testing in either the feasibility or the stability programme also needs careful evaluation, as changes in the pack may occur that will lead to incorrect interpretation of results. For example, a closure on a pack may loosen and/or tighten under broad cycling conditions due to dimensional changes associated with temperature and relative humidity. Similarly, in a static condition test where samples are prepared at, say, $18\,^{\circ}\mathrm{C}$ and then stored for a prolonged period at a higher (e.g. $40\,^{\circ}\mathrm{C}$ 75% RH) or lower temperature (refrigerator), differential expansion and/or contraction between container and closure may cause loosening or tightening of the closure. Measurements are essential at all temperatures as too often packs are allowed to equilibrate with the laboratory environment before being checked. The use of temperatures above $45\,^{\circ}\mathrm{C}$ or $50\,^{\circ}\mathrm{C}$ also tends to cause some changes, both physical and chemical, with many packaging materials, any of which may subsequently lead to product deterioration.

It is therefore important that all packaging support work is meaningful, as inadequate attention to detail can totally invalidate even the most technical and scientific stability programmes. When stability work is carried out by an area well divorced from packaging development there is an inherent assumption that packaging work has been adequately and effectively done. A list of this work, taken from the introduction to packaging development given earlier, therefore bears some expanding, since this clearly identifies further areas of possible weakness where a 'company' may be caught out.

Packaging and stability (the formal estimation of shelf life)

Companies frequently see a 'formal stability test' as the ultimate stage which confirms that there is a satisfactory product–pack with an established 'shelf life'. It must therefore be stressed that this approach is only relevant if all the supporting activities have been adequately covered. Although the stages identified below make major reference to plastics, similar detail is essential for the approval of any (primary) material. This is particularly relevant when ICH and EU guidelines are considered, as these make assumptions that the activities listed in the remainder of this section have been effectively carried out.

The formulation and packaging disciplines have carried out adequate investigation or feasibility support work to establish the functional and aesthetic aspects of the pack, both primary and secondary. The primary pack (US terminology – immediate pack) may be defined as the pack which is in immediate contact with the product, and the secondary pack as the ancillary materials required for presentation, information, warehousing and distribution purposes. Feasibility or investigational work may involve information-gathering on the pack and its components, etc. (i.e. basic research into materials, packs and processes) and compatibility studies, accelerated or otherwise, on the product and pack.

The materials used for the primary (and secondary) pack, even if constituents are non-migratory, are non-toxic and non-irritant and this information can be adequately supported by the study of:

1   the constituents in the materials (the material itself)
2   toxicological data on the constituents
3   the availability of adequate analytical methods to detect migration, or surface removal should it arise.

It should be noted that constituents in terms of plastics could include *residues* (from the polymerisation process), *additives* (ingredients added to enhance or modify certain properties), *processing aids* (ingredients added or used to assist in a fabrication or conversion process, e.g. mould release agents, lubricants), and *master batch* constituents (if a master batch is used).

Sufficient in-depth extractive and compatibility investigations have been carried out to establish likely level of extractives with conventional simulants and the actual product(s). Note that exchange between product and pack may occur in either direction (and with materials other than plastics).

Note also that although EP, USP and WHO extractive procedures (see also BS 5736 parts 1–10) give only limited information and are usually mandatory only for eye products and injectables, this type of test may be useful for company assessment of various types of plastics. Compatibility tests at the feasibility stage may involve so-called accelerated or stress conditions. It should be recorded that higher temperatures may in some way either destroy the pack or make it less effective, with the result that the product is no longer fully protected by the pack. Thus, unless these higher temperature conditions are to be found in practice, some accelerated tests may not provide realistic extrapolations.

Provisional specifications have been created for all packaging components, and these are subsequently used to clear all materials through a QC plus type operation prior to use in any tests, irrespective of whether these are feasibility or formal stability studies. Procedures should include (for plastics) material identification (by IR, UV, differential scanning calorimetry (DSC), etc.), physical assessment including dimensions and functional tests, and should be of greater technical and scientific depth than the QC procedures used for subsequent regular incoming production materials (hence the use of the phrase 'QC plus').

Repeat the previous paragraph creating a provisional product specification and in particular have complete and comprehensive records of how the drug entity was produced and the formulation processed into a product. Note that any subsequent changes may not only require monitoring but possibly lead to further stability work to support the product stability profile (i.e. scale-ups).

Accurate details are kept and recorded on how the product–pack was processed and assembled. This detail should include reference to environmental conditions, machine types, speeds and settings, heat seal strength, cap torque, fill volumes, etc. and where, when and by whom the operation was performed, etc.

One should constantly recall that a static stability test does not cover those effects likely to be associated with warehousing (in bulk), handling, transportation, display or use. It is essential that other tests cover these aspects to ensure that stability data is not invalidated. This may be done by the use of either laboratory simulated tests or actual 'field trials'. Top pressure (compression) and/or vibration is likely to present one of the more serious hazards.

One should ensure that packaging evaluation work where possible includes 'control' packs and involves recognised test procedures in order to provide good comparative type data, e.g. tests to show moisture loss or moisture gain, changes in closure torque and heat seal strength on storage. Test procedures should involve adequate analytical and instrumental support. Remember that, even in a scientific society, the use of observation to detect visual and organoleptic changes is still invaluable (e.g. touch, sight, taste and smell). This work should cover not only the primary pack but the secondary packing (effects of storage, stacking, vibration, etc.).

One should ensure that in use testing, patient acceptability and possible abuse and misuse aspects are adequately covered and interpreted, since most formal shelf-life testing does not involve any 'use' of product and pack. It is possible that the product–pack may have a restricted shelf life once the pack is opened and is in use, i.e. it may occasionally be necessary to have two shelf-life periods, e.g. for reconstituted and/or over-wrapped products:

- for the unopened pack, e.g. 3 years plus
- for the opened pack, e.g. 'use within 4 weeks' or 'the contents should be discarded after one month', etc.

There may be differences between the product–pack formally stability tested and the pack to be sold. It is essential that all 'differences' are considered and, where relevant, investigated. Although there may be a firm intention to test the pack to be ultimately sold, there are frequent (and almost invariably subtle) differences either from the primary pack or arising from the fact that the primary pack is rarely tested together with the secondary (warehousing, transit or display) packaging materials. A typical example is where an entirely new pack is to be produced and the 'economics' do not permit the laying down of production moulds until the initial concept has been proven. The options then are:

- to test in the 'same materials' using a similar design of pack
- to test in the correct design using packs produced from a single impression prototype tool (using the materials of choice)

- to test in similar materials using the nearest size which may in fact be significantly different in design (i.e. product to pack surface area to ullage is different).

If tooling is required for both a bottle and a closure, then the situation is further complicated by even higher tooling costs. Also, if a pack either acts as or incorporates a delivery system, often tooling may become even more complex and costly, particularly as the number of components involved increases. However, as the pack becomes more complex there is a greater need to complete stability work on the pack to be ultimately used, as this decreases risks associated with possible anomalies.

Stability samples and any samples used in evaluation programmes (including clinical trial supplies) should be subjected to QC evaluation inspections:

1 at commencement of programme
2 at various stages during any lengthy storage period (e.g. roving inspections)
3 on removal from test condition for assessment
4 during opening
5 after use or evaluation of product.

An adequate number of additional samples should be included in each programme to allow for 'destructive testing'. In the case of samples withdrawn for analysis, these should be examined visually, any critical parameters recorded (e.g. cap torque, if relevant), and then examined in detail prior to disposal.

The data generated from any programme, whether formal or otherwise, should satisfy both the company and the regulatory authorities. It is therefore important that all testing procedures leading to a 'decision' be well recorded in notebooks (GLP) and then, when written up as a formal document, checked and signed by a responsible person. These will form part of the 'Validation' archive.

The data leading to final product and pack specifications, with accompanying standard operating procedures, should support all the work earlier carried out to approve the product and pack.

All companies should work towards a total data philosophy, whereby all data, literally from inception of drug to ultimate discontinuation of product, should be used to justify not only stability, but also safety, efficacy, quality and integrity, in order to safeguard both the position of the company and the ultimate patient/user.

Drug substance

There is one important stage which must occur prior to the start of any work where stability on the drug entity, now referred to as the 'drug substance', must be performed. This work, carried out by a research or development function or an external laboratory, is now likely to follow the guidelines issued by the EU or ICH (harmonisation), which provide details on scale of batches, number of batches, environmental storage conditions, information on packs, etc. Since this work also needs input from 'packaging', a further check list is advised along the previous lines to make certain that nothing is overlooked. It must be noted that the pack, although not destined for a patient and not primarily for sale, may in the long term be sent to another factory, a contract packer or another company.

In the case of established drug substances (as used for OTC products), the formulator must be satisfied that adequate stability data exist (by reference searches) prior to using it in a formulation. These data also become part of any regulatory submission, independent of the source. It is too easy to assume that every other company's product has been thoroughly tested. Some examples of where problems have occurred, with reference to the above, are given below:

Example of inadequate monitoring between the pack tested and the pack adopted

(See the paragraph commencing 'There may be differences' (p.45).) A device (separate to a pack) which used a rubber bulb was stored under a range of conditions and observed for deterioration (visually and performance). None was detected. It was subsequently packed in a dark-coloured carton, marketed, and no problems occurred. It was later packed in a printed white carton with a polypropylene film overwrap (to give a degree of tamper evidence). The white carton changed slowly to a yellow-orange colour as a volatile organic copper ingredient from the rubber bulb, retained by the polypropylene film, caused carton discoloration. This was lost through the previously non-overwrapped carton, without detection, partly due to the printed dark colours and partly because it escaped into the atmosphere.

Example of where low temperatures gave an accelerated effect

Zinc and castor oil cream was tested in a polystyrene jar using a four start lug finish to simplify removal of the closure (mother holding baby). Samples were stored at 4°C, 20°C, 30°C and 37°C. Jars cracked at the four stress points created by the four lug closure, first at 4°C then at the higher temperatures in ascending order of temperature (i.e. 6 weeks, 3 months, 7 months, 10 months). The subsequent use of an impact modified polystyrene with the return to a conventional continuous screw thread and screw cap ultimately provided a satisfactory pack.

Example of use of incorrect material and lack of initial specification detail

A strip pack using an aluminium foil/low density polyethylene laminate was used for a tablet containing volatile oil constituents. Delamination between foil and film subsequently occurred as the volatile constituents passed through the polyethylene and softened the adhesive bond. It was not known that the bond was an adhesive at the time, and subsequently an extrusion-coated laminate provided a satisfactory answer.

Example of insufficient investigation prior to formal stability

A neutral unbuffered aqueous solution was stored in a polyethylene bottle. The pH reduced on storage to 4.3–4.5 but reverted to 6.5 when the solution was heated. The change was identified as carbon dioxide permeation with the formation of carbonic acid. Possible solutions include change of plastic, an overwrap or possibly a buffered formulation.

Example of adequate investigations prior to formal stability
(problems discovered then overcome by pack choice)

It was required that a veterinary iron injection be packed in a collapsible (for withdrawal of multiple doses) flask, and LDPE was chosen as a possible contender as this gave good collapsibility. However, the product was susceptible to oxygen permeation and a pH shift, and the phenol preservative system was apparently readily lost through LDPE. This information, given in a literature search, challenged the use of LDPE. Subsequent investigations showed that phenol loss into LDPE was very low and that the loss of the volatile phenol had been judged by the nose (external aroma). The flask, when packed in a paper/foil/polythene sachet, which restrained phenol loss, prevented oxygen permeation/degradation, pH change, etc., and subsequently provided a 3 year plus shelf life.

Example of ineffective monitoring of environment

(See the paragraph commencing 'Accurate details are kept and recorded (p.45).) A part of a batch of an effervescent tablet packed in a foil strip pack subsequently 'ballooned' due to release of CO_2 within the pockets. A searching investigation showed that the dehumidification of the room where the product had been packed had not functioned properly for a short period, and that a reaction had resulted from the introduction of moisture to the product via higher RH. Although this change had been recorded on temperature–humidity charts, these had been filed as a record rather than read (reason: previous charts had not shown problems).

Lack of process monitoring

A sterile product was prepared for stability using a hand plugging, capping operation due to the non-availability of automatic equipment. The team doing the plugging and capping used rubber gloves, lubricated with a sterile glove powder based on starch. Examination of the product prior to placing under test revealed a 'haze' in some samples which was subsequently identified as grains of starch that had become detached from the gloves. Procedures to clean gloves prior to use had not been followed. The batches had to be remade, thereby causing delay in registration and launch.

Although these examples clearly identify some of the risk areas associated with packaging and the need for good laboratory practice (GLP) and GMP covering adequate records of all activities, this type of thinking may well have to be extended outside the true development area. For example, many companies tend to assume that bought-in materials are adequately packed and are stable for, frequently, an indefinite period. This assumption needs to be questioned and if an ingredient is to be stored for prolonged periods some allowance for re-analysis is always advisable, particularly as some products and packs may never have been subjected to any formal assessment (now being advised in guidelines). Equally, data produced 10 years ago may be inadequate.

Most companies have systems involving retention samples of ingredients, intermediates, completed formulation, etc. which are sometimes based on the assumption that all retention packs are perfect. The author has on a number of occasions discovered totally unsuitable packs being used, i.e. small polyethylene bags, polystyrene tubes and

PVC bottles or glass with an unsuitable closuring system. Even such packaging systems therefore need monitoring, if reference to an analysis of retention samples is to be meaningful should complaints arise. One further aspect is the handling of materials in house. It has been noted that ingredients may occasionally be transferred and stored in polyethylene bags, or formulations or intermediates in a process stored for unexpectedly long periods, in containers which have not been shown (or proved) to be suitable. Instances have also been known where changes to equipment (e.g. the introduction of plasticised PVC tubing or the use of non-approved filters) have introduced migratory ingredients or particulate matter into the product. Validation procedures should prevent such occurrences in the future.

Shelf life

The ultimate shelf life of any product may, in certain instances, depend on and be influenced by how and in what containers and materials the ingredients and the intermediates are stored, prior to and during processing, including bulk storage of the product, until the time when it is packed into the pack for sale.

. It can therefore be inferred, having identified some of the possible areas of weakness/risk associated with establishing a product–pack shelf life, that no company has yet found the ultimate means of estimating and approving the 'best' pack which will guarantee optimal shelf life for all times and conditions. The latter part of this chapter will enhance this point in that all packs finish up as a compromise of a number of often conflicting factors.

However, before moving on to these aspects, the converse of the above examples of 'risk' could be counter-balanced by asking how realistic is your predicted shelf life as identified by initial investigative tests.

Shelf life based on moisture loss or gain

The rate of moisture transfer via a pack by permeation or the seal/closure depends on a number of possible variables, including the following.

1   The vapour pressure gradient between the environment inside and outside the pack (the greater the gradient, the greater is the potential for moisture transfer detected as loss or gain).
2   Whether the external environment is 'static' or has a constant air circulation (which encourages maximum gradient conditions).
3   The presence or otherwise of temperature changes which will cause changes in vapour pressure and gradient, plus such other factors as:

- material gauge or caliper
- effectiveness of the seals
- nature of the barrier material and how it absorbs moisture (i.e. whether it has a low or high moisture content at equilibrium)
- nature of the product and level of moisture content (which again will reflect on the vapour pressure exerted for a given temperature).

Although each of the above (and other) factors will contribute to how a product in a pack may lose or gain moisture, factors (1) and (2) will have a major influence. This is supported by the following example.

Example

If a moisture-sensitive product is packed in a UPVC blister pack lidded with 18–20 μm hard foil, it is likely that this pack will be 'proved' unsuitable if samples are exposed, naked in a climatic cabinet, at 25°C 75% RH or higher conditions, e.g. 38°C 90% RH, using a fan-driven environment. Therefore let it be assumed that the product shelf life under say, 25°C 75% RH conditions is 6–8 weeks. (Note that using more protective PVC + barrier combinations might give 24–30 weeks with 100 g/m² coating of PVdC and $1\frac{1}{4}$–$1\frac{3}{4}$ years with an Aclar/PVC combination.) However, this does not take into account

1   the fact that the environment transfer can be slowed down by considering various 'overwrap' options
2   the fact that placing blisters in a carton, twelve cartons in an outer, four outers in a shipping outer, 240 outers to a pallet and then adding a shrink hood could extend the shelf life to over 2 years (even at 25°C 75% RH), if held for that period as a full pallet load.

The additional overwraps which might be considered could include:

- a PVdC coated PP flow wrap for x blisters
- a carton with a PVdC/PP overwrap
- an outer pack of x units (e.g. six or twelve) fully shrunk or overwrapped
- a pallet load of outer packs fully shrunk or stretched wrapped.

Basically each overwrap changes the gradient around the pack (between the inside and outside of the pack) and adds an additional barrier through which moisture has to permeate. Theoretical calculations for a multiplicity of barrier layers need a fairly complex mathematical appreciation and practical estimates may be equally difficult, as either a pallet will not enter a climatic cabinet or the cost of samples could be prohibitively high, with an expensive product kept on test for a prolonged period.

Table 2.1 must inevitably raise some queries, e.g. how does continuous exposure to 25°C 75% RH equate with actual *fluctuating* conditions, i.e. is it an accelerating or decelerating effect? How does 25°C 75% RH equate with 48 months under normal warehouse conditions where both the mean temperature (say 14–17°C) and the RH (40–55%) will be significantly lower? How effective are the overwraps, particularly with reference to seals and as a barrier to moisture? This will also depend on tightness of wraps and airspace therein. How does one know the period that each (1–5 in Table 2.1) will be stored for, and the climatic conditions involved?

These unknowns can partly be covered by shelf-life declarations, particularly when the final blister is removed from its last overwrap, e.g.:

- 'This product should be used within x months following removal from . . .'

Table 2.1 Variation of shelf life with packaging and conditions

	Pack A (with flow wrap)		Pack B (no flow wrap)		Storage
	Description	Shelf life	Description	Shelf life	
1	PVC blister foil lid	6–8 weeks	PVC blister foil lid	6–8 weeks	at 25°C 75% RH
2	+ Flow wrap	25–30 weeks	Excluded		at 25°C 75% RH
3	+ Overwrap in carton	80–90 weeks	+ Overwrap in carton	25–30 weeks	at 25°C 75% RH
4	+ Overwrapped outer pack	$3\frac{1}{2}$–4 years +	+ Overwrapped outer pack	$2\frac{1}{2}$–3 years	at 25°C 75% RH
5	+ Shrink wrapped pallet	$4\frac{1}{2}$–5 years + (no change detected after first 60 months' storage as a full pallet)	+ Shrink wrapped pallet	$3\frac{1}{2}$–5 years (no change detected after first 48 months' storage as a full pallet)	Normal warehouse conditions

- 'x will normally be either equal to the 25°C 75% RH shelf life (tropical, subtropical conditions) or greater than this, e.g. $2x$ (for temperate markets).'

It can be concluded that a series of overwraps will significantly extend the shelf life of, for example, a moisture-sensitive product as moisture permeation is considerably reduced and/or a low barrier primary material may give adequate protection. This counters any need for an improved pack as found under the ICH 40°C 75% RH conditions.

Thus if one tests blister packs in a carton (possibly overwrapped with a protective film) and from this predicts a shelf life, under actual conditions it could be expected that a much longer life could be achieved, i.e. the prediction has probably built in a significant 'safety factor', e.g. 6–8 weeks (no shelf life) has been extended to up to 60 months.

It should be noted that formal shelf predictions can be checked in the long term by withdrawing samples for analyses from various marketing conditions (home, export, warehouses, hospitals, etc.) and from home storage points. This is usually considered to be part of an ongoing stability activity.

Under the earlier definition of packaging as the *economical* means of providing *protection, presentation, information/identity,* and *convenience/containment/compliance* for the full life of the product during storage, carriage, sale, display, and use and until such time as the product has been used, or administered or simply disposed of, most packs inevitably finish up as a compromise. Since no compromise can ever be considered as perfection, it has to be recognised that in a human judgement reached by humanly devised evaluation (tests), some risk of failure (even if by misuse by the ultimate user), however small, is invariably present. It can, therefore, be concluded that even the apparently 'best' pack may not guarantee the optimal shelf life at all times.

For example, in this context, any pack which involves multiple opening and reclosuring almost always evoke the question, 'how often is the pack effectively reclosed during use?'. Since the answer may at least be 'not always', this can immediately create a case for an alternative unit dose pack which provides individual protection right up to the time of use, albeit in some instances at a higher cost per dose. There has also been a tendency towards introducing microbial limits for many types of product, and any support for these limits may be difficult to substantiate if gross contamination can occur during the product in-use period. Although it may be relatively easy to justify the absence of certain pathogens, it is more difficult to accept, for example, an argument for a sterile nasal preparation, especially as we do not continuously breath 'sterile air'. The *protective* aspects of the pack will therefore vary from product to product with differing emphasis on chemical (including compatibility), biological, climatic and mechanical protection.

With many pharmaceutical products the protective aspects of the pack may be both critical and diverse. It is therefore essential to identify clearly a range of hazards against which some products may require *protection*, especially as those of an obvious nature can easily be overlooked on the basis that 'familiarity breeds contempt'. The author therefore advises even the most knowledgeable to use some form of check list under the headings given in Chapter 1. It is also important to remember that hazards tend to work in combination rather than in isolation.

The above should clearly establish that the many important functions of the pharmaceutical pack can be variable and complex. To emphasise this point, two further examples are given.

A sterile product incorporated a preservative system to cover withdrawal of a multi-dose liquid product. The product passed the USP XX microbial challenge test when first made and packed. After six months it was noticed that the level of ethylenediamine tetra acetate (EDTA) had significantly reduced, possibly by chelation with heavy metals + surface adsorption onto the plastic. A repeat microbial challenge test was not passed. It was 'theorised' that this was due to slight preservative loss coupled to the loss of EDTA which tended to enhance the preservative efficacy, i.e. a chemical + physical change (preservative adsorption) had created a drop in preservative efficacy. Changing the EDTA/preservative levels was subsequently necessary in order to meet the microbial challenge test over the full shelf-life period.

A powder formulation, diluent plus active of differing particle sizes designed to give an accurate dose when dissolved in water, was packed in a sachet. Immediate analysis indicated no problems. Subsequent analysis after transportation to a different site showed a drop in the active drug by approximately 5%. This was traced to preferential adhesion of the drug of the finer particle form (not the excipient) to the inner plastic layer of the sachet. The situation was corrected by an overage whereby the full dose could then be delivered at the drug solution stage. Sachet vibration tests could have established the above at an earlier stage, and avoided a new packing operation, which delayed the product launch.

If the phases covered above are considered as normal development procedures, then it is necessary to state that any packaging development operation has recently had to consider two newer aspects, i.e. patient compliance and the pack's relationship to such environmental issues as pollution, disposal and conservation of energy and the world's natural resources. It is obvious that a pack can either assist or deter patient compliance, and therefore greater emphasis may be placed on this by investigational research in the long term. The environmental aspect will also need more consideration in the future, particularly as some patients will see this as an additional emotional issue if the anti-packaging lobby continues to be publicised, without the advantages which packaging contributes to today's society being fully explained, to the public in general. The EU Packaging and Packaging Waste Directive, 94/62 will apply to pharmaceutical packaging.

It must be re-emphasised that a company, in generating data to satisfy itself and the regulatory authorities, should consider the former to be initially more important. A company must therefore try to stand back and ask whether the data generated can withstand challenge; only then should the data be submitted externally to the authorities. The use of experts and expert reports should assist such needs. Frank, early discussions with regulatory authorities may also help to give confidence that a likely successful and acceptable approach is being adopted and followed.

The total data philosophy approach mentioned earlier, which embraces information collected from product inception to final withdrawal from the market (cradle to grave approach), is receiving greater regulatory attention and acceptance. To achieve this, monitoring, validation and co-ordination are essential both at the initial research and development phases and during subsequent ongoing production and sale. The activities leading into this total accumulation of data will usually cover the following.

1 Full knowledge of the drug entity or active substances (from initial research phase) related to identity, purity, process residues, degradation routes, crystal structure, polymorphism, etc. and changes which may occur when challenged by light, oxygen, moisture/water, acid, alkali, carbon dioxide, temperature, etc., plus interrelated safety and toxicological (toxicity/irritancy) studies. The above is now frequently covered by preformulation work. (See (3) below)

2 Initial drug entity scale-up and a recheck leading to a comprehensive provisional specification, which is likely to be used for the activities below.

3 Preformulation studies including interaction, challenge (similar (1) above), dissolution studies, polymorphic form, release, bioavailability, etc.

4 Stability studies on drug entity (i.e. drug substance) in various packs are now strongly advised under EU guidelines and international harmonisation programmes.

5 Clinical trial supplies which include full QC and supporting stability studies to show that product–pack is satisfactory for issue (i.e. IND stage in the USA). See also (8) below, paying usual attention to GMP, effectiveness of standard operation procedures (SOPs), etc.

6 Formulation studies/feasibility investigational work which are part of or an extension to clinical supplies, leading to final formulations. Accelerated stability and longer term stability tests on pharmaceutical development batches and scale-up batches, leading to a full product specification.

7 Packaging studies – investigational work usually carried out in conjunction with (5) above. Provisional pack specifications, backed up by in-depth recording of all information and data.

8 Formal stability, preferably using three production scale batches (or initial semi-production scale) in final pack where possible, using internationally acceptable protocols. ICH requires 12 months at $25\,^\circ$C, 60% RH, 6 months at $40\,^\circ$C, 75% RH or 12 months at $30\,^\circ$C, 60% RH prior to submission.

9 In-use tests with patients. May be part of clinical evaluation or an extension to it. Most important with devices or where pack acts as an administration aid.

10 Initial production batches for first launch supplies – additional stability work on first three production batches, using ICH storage conditions to verify shelf life if formal stability batches were not representative of final production scale.

11 Ongoing production, ongoing stability tests. Batches representative of production placed on confirmatory stability tests at regular intervals.

12 Warehousing inspections (own and wholesaler's), drug store inspections and end user checks (professionals and patients).

13 Monitoring all complaints – product and pack, adverse reactions, etc.

14 Updating records, leaflets, specifications by constant review of accumulated data.

At all stages attention must be paid to GLP, GMP and validation. Having surveyed the broad functions of the pack, further emphasis should be placed on the role of the packaging specification and the method of pack assembly. Attention to these two factors is highly important to both the development and the ongoing production situation.

The packaging specification (purchasing)

One ultimate purpose of a specification is an agreement document between purchaser and supplier. A provisional or outline specification is, however, essential, even when initial development samples are being surveyed, since it provides both a disciplined approach to the examination of materials and components and a record of exactly what was received, used, etc. A specification is usually documented under the following layout headings:

- standard title (bottle, cap, laminate, etc.)
- specification reference number and date written
- previous edition/specification ref. no.
- general description of item.
- materials of construction – types, grade, colour, etc.
- construction, the process by which constructed; size/weight/capacity, with tolerances (may be under a drawing reference)
- drawing ref., date, details of dimensions and tolerances
- decoration, detail of print, method of decoration, colour target(s), artwork reference, etc.
- performance tests (with reference to test method, number, etc.)
- how to be delivered and identified
- signatures of approval: supplier/purchaser.

Inspection procedures, and acceptable quality levels (AQLs) related to critical, major and minor defects may be part of the specification document but are more likely to be in a general information support manual, unless these are specific to the item concerned.

An alternative approach involving a master manual which contains the basic features for a selected type of component, i.e. glass bottles, plastic bottles, collapsible metal tubes, etc., has much to recommend it. This, together with a simpler description-type document, then becomes an agreement specification between the supplier and the user.

It is therefore advised that prior to the commencement of any product–pack tests, materials should be clearly identified, quantified, measured and checked for performance, etc. In this way the components used for any test can be employed more confidently and better comparisons can be achieved between a series of tests irrespective of whether the tests are investigational, feasibility, formal stability, travel test, etc. If materials, product and pack cannot be properly quantified, then obviously test results may verge on being meaningless. Aspects of quality are further explained in Chapter 4.

Performance specifications

Some companies have specifications which define the performance of an item, rather than specifying it in full detail (e.g. this could apply to shipping outers). However, in the pharmaceutical industry, certainly for primary packs, it is normal and often essential to follow details established in pack approval tests exactly.

Pack assembly detail (assembly procedures for packing operations), i.e. (SOPs), works instructions (WIs), etc.

Full pack assembly detail follows the philosophy of knowing what you are testing and what is to be ultimately produced in a final production situation. The establishment of comprehensive records of both how a pack was assembled and the tests performed to show that the pack was recorded as satisfactory is likely to cover the points detailed below, most of which can be related to GLP or GMP. Data obtained from this initial pack assembly detail ultimately lead into the documents which cover the final product in a production situation. These must, therefore, cover any assembly operations in sufficient detail to ensure that a consistent quality of output is achieved.

Some pack assembly features

The points to consider in activities prior to the final production operation so that a pack assembly detail can be derived include the following.

1   Batch references and batch numbers of the components and product used. Any previous history of components and product, previously unrecorded traceability.
2   Date assembled, where assembled, how assembled, responsibility for assembly.
3   Quantity of material/components issued, used and recovered, i.e. accountability and reconciliation.
4   Equipment used for assembly operations (assembly speed/output). Product–pack specification.
5   On-line target figures associated with fill (volume, weight, number), cap torque, heat seal strength, etc. Figures achieved.
6   Problems encountered during assembly.
7   Environmental conditions etc. in assembly area(s).
8   Results of any special functional tests applied to finished pack.
9   Judgements on visual appearance (i.e. attributes which may be critical to ongoing production).

Only when detail such as that given above is recorded and studied can ultimate confidence be expressed in any test results and the pack assembly document created from them. This becomes particularly relevant when responsibilities become split, i.e. production packed, QC tested, third party evaluated, where each may adequately perform their own functions, but no one area accepts full responsibility for co-ordinating and assessing the total data.

Although emphasis has been placed on specifications and the examination of all test materials prior to the initiation of any tests, the more formal QA/QC approach in a continuing production situation also needs a mention. Records acquired from such ongoing examinations may yield valuable data on changes to incoming materials, process modifications, changes in pack assembly procedures, which in turn may result in a modification to the product shelf life. It is therefore important that QC records are constantly monitored so that any trends may be recognised, as even in today's climate technologists can be overcome by the simple pass or fail syndrome rather than using data to sense change. For instance, one company introduced an apparently impressive supplier or vendor rating system which ultimately graphed each supplier on a points system every few months. Suppliers at the top of the table were naturally considered good and those at the bottom bad, with constant efforts being made to upgrade the latter through a more rigorous and critical approach to defectives. However, a quick assessment by an outside consultant immediately indicated that some of the top suppliers had items of good design and those at the lower end of the scale had poor or difficult designs. The table, therefore, gave a general design rating in addition to being a vendor rating system. Technical discussions which concentrated on the design were able to upgrade the ratings of some of the poorer suppliers. As suppliers occasionally introduce minor or even major modifications which they regard as improving the process or the item being produced, it is essential to insist that any change is notified to the user company. A phrase to cover this is normally incorporated into the specification. Once a company has been notified of an impending change, judgement has then to be made as to whether any further tests are required to establish whether the change has any significance.

As indicated earlier, formal stability work is only of relevance if it is backed by an effective team which studies the project and the product–pack in total. Within this team there must be a high level of packaging expertise and effective co-ordination between formulators, analysts, engineers, statisticians, packaging technologists, etc. Even when a shelf life has been initially established, this must be supported not only by ongoing stability, by sampling production batches, but also by a monitoring system that ensures that the product and pack continue to meet the requirements essential to guarantee efficacy, safety, integrity, uniformity, etc., and confidence of the ultimate user. Only by this approach can a product and the industry as a whole be assured of consistent quality. The need to improve quality constantly is also essential to the industry.

It can therefore be concluded that those carrying out formal stability work must not only be supported by an effective pack examination system but also have adequate knowledge of the total supportive role which the pack plays.

Clearance of a pharmaceutical pack or device

In order to provide a greater appreciation of the in-depth knowledge required for the above packaging development operation, it would perhaps be useful to look at the steps involved in the clearance of a pharmaceutical pack/device. This type of activity is becoming increasingly important in terms of both the expertise required and the need to support the significant growth in the use of plastic. This growth has frequently been associated with user convenience features (e.g. squeezability), a more modern hence psychologically acceptable image, a greater ability to produce packs and devices in functional and complicated shapes involving less weight and frequently lower volume, at competitive and economically acceptable prices. New concepts, which would not be practical in glass and metal, have also assisted the progress of plastics for both packs and devices in the pharmaceutical industry. Thus plastics now stand a high chance of being used for new pharmaceutical products in spite of the fact that all are to some degree permeable to moisture, oxygen, carbon dioxide, etc. and may not be as 'inert' as the other longer established competitive materials such as glass and metal.

The fact that plastic packs have undoubtedly received greater scrutiny than many other longer established types of material has to be noted and accepted. Although the author would stress that in many instances this might be considered unfair, plastic can at least be used as an example of how a material can be thoroughly 'cleared' in the widest pharmaceutical context.

It is for this reason that Chapter 8 traces the development of a plastic pack, covering:

- functional and aesthetic design
- process of manufacture, as this may influence the grade of plastic required
- selection of plastic type – general physical and chemical properties
- selection of plastic grade – detailed physical and chemical properties, plus knowledge of constituents including toxicity and irritancy aspects
- compatibility requirements, involving both the feasibility and formal stability stages identified previously
- performance requirements associated with warehousing, distribution, display, use, including closure efficiency and durability of identification/decoration/print.

Differences between development and production packs need to be recognised, plus any possible special test requirements for such deficiencies as environmental stress crack resistance, surface changes and static charges, panelling/cavitation, etc., which should be established at an early stage.

Although the above items have been listed separately, in actual practice several have to be considered in combination. For example, the practicability of any design has to be related to the process of manufacture, the grade of plastic employed and the constituents found in the plastic.

The early part of this chapter indicated a number of different scenarios where package development activities might be involved. These are now expanded.

Changes to product and pack (after initial launch)

The means of proving product or pack equivalency when either the product or the pack is altered or modified in terms of size, materials, shape, closure, etc. is a constant discussion point. Of these a change in pack size using the same container, materials and closure size should be the easiest to prove in equivalency, particularly when the product has been shown to be highly stable. Products sensitive to moisture (or gases) can be evaluated against the moisture (or gas) lost or gained per product (i.e. per item, volume or weight) and, provided this is similar or not significantly greater than the previously used pack, a case could be made for a change in pack size, even if the closure was also altered. Although similar reasonings could be put forward for changes involving different pack types and packaging materials, additional factors such as compatibility have to be considered. This may be covered by short-term, possibly accelerated studies which can then be backed up by longer term formal stability tests. The time at which change can be released must largely depend on the complexity of the alterations. Arguments have been put forward that provided a series of packs has been proven equivalent and the product has good stability, interchange should be readily acceptable to both the company and the regulatory authorities. This approach, although very dependent on the phrase 'proven equivalent', goes back to a philosophy that if a company is satisfied with the data and is thereby happy that a commercial risk is justifiable, this should prove adequate, with discussion if necessary, for clearance by any regulatory authority. In virtually all cases any change will have to be supported by longer term stability tests (possibly covered by established product/ongoing product stability procedures) which in certain instances can be carried out in parallel with production and 'sale' of the product–pack change. Internally within a company, any proposed alteration should involve all those who could possibly be affected, i.e. purchasing, development, production, quality control, warehousing, customers, etc., as occasionally a change which seems excellent to one area may have significant disadvantages to another. Each proposal should, therefore, be fully reviewed in its own right before any resources are allocated to the more expensive testing procedures which 'prove' equivalence. More formal guidelines are provided by Japan, where 40°C 75% RH is offered as a condition under which both the existing and new/modified pack are compared. Provided both packs can be shown as equivalent (or better) over four analytical periods during 6 months (e.g. 0, 2, 4, 6 months), a change may proceed. Some examples of the more usual types of change are provided, with discussion, below.

Pack change examples

Example

The current pack of 100 tablets is an 80 ml rectangular amber glass container fitted with a 28 mm metal screw cap with pulp board/PVdC faced wadding. An additional pack size is required involving a 125 ml cylindrical amber glass pack holding 150 tablets. At this size the screw neck is increased to 33 mm but has identical wadding. Points to consider are as follows.

1 Glass and closure system use identical materials, hence there should be no major compatibility issues.
2 Moisture (gas) ingress/egress is likely to be proportional to circumference of the screw finish provided a proportionately similar torque is used (i.e. higher torque for larger bottle orifice). The effectiveness of the closure seal can be quickly checked by desiccant tests, or other tests which are coupled with confirmation of screwing-on and screwing-off torques. (Note – 28 mm:33 mm in circumference are of the ratio 1:1.5 (i.e. ratio of 100:150 tablets), hence in this example moisture ingress/egress should be similar per tablet assuming sealing surfaces are of similar quality.)
3 A cylindrical bottle will rotate (due to vibratory effects) in transit and therefore has a greater chance of label rub or loosening of the closure than a rectangular pack. Some form of assessment of this factor is therefore advisable.
4 Checks should also be made on ullage volume, i.e. whether headspace to content volume is similar or whether product could suffer greater physical change if differences occur.

Likely conclusions

Any risks are very much related to the physical nature of the product and journey hazards; otherwise 'equivalence' should be relatively easy to establish.

Example

Rectangular glass bottle 80 ml with 28 mm closure and 100 tablets as above. Change is required to high density polyethylene bottle involving a similar size (capacity) and the same closure.

1   HDPE is permeable to both moisture and gases, hence exchange via the container walls may be more relevant than the closure, dependent on container wall thickness and uniformity of distribution (including desiccant tests).

2   Closure may react differently on plastic, i.e. change of torque, back off, under variable conditions of temperature and humidity (humidity less significant). Thread form may not be ideal for a metal closure, e.g. buttress thread form is preferred for a plastic-to-plastic closure fit and is more likely to be used on an available stock container. Additional tests necessary to confirm suitability of metal to plastic fit and effectiveness of closuring systems. Cycling conditions useful. Tests may show that a closure change, including an addition of a foil diaphragm might be advisable. This may involve another potential contact material.

3   Dimensional assessment of drawings essential – particularly bottle-to-closure tolerances.

4   Detail of plastic and constituents. Incompatibility unlikely unless volatile constituents are present, but some form of accelerated test probably essential if there has been no previous experience with the material. Check odour and taste, plus degradation.

5   Moisture ingress tests – use glass as a control to establish combined closure and container permeation differences.

6   Light penetration may be greater with plastic (compared with amber glass). Additional checks advised, both with and without a carton.

Likely conclusions

Decision largely dependent on the stability of the formulation and whether any degradation, physical/bioavailability changes related to moisture, oxygen, light, carbon dioxide, etc. could occur. Long-term stability data on pack appears essential and could be part of procedure prior to agreed release, i.e. check via the above tests, then do 3–6 months of a formal stability test prior to release. A change in closure may become necessary, as a metal cap on plastic container has certain limitations. A plastic cap incorporating a diaphragm induction seal may provide an ideal solution.

Example

Change from an amber glass bottle to a foil strip pack. An aluminium foil strip (i.e. paper/foil/polyethylene or foil/polyethylene) should, in theory, give as good or superior protection against moisture ingress to a glass bottle with an effective closuring system provided machine problems are absent (i.e. good heat sealing, no excessive extension of pockets by size or location of item in the pocket, etc.). There will, however, be a new contact material with the product, namely the heat sealing ply. Product headspace (air) may differ from that of a glass pack. The factors to consider include the following.

1   General machine efficiency – delivery and location of product in pocket, extension of pocket area, strain on seal area, etc.
2   Does heat sealing operation raise any product problem with heat retained by pack and transferred to product?
3   What is material in contact with product (heat seal material)? Query compatibility against material specification including any constituents in plastic.
4   What are seal requirements etc.?

- Elimination or avoidance of capillary channels in seal margins (possibly due to creases in seal area).
- Peel strength of seal (i.e. related to temperature, dwell and pressure).
- Vacuum testing requirements, or alternative leak detection.
- Moisture ingress/egress (weight change on product or desiccant tablets).
- Does heat seal pattern avoid perforation of pack?

Likely conclusions

Not so simple to prove total equivalence – some stability advisable prior to acceptance. Strip pack should, in theory, be superior. Flavoured type tablets need additional checks. Formal stability tests essential.

Example

A product (aseptically produced and filled) in a multidose vial (20 ml) uses a natural rubber stopper through which the volatile preservative system is lost. As a result a 3 year shelf life (predicted and assumed previously) cannot be achieved. An alternative rubber stopper is advised. The supplier recommends a chlorbutyl synthetic rubber stopper. Actions advised are as follows.

1   Check new stopper for fragmentation, resealing (following multiple penetration) and force for needle to penetrate – note that synthetic stoppers are generally inferior in these properties. (Repeat after ageing period.)
2   Check extractives before and after autoclaving of stoppers – chemically and toxicity.
3   Check preservative absorption and moisture loss via stopper (synthetic stopper should be significantly superior with regard to both).
4   Check if washing and sterilisation process (i.e. autoclaving of stoppers) generates any particulate matter.
5   Consider stability test parameters, including analytical methodology (if product has been marketed for a number of years methodology may be out of date and non-specific).
6   Make up necessary batches for stability and place on test (check stopper insertion and subsequent seal); 12 months' data advised prior to submission.

Likely conclusions

Formal stability-type tests essential before clearance can be given. Release most likely after a 6 month or longer period, depending on quality of previous product data. Even if certain accelerated conditions are used, there is no room for error on an injectable product. Level of testing likely to be intensified when compared to programme used to achieve a launch on the same product previously.

Note

The number of batches required for formal stability data to support changes varies between regulatory authorities. In certain cases there may appear to be good reasons to support a one or two batches approach rather than the more conventional three batches. The latter provides a higher confidence level and is essential according to ICH guidelines.

Having provided a number of examples of specific roles of the pack, the hazards which a product may face and how the pack may cope with these factors can be further expanded under a check list. Such a list is essential as frequently the risk of errors is associated with the most obvious observations.

The expanding role of the pack (e.g. where pack acts as an administration aid or is used in a device)

In an early definition, packaging was defined as the economical means of providing protection, presentation, information, identification and containment of a *product* during storage, distribution, display and use. Today this definition is changing as the role of the pack expands with more emphasis on factors of convenience, compliance, improved drug delivery, associated with use as an administration aid, or as a component within a device, etc. Although this trend produces more sophisticated forms of pack, and a need for greater innovation makes the clearance procedures for a pack more complex, the future environmental issues will need additional consideration.

Before discussing examples of the more sophisticated forms of pack which are involved in improving 'compliance', brief mention should be made of increasing emphasis on user–patient protection which may be included under the broad heading of 'product liability'. This other protective role can include aspects of integrity and security associated with such factors as tamper-evidence, tamper-resistance, child-resistance, etc. However, as with innovation and the environmental issues, these safety aspects may conflict with other issues, i.e. concern for the increasing elderly population. As a result, the latter may experience difficulty both in gaining access to and reclosing their medication and in coping with infirmities, rheumatism, weakness of grip, poorness of sight, etc. when using these more complex administration systems. This all means that the tests necessary to establish pack acceptability have to be extended beyond basic product–pack compatibility into areas of use, long-term performance, misuse, abuse, interpretation of instructions, general hygiene, cleaning procedures and their microbiological significance, etc. As an aid to working out the intensity of testing necessary to achieve this, the author offers in Chapter 8 a league table based on the product, the route of administration, and the risk to patient. The products at the top of the list, which include IV preparations followed by injections, involve significantly higher 'risks' than those at the foot of the table, e.g. oral solid products, particularly in terms of compatibility between pack and product. However, no position in such a table is fixed, as the 'risk' will vary due to a number of factors (see Appendix 8.8, Chapter 8).

Defining the type of tests which may be required will depend on the types of material involved, i.e. glass, metal, plastics, etc. However, as packs become more complex and more innovative, plastic becomes the more favoured material for sound economic reasons (frequently associated with fewer components which provide simpler assembly procedures).

The types of test to be applied may be influenced by the role of the pack, as follows.

1 Pack where administration component forms part of the primary or immediate pack and where some components are in intimate contact with the product (examples: aerosols, pumps, etc.).
2 Pack where some of the administration components are in contact with product only during in use period (i.e. possibly act as a transfer system, e.g. IV transfer of additives).
3 Pack that is used in a device but is otherwise separate from the device in which it is used (e.g. Glaxo Diskhaler system).
4 The actual type of test(s) are likely to be selected from the following.
   (a) Identifying that the plastic, meets food, toy, FDA, etc. approval requirements.
   (b) Identifying constituents covering polymer residues, additives, processing aids, and master batch components, together with toxicological/irritancy risks, methods of analysis, etc.
   (c) Carrying out extractive-type tests to USP, BP 80, WHO, EP, BS 5736 procedures, etc. and establishing chemical and biological acceptance.
   (d) Carrying out investigational tests on device/packed product using accelerated and normal conditions to indicate suitability/compatibility.
   (e) Carrying out formal stability tests using control, EU climatic and accelerated test conditions to meet EU and international/national standards with emphasis on Europe, Japan, USA, etc. including ICH guidelines.
   (f) Carrying out preservative efficacy challenge procedures, i.e. test initially, and at appropriate condition–time intervals to check that preservative efficacy (chemical v. microbiological change) still provides adequate protection against microbiological challenge. i.e. if preserved.
   (g) In tests (e) and (f) check that product when dispensed via 'device' does not significantly change or remains acceptable (i.e. combined product–device tests).
   (h) If device is separate to pack, check storage against accelerated and typical conditions to ascertain that performance does not change. This may be covered by batches of product (as initially produced), some derived physico-chemical test procedures, etc. and involves batches of product from (d) and (e) above to ascertain whether changes in performance have occurred.
   (i) Clinical trial assessments or special user tests (actual patients or simulated laboratory tests) to check how:

   • effective are the proposed instructions
   • abuse or misuse may occur, and the effect on product–device efficiency.

   (j) Check microbiological contamination risks of device:

   • in use
   • by grow back experimentation
   • from recommended cleaning procedures, where applicable.

   (k) Check safety aspects of cleaning, particularly where cleaning solutions are recommended (i.e. using chlorine, peroxide or other antimicrobial systems), i.e. do residues occur; are residues a hazard; can residues affect or inactivate drug actives? etc.

(l) Where devices and product are critical to the particle size delivered (i.e. inhalation-type drugs), check initial and ongoing particle size distribution as affected by storage of product and device.

(m) Check 'dose' delivered from device:

- initially
- during storage tests on product and device
- and define any losses which may occur due to
    (i) impingement/impaction
    (ii) environmental conditions, e.g. temperature and RH
    (iii) air flow velocity (e.g. inhalation rate 15 to say 120 l air flow per min)
- under specific environmental and user conditions (humidity can affect powder particles which attract moisture).

(n) Identify likely 'dose' to patient and confirm whether this can be quantified via urine, blood, plasma, breath analysis, etc. Check (d), (m) above by mass balance estimations to ascertain whether total device output has been explained. (This also involves any residues remaining both in the pack and in the device components.)

(o) Having established (d), (m), (n) above, total dosage delivered can then be quantified:

- as—
- with a dosage range in standard deviations etc., paying attention to whether this varies according to storage of device/product/pack and at beginning, middle and end of pack use together with any residues remaining (as losses).

(p) Quantify expected 'doses' delivered from each pack, taking due allowance of fill accuracy and variations of fill.

(q) Carry out accelerated usage tests – to define shelf life of device using likely, actual, and excessive usage, checking performance, appearance, wear, at all stages, etc., i.e. can device performance change?

(r) Sterile products – involve the validation of the process of sterilisation, and sterility of components. Validation of maintenance of sterility of closure system(s), retention of sterility during storage and use, including any grow back tests (see also (j) above).

(s) Measurement of loss or gain via the total system, i.e. by permeation or seepage–leakage via the closure system or the container.

Note that in the case of aerosol valves, the effectiveness of the valve system is likely to depend on how the propellants cause swelling (or shrinkage) of the rubber components, i.e. gaskets. Initial loss and steady loss may therefore have to be quantified, with loss usually reducing after the rubber components have expanded. Since all plastics are to some degree permeable to gases, solvents, moisture, etc., the significance of these losses or gains will probably have to be checked to establish relevance to shelf life.

Note that although plastics are emphasised in the above list, some of the tests are equally relevant to other materials (metal, lacquered metal, glass, etc.).

Some historical device-oriented products

Packs acting as devices began many years ago in relatively simple ways. The author recalls menthol cones in thermoset plastic cases, lip salves in special push-up cases and spirally operated godets, smelling salts in special glass-stoppered bottles, rubber-teated dropper screw-necked glass bottles for eye and nasal drops, which date back over 50 years. The Second World War encouraged the invention of some early innovative packaging. One of these items was a collapsible metal (tube) syringe fitted with a metal needle used for injecting morphine (Omnopon). The dental syringe which took a glass cartridge tube, with a rubber diaphragm fitting at one end and a rubber plunger internally, is an early example of a pack used in an administration device. Following initial use in dentistry anaesthesia, its use was extended to a range of injectable medications (e.g. Boots' 'Viule' range). Medicated dusting powders, with sprinkler–sifter type tops, are another example of administration aids within a pack.

At that time, other than syringes and a few spray systems for throat usage (based on the Bernoulli principle as used in the 'Flit' fly spray) and the Rybar inhaler, separate device systems were virtually non-existent.

These early examples of pack–product device systems were made from glass, rubber, metal and thermosetting plastics such as urea and phenol formaldehyde. As mentioned earlier, a steady growth of pack administration systems was not possible until the arrival of thermoplastics in the 1950s.

Since the first thermoplastics on the scene involved polyethylene (and to a lesser extent polystyrene), it was the soft, flexible nature of the former that was initially exploited. Squeezee bottles, dropper plugs, followed by nasal spray packs, therefore appeared. These passed through a fairly traumatic learning period which lasted for nearly 10 years as various adverse effects related to the use of plastics were identified and overcome. These included poor closure systems (leakage, seepage, overriding of threads, loss of torque, etc.), changes in drop size due to orifice closure or distortion, plugs flying out when bottles were squeezed, stress cracking, dust patterning due to electrostatic build-up, constituent degradation due to oxygen permeation, moisture loss or gain due to water vapour permeation, preservative loss due to absorption and adsorption, loss of other volatile and permeable constituents, etc., and the disintegration of polystyrene caps when in contact with isopropyl myristate. Virtually all these problems, together with others, were identified in the period up to the late 1960s. At one time it appeared that the exciting predictions on the use of thermoplastics would never be fulfilled. However, the adage that a problem identified is the first stage to finding a solution proved true. These problems were not only overcome, but the positive features of plastics were identified and then further exploited. Unfortunately much of this historical information is not always in textbooks, and a visit to Third World countries can frequently show that the problems are happening once again. Those who believe that the above list of negative features is purely historical and that 'I don't need to know either the problem or the solution' may therefore be caught out if other parts of the world are visited.

Having briefly given the historical background, the development of pack–device systems can be brought up to date and the current state of the art considered. This will indicate that as systems have progressed, with many having a high degree of complexity, a greater level of testing has become necessary to satisfy both the company and the regulatory authorities as a safeguard to the ultimate user, i.e. the patient.

This growth into modern technology has seen new product and pack trends, involving both sterile and non-sterile products. These include developments in multidose and single (unit) dose product forms covering both preserved and non-preserved products. The latter has brought a growth in sterile products for such preparations as oral liquids, eye drops and nasal preparations, where preservative systems are possibly undesirable due to sensitising effects.

Typical examples of product–pack 'devices' and packs which are used in devices include:

- aerosols (delivering a range of product forms)
- pump systems (delivering a range of product forms)
- powder insufflators (nasal, wound care, etc.)
- powder inhalation systems for delivery to the lungs
- nebulisation systems for delivery of liquids to the lungs
- multi-port IV packs
- IV additive systems
- dermal patches
- pump systems including electronics to provide a timed delivery
- insulin 'pens' and other automatic injection systems
- prefilled syringe systems
- enema (large volume and 'micro')
- intra-uterine devices etc., and recently needle-less syringes.

It should be immediately apparent that this is only a starter list, and a few of these options will therefore be expanded as an indication of the total complexity, remembering that the additional influences of the environmental issues, use by an ever-increasing number of elderly people, needs for tamper-evidence/resistance, child-resistance, etc. still have to be considered.

At this stage there may be some difficulty in defining what is a pack. Is a soft gelatin capsule containing vitamins in an oily base – a pack? Is a hard gelatin capsule containing a fine powder for lung inhalation, e.g. spincaps and the Spinhaler (Fisons), Rotacaps and the Rotahaler (Glaxo), a pack? In the author's opinion these are open to interpretation either way.

At the other extreme are aerosols, where neither the product nor the pack can exist without the other. Aerosols can be used to dispense powders, liquids, sprays, gels, true aerosol clouds, etc., either as a continuous delivery or as a controlled or metered dose. The main container component can be fabricated from metal (aluminium or tinplate), glass or plastic coated glass, or plastic (e.g. polyester), and the valve components from combinations of plastic, metal and rubber. Depending on the product usage, the majority of the tests listed earlier may have to be involved in the clearance of an aerosol, particularly if it is a metered dose aerosol for administration of a product to the lungs (a critical administration route).

Since certain aerosols can be sterile and non-preserved, microbiological risks may have to be checked at the dispensing orifice, including the possibility of 'grow back'. Special double valve systems and other alternatives are being continuously evaluated for such applications. Innovation related to aerosol adaptors for nasal, ear, eye, etc. applications are typical examples of evolving technology.

For aerosols delivering products to the lungs, patient compliance associated with firing and breathing has brought about the introduction of 'spacers' (yet another component needing investigative procedures) and breath-activated aerosols (e.g. 3M (Riker) – Autohaler).

The virtual condemnation of CFC propellants has put new challenges to aerosols in general and to the pharmaceutical industry in particular, when cloud break-up into small (less than 10 μm) particles is critical to product success. The latest date for the withdrawal of CFCs for pharmaceutical products is 2005, with HFAs 134a and 227 being the main replacement candidates.

Powder inhalation devices

The mid-1960s saw the first development in fine powders destined for the lungs, with particular emphasis on the invention of the Spinhaler (Fisons/Aventis) and its successful use with sodium cromoglycate (Intal – Fisons). Investigations into actual devices and ideas (patient searches) will indicate that there are now over 200 options available for powder delivery systems. Successful examples include the Rotahaler (Glaxo), Turbohaler (Astra Zeneca), Diskhaler (Glaxo), Accuhaler (Glaxo), etc.

As with aerosols, the effective dose to patient is difficult to quantify and validate, as this depends on a range of factors. Although when questioned patients generally prefer the apparent convenience of metered dose aerosols, the dose is very much dependent on the use of correct techniques and procedures. Since powder inhalation systems more readily couple 'synchronisation with use', the more complex operating procedures may be more than compensated by a more effective dose guarantee.

A continuing competition between aerosols and powder inhalations can therefore be predicted.

Small and large volume parenterals

Both SVPs and LVPs have been subject to an active area of innovation to improve administration and compliance. LVPs have offered packs with a range of 'ports' either as preformed containers or as packs produced as a form (blow)–fill–seal operation (e.g. as equipment offered by Rommelag and ALP). Modifications to giving sets and transfer aids (for the production of IV 'cocktails') also fall into this category. Examples of the latter include the Abbotts system (ADD-Vantage) and the Kendall McGaw (Add-A-Vials) transfer device.

SVPs are meeting similar challenges, e.g. plastic ampoules via form–fill–seal (Braun Mini-plasco), prefilled syringes (using single or bicompartmental systems), etc.

Closures

Closures have for the past 30 years been a major area of innovative changes either to improve product removal administration or to meet some specific challenge to safety. The options related to the former are enormous and could constitute a book in their own right.

Safety challenges have, since the introduction of the Poisons Prevention Act (1970) in the USA, seen a steady increase in the use of child-resistant closures (which meet BS

6652 1989 in the UK or DIN 55559 in Germany or ISO 28317). The Extra Strength Tylenol poisonings of 1982 also put new emphasis on tamper-evident and tamper-resistant packaging, and, it is hoped, the disappearance of the word 'tamper-proof' or 'child-proof' from any of the packs just mentioned. For example, a CRC may actually be less safe if it is not properly or correctly reapplied. As mentioned earlier, many of these safety features cause difficulty to the elderly population either in the opening of the pack or in the correct replacement after use. Providing elderly user-friendly packs is therefore a recent trend. Among these one finds the monitored dosage systems and medical event monitored systems (MEMS).

Other systems and examples

The above examples have only scratch the surface of the expanding role of the pack. What about dermal patches, implants, insulin pens, pump systems, suppository and pessary delivery systems, nebulisation, puffer packs, 'Ocuserts', a review of unit dose applications, etc. Systems are now so numerous that doing a paper search and review would take several weeks. However, they do indicate the new roles which are being undertaken by the pack. Each new system challenges new sets of tests in order to evaluate performance and efficiency.

Conclusion

The information given in this chapter, together with that in Chapter 8, should provide a good basic understanding of the broad role of a packaging development activity, and the supporting role associated with other relevant disciplines. All activities must support the ultimate task of the pack, i.e. to provide confidence in the product in terms of convenience, presentation, protection, etc. while ensuring that the product remains satisfactory in the fullest sense, i.e. in terms of integrity, identity, uniformity, safety, effectiveness, etc., all at an economically acceptable cost. Undoubtedly pharmaceutical packaging does receive and demand greater attention to detail than any other form of product. With the advent of product liability and the expanding administrative role of the pack, investigations will not relax but rather will intensify.

Although the types of test procedure will broadly continue to follow the stages identified in this and other chapters, the ultimate intensity of the procedure must be related to (and vary with) the type of product and the route by which it is administered etc. The use of a declared 'food grade' plastic is usually the minimum standard that would be used for a pharmaceutical product, either for a secondary packaging component or where extraction between product (solid items) and the plastic may seem unlikely. Reference to toy regulations may also provide useful information, especially where coloured materials are employed.

As the cost of clearing any product–pack combination is inevitably high, it is extremely important to define adequately the product, the pack and the processes involved in these original clearance schedules and to finish with a total clearance programme which is ultimately supported with full specifications.

The future control of the product and pack then revolves around these documents. In the case of a plastic pack or plastic components, it may be necessary not only to define certain critical factors in the specification tightly, but also to purchase under a certificate of warranty, as exhaustive QC procedures (particularly biological tests), which might be necessary to detect change, could involve prohibitive costs. Regular QC checks are likely to include melt flow index, density, IR or DSC identity, etc. The last two are a particularly useful means of providing plastic identification, with DSC now more widely used.

As an additional insurance, a selected number of production batches are placed on an 'existing' product stability test annually. This monitoring system ensures that the stability profile (and shelf life) of the product does not change with the passage of time. Any changes in product, pack or process inevitably involve some form of retesting schedule, the intensity of which varies according to the nature of the change. In all such support programmes it is still important to thoroughly re-inspect all packs before, during and after chemical and biological analysis.

It can therefore be concluded that packs and devices supplied by the pharmaceutical industry which utilise plastics (and any other material) normally have to pass through a thorough and rigorous test procedure, but such procedures must still be improved upon with progress. If possible loopholes in the present systems are to be identified, more attention will be required on the internal storage containers which are usually found in factory production areas and the bulk containers used to supply the industry with drugs and other excipients, as these receive far less attention than the pack destined for the patients. Validation and traceability are current key words, but undoubtedly others will arise.

The work related to the clearance of the pack, the establishment of total integrity and GMP cannot be isolated into apparent water-tight compartments such as product development, pack development, production, marketing and QC, as all must operate as an effective team with a high degree of communication and co-ordination. A packaging co-ordinator with an ability to give an overview is virtually essential to success but to date this has been recognised by only a few companies.

It should be stressed that the latter part of this chapter has been written in such a way as to encourage a degree of both alertness and understanding. It does not set out to say that any one approach is the ultimate. Test procedures must be constantly reviewed and updated. Virtually all the stages identified must be treated as long-term information gathering. Extractive tests fall into this category; they provide the best information available at this time and therefore must not be treated as the ultimate. To date there are no records of people dying from plastics, but rather of deaths from the processes by which they are synthesised (e.g. the vinyl chloride monomer saga). However, the industry must remain responsible, particularly in terms of product–pack liability, and at the same time remain commercially viable.

To complete this chapter a final section is required, i.e. consideration of tests and test schedules which may be used for the evaluation of materials and completed packs. This represents the area where information tends to change the most, and the subject is so diverse that it would only be effectively covered by a full textbook. It is therefore not practical to cover all tests and methods in detail but only to provide broad reference to possibilities. Tests can be applied to materials (e.g. water vapour permeability), on components or completed packs. Tests generally fall into three categories, i.e. those required:

1   to gain information where no previous information exists or information is scant
2   to control quality – usually fairly simple tests that can be carried out rapidly, giving numerical results which can be readily interpreted and compared

3   to predict performance – used where some relationship has clearly been established between field performance and a laboratory test.

The standard of these tests may be related to in-house company standards, industrial or national/international standards.

Typical standards bodies include:

- ISO (International Standard Organisation)
- BSI (British Standards Institute, which issues British Standards)
- ASTM (American Society for Testing and Materials, which issues ASTM Standards)
- FEFCO (Federation Européenne des Fabricants de Carton Ondulé (test methods))
- BPBMA (Technical Association of the British Paper and Board Makers Association)
- TAPPI (Technical Association for the Pulp and Paper Industry (USA), which issues TAPPI Standards).

Standards are generally applied to the following applications:

1   dimensional standards
2   performance or standards of quality
3   standard methods of testing
4   standard technical terms and symbols
5   standard codes of practice.

Table 2.2 Tests on plastics (general) (see various parts of BS 2782)

Test	Standard
Melting temperature (°C)	BS 2782 part 1
T_m (crystalline)	BS 2782 part 1
T_g (amorphous)	BS 2782 part 1
Specific gravity/density	D792, BS 2782, ISO 1183
Tensile strength	D638, BS 2782, ISO 527
Elongation (%)	D638, ISO 527
Compressive strength	D695
Flexural strength	B790
Impact strength (Izod)	D256, BS 2782, ISO 180/1AR
Hardness (Rockwell)	B785
Impact strength (Charpy)	ISO 179/1
Vicat, softening point	D1525, ISO 306
Modulus of elasticity	D790, BS 2782, ISO 527
Thermal conductivity	C177
Thermal expansion	D696
Refractive index	D542
Transmittance	D1003
Haze	D1003
Water absorption	D570
Flammability	D635
Water vapour transmission	ASTM C355, BS 3177
Melt flow index (g/10 min)	D1238, ISO/R 1133
Stress cracking	ASTM D1693–70, BS 2782–832A

Table 2.3 Tests on plastics (films)

Test	Standard
Specific gravity/density	D1505
Tensile strength	D882
Elongation (%)	D882
Bursting strength per 0.001 inch thickness	D774
Tearing strength	D1922 (Elmendorf), BS2782 360A–360C
Tearing strength	D1004
Folding endurance	D2176
Water absorption (24 h/%)	D570
Resistance to acid/alkali	D543
Resistance to grease/oils	D722
Resistance to organic solvent	D543
Resistance to heat and cold	D759
Change in linear dimensions	D1204
Flammability (burning rate)	D1433, CS192
Rate of water vapour transmission	E96 ASTM, BS2782–820A/822, DIN 5312L, BS 3177
Oxygen permeability	DIN 53380, BS2782–821A, ASTM D1434

Table 2.4 Tests on plastics (optical)

Test	Standard
Gloss	BS 2782 520A, ASTM D2457 (Gardner 45°)
Haze (wide angle) (%)	ASTM D1003
Haze (clarity)	ICI test (Gardner), BS 2782 521A
Coefficient of friction	ASTM D1894, BS 2782 824A
Dart impact	D1709

Table 2.5 Tests on plastic containers and mouldings

Test	Standard
Screw-neck finishes	BS 5789
Environmental stress cracking	BS 2782–832A
Permeability (moisture)	BS 3177

Table 2.6 Standards related to other specific containers

Item	Standard
Collapsible tubes	BS 2006
Glass bottles	BS 1133 section 18, BS 1918 glass container finishes, drop test, impact, thermal shock, hydrostatic pressure
Fibreboard	BS1133 section 7, FPCMA
Timber and plywood cases	BS1133 section 8
Aluminium foil	BS1133 section 21
Metal containers	BS1133 section 10
Metal collapsible tubes for eye ointment	BS 4230
Printing inks, resistance testing	BS 4321

Table 2.7 Tests on sterile products

ISO 8362:	Injection containers for injectables and accessories.
Covers:	hardness, fragmentation, self-sealability, needle penetration, seal integrity, etc.
ISO 8536:	Infusions
ISO 8871:	Elastomeric parts
Covers:	extractive tests including chemical and biological assessment, UV, reducing substances, ammonia, non-volatiles, pH, zinc.

Tables 2.2–2.7 provide some 'lists' on the types of standard tests available. None of the lists are anywhere near inclusive of all the tests which are available. Tests are particularly useful for the comparison of materials, usually to assist the selection of a material or materials for further evaluation. The ultimate selection phase usually stems from the investigational tests in contact with the product, and is finally supported by formal stability programmes. In all these data must be adequately detailed, properly recorded and, where necessary, relevant conclusions must be drawn.

Examples of tests for specific materials

For tests on paper and board, see Chapter 5.

Tests other than those quoted in this chapter can be found as ISO, ASTM, TAPPI and BSI standards. In most tests on paper and board, the materials have to be conditioned prior to testing, otherwise compatible results will not be achieved. See Tables 2.2–2.7.

3

REGULATORY ASPECTS OF PHARMACEUTICAL PACKAGING

J. Glasby

Introduction

The pharmaceutical industry is one of the most highly regulated industries in the world, the aerospace industry perhaps being the only one more highly regulated. Control is imposed on:

1 how the product is developed (toxicology testing is controlled through good laboratory practice (GLP); clinical testing is controlled by good clinical practice (GCP))
2 how the product is manufactured (through good manufacturing practice (GMP))
3 how the product is sold (through controls imposed through the Product Licence Application (PLA))
4 how the product is labelled (in Europe through the Labelling Directive and summary of product characteristics (SPC))
5 how the product is advertised (in Europe through the Advertising Directive)
6 how the product is disposed of (in Europe by the Packaging Waste Directive).

Thus, from the origination of the first idea to the final sale of the product, the legal system plays a key role in shaping and controlling the product. In this chapter we are particularly interested in how regulatory demands affect packaging.

Definition of the pack

The packaging technologist defines the pack as 'a device for carrying and protecting the product from producer to user', thus it is involved in containment, convenience, compliance, and confidence. The regulator, however, is interested in only some of these aspects (Table 3.1). In particular, the regulator sees the pack as having the following characteristics:

1 containing the product
   - protection of the product
   - protection of the consumer
   - dosage control
2 carrying the label
   - legal control of the product
   - informing the recipient

Table 3.1 Respective areas of interest of pack definition technologist and regulator

Area of interest	Technologist	Regulator
Economics	X	
Protection	X	X
Identification	X	X
Containment	X	X
Convenience	X	
Market appeal	X	
Presentation	X	
Disposal	X	X
Compliance	X	X
Primary pack	X	X
Secondary pack	X	
Tertiary pack	X	

3   contaminating the environment

- packaging waste
- ozone depletion

4   protecting the consumer

- child-resistant closures
- tamper-evidence.

The pack as a container of the product

At one time the container excited little interest since, it being invariably made of glass, there was little potential interaction with the product. The glass bottle was regarded as little more than an inert receptacle. Since there were also severe limitations on the form of the glass bottle there was little scope for ingenuity, thus packaging development tended to be considered as a separate topic tagged onto the end of the development programme, i.e. almost as an afterthought. Now the situation is different, and product development is totally integrated with packaging development. Of course, the packaging technologist had been saying for years that packaging development cannot be separated from product development, insisting that it was not possible to separate the pack and product. Why then has the attitude of industry and the regulators changed? There are several factors, as detailed below.

Increasing sophistication of the pack

Glass, being so inert, does not present a very interesting problem to the packaging technologist. Once plastics are involved, however, the situation changes and there is much more scope for interactions between product and packaging. Packs can also be designed to be more closely tailored to the needs of the patient. Like all advantages, however, there are associated disadvantages to the use of plastics, for example the extraction of materials from the plastics into the product. Once the possibility of contamination arises, regulatory authorities become much more interested in the selection, composition and performance of the package.

Increasing sophistication of the product

New chemical entities are so few and far between these days, and are so expensive to develop that companies regularly look at their ageing products with a view to revamping them by means of new presentations. One way to do this is to repackage the product in a more sophisticated way. Once there is more complexity, there is greater potential for problems to occur between the pack and product.

Incorporating a device into the pack

Control of dosage and administration has always been interesting both to pharmacists and to regulators, but it can be a major problem with pharmaceutical products. The pack can play a key part in controlling the dosage, for example in the use of a pressurised aerosol for dispensing powders or solutions. Once the pack and product administration system are integrated in this way the development cannot be separated and neither can they be separated in regulatory terms. A drug is thus affected by its packaging, both in practice and in the eye of the regulatory authority. For example, in the USA a parenteral drug product, even if it is an old drug such as sodium chloride, when produced in a plastic container does not fall within the category of 'generally recognised as safe' (GRAS). It is regarded as a new drug (Federal Food, Drug and Cosmetic Act S201(P)).

Cost of development

It is not only the development of new chemical entities that is becoming more and more time-consuming and, thus, expensive (Table 3.2). The cost of development of any product is now so high that a company must look to worldwide distribution in order to recoup the development costs. Ideally the same product should be used worldwide. However, while the pharmaceutical development department will be trying to develop a single formulation, the packaging development department's aim must also be to try and develop one single pack for worldwide use. This trend, however, will be countered by marketing departments trying to obtain precisely the right presentation for each market, insisting that markets differ in their needs.

Just as market needs differ, local regulatory agencies also have different requirements. While it may be possible to convince marketing departments at least to reduce the number of variants required, what about all the different regulatory agencies, of

Table 3.2 Time to develop new drug

Activity	Time (years)
Research	2
Toxicology	3
Development	3
Clinical	4
Registration	?
Total	12+

which there are over 150 in the world? How can they be satisfied by the same product and data?

In regulatory terms the situation is not quite as bad as it might appear. If we look at the world market (Figure 3.1), the EU represents approximately 30% of the market, the US approximately 27% and Japan approximately 18%. In total this represents 75% of the total market. Therefore, in commercial terms if one can satisfy these countries then a large step has been made towards meeting the commercial goal.

This situation has been improved through the International Conference on Harmonisation (ICH) between these three areas, since agreement has been reached on stability testing, impurities of active materials and others. As this expands, the multiplicity of data requirements will be significantly reduced. However, although there is some harmonisation between the three major regulatory areas in terms of the data required, it is likely that in regulatory terms the world will continue to be split into three different types of regulatory system: EU, USA and Japanese. Other countries will tend to follow one of these approaches with local modifications.

Regulatory authorities – background

The EU, although under criticism in many areas, has been fairly successful in the pharmaceutical area, with the following achievements:

- centralised system in place
- decentralised system in place
- harmonisation of format
- expanding acceptance of format outside EU
- harmonisation of standards (PH EUR).

A standard format of product licence application has been adopted, making the preparation of regulatory documents much simpler. The format and data requirements of

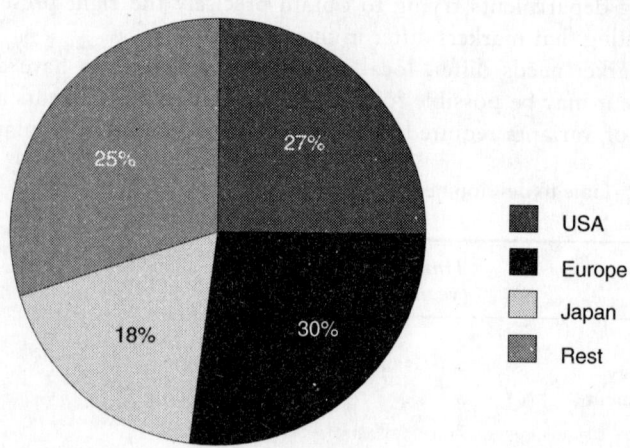

Figure 3.1 The world pharmaceutical market

the EU are being adopted by several countries outside the union, so reducing the number of types of application necessary.

The Food and Drug Administration (FDA) is finally recognising the competence of certain overseas agencies and the skill of scientists, and accepting more data that has been generated overseas (Figure 3.2). Even Japan is becoming more international, with several initiatives suggesting, in theory at least, that data from overseas should be acceptable within Japan.

In order to understand the approach of regulatory authorities, it is necessary to understand their attitudes and for this it is necessary to look back into history.

The history of pharmaceutical products is, in fact, rather short (Figure 3.3). Before the nineteenth century there were few really effective drugs apart from a few herbal remedies such as digitalis from foxglove. In general, only herbs and spices were used in treating disease. Since they had variable and unproven efficacy, the main perceived problem was that herbs and spices were expensive. Certain unscrupulous dealers tended to dilute the material in order to maximise profit, and this led to the introduction of the first control of drugs. First local pharmacopoeias and then country-wide pharmacopoeias were introduced which defined the specific composition and quality to be applied to drugs.

In the nineteenth and early twentieth century, with the increased urbanisation and industrialisation of the UK, the majority of medicines were the so-called patent medicines which contained few active ingredients but had extensive claims for their curative actions. Thus, the controls that had to be applied were on the advertising and claims for the product. It was only after 1935 that the 'therapeutic revolution' brought products which actually had some proven and consistent efficacy. Unfortunately, along with the efficacy came side-effects and problems, since for every pharmacological activity which is beneficial there will inevitably also be side-effects. If we look back at the introduction of controls on medicines, it is generally a problem or disaster which leads to introduction of the specific control.

In the USA, the death of a large number of children from a sulphanilamide preparation led to the Food, Drug and Cosmetic Act (1938). For the first time, proof of safety was required before any product was introduced to the market. It was not until the 1962 thalidomide tragedy that proof of efficacy was required in the USA through an amendment to the FD&C Act, the Kefauver Amendment, and this led to the

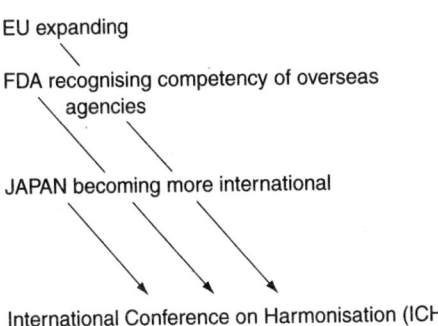

EU expanding

FDA recognising competency of overseas agencies

JAPAN becoming more international

International Conference on Harmonisation (ICH)

Figure 3.2 The worldwide regulatory split

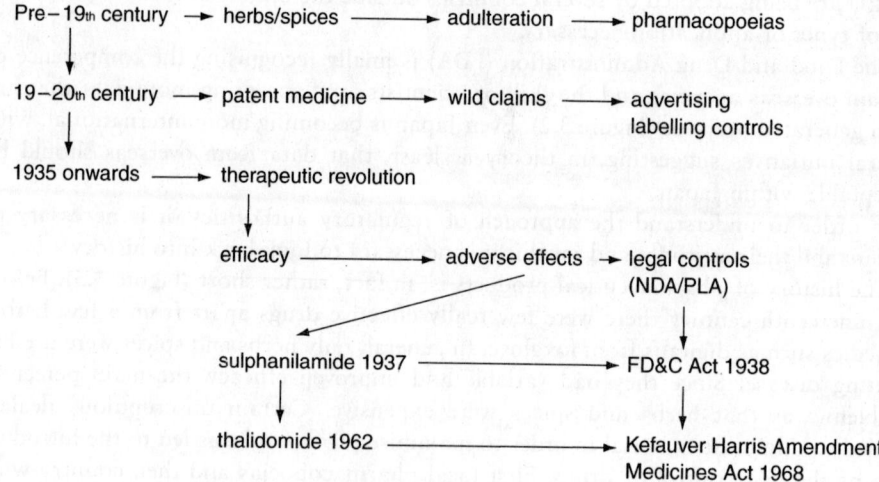

Figure 3.3 Outline of pharmaceutical history

introduction of other regulatory controls worldwide including the Medicines Act 1968 in the UK. Such problems, together with other factors such as political pressure, public pressure, consumerism and bureaucracy, have created the regulatory agency attitudes we see today.

Despite the differences in regulatory agencies, the actual registration approach is very similar (Figure 3.4). The process starts with the research area producing compounds for evaluation, followed by toxicology testing, first in animals and then the first introduction into human volunteers to determine safety and tolerance. This is followed by small clinical efficacy studies and finally the Phase III full efficacy studies involving large numbers of patients. In parallel to these clinical programmes the product development progresses with finalisation of the formulation and pack, and stability testing. Once sufficient clinical and pharmaceutical data are available, the product licence application can be prepared and submitted to the authorities. For review, it is generally

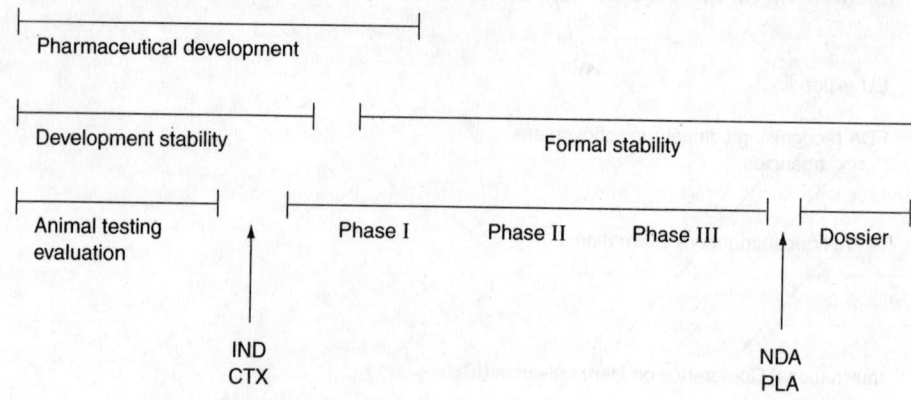

Figure 3.4 The development process

78

split into the three different sections, chemistry and pharmacy, pre-clinical studies and clinical data, so that these separate parts can be examined by specialist reviewers. It is almost certain that reviewers will have questions during their review which have to be circulated back to the company while the application is put on hold, pending suitable replies. This circuit may be followed several times and, in part, explains why the review cycle can be so long and variable. Finally, once all the questions have been resolved and the precise labelling agreed, a licence is issued and the product can be launched.

European Union processes for drug evaluation

Within the EU there are currently three processes by which a drug can be approved for marketing (Table 3.3). These are individual local applications to specific countries, the decentralised system, (mutual recognition route), and the centralised system.

Local applications

For products intended for a single country a local application can be made. Since 1 January 1998 any subsequent application to a second country must be made through the decentralised system.

Decentralised system (mutual recognition)

The decentralised system is, in effect, a system of mutual recognition. An application is first made in a single country and when approved the application, translated in certain aspects, along with the assessment report prepared by the regulatory agency, is sent to the other countries. Each country then has a limited time to accept the application and assessment report or to provide reasoned objections. If the objections cannot be resolved by bilateral discussion then the application is referred to the CPMP for a binding recommendation (Figure 3.5). Alternatively, the country or countries with objections can be withdrawn from the procedure. Although not without its problems, the system is working and products are receiving approvals in many European countries by this route. At present however, individual countries tend to be carrying out a full review of the applications despite the availability of the original approval and assessment report, and have not yet fully embraced the idea of mutual recognition.

Centralised system

It was recognised that certain products, such as biotechnology products, were taking a considerable period to become registered in Europe because of their complexity and

Table 3.3 EU processes

Local applications	*After 1998 for one country only*
Decentralised applications	Mutual recognition Majority of applications
Centralised applications	Innovative products and biotechnology Single licence for all EU

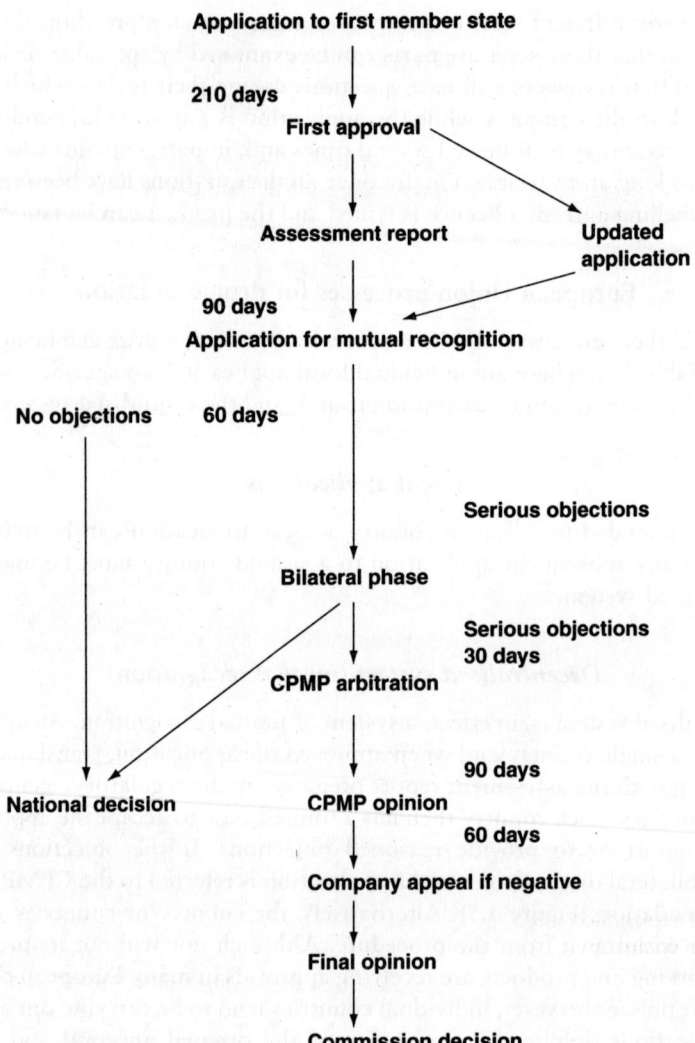

Figure 3.5 The mutual recognition process

the absence of skills to evaluate them in certain countries. A central scheme was therefore set up where by a single evaluation of the application is made and a recommendation for approval issued by the CPMP followed by issue of a single licence issued by the London-based European Medicines Evaluation Agency (EMEA) for all the EU (Figure 3.6). Since 1 January 1995 this centralised procedure has been mandatory for all products of biotechnology and optional for projects which are very innovative such as new chemical entities or new presentations of drugs. CPMP appoints one or two of its members to act as rapporteur to co-ordinate the assessment using the facilities of the various regulatory agencies within Europe. Once the evaluation reports are available the CPMP makes an opinion within 210 days of receipt of the application and a single licence is then granted, valid throughout the Union.

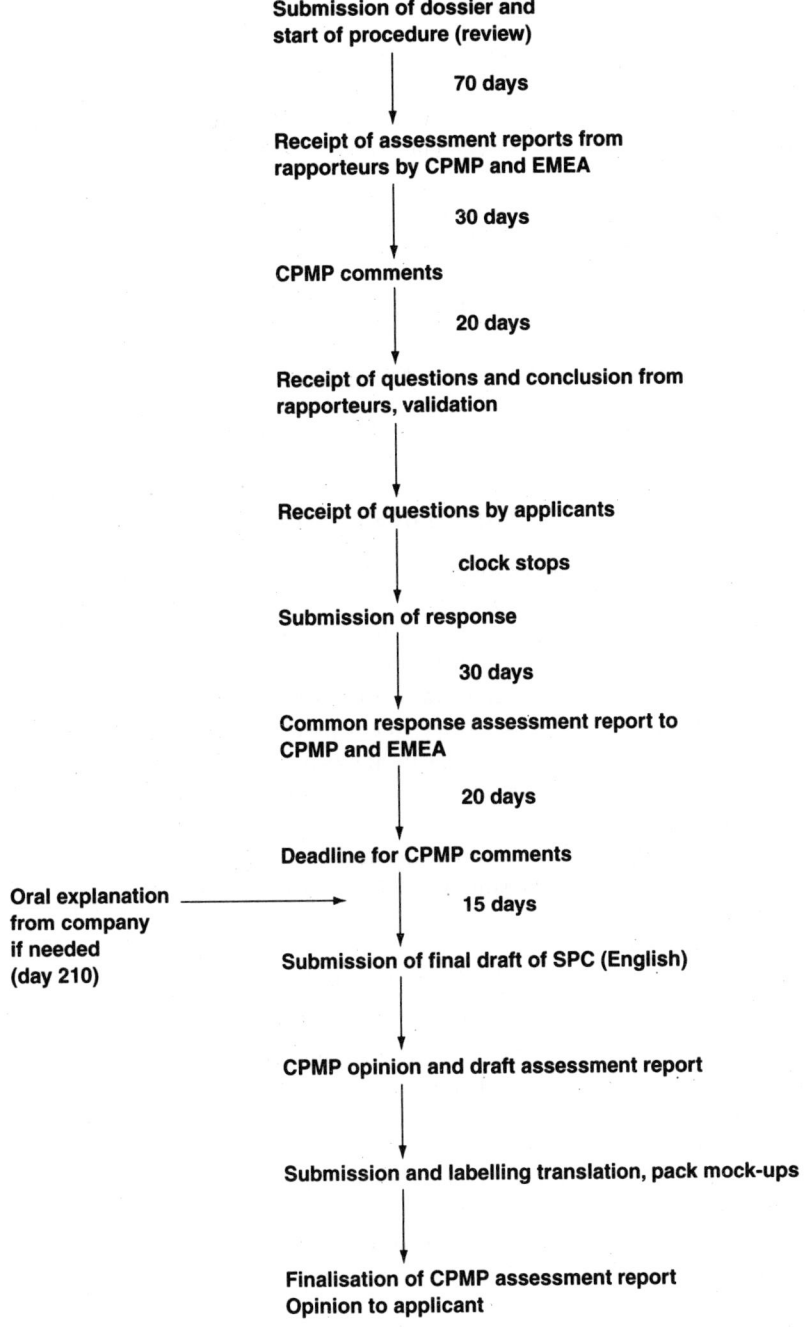

Figure 3.6 Outline of the centralised procedure

Product licence applications – data requirements on the package

A few years ago there was almost no legislation concerning packaging. The 1968 Medicines Act in the UK, for example, makes almost no mention of the subject. However, for the reasons discussed earlier, certain specific EU guidelines applying to packaging have now been published. These are:

- CPMP List of Allowed Terms (III/3593/91) (new list issued in February 1998)
- Notice to Applicants (Updated 1998)
- Plastic Container Guidelines (III/9090)
- Plastics in Contact with Food Directive (90/128).

These, along with the requirements of the European Pharmacopoeia, provide guidance for the data requirements for packaging and its format for presentation in the product licence application.

CPMP list of allowed terms

Descriptive terms for pharmaceutical forms, routes of administration, and packaging and delivery systems allowed to be used in a Product Licence Application are now prescribed by EU Regulations (Table 3.4). It is hard to understand the value of this legislation except in terms of the legal nature of the Product Licence Application. It must be remembered that a product licence is more a legal than a truly technical document. As with all legal documents, it is necessary to ensure the definitions are consistent wherever the application is made. It is not clear, however, how much attention is being given by regulatory agencies to this list, although experience has suggested that they do insist on using the appropriate terms in at least the application form part of the submission, since this becomes the legal body of the licence. The official terms should also be used in the labelling, particularly the summary of product characteristics.

Notice to applicants

The main pharmaceutical Directives 65/65 and 75/318 do not actually spell out in detail what is required in a Product Licence Application. These key directives require that applications be made, and define only in outline the data requirements. It is therefore necessary to expand the guidance and this is done in the Notice to Applicants (1986) and its subsequent amendments. The Notice to Applicants prepared by the European Commission has no legal standing, but gives additional advice over and above that given in the various EU Directives. The notice actually forms volume 2 of 9 volumes of the Rules Governing Medicinal Products in the European Union, and has two parts:

- 2A deals with the legal procedures for marketing authorisation
- 2B deals with the presentation and content of the application dossier.

In these documents the Marketing Authorisation Application is defined in the following sections.

Table 3.4 Standard terms for marketing authorisation applications, Notes for Guidance III 3593/91 EN final (updated February 1998)

Covers standard terms for:
- pharmaceutical dosage forms
- route of administration
- container
- closure
- administration device.

Containers	Drench gun	Oral syringe
Ampoules	Dropper applicator	Pipette
Applicator	Gas cylinder	Pour-on container
Automatic injection device	High pressure transdermal	Pre-filled syringe
Bag	delivery device	Pressurised container
Balling gun	Implanter	Sachet
Barrel	Inobo injection device	Scarifier
Blister	Injection needle	Screwcap
Bottle	Injection syringe	Single dose container
Box	Internal graduated calibration	Spatula
Brush	chamber	Spot-on applicator
Brush applicator	Intramammary syringe	Spray container
Cannula	Jar	Spray pump
Cap	Measuring spoon	Spray valve
Cartridge	Metering pump	Stab vaccinator
Child-resistant closure	Metering valve	Stopper
Cup	Mouth piece	Strip tablet container
Dabbing applicator	Nasal applicator	Tube
Dart	Nebuliser	Vaginal sponge applicator
Dredging applicator	Needle applicator	Vial
Dredging container	Nozzle	

- *Section I:* application form, administrative details, labelling and expert reports (chemistry and pharmacy, toxico-pharmacological, and clinical).
- *Section II:* chemistry and pharmacy data.
- *Section III:* toxicology data.
- *Section IV:* clinical data.

For most of our purposes, the data on packaging is included only in the chemistry and pharmacy section and in the pharmaceutical expert report, although if a new plastic or polymer material is used, toxicology data may be required along with comment in the toxicology expert report.

With Section II, data is required on the packaging in four areas:

- *Section IIA2:* composition – immediate package
- *Section IIA4:* development pharmaceutics
- *Section IIC3:* control of starting materials
- *Section IIF2:* stability testing.

The Notice to Applicants remained the only guidelines available until 1990, when the draft Plastic Container Guidelines III/9090 was published which expanded the requirements in these four areas (Table 3.5).

Table 3.5 CPMP Guideline III/9090 EN final, plastic primary packaging materials

Take account of:
- Directive 90/128/EEC – plastic materials intended to come into contact with foodstuffs
- European Pharmacopoeia
- Notice to applicants
- Volume IV of Rules Governing Medicinal Products in European Community. Parts covering packaging:
  - IIA2 immediate packaging
  - IIA4 development pharmaceutics
  - IIC3 packaging materials
  - IIF2 stability.

MAA application section IIA2 – container

This requires only a brief description of the nature of the container and of the components, with a qualitative composition and details of the method of closure and opening (Table 3.6).

MAA application section IIA4 – development pharmaceutics

The development pharmaceutics area is often neglected, but is proving to be a key area in submissions. In this section the applicant must justify the choice of the formulation and of the packaging. Thus, the selection of the resin must be discussed and data provided on the interaction or compatibility between product and pack. If there is processing involved, such as sterilisation, then the influence of the process on the product and container must be studied and reported (Table 3.6).

MAA application section IIC3 – control of starting materials

The container is regarded as one of the starting materials for the product along with the other ingredients of the formulation. For this reason the specification, testing regimen and details of any tests carried out must be provided for both the plastic resin material and the container (Table 3.7).

Resin

The name of the resin material, the name and address of the manufacturer, the chemical name, the complete formulation, characteristics and quantity of all ingredients and the function are required where the material is to be used in a container which will be exposed very intimately to the product, such as a large volume parenteral solution or eye drop. The identity, using IR absorption along with a reference spectrum must be provided. Additives, particularly those likely to migrate, including antioxidants, plasticisers, catalysts, initiators and materials such as phthalates, adipates and organic tin in PVC or any dyes used in the resin must also be identified.

Tests on plastics should include physical, mechanical, dimensional, purity in terms of monomer and additives, buffer potential, reducing substances and UV absorption.

If the material is not listed in the European Pharmacopoeia then its status as a food-approved plastic must be described with reference to the EU Directive. If these data are

Table 3.6 CPMP Guidelines III 9090

IIA2 Immediate packaging
Description container including:
- nature of material (qualitative)
- description of closure
- method of opening
- information on container
- Description of tamper-evidence and child-resistant closure.

IIA4 Development pharmaceutics
Justification of choice of containers in terms of:
- stability of active ingredient and product
- method of administration
- sterilisation procedures.

Choice of plastic including information on:
- tightness of closure
- protection of contents against external factors
- container–contents interaction
- influence of manufacturing process.

Table 3.7 CPMP Guideline III 9090, IIC3 – packaging materials

Specification and routine tests
- Container construction, list components
- Nature of polymers used
- Specification of material:
  – identification
  – visual inspection
  – dimensional test
  – physical test
  – microbial tests.

Scientific data collected during development
Plastic:
- name/grade
- manufacturer (parenteral and ophthalmic)
- chemical name
- monomers used
- qualitative composition of interaction
- description and solubility in solvents
- identification material
- identification additives
- Tests (general and mechanical).

Container:
- Name converter (ophthalmic and parenteral)
- Reproducible process
- No changes in composition without verification

not available then toxicology data may be required, along with an assessment by a toxicologist. Where there is less contact, such as the case for a solid dosage form, it may be possible to reduce the amount of data supplied, particularly if the plastic is of pharmacopoeial grade.

Container

The container must be described in terms of the plastics used and the name of the manufacturer, along with an evaluation of its suitability and risk of toxicity through extractives. Consistency of the container quality is a key aspect and data must be provided on containers tested in conditions similar to those to be used, including sterilisation if this is part of the process.

Once the resin and the container have been fixed there should be no changes in materials or manufacturing process. If a change is made then further testing and approval of a product licence variation by the regulatory authority will be necessary. This means that pharmaceutical companies look to resin and container suppliers to maintain supplies for many years without making changes to processing or composition.

MAA application section IIF2 – stability

The final section of III/9090 covers the stability data required (Table 3.8). It does not provide a comprehensive coverage of the subject but relies on the existing general stability guidelines, adding extra points which specifically cover the package.

The guideline makes the key point that the choice of test conditions is influenced by the compatibility and protectability of the resin and the product type involved. In setting up stability tests, both normal and stress conditions are required. Normal conditions look at interaction between pack and product, migration of components and protection of the product under normal temperatures and humidities. Stress testing is carried out using higher temperatures, light, high humidities and increased surface ratio to highlight the migration and interaction potential of the components.

Table 3.8 CPMP Guideline III 9090, IIF2 – stability

Choice of plastic based on protective effect and compatibility
Compatibility study part of product stability test
Solid forms:
- migration risk low
- no interaction' study needed

Semi-solid:
- migration of additives or dyes
- study with actual formulation

Liquid:
- migration risk for formulation
- O&P – active and preservative
- studied under simulated use conditions

General
- Study at least one batch of finished product
- Normal and accelerated conditions
- Extraction tests with solvents (as foods) only predictive
- Migration studies should include technological characteristics, leaching antioxidants, monomers and oligomers, plasticisers, mineral compounds
- Sorption of formulation components to be studied

Study methods should include technological characteristics, the leaching of antioxidants, plasticisers, minerals (calcium and barium), and absorption of the active component of the product into the plastic.

For solid products the risk of migration is low and therefore interaction studies are not required over and above the normal stability test results. For semi-solid products it is necessary to look particularly at the migration of additives, vapour permeation and the effects of the product on the physical parameters of the pack. For liquid products the migration potential for the specific formulation is required, and the determination of active ingredient content under simulated use, along with extractives data is required for parenteral and ophthalmic products. Moisture permeation is important, particularly for solid products packaged in blister packs.

In the past it has been difficult to satisfy in a single test programme the requirements for the EU, the USA and Japan. However, following the 1992 International Conference on Harmonisation, tripartite stability recommendations have been produced which have considerably simplified the situation (Table 3.9), laying down storage conditions and means of evaluating results.

Expert reports

The major difference between an EU dossier and that for other regulatory authorities, such as FDA, is the requirement for expert reports. These documents play an important

Table 3.9 ICH tripartite stability guidelines – final product

Test frequency
- 3 months for first year
- 6 months for second year
- 12 months thereafter
- continue to test to shelf life

Packaging
- final marketed pack plus unprotected product (useful)

Evaluation
- systematic approach (protocol)
- matrixing possible
- variability affects protocol
- shelf life is suggested as 95% confidence of the mean reaching the specification limit
- can combine batch results to determine shelf life if variability low
- if variability high, use minimum values
- if little degradation, no need for stats
- mass balance

Extrapolation
- limited extrapolation can be done – must be justified (e.g. linear and mechanics)

Labelling
- as national requirements, e.g. store below 25°C in UK (cannot use room temperature)

Storage conditions
- $25°C \pm 2°C/60 \pm 5\%$ RH
- $40°C \pm 2°C/75 \pm 5\%$ RH
- if 40°C fails, test at $30°C \pm 2°C/60 \pm 5\%$ RH

part in the assessment of the application. Three expert reports are provided, covering chemistry and pharmacy, toxico-pharmacology and clinical aspects of the product. Only the chemistry and pharmacy expert report will cover packaging aspects, unless a new packaging material is involved. The expert report must provide a balanced evaluation of the data and therefore may be critical of the data presented. Many companies find this difficult to accept, but regulatory authorities expect criticism and thus even a critical expert report need not prejudice the review of an application. If done properly the expert report can, in fact, assist the company since it allows some flexibility. It can, for example:

- justify a temperature other than 25°C having been used for room temperature storage
- provide a shelf-life prediction at 25°C based on overall data from various temperatures
- justify fewer than three batches having been used in the stability tests
- justify the use of non-production batches
- explain different stability profiles between batches
- provide a materials balance if decomposition appears
- justify the statistical methods or explain the absence of a statistical method.

Thus, the guidelines need not be followed absolutely providing the expert can justify the alternative approach taken.

USA procedure for drug evaluation

The New Drug Application (NDA) is the formal request that the FDA review and approve a drug for marketing in the USA. FDA has the responsibility to determine that the drug is safe and effective, the proposed labelling is appropriate, and the methods used in the manufacturing are adequate to control the drug's identity, strength, quality and purity. Thus, all new drugs must be subject to an approved NDA before they can legally be marketed or transported across state lines. The NDA was introduced in 1938, and required only proof of safety for the product until 1962, when the need to prove efficacy was introduced. A 1985 rewrite of the NDA procedure modified the content of application, the format and the review procedures to make them more effective and logical to review. The NDA currently contains the following sections:

1   application form
2   index
3   summary
4   chemistry and manufacturing controls
5   non-clinical pharmacology/toxicology
6   human pharmacokinetics/bioavailability
7   microbiology (for anti-infectives)
8   clinical
9   statistics
10 case report forms and tabulation section
11 samples and labelling.

The content of the various sections is identified in very detailed guidelines which contain much more guidance than the more outline type of guideline issued by the EU. In terms of packaging the data requirement is covered in the 'Guideline for submitting documentation for the manufacture of and controls for drug products' and, more specifically, in a guideline reserved for packaging, the 'Guideline for submitting documentation for packaging for human drugs and biologics (February 1987)' (Table 3.10).

FDA packaging guideline

An applicant may rely upon the guideline in preparing the application or, alternatively, can follow a different approach, although if the latter is chosen, FDA encourages the sponsor to discuss the matter in advance with it in order that an unacceptable approach is not taken. The role of the drug packaging in maintaining the standards of identity, strength, quality and purity of the drug for its intended shelf life is stated in the guideline and reference is made to the pharmacopoeia for guidance on the type of packaging to be used and the test and procedures to be applied.

Much more detailed information on the package is required by the FDA than is generally required in the EU, but the data may be submitted in the form of a drug master file, which allows container or resin manufacturers to supply the FDA directly with detailed confidential data.

The guideline defines the types of container to be used, dividing into parenteral (glass or plastic) or non-parenteral containers (glass, plastic and metal), along with pressurised containers and bulk containers for active ingredients and drug products. The information that must be submitted for each of these categories is defined.

Closure types are also listed, including tamper-resistant and child-resistant caps. Liners are also given prominence, along with inner seals and elastomers when used as closures. Aerosols are given specific coverage since they affect both the rate and the amount of drug delivered.

The suitability of packaging components is discussed in terms of their physical, chemical and biological characteristics, specification and tests to be applied, stability and compatibility considerations and the involvement of adhesives and inks. In selecting a package it is recognised that ingredients added to the resin such as plasticisers, lubricants, mould release agents, pigments, stabilisers, antioxidants and binding or anti-static agents may be leached from the plastic. Certain ingredients of the drug

Table 3.10 FDA Guideline for submitting documentation for packaging for human drugs and biology

1	Purpose
	• Package must maintain standards, identity, strength, quality and purity of drug for shelf life
	• Full information needed
	• USP provides guidance
2	Type of containers/closures
3	Suitability for intended use
4	IND needs
5	NDA needs
6	Submission of packaging information and data (format)

preparation may bind to plastics or be absorbed by them. It is also possible for a component of the drug to migrate through the walls of the container and for oxygen, carbon dioxide and other gases to permeate through the plastic into the drug system.

Clear reference is made to the USP/NF for definition of the specifications and tests required for the package. Such tests can involve extractive testing, IR or UV spectra, thermal analysis, melt viscosity, molecular weight, molecular weight distribution, polymer linearity, degree of crystallinity, permeability, stiffness, softening temperature, ash and heavy metal content. It also may be necessary to carry out biological testing where appropriate, using the specific USP/NF tests.

As in the EU, the basic details of stability testing requirements are not given, since reference can be made to the general guidelines on stability testing. Instead, the packaging parameters that must be added to them are described. Special note is made that formal stability studies should be carried out in product packaged in the container/closure system in which the drug is to be marketed. Tests should be performed to check the absorption of toxic impurities from the container/closure system so that appropriate tests can be defined to control the problem. Leaching studies should be carried out in accordance with the USP procedure and, where appropriate, checks should be made that contamination with micro-organisms will not occur through the container or closure.

Attention is given by FDA to the fact that cements and lacquers used as label adhesives are often dissolved in organic solvents which may allow migration of adhesive components into the contents of the packaging. Appropriate testing should, therefore, be performed to determine whether this occurs (also being considered by the EU). In addition, testing should be conducted on the effectiveness of the adhesive under appropriate challenge conditions of temperature and humidity.

Format of NDA application

Information necessary for the various types of packaging is detailed in the guideline and should be submitted in the following order:

1   name of manufacturer
2   description of packaging components and processes
3   sampling plan
4   acceptance specification
5   test methodology.

Although the NDA requires a summary, this should be strictly factual and should not contain the evaluation and opinion found in the European style expert report. In the USA it is the FDA that draws the conclusions based on the factual data and summary provided by the applicant.

Packaging for clinical trials in the USA

Before any clinical study can be carried out in the USA, an exemption from the need to hold an NDA must be obtained from the FDA. The detail required on the packaging provided in the Investigational New Drug Application (IND) depends on whether the study is in an early phase (Phase I) of testing or in the late phase (Phase III). It is recognised that at the early phases, an outline of the packaging used and an indication of the appropriate stability studies which have been initiated may well suffice, but at Phase III the information supplied should be directed towards fulfilling the requirements of the full NDA.

Comparison of EU and FDA data requirements for PLA or NDA

In general the data required for packaging, as in other parts of PLAs, is basically the same. The differences lie in the format of the application and the depth of information provided. This is mirrored by the type of guidelines issued by the respective organisations. FDA guidelines are very detailed, providing reviewers and applicants with the detailed basic requirements for the application. In addition, the FDA requires and encourages companies to consult it at various stages during the development programme, since the period between IND submission and final NDA approval is seen as a continuous process. The FDA sees this advisory role as an important part of its work, and as development progresses additional data is generally filed to the IND with the aim of increasing the data held within the IND such that, by Phase III clinical testing, the amount available is almost that required for the NDA, and has already been FDA reviewed.

In Europe the two phases are kept separate, although some guidance is given during the clinical testing procedure as to future requirements for the PLA. The guidelines are less detailed and the applicant is encouraged to formulate its development plans and to justify them through the vehicle of the expert report without the considerable interaction that goes on between company and FDA.

Pharmacopoeias

The main guidance on package requirements can be found in pharmacopoeias (Table 3.11). Of the three key pharmacopoeias of the world (USP/NF, Ph Eur and Japanese Pharmacopoeia), it is the European Pharmacopoeia that is the main reference source in the EU, being set up by the Convention of Elaboration of European Pharmacopoeia of the Council of Europe. Once a monograph is accepted, EU members are charged to make the monographs official standards in their own countries. However, this does not

Table 3.11 Pharmacopoeias and their contents

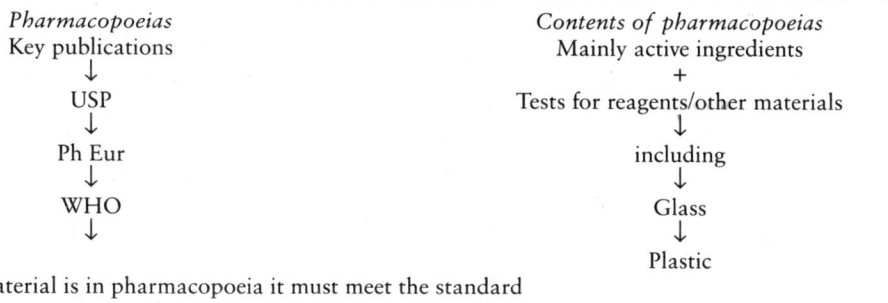

Pharmacopoeias Key publications	Contents of pharmacopoeias Mainly active ingredients
↓	+
USP	Tests for reagents/other materials
↓	↓
Ph Eur	including
↓	↓
WHO	Glass
↓	↓
	Plastic

If material is in pharmacopoeia it must meet the standard

mean that compliance with a pharmacopoeial monograph automatically makes the substance acceptable to the regulatory authority, since there is always the option for the regulatory authority to require additional testing over and above that in the monograph. Nor does it mean that all the tests in the pharmacopoeia necessarily have to be carried out. Alternative methods can be used, providing that comparative data are provided to show equivalence. If there is a dispute, however, the pharmacopoeial method becomes the reference standard.

In terms of packaging, the European Pharmacopoeia provides a list of plastics that are permitted for use in pharmaceutical containers. These are:

- PVC for containers for human blood, blood components and aqueous solutions for IV infusion
- PVC for components used in blood transfusion
- polyolefines
- polyethylene (low density) for parenteral and ophthalmic preparations
- polyethylene (high density) for parenteral preparations
- polypropylene for parenteral preparations
- ethylene–vinyl acetate copolymer for total parenteral nutrition products
- silicone oil as lubricant
- silicone elastomer for closures and tubing.

For each, appropriate specifications are given, along with the test methods and permitted additive levels.

Although the main packaging material covered is plastic, it must not be forgotten that glass is still often used. Type I, Type II, Type III and Type IV grades of glass are described in the pharmacopoeia. In this chapter, however, we will concentrate on plastics.

The section on plastic containers states that the plastic material can consist of one or more polymers along with certain additives, but must not contain any substances that can be extracted by the contents in such a way, or in such quantities, to alter the efficacy or stability of the product, or increase its toxicity.

The monograph states that the nature and amount of additive used will depend on the type of polymer, the process used to convert it into a container and the intended purpose of the container. Approved additives include antioxidants, stabilisers, plasticisers, lubricants, colour and impact modifiers. Anti-static and mould release agents can be used only for containers for oral and external preparations. Specific permitted additives are given in the specification for the material within the pharmacopoeial monograph.

In selecting the appropriate polymer material the key aspects are that the drug is not absorbed, that it does not migrate through the material and that the plastic does not yield any material in a quantity sufficient to affect the stability or the toxicity of the product. Tests of compatibility should include physical changes, permeation, pH change, effect of light and chemicals or biological testing as appropriate for the type of product involved.

The method of manufacture must ensure reproducibility between batches and the conditions should be chosen to preclude the possibility of contamination with other plastic materials or their constituents. Containers made should be similar in every respect to the type sample. For the testing on the type sample to remain valid, there must be no change in the composition of the material or in the manufacturing process, particularly with regard to temperature to which the plastic material is exposed during conversion or subsequent procedures such as sterilisation. Scrap materials should not be used. Recycling excess material of a well-defined nature and proportion may be permitted if the appropriate validation is carried out.

Plastic material in contact with food (90/128 and amendments)

If a material is not listed in the pharmacopoeia then reference must be made to a further Directive dealing with plastic materials in contact with food. Materials authorised for use in contact with food are generally acceptable for contact with pharmaceuticals (Table 3.12), but if this approach is taken it will also be necessary to provide a list of countries where the plastic has been approved for pharmaceuticals. If these two aspects can be covered, then toxicology data should not be required in the application. The Plastic Material in Contact with Food Directive lists, in an annexe, the monomers and starting materials which can be used for food purposes after January 1997. A second annexe lists the monomers which can be used, but which may be deleted if data were not supplied to enable the Scientific Committee to evaluate the product before 1 January 1996 (since then amendments have been inserted updating Annexe 1 as the data have been provided). Finally, specific migration limits are given for each material listed.

There is no doubt that the regulatory authorities are now requiring much more information on plastics and plastic containers than was required previously. At the same time reviewers are beginning to become more knowledgeable in the area of resins and containers. However, they are not yet packaging experts and, as such, some of the regulatory requirements may not be strictly logical when reviewed by an expert in the area. However, the requirements stem from guidelines which are suggestions rather than

Table 3.12 Plastic materials and articles intended to come into contact with foodstuffs – Directive 90/128 and amendment Directives

---

Framework Directive 89/109
Legal basis (framework Directive for future Directive)

Food contact materials must be inert and have no transfer constituents
Scientific Committee for Food (SCF) will set criteria
↓
Plastic materials in contact with food directive 90/128
- Defines plastics
- Sets overall migration limits 10 mg/dm^2 or 60 mg/kg food where container capacity > 500 ml or for caps
- Sets standard test conditions amended or extended in Directives 82/7118, 85/5728 and 93/8
- Specifies overall migration limit (amended in Directives 92/39, 93/9).
- Lists permitted monomers and starting materials
↓
Annexe IIa – sufficient data to evaluate
Annexe IIB – insufficient data (to be deleted January 1997 if data not provided)

---

mandatory requirements and, therefore, in the EU at least it is possible to argue for an alternative approach using the vehicle of the expert report, provided the case is well documented and reasoned. In the USA the same result can be obtained by discussions with the FDA. If a good case is made, backed up by sound data, then experience would indicate that authorities are still prepared to review specific cases according to specific data available. (Care must be taken not to over-interpret European flexibility, since mutual recognition reviews could introduce fifteen different viewpoints.)

The pack as carrier of the labelling

Just as the container cannot be separated from the product in regulatory or technical terms, the container, label and leaflet are also intimately connected, and in pharmaceuticals the term 'labelling' generally includes both the labels and any leaflet included with the product.

The term 'label' can mean the label on the immediate container, the carton label, the outer label or the label on the case or pallet. Each label has a different function. A leaflet, enclosed within the carton, can be a patient leaflet or a professional user leaflet, or in some cases a summary of product characteristics (SPC).

The function of labelling

The function of the label and leaflet is to inform the patient, to inform the pharmacist/wholesaler/manufacturer, to control the product in terms of its distribution and medical aspects, and to reduce the risk of product liability claims.

For a prescription medicine the patient wants to know about the treatment being given, to supplement that given to him or her by the doctor or the pharmacist and possibly to counteract information provided by the media, friends and family.

The pharmacist, in making up the product to the doctor's order, needs to identify the product and detect any gross prescribing error in order to advise the patient where required. The wholesaler needs to identify packs and outers readily and quickly and thus needs access to the name, strength, pack size, storage and handling conditions, expiry data and batch details.

The doctor who has prescribed the medicine does not generally handle it personally. He or she does, however, require reliable information on the name, presentation and strength, indications, contra-indications, dosage instructions, precautions, interactions, side-effects and pack sizes which must be absolutely consistent with the details on the immediate label, carton label and any package leaflets enclosed. Since he or she does not handle the product, some other mechanism must be found to provide him or her with this information separately from the product. This is probably the SPC or summary of major product characteristics (SmPC, see below) data sheet.

Thus, the patient has the label on the primary container and package insert, the wholesaler has the carton and pallet labels, and the pharmacist has the immediate container label, the carton label, package insert and possibly the SPC. The doctor looks at the SPC or equivalent document, probably in a compilation of such documents, such as the data sheet compendium in the UK.

All this information must be accurate and consistent both scientifically and legally.

The SmPC

The key document from which all other text is derived, is the summary of product characteristics (SPC), sometimes referred to as the summary of major product characteristics (SmPC) to differentiate it, as abbreviated, from the supplementary protection certificate which is concerned with patent protection.

The purpose of the SmPC is to set out the agreed position of the product between the regulatory authority and the company. It thus controls all the labelling and advertising of the product. Any changes to the SmPC must be approved by the regulatory authority before they are introduced (Table 3.13). The SmPC also provides a vital document in the harmonisation of products within the EU. The centralised procedure results in one licence and one SmPC and is, therefore, relatively straightforward, but the decentralised procedure involves gaining approval in one country and then seeking mutual recognition in other member states, based on that first approval. In this case, it is recognised that complete harmonisation of the SmPC throughout Europe would be very difficult and discussion continues, particularly for generic products.

The information to be provided in the SmPC is clearly defined in the CPMP Notes for Guidance document (III/9163/90) (Table 3.14) which defines the sequence of data and then gives some explanation as to what is required under each heading. In addition to III/9163/90, the key EU legislation for labels and leaflets is as follows.

- Directive EC 65/65 provides the particulars required for labels in outline.
- Directive 75/319 provides the particulars for leaflets in outline.
- Directive 89/341 makes a leaflet compulsory if all the details required are not displayed on the label.
- Directive 92/27 consolidates and provides greater detail on the requirements for labels and leaflets.
- Directive 92/73 makes similar provisions for homeopathic drugs.

European Directives do not actually make local law, they merely place an obligation on countries within the EU to introduce specific legislation to fulfil the requirements of the directive. For example, the requirements of Directive 92/27 have been achieved in the UK through Statutory Instruments (1992) 3273 and (1992) 3274.

Table 3.13 SmPC

Role and summary given in 65/65 article 4(A)

Purpose:
To set out agreed position of product
- between competent authority and company to provide common basis of communication
- between competent authority and all member states

Controls the product:
- All labelling, advertising must be consistent
- Any changes must be approved by regulatory authority
- Must be presented to doctor by representative
- Must be supplied with any samples

Table 3.14 CPMP Notes for Guidance III/9163/90; SmPC – content and sequence

1   Name of the medicinal product
2   Qualitative and quantitative composition
3   Pharmaceutical form
4   Clinical particulars
    4.1 Therapeutic indications
    4.2 Posology and method of administration
    4.3 Contra-indications
    4.4 Special warnings and special precautions for use
    4.5 Interaction with other medicaments and other forms of interaction
    4.6 Pregnancy and lactation
    4.7 Effects on ability to drive and use machines
    4.8 Undesirable effects
    4.9 Overdose
5   Pharmacological properties
    5.1 Pharmacodynamic properties
    5.2 Pharmacokinetic properties
    5.3 Pre-clinical safety data
6   Pharmaceutical particulars
    6.1 List of excipients
    6.2 Incompatibilities
    6.3 Shelf life
    6.4 Special precautions for storage
    6.5 Nature and contents of container
    6.6 Instructions for use/handling
    6.7 Name or style and permanent address or registered place of business of the holder of the marketing authorisation
7   Marketing authorisation number
8   Date of approval revision

Label and leaflet directive 92/27

Directive 92/27 starts with a definition of name of product, common name and strength of product, immediate packaging, outer packaging, labelling and manufacturer. It then defines the particulars which must occur on the outer packaging (Table 3.15). When the immediate packaging takes the form of a blister pack which is placed in an outer package that complies with the provisions above, then the blister pack (Table 3.16) can show reduced particulars, but must show at least the name of the product, the name of the holder of the authorisation, the expiry date and batch number. Some other immediate packaging may be so small that it is impossible to display all the requirements. In this case it is possible to reduce the number, but all packs must display at least the following: name of the product, method of administration, expiry date, batch number and contents by weight, volume or unit. There is no specific definition of 'small' in terms of the pack, although 10 ml is generally regarded as a good guide for the limit.

The presentation of the particulars on the label should be easily legible and clearly comprehensible, indelible, and must appear in the official language of the member state. Other items which may be required locally, such as price, reimbursement conditions and legal status, can also appear.

Table 3.15 Labelling and packaging Directive 92/27/EEC

Immediate packaging must contain:
- product name
- active ingredients
- pharmaceutical form and contents
- list of excipients
  (all for ophthalmic or parenteral)
  (any with recognisable effect)
- method and route of administration
- special warnings
- expiry date
- special precautions
- name and address of authorisation holder
- authorisation number
- manufacturing batch number
- instructions for use for self-medication product

Table 3.16 Directive 92/27, exemptions from full labelling

Blister packs:	Small units:
• product name	• product name
• authorisation holder's name	• strength (if necessary)
• expiry date	• route of administration
• batch number	• expiry date
	• batch number
	• contents

Leaflets

All products must contain a patient leaflet unless all the information can be conveyed on the outer packaging label. The content of the leaflet and order of presentation are defined in Directive 92/27 and must be as follows.

1 Identification of product.
2 Name of product, statement of active ingredients, pharmaceutical form, pharmaco-therapeutic group, name and address of authorisation holder.
3 Therapeutic indications.
4 Information needed for taking the product.
5 Contra-indications, precautions for use, interactions, special warnings, including use in pregnancy, elderly, effect on ability to drive vehicles and details of any excipients which may be important for the safe and effective use of the product.
6 Instructions for use.
7 Dosage, method and route of administration, frequency of administration, duration of treatment where limited, action to be taken in the case of an overdose or lack of dosing and risk of withdrawal effects where possible.
8 Undesirable effects.
9 Effects that can occur under normal use of the product and action to be taken.
10 Expiry date.
11 Warning against use of the product after the date, appropriate storage precautions and warning against visible signs of deterioration.
12 Date on which package leaflet was last revised.

The leaflet must be written in clear, understandable terms, be legible and be in the official language of the member state. Inclusion of symbols or pictures is permitted if in compliance with the SmPC. Since this is a user leaflet the language must be understandable to the lay person.

At the time the Directive was issued there were a number of tasks that the Commission had not yet undertaken and items that were to be introduced:

1   special warnings
2   special needs for self-medication products
3   legibility of text
4   identification and authentication of medicinal products
5   list of excipients which must appear on the labelling.

The above information relates to a package insert designed for the patient, but in some cases further information is required for use by the doctor, dentist or nurse in supplying or administering the product. To cover this need a professional user leaflet may be included provided it is within the scope of the SmPC, but even if the product is administered by a professional a patient insert must also be provided.

The package as a contaminator of the environment

Packaging waste

Just as public and political pressures have increased the amount of information required by regulatory authorities on packaging as a result of concern for the safety of drugs, the same changing attitudes have made the environment of greater concern. Hence there has been considerable pressure to reduce contamination of the environment through waste products (Figure 3.7). Of particular concern is the amount of packaging used today and how it is disposed of. Of course the amount of pharmaceutical packaging waste is small compared with the total amount (probably less than 1%), so that any reduction will have little impact on the environment. The industry, however, must comply with any regulations made, and experience has shown that it will not be regarded as a special case.

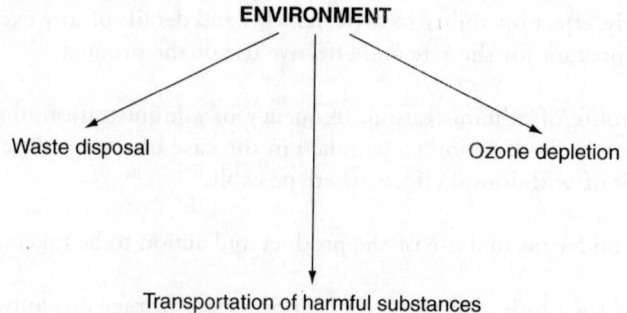

Figure 3.7 Environmental concerns

This increase in concern has led to the EEC Packaging Waste Directive 94/62 (Table 3.17) which requires:

- reduction in the quantities of waste
- reduction in harmfulness of waste
- promotion of reuse of packaging
- recycling and recovery of packaging waste
- reduction of the total packaging to be disposed of.

Since the first Directive there have been several amendments increasing the scope and reducing the time scale for achievement of targets of recycling and reuse. Targets of 50–60% waste recovery in 5 years and 25–45% recycling with a minimum of 15% for each material have been set, and tightening of the targets can be anticipated at any time (Table 3.17). Return, collection and recovery systems for packaging must be set up and there must be a marking system on the pack to allow the nature of the plastic to be identified.

All new packaging introduced must now meet the Directive, and to avoid differences between countries the elements of standardisation are outlined. With recycling there is likely to be an increased concentration of heavy metals, and this aspect is also covered.

Table 3.17 Directive 94/62, packaging and packaging waste

Objective
To harmonise national measures for management of packaging and packaging waste by
- prevention of production of waste
- promotion of reuse and recycling
- reduction of disposal

Scope
All types of packaging

Definitions
Packaging, levels of packaging, waste

Reuse
Postpones creation of waste

Recovery/recycling (5 years from implementation)
- 50–65% recovery
- 25–45% recycled
- minimum 15% each material recycled
- return, collection and recovery systems

Marking and identification systems
To identify material used

Heavy metal content
- 600 ppm by 30 June 1998
- 250 ppm by 30 June 1999
- 100 ppm by 30 June 2001

To ensure that progress is properly monitored, a database on packaging use is prescribed and the information that should be supplied to users defined.

At first there was hope that pharmaceutical products would be exempt from the Directive, and considerable pressure was applied. However, most representations were unsuccessful. It is not easy for the industry to meet these requirements and, at the same time, meet the requirements of GMP which, for example, restricts the amount of recycling of plastics that can occur and generally prevents the use of scrap material.

The industry may have to produce new materials for packaging since several of the current ones, such as PVC and foil laminates, have limited scope for recovery or recycling. The packaging development department must take account of these factors since the waste Directive must be a key factor in choosing packaging for new products.

Ozone layer depletion

Pressurised aerosols play a major part in modern pharmaceuticals and in many ways are a perfect pack in efficiently protecting the product and dispensing an accurate dosage of the contents when required. They are, therefore, clinically effective and convenient to use. Unfortunately, the propellants originally used (generally a mixture of chlorofluorocarbons (CFCs)) were shown to be depleting the ozone layer. As a result, an international agreement was reached in 1987 that CFC production and consumption should be curbed. This agreement, the Montreal Protocol, was signed by 27 nations and originally called for a 50% reduction in CFC consumption by 1999. In the EU the proposals were incorporated into Regulation 594/91 which required that there be no production of CFCs by 30 June 1997. Controls have also been introduced on exportation and importation of CFCs from the EU, and the original Directive has been expanded to cover such substances as methylbromide, hydrobromofluorocarbons and hydrofluorocarbons.

To overcome the non-availability of CFCs for use in metered dose aerosols, alternative propellants have been developed and are being introduced progressively. The process is complex, requiring first long-term toxicology studies in two animal species on the propellants themselves, followed by pharmaceutical work using the propellant and product to determine compatibility and stability of product and propellant in combination. Normally a new propellant can only be approved by regulatory authorities as part of a marketing authorisation for a product, but in this case applications were made in the EU to cover the propellants alone so that the safety issues could be cleared prior to review of individual applications for specific products. The first stage has been achieved for two alternative materials, and products containing them are now reaching the market.

Classification, packaging and labelling of hazardous materials

In discussing the environment a further Directive should be considered which specifically excludes medicines, but still may impact the pharmaceutical industry since companies package and transport hazardous intermediate materials between production sites (Table 3.18). Such intermediate materials are often toxic, inflammable, oxidising or irritant and, therefore, are caught by Directive 67/548. Because of the increased pres-

Table 3.18 Directive 67/548 (and amendment), classification, packaging and labelling of dangerous substances

Excludes:	Medicines
Includes:	Explosive, oxidising, inflammable, toxic, irritant substances
Classifies:	Very toxic, toxic, harmful
Testing:	Obligation to investigate properties
Safety data sheet:	Needed to protect operations
Notification:	Technical dossier needed, detail depends on quantities produced
Packaging:	Must avoid loss of contents
	Materials of construction not attacked
	Strong and solid to meet normal stresses and strains
Labelling must include:	Name of substance
	Origin (name and address of manufacturer)
	Danger symbol
	Special risks
	Precautions

sure on costs and profit margins there is an increased trend today for the centralisation of production worldwide, which means that more and more intermediates must be transported.

The original Directive covered:

1   inclusion and exclusion of materials
2   selection of packaging which avoids loss of content, is not attacked by the product, and is strong and solid enough to meet the nominal stresses and strains of handling
3   labelling, including the use of specific danger symbols
4   notification of the competent authority of new materials by use of a technical dossier.

Since 1967 there have been many amendments to the original Directive. For example, Directive 88/379 shows how the physico-chemical properties of the compound must be determined to evaluate the health hazard. Directive 67/548 reiterates the requirements for packs requiring the pack shape not to attract children. For certain substances, child-resistant or tactile warnings are required and the labelling is covered in great detail, including the dimensions and colours to be used. Directive 91/115 requires that a data sheet be produced which covers identity, composition, hazard identification, first aid, fire fighting, accidental release measures, exposure control, personal protection, physical and chemical properties, stability, disposal, transport, regulatory and other information. Directive 72/32 (amendment 7) pulls together many of the earlier amendments covering testing, classification and notification, describing the technical dossier that must be submitted, covering unfavourable effects, classification, data sheet and notification requirements. The amount of data that must be supplied increases as the production/supply quantities increase, from smaller amounts of data if the quantities are less than 1 ton per annum, increasing at over 1 ton, over 100 tons and over 10,000 tons. After submission of the dossier the material can be placed on the market after 60 days if no response is received.

Polymers (Directive 92/105)

Directive 92/105 provides special notification needs for polymers. The Directive states that the notification should contain the information necessary to evaluate the foreseeable risk to man and the environment. It is possible to avoid preparation of several dossiers and to group polymers and produce representative tests covering the whole group. A reduced package of data is possible for high molecular weight materials if they meet certain criteria. In an annexe to the Directive, homopolymer, copolymer, polymer (RTP) and family polymers are defined, and the standard test package required is defined, the amount of data varying according to the annual production level.

Protecting the public

Child-resistant closures

As well as protecting the product, the package can also protect the public through the use of child-resistant closures (CRCs) or tamper-evident packs.

There has been criticism that child-resistant closures are difficult to remove by the elderly. This is true for many of the devices, but on the other hand there is no doubt that CRCs have been effective in preventing poisoning in children. For example, the number of analgesic poisonings in children in the UK reduced from 626 in 1974 to 181 in 1977 after introduction of the requirement for use of CRCs.

Although there are no EU requirements for child-resistant closures for medicines, there are directives (91/442 and 90/35) which require containers for products that are toxic or corrosive to be made child-resistant. For pharmaceutical products individual countries have introduced requirements; for example, the Pharmaceutical Society of Great Britain requires in its code of practice that all solid and liquid preparations be dispensed in reclosable child-resistant containers, unless:

1   the medicine is in an original pack such as to make this inadvisable
2   a specific request is made that it not be so dispensed
3   no suitable child-resistant container exists for a particular liquid preparation.

Tamper-evidence

Tamper-evident and tamper-resistant packs were few and far between until the Tylenol incident in the USA, when such packaging became the rule for OTC products almost overnight. WHO, in its guideline on the assessment of medicinal products for use in self-medication, recommends that such packages are highly desirable.

Child-resistant, tamper-evident and tamper-resistant closures are dealt with in detail in Chapter 11, and therefore will not be dealt with further here.

Summary

In this chapter, I have tried to cover the registration requirements for packaging, along with other regulatory constraints imposed on the pack. There is no doubt that the regulatory climate is getting more restrictive for pharmaceutical products and it is likely that packaging for pharmaceuticals will have more and more constraints placed upon it

In terms of the regulatory attitude, it must be remembered that the product licence is a legal document and that regulators are bureaucrats. Regulatory agencies were set up generally following disasters and as such they are very cautious and open to both political and public pressure. In approaching data requirements, therefore, it is necessary to look at the guidelines, but also to try to think not only as a packaging technologist but also as a regulator. Data needs are increasing and the regulators, although not yet packaging experts, are increasing their expertise, so increasing demands for the volume of information.

The data needs on packaging required in a product licence are becoming more clearly defined and more consistent worldwide with such initiatives as ICH. However, as the needs become clearer, they become more restrictive. Industry, thus, has the choice between having some open general guidelines which do not provide a great deal of help, but are not over-restrictive as we find for the EU, and much more detailed guidlines similar to those of the FDA which are clearer and more helpful, but become more restrictive.

4

SPECIFICATIONS AND QUALITY

E. R. Evans

Quality – a philosophy

In a cost-conscious world, companies have to be efficient to survive, and products need to be competitive to satisfy the consumer. Where two products compete for the same market, and in the same price bracket, the consumer will search for some advantage to aid the final product choice. Quality is the advantage normally chosen, and this fact is as relevant to the purchasing and selling organisation of the large national and international company as it is to the domestic consumer.

The lesson that quality sells (in particular, realistic quality sells) is, and has been, a hard lesson to learn, particularly when domestic markets become the targets for imports. However, companies that survive the attrition of more quality-conscious competition will themselves eventually develop and exhibit the same superiority in their marketing and manufacturing operations.

The evolution of quality assurance (QA) and quality control (QC) in industry has been a blend of the legally and regulatory imposed standards (since legislation is a quality control over national standards), together with the competition from the occasional far-sighted company, which imposes on the market its own advanced quality standards, leading to imitation by other companies for commercial purposes.

Any examination of the development of QC technology, which now falls under the broad umbrella of QA, will reveal that it closely parallels the history of the mass production industry. This is not difficult to explain, since the simplified, long-running processes that are the efficiency of automation remove the individual craftsmanship and skill that were once required for 'quality products'. Once this step was taken, the need for an independent responsibility for quality was an obvious reaction, and most of industry now operates with a quality check 'separate' from the production process (in the same way, responsibility for machine setting, repair and maintenance has been delegated to specialist departments).

In recent years it has been recognised that it was perhaps impetuous to divorce QC completely from the production process, not because the concept of an independent QC function was itself wrong, but because:

1   QC operates retrospectively to check the quality of what has been made
2   quality cannot be 'inspected' into a product after it has been produced (i.e. its immediate actions are limited to the release of conforming product and the recovery and investigation of defective batches)

3   production should be encouraged and organised through formalisation of good manufacturing practice (GMP), proper work training and staff motivation to manufacture to the agreed quality standard, i.e. 'make right first time'

4   the quality organisation (QC and QA) must be proactively involved in material, product, process and staff development to ensure that quality and process efficiency are not just fully compatible, but are mutually self-fulfilling.

Close liaison between QA and production will more efficiently blend the reliability of an independent QC operation with the higher initial manufacturing standards of the positively motivated manufacturing operator. This degree of motivation has proved achievable using the well-documented techniques of quality circles and company programmes of continuous improvement i.e. parts of 'total quality'.

The intention and purpose of a correctly organised QA operation must be to aid the company in efficiently producing a specified product which is cost-effective (to the company) and meets the desired requirements (of the customer). This purpose should not be limited by the boundaries of a normal production environment, but be free to co-operate in all phases within the company (development, marketing, etc.) and outside (supplier, sales, customer reports and complaints, etc.).

This approach automatically leads to a quality examination at two levels:

1   quality of design
2   quality of conformance.

Quality of design

This term has been defined as 'the quality specified or required by the customer', and requires active participation between the quality management and the total development function to finalise design standards which will allow and aid manufacturing compliance (with the supplier or sub-supplier organisation as well as with the customer). Additional attention has to be directed to the manufacturing facilities, documentation systems, process and staff training, which together will prevent quality deviations at source.

The quality of design is normally associated with the responsibility of QA, and an important element is the practice of validation and qualification.

Quality of conformance

The assessment of component quality once the manufacturing process is partly or fully completed allows only for a measurement of product conformance and, if a problem is revealed, some remedial action. Limited conformance testing lacks the essential anticipation that prevents problems and does not merely detect them. Therefore, as means of 'controlling' quality, this simplistic regime of QC is a very poor tool.

This does not mean that the role of conformance testing in a practical QC organisation can be minimised, or that effort need 'only' be directed into designing systems. On the contrary, any efficient organisation must employ conformance testing in maximising the quality of production. Close co-operation between production and quality control, with production technicians carrying out multiple scheduled product checks, supported by the QC conformance test, ensures effective process controls, maximises production efficiency, minimises wastage and provides feedback to management and development. However, QC is the final release authority in meeting the standards required by the customer or legislation.

Within a company, QC action is directed at three areas: raw material control, process control, and finished product control. The approach in setting up a system will be very similar in each case, i.e. design into the operation all the parameters that will bear on the manufacture of quality, followed by a means of establishing that conformance has been achieved. (An important element of this is the continuing revalidation that processes continue to perform as specified.)

To generalise by using the examples of raw material/component control: once the product has been made faults either cannot be, or are expensive to, put right or remove by sorting. QC must therefore be involved with the design and development of the raw material/component, the choice of supplier (by evaluation), the pre-production trial of components, the setting of universally acceptable/achievable standards, the testing of components (at the supplier and in-house) and the in- house efficient use of those components with referral to the supplier of any defectives. Unnecessarily high-quality components are expensive and wasteful of resources, to the customers and suppliers, while supposedly high-quality components can justify their sometimes higher initial purchase cost by increased in-house usage efficiency and the avoidance of customer complaints.

It is without argument that low-quality components (i.e. those that do not fully meet the desirable requirements), while sometimes being initially cheaper to purchase, will eventually produce lower in-house efficiency, coupled with lower finished product quality.

Priority of the QC resource will usually be directed at the more 'important' component, but this attention should be balanced by consideration of the ultimate usage (see Figure 4.1). The example shown in Figure 4.1 illustrates several points.

1   It is necessary to know the in-house requirements plus the supplier's abilities before setting component standards.
2   A supplier of variable quality can meet the requirements of a customer whose rejection threshold for defectives is high.
3   A supplier that lacks in-process controls or pre-release inspection will invariably fail acceptance by a customer that requires exacting standards for either product or process efficiency.
4   A supplier with in-process controls and/or release inspection sympathetic to the customer requirements will invariably meet expectation.
5   A customer with an approved quality systemised supplier can employ reduced levels of component inspection, supported by low-level supplier audits.

This fairly simple example illustrates the need to review the quality route between design and conformance. Similar examples can be found in the QC role for process quality as well as finished product quality, but the following discourse, in order to be comprehensive, will concentrate on raw material control.

To conclude this introduction, it is perhaps necessary to generalise on a philosophical level.

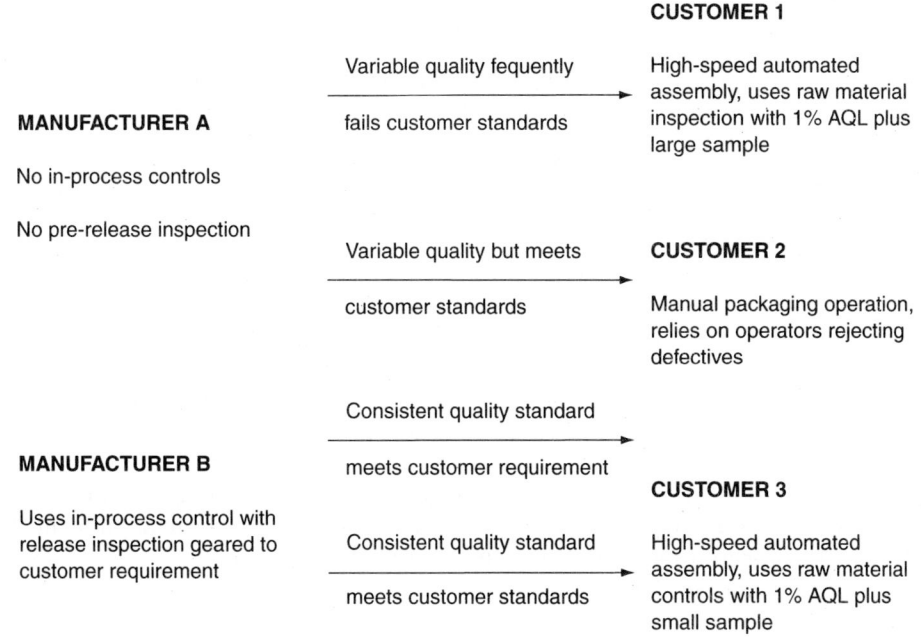

Figure 4.1 Manufacturers' quality policy and customers' standards

1   All personnel employed in a manufacturing organisation will have an impact on product quality. In some areas this is a direct effect, as in production or the support areas of QC and engineering. The impact from the areas of marketing, sales, development, training, purchasing, etc. may be less direct, but it is no less fundamental to the total product quality.

2   All manufacturers are both suppliers and customers and should maintain the same consistency of policy over quality whether they are dealing with internal or external sources.

3   Suppliers and customers must appreciate that they are simply opposite ends, and not opposing ends, of the same quality chain. To achieve the maximum potential of their combined product resource, it is necessary to work together as one development and quality team.

The first part of this chapter therefore concentrates on the QC function and the statistical appreciation required to progress a QC operation successfully. QA, which aims at building-in quality and defect prevention (rather than defect detection), although involving statistics to obtain data (e.g. statistical process control), relies more on regimented procedures and documentation to keep validated processes under control.

Material specifications and quality standards

In discussing packaging quality standards it has to be agreed that no component quality examination can start before construction of the material specification, and the reverse is equally true. The final component specification and the quality inspection procedure must be viewed together, and completed to a similar time scale to realise maximum component potential fully.

In the pharmaceutical industry, while drug research or R&D is formulating the active product, basic packaging presentations will be vetted as primary containers (i.e. for material stability and compatibility). However, once the drug moves into the production development interface, its total packaging design and application for production, distribution, market (and supplier) necessitates close formal liaison between the writers of the component specification and the quality inspection procedure.

Acceptance of this formal liaison introduces the concept of the 'quality project team', in which the original research container can be transformed into the viable component which is designed and manufactured to meet the needs of all parties.

The team should comprise delegates from marketing, development, production, engineering, purchasing and QC. This should be formed once drug research and marketing research have completed their broad packaging brief and have clearly established a viable project.

Responsibility for the final specification must still reside with the specific functional heads responsible for component design and QC test and standards. Hence, if formally required, these functions would provide the project's co-chairmen.

The team activities would concentrate on:

- *aesthetics*: acceptability to ultimate customer or patient
- *component dimensions*: interrelationship with other components, machine, etc.
- *machine requirements and limitations*: line speeds, tolerances, setting ranges, reliability
- *marketing/production*: batch sizes, frequency schedules
- *stock policy*: availability/cost, storage temperature/humidity, shelf life
- *distribution*: unit/collation size, weight, fragility, environmental
- *legislative regulations*: pack size, fill weight, number of items, print labelling
- *supplier*: abilities and limitations.

Although it is not always included as a direct member of the project team, decisions and actions must be agreed with the supplier (see below), since it is the supplier that has the specific technology to make or break the specification.

It cannot be over-stressed that the long-term suitability of the component and the efficiency of the production operation depend on the relevance of the component design. Deficiencies in design can be partially offset by extensive testing and sorting during or after manufacture, but full compensation will never be entirely feasible without redesign. It is for this reason that the importance of design must be recognised and accorded the resources of the project with a realistic time scale concurrent with the actual drug project.

It should be noted that quality audit and vendor rating systems need not only assess the manufacturing capability of a supplier, but may reflect on the quality of its design capability. A poor design, or a design with inherent deficiencies, has a lower chance of achieving high quality. A supplier desperate for new orders has been known to accept knowingly a poor design from an aggressive customer.

The project team should progress design studies through hand-made samples (produced in connection with the supplier) to a first machine sample. Where practical the first machine sample should be used to confirm the supplier's technical ability to quantity-produce the component, as well as the purchaser's design theory. To this end the machine sample for a plastic or moulded glass component should be from a single cavity tool, or for a folding box board carton, from a one-up die (as an intermediate stage to multi-cavity or multi-die production).

Samples should be assessed by laboratory, production, and marketing with the conclusions and recommendations recorded in the minutes of the project team's report.

A useful tool during component design is a failure mode and effect analysis (FMEA). This involves a detailed examination of the design, its uses and application, to determine how it can fail and the consequences of failure. By eliminating potential risks at that stage it is possible to produce a robust design meeting all design requirements, without the eventual need for in-production cures and delays involved in a design revision.

Once all departmental activities are satisfied, with redesign and resamples if necessary, metal should be cut for the full production tool, but on the understanding that further purchaser evaluations must be completed before tool acceptance (or, for example, before a mould is finally plated or hardened).

A component is more likely to complete a satisfactory working life, to the purchaser's and the supplier's benefit, if the project team co-ordinates design study and component trial before commitment to production use, i.e. the purchaser's production use of the first consignment of components should not be the first time that newly developed components have been tried under production conditions.

The component specification

Unlike many commercial operations, most pharmaceutical components are special to each and every pharmaceutical company, although fortunately some commonality will occasionally occur. In fact, distinct technical and commercial advantages exist when a universally common component can be standardised, either by demand or consent of supplier, purchaser or market legislation. These can be to industrial standards (TAPPI), national standards (BS, British Standards; MIL, Military Standards; USP, United States Pharmacopoeia) and international standards (ISO).

For either situation (i.e. of a special or common standard component) the purchaser must document the component specification. The specification must be approved and authorised by the relevant departments of the organisation and accepted by the supplier as the contract specification.

It is now fairly normal procedure to have a general support document, i.e. packaging material manual, issued under specific headings such as bottle glass; bottle plastic; laminations; labels; leaflets. These broadly describe the requirements of the items including reject (defect) terminology and possibly associated AQL. Such manuals provide suppliers with a broader view of the quality expected, and may cross-reference the details of the test procedures, including performance, to be applied (see below).

Quality standards

Policy

No one will argue with the statement that the purchaser has the right to obtain what he or she has contracted for. The initial basis for this expectation must be the agreement between supplier and customer to use the formal component specification. Although the component specification is intended to be contractual, it is sometimes misinterpreted as merely stipulating the intentions, the expectation or the target.

All manufacturing processes have a natural variability, through drift in machine settings, variable raw materials, variable operator standards, etc., and will therefore yield components which also vary. The quality project team, with the supplier, must assess the process capability of the component manufacturing process to ensure that it is capable of producing to the desired quality which always meets the customer's requirements. It is only to be expected that indifferent quality will result if the manufacturing process capability does not match the specification requirements.

The quality control procedure can be viewed as the framework built around the component specification which will translate the development laboratory target (ideal) into the mass production consumables (practical). The quality procedure is devised to achieve consistency of component deliveries by realistically:

1 identifying the total component requirements (of marketing, production, etc.) by correlating practical background experience with the same or similar components against tolerable variability both within and outside the specification, i.e. with relevant defect definitions, AQLs, etc.
2 producing a realistic test regime under which materials can be tested and assessed at both the supplier and the purchaser
3 establishing, and if necessary developing, the supplier's ability (through audits, training programmes, inter-company visits, lists of 'acceptable' suppliers, etc.) to meet the quality demands (see below).

To realise the optimum quality requires a total understanding of the handling and manufacturing processes of supplier and customer. Too high a quality will prove financially expensive to the purchaser, but will also be punitive or restrictive to the supplier that tries to achieve it. Too low a quality can result in purchaser rejections, greater machine downtime and running inefficiency, extra wastage in sorting and in-use complaints.

Optimum quality standards necessitate early involvement between development and QC and close liaison with the supplier (which must be compatible with the full production schedule). A variable-quality product (through design or conformance defects) can interfere with or interrupt the efficient operation of the purchaser's entire production line, possibly leading to variability with associated components (e.g. closures that do not fit containers) and with the pharmaceutical product (e.g. capping difficulties leading to machine stoppages will increase the fill variability of a liquid filling line). This cannot but reduce the ultimate quality of the pharmaceutical presentation as received by the user (hospital/doctor/patient).

Suppliers, particularly of a newly designed component, must be encouraged to participate in fault-finding/debugging of the component, both during the initial trialing period and in early manufacturing batches. This can be greatly aided when a supplier incorporates statistical process control (SPC) into its routine process controls, which relates defects to causes and then removes those causes.

It is to identify and emphasise the fact that, in spite of the efforts of quality project teams, defects can occur, and specification details can be unrealistic, that the first component specification and the first QC procedure must be considered provisional. A review of both documents should be the last operations of the quality project team within an agreed time scale, say after the first five deliveries, or 6–12 months. This will allow practical experience through manufacture, distribution and use to be applied to the final specifications.

The regular review and updating of all specifications and test procedures must be a normal part of the internal disciplines of technical departments. This is separate to the specific responsibilities of the project team engaged on a new component, and tends to expand specification details as specific points arise. Although this may be the inevitable way of quality progress as knowledge grows, the reverse may also be true, e.g. unique quality parameters included in the original specification may be redundant through production, process or market changes. While the review should include opportunities to expand or contract the specification, the updated document must cross-reference all changes.

Procedures/specification

The purpose of QC is to determine compliance with an agreed standard, i.e. whether it passes or fails. Ideally this simple approach maintains the independence of QC and keeps it separate from any commercial expediencies. This does not imply blind adherence to the specification, but simply that if standards are correctly devised, then apart from a 'crisis' any failure against the specification must by definition be unacceptable.

It is for this exceptional crisis that the quality procedure must include a route for concessions, whereby material normally considered unacceptable can (after full inter- or intra-department agreement, possibly involving machine and distribution trials, product functional tests, etc.) possibly be given a qualified release. The decision to release must not be the sole responsibility of QC, but a group decision in which QC is one member (the one with the initial data on the problem).

Following this concession two actions are implied:

1   to determine the causes, with the supplier, of the reason for the defective consignment, and to introduce supplier remedies which prevent repetition
2   to monitor the 'released concession batch' through the company and assess its effects.

If a concessionary batch performs satisfactorily in all areas, this information could allow permanent modification to the specification, or revision to the defect rating of that particular fault. This will not always be desirable when the production requirements are for a 'tight' specification to aid high-speed line performances.

All opportunities presented by defect detection in incoming materials should be taken to monitor the validity of the QC standards. This, as stated earlier, should be a formal procedure, say within 6–12 months or five deliveries of a new component, but can also take place outside this convention.

With the exception of a 'concession', the quality procedure needs to be as precisely defined as the component specification. It will, of necessity, follow a similar format (Table 4.1).

Conformance testing

The QC testing programme for component assessment can be simple or complicated, depending on:

1   the Company's policy on product and market risk (this policy is sometimes qualified by national and international regulatory requirements)
2   the degree of QC resource available
3   the type of material under examination (e.g. moulded glass containers where random samples are feasible versus reel-fed laminate materials where only 'spot' samples can be taken, or sterile versus non-sterile components)
4   the degree of confidence in the supplier (e.g. has it documented systems of process control and quality control?)
5   the production application and required line efficiency, e.g. components for a manual or semi-automatic, low-speed packaging operation need not be as demanding as those for an automated, high-speed one.

The specific requirements of a common component can therefore vary from purchaser to purchaser.

For these and other reasons, it is not always possible to describe a universal system and standards of QC. A basic approach to inspection can, however, be formalised which should ensure compliance with the component specification.

Identification

All batches of components (routine deliveries or trial batches) should on receipt be allocated a unique lot number for future traceability purposes and then subjected to a formal identification on two counts:

1   that the material is as ordered
2   that the material is as specified.

For the first identification, this can amount to a simple comparison with the purchasing order. For the second, identification can be as simple or as complex as procedures demand, i.e.

1   checking the printed identification code on a printed carton or label
2   using IR/DSC techniques to identify the thermoplastic in a moulding or laminated composite.

However tested, the results should record positive component or material identification, as 'does/does not comply'.

Table 4.1 Quality procedure

1. Title	The term by which the procedure is identified.
2. Reference no.	The code number, usually computer-derived, which identifies the procedures. (It should cross-reference the supplier's code number, if different.)
3. Sampling details	How the material is packaged. How it is to be sampled, i.e. the system for establishing the number of pallets and containers to be opened, as well as the number of components to be taken. The details for sampling, should call for a visual report on delivery presentation.
4. Physical examination	(i) Component identification. (ii) Visual standard of presentation, e.g. (a) print defects (b) moulding defects (c) constructional defects (d) contamination defects.
5. Dimensional examination	The critical dimensions to ensure acceptability on: (a) The production line (b) assembly and performance with other components (c) use with the product (d) distribution handling (e) patient empathy.
6. Functional examination	Tests involving compatibility with production use, product use, distribution, etc.: (a) assembly tests (e.g. capping torques, scuff-resistance of inks, heat seal strength of lacquers) (b) capacity tests, whether to shoulder or brim under specified temperature or pressure conditions (c) leakage tests, moisture vapour permeability of laminates, etc.
7. Analytical tests	Tests involving the chemical/physical nature of the component: (a) glass neutrality (b) pyrogens/toxicity of rubber (c) light transmission of glass (d) heavy metals in glass or plastics (e) IR/DSC identification of plastic materials.
8. Defect classification	Definitions of faults and their significance, i.e. (a) critical defect – tight AQL (b) major defect – medium AQL (c) minor defect – lax AQL.
9. Defect types	Examples which constitute all fault categories: critical, major, etc.
10. Defect action levels	Action/reject numbers which relate batch size versus sample size versus AQL.
11. Statistical reference	The identification references of the scheme, e.g. BS6001, MIL-STD-105E, normal inspection, inspection level II, Table IIA AQL levels, x, y, z.
12. Defect concession	The basis for using non-standard deliveries.
13. Supplier/purchaser obligations	Contractual obligations, e.g. (prior to change) (a) the supplier to notify the purchaser of any changes to its process/materials or system of control (b) the purchaser to notify the supplier of any changes to its process, product application, or system of control.
14. Authorisation	• Signatures of issuing departmental function, e.g. laboratory head, department head, QA director. • Supplier agreement.
15. Changes	Revisions history.
16. Date of issue	The date on which the specification was issued.

When it is considered useful, suppliers should include their manufacturing batch numbers or production dates with each delivery and these should be recorded.

Quantity

Quantity does not usually constitute a QC responsibility, although there are occasions when it may be relevant and require QC actions.

1   Where substance weight of foils, films and foil/film/paper laminates are involved, yield calculations require 'quantity' QC measurements.
2   Where component reconciliation, in warehouse and production, requires a knowledge that labelled 'box quantities' have been QC validated.

Physical inspection (visual, odour, texture, etc.)

Quality control of packaging components does not always require sophisticated measuring equipment to rate variable quality. Detailed visual examination by a trained QC inspector can often identify the unusual or low-level per cent defectives.

Visual inspection is a classical example of quality by 'attributes', where the batch is compared with a 'standard', which can be a quality 'perfect' example of the component or a quality check list. It should be noted that the physical senses of smell and taste, where safe, are often more sensitive than many sophisticated analytical methods, but equally require validation and standardisation.

For attributes, quality training is essential, since the QC inspector (in a pharmaceutical environment) will be challenging the release of material produced by a 'foreign' technology. It can sometimes be advantageous for the QC training programme to acquire, via involvement with the company's own packaging development technologists and visits from suppliers, some specialist technical knowledge of the supplier industry and technology. Additional training, as with testing, can be based on national or industrial testing and safety standards. These points are best clarified by a few examples.

Example 1 – printed secondary components (cartons, labels, leaflets, etc.)

The most important characteristic of any printed component is its text, since this provides the user with critical identification of and information on the product. Text is therefore too important to leave proof checking to the time of first delivery, so QC involvement must commence with artwork origination and approval, and be confirmed by batch deliveries.

All printed components should contain a specific artwork reference code, to allow reference between artwork and cylinder or plates. In addition, a general code should identify cylinder/plate positions which will aid QC positional proof checking as well as assisting supplier fault rectification.

Since QC relies on random sampling, complete coverage of every print station in a multi-station cylinder or plate cannot be guaranteed. It is sometimes useful for a printer to supply the customer with a 'first' and 'last' sheet (often termed 'gang' pulls) to show that text did not change between start and finish.

Unless the risk is contractually agreed as acceptable, no printer should print composite sheets, containing examples of several different products, drug strength or one product for different markets. Composite sheet printing introduces the hazard of 'rogue' mixes, and contravenes the basic rule of never allowing two different components to be mixed, since separation (unless automatic with double redundancy) cannot be 100% effective at all times. (Imaging can be used with optical character recognition (OCR) to check automatically the correctness of design and typography.)

For quality checks on colour or graphics, controlled lighting conditions are virtually obligatory. Eyeball colour comparison, by trained inspectors, is still a valid quality tool, although colour comparators or densitometers will provide recordable measurements.

All equipment should be standardised between supplier and purchaser, although some equipment (like electronic code reading) may, because of its sophistication or expense, be delegated to only the supplier.

Example 2 – primary components

MOULDED GLASS CONTAINERS

Glass is generally considered to be the oldest form of packaging material, and the glass industry is probably the most quality documented and systemised of component suppliers (e.g. its list and descriptions of defect types are extensive).

As with most technologies, some technical deviations or defects obvious to the 'expert' are sometimes barely detectable to the non-qualified user, and will not present any impairment to use. Alternatively, several defects are liable to affect use on the purchaser's production line (e.g. capacity variation), while some could hazard product and patient (fragmentation of glass particles from the rim on cap application).

It is essential for QC to acquire the skills to differentiate between grades of defects and to be able to classify their usage implication, e.g. splits in bottles can be significant according to their length or depth as well as their position (in the neck, ring, shoulder, body, base, internal or external surface, etc.) and whether product is hot or cold filled etc.

Most faults should be categorised according to their secondary implication (i.e. 'what it does') as well as its primary rating ('what it is') e.g. lubricants are frequently employed to aid the moulding operations, and components produced immediately after lubricant application will be surface contaminated and usually removed by sorting. Contaminated bottles that reach the purchaser must be considered as visual defectives (i.e. the primary rating). However, since lubricants are normally detectable only on 'white flint' glass (not amber), a normally unacceptable level of defectives could be tolerated if in amber glass and on the outside surface only.

Acquisition of these necessary skills is easier through co-operation with the supplier in an agreed training programme and cross-comparison of defect types and ratings, e.g. purchaser-detected defects to be independently reference-classified by the supplier.

MOULDED PLASTIC COMPONENTS

Plastics have probably changed the packaging industry more rapidly than any other type of material. Their versatility is well appreciated, but limitations such as mould flash, stress cracking and shrinkage can seriously affect compatibility with other components. Fortunately, most defects of the type likely to impair pack performance can normally be visually detected, and then dimensionally and functionally tested before confirming the defect rating.

As described for glass mouldings, training to acquire the necessary specialisation skills must involve the supplier and supplier technology, particularly since the development of plastics is still expanding and the pharmaceutical industry must maintain quality comparability.

A simple disadvantage common to most plastic material is the susceptibility to static dust attraction, and all suppliers should control their manufacturing environment as well as their handling/packaging operation to minimise particulate contamination. Once a component is contaminated, both the product and final process including the operators handling the components can be cross-contaminated and product recovery can be difficult as well as costly. 'Clean' production in a controlled environment is an essential means of avoiding particulates as well as maintaining a low bioburden.

Dimensional inspection

When one is dealing with complex components, or high-speed equipment, it is the subtle dimensional variation between components that can often produce the greatest variability in quality.

Component variation within a batch, or from batch to batch if batches are mixed, can affect compatibility with associated components and lead to reduced running speeds as well as reduced shelf life. Similarly, variability can introduce line running peculiarities which can widen the normal process capability distribution in other machine operations (e.g. the volume range from a liquid filling line can be greatly extended under stop–start operations).

Great emphasis must be placed on the laboratory assessment of dimensional compliance, and the relevant measuring equipment. All measuring equipment should be reviewed in terms of the initial purchase cost, its ease of use (and any training) and its accuracy, precision and reliability. This should then be balanced against the value of the results. The following are examples.

GO/NO GO GAUGES

For basic compliance testing, where there is no requirement to record values, these gauges provide rapid, positive information. Results can be obtained very easily, and training is usually minimal.

The disadvantages are that the gauges are usually one component specific (i.e. they lack versatility) and treat variables (measurements) as attributes (good or bad).

There are several types of go/no go gauges, but the most common are those used on primary components:

1 *ring gauges* – body, neck, ODs
2 *plug gauges* – both IDs, internal depth
3 *combination gauges* – constructed to meet special requirements and often combine diameter and height/length checks.

Non-primary components such as cartons can also employ gauges, although obviously the type of gauge will be somewhat different, e.g. a transparent plastic line drawing of the carton profile, creases and scoring will show specification compliance if simply laid over the test carton. They can also show positional variation of identification and register code bars.

A weakness of gauges is the usual need for further accurate dimensional measurement of components that fail the gauge. The information then provides fuller understanding of the range of the problem and the possibility of a concession to use, as well as feedback to the supplier.

MICROMETERS/CALIPERS ETC.

Most precision dimensional testing procedures utilise micrometers, vernier calipers, optical comparators, measuring microscopes, etc. This equipment provides accurate as well as precise measurements, and offers the versatility to encompass a wide range of component sizes and types. Its disadvantages include the need for perhaps complex training and assessment rating of skills, as well as occasional slowness of obtaining results. The following comparison illustrates the need for understanding the merits of both gauges and calipers.

In testing the body OD of a bottle, a single ring gauge check will confirm whether it passes and, if it fails, the position along the body of the deviation. A single check with a vernier caliper will only establish the dimension of one diameter, at one point of the body. Further repeat measurements are necessary if the maximum or minimum body diameters, and their positions along the body, are required. These manual measurements can, however, be recorded and interpreted statistically (standard deviations) and graphically (histograms) to provide trend plotting.

There is now also equipment that uses electronic gauging, computer controller optical comparators and video image analysers to measure component dimensions automatically. Once this type of equipment is correctly calibrated and programmed, it can relieve pressure on staff operatives while providing an enormous increase in accuracy, statistical data and overall value of examinations. It is only to be expected that it suffers the major disadvantage of being expensive, and probably outside the normal laboratory budget.

As with visual faults, all new dimensional deviations should be functionally tested (in the laboratory where possible, or by machine and process trial under normal operating conditions). Results should be judged as follows.

1   If the components perform normally, and/or to the satisfaction of production/development /QC, they should be accepted. The laboratory results and machine trial should be considered by the component specifying department for possible specification revision, in consultation with the supplier. The supplier should be separately notified, by QC, of the deviation and its consequences, i.e. the concession to accept. The supplier should establish and circulate details of the process variation causes which produced the deviation in order to provide greater process understanding, and the steps taken to avoid recurrence.

2   If the components can only be made to perform normally by extensive line adjustments which cannot be tolerated as a long-term measure (e.g. reduced line

speeds/semi-manual handling), a partial concession to use a proportion of the batch may be allowed. This will normally depend on commercial attitudes.

3   If the components cannot be made to run, the batch should be rejected for possible sorting and re-submission.

All 'failed' batches should be fully investigated with the supplier, to assess the route of manufacture, with the intention of preventing further deliveries of defective materials. This also applies when problems are identified during production use, or during a patient complaints investigation.

Any use of precision equipment, even simple gauges, requires formal and regular recalibration to ensure that it still meets the performance requirements. The choice of equipment should be discussed with the supplier (and internal colleagues) to ensure commonality of ability as well as fitness for the purpose. Such routines need clear documentation and records as part of site-wide GMP.

Functional/performance tests

Components and component assemblies identified as critical should be functionally tested as part of the QC test operation. This should include compatibility between components (i.e. do they assemble correctly, perform satisfactorily) as well as suiting the production requirements.

To survey all possible functional tests is beyond the scope of this chapter, but the following are examples.

CAPACITY

This measurement must be made under standard conditions (e.g. water at 20°C) using preset rating points (e.g. to the shoulder or to the brim).

RUBBER HARDNESS

Samples can need conditioning (e.g. 20°C/65% RH for 12 h) and be tested according to national or industrial standards using specified equipment and units (e.g. durometer/shore).

HEAT SEAL STRENGTH

Where components include heat seal lacquers or coatings, laboratory tests should subject the material to agreed (supplier/purchaser) sealing conditions of temperature, pressure and dwell time using approved equipment. Once sealed, a section of stated size should be subjected to a strength measurement, again using approved equipment and specified rates. The test, in addition to establishing the strength of the bond, should also (where applicable) confirm the presence or absence of delamination.

PRINT SCUFF TEST

Since patient/market/legislative data have to be incorporated in modern product presentation, it is essential that the text remain legible throughout the shelf life. Printed material should be scuff abrasion tested, under agreed conditions, to meet visual standards of performance.

CHEMICAL TESTS

Compatibility between product and pack is assessed before final component specifications are issued. As a consequence, some materials are coated, or treated, to ensure surface inertness.

1   When aluminium containers are lacquered, the integrity of the coating can be ·conductivity tested using a copper electrolyte solution. Increased conductivity indicates a poor coating, and results can be referred to standard tables for acceptability.
2   Neutral glass is normally specified when injectable products are involved. Tubular glass neutrality may be affected by the supplier's forming conditions (too hot, too slow, etc.) and chemical testing, to pharmaceutical standards, is a prerequisite of QC acceptance. Failure must result in rejection, with possible supplier treatment (sulphating) to bring the components into specification. (Note that this is only possible with some products in some markets.)

ASSEMBLY

Packs that require mechanical assembly should be tested to assess ease and consistency of fit (e.g. against a maximum force/torque requirement) and to ensure that they function correctly when assembled.

1   A pressurised dispenser (e.g. a material dose inhalation system) should spray the correct quantity versus time, with the correct spray pattern.
2   Hermetically sealed packs should not leak under normal conditions, so laboratory testing could include a vacuum/vibration cycle, in vertical, inverted or horizontal pack modes, if relevant to the product, the market, or the distribution system (e.g. in the pressurised freight hold of an aircraft).

In addition to the normal routine functional/performance testing of components, all deviations which could have an influence on the in-company or in-market use of the product should be similarly assessed.

Defect classifications

Deviations from the specification must be classified according to their effect on patient, product, pack or production operation. This will require laboratory as well as possibly production and market application testing, since it is essential that a defect/defective is accurately defined and quantified.

The normal defect classification is into three categories which are allied to progressively tighter acceptance levels (limits) or AQLs, as follows.

• *Category 1:* minor defect, high percentage AQL.

- *Category 2:* major defect, medium percentage AQL.
- *Category 3:* critical defect, low percentage AQL.

Pharmaceutical packaging, because of the medical risk attached to its products, probably requires a fourth category, possibly termed 'intolerable defect'. This category fulfils the need for the type of fault which, by definition, results in batch rejection and quarantine if one example is found anywhere at any time. It is therefore not necessarily related to any AQL.

- *Category 4:* intolerable defect, 0% AQL (accept 0, reject 1).

This category must only be used for a defect which hazards the patient. For example a 'rogue' printed component mixed within a batch of other products misidentifies and misinforms the user of its contents. This is an intolerable defect and a batch cannot be used until after a 100% fail safe sorting operation (if possible).

It is not possible to include a list of universal defects versus AQLs, since this must be the prerogative of each purchaser and must take into account the ability of its supplier and the requirements of its own production/marketing organisation. This point can be illustrated by the following example.

1   Supplier manufactures and supplies identical closures and bottles to two customers, B and C.
2   Customer B uses these components on a high-speed, automated line, where capping defectives will result in component damage, breakage, contents spillage and line stoppages. Defects which affect capping efficiency (i.e. bottle or closures) are categorised as major defectives with a corresponding AQL of 0.65%.
3   Customer C uses these components on a low speed, manual and semi-automatic line, where capping defectives can be individually rejected and satisfactory replacements used. This results in all unusable components being easily scrapped with minimal loss in efficiency and no line stoppages. For the sake of long-term line efficiency (as well as purchasing standard), a nominal AQL of 4% is applied, and capping defectives are considered as minor.

This example assumes no other functional effect caused by capping defectives (e.g. long-term product leakage), but indicates that identical supply faults need not be rated by two users with the same degree of criticality.

However it is devised, the QC inspection procedure must include:

1   definitions of every defect classification, with corresponding acceptance levels and/or AQLs
2   examples which clearly illustrate each defect classification
3   the route for classifying previously unknown defects, i.e. according to primary definitions in (1) above, plus component trials
4   the possible route and mechanism for component concessions.

Action

Each batch examination calls for a conclusion on the acceptance or rejection status of the materials. The route for establishing this status needs to be simplified into a presentation which immediately relates batch size to sample size and defect AQL to the acceptance number, as shown, for example, in Table 4.2.

The statistical relevance of the action plan should be included for cross-referencing between organisations, i.e. that the plan is based on MIL-STD-105E, Inspection Level II, Normal Inspection, Table IIA AQL 1% (single sample).

All users of the plan should ideally be aware of its derivation and the obligations in following it, i.e. that the agreement to use the plan only allows batch acceptance when the number of defectives found in the sample is less than or equal to the acceptance number. Interpretation outside this constraint is not allowed within the internally delegated responsibility of QC. A batch fails when its acceptance number is exceeded. (As previously explained, the purchasing company can allow a concession, but this is a decision taken by the entire organisation and not independently by QC.)

Records

It is sometimes assumed that QC responsibility for a batch ends once the status has been assigned, and the usefulness of records can be overlooked.

With a pharmaceutical component, inspection can be just the beginning, particularly with modern means of electronic data analysis, storage and retrieval. Records can be used to:

1   build material performance trends into user–supplier relationships (a function of QA)
2   relate in-company production and market performance to the quality specification (e.g. are the quality standards too high/too low?)
3   aid problem-solving during the life of the design/product (e.g. historical data used in future developments of components and component handling equipment etc.), as a part of SPC
4   meet legislative/market requirements.

Records should faithfully represent the tests that have been carried out, and the results that were obtained. They should include all qualification assessments such as repeat samples, machine trials, and batch specific actions by the supplier. The final record should be signed as correct by the examining QC inspector (with his or her numbered stamp, if applicable) and then countersigned by the functional laboratory head. They should be retained for a defined period of time (generally 10 years).

Table 4.2 Establishing acceptance or rejection status

Batch size	Sample size	AQL 1%	
		Acceptance no.	Rejection no.
50,000	500	10	11

Authorisation

The QC procedure is an official company document and forms part of the formal company quality plan (the total company policy on quality). Qualified authorisation is therefore essential and this should ideally include such persons as:

1 the QC laboratory head
2 the QC department head
3 the component supplier
4 persons from the development department responsible for the component specification.

All inspection must be to the approved procedure and temporary revisions cannot be expediently introduced without similar formal approval.

Sampling

It has already been stated that the purpose of QC, in its strictest interpretation, is to determine compliance of a component, a product or service, etc., with an agreed standard. This assessment will form the basis for the decision on acceptability.

When the examination can be restricted to just an individual unit (e.g. examine one item, establish its acceptability, then pass or fail just that one unit) then we can ignore the necessity for random sampling. However, most multiple or mass production involves large quantity batches where the checking of all individual items is not practical. Under these circumstances, sampling of the batch, and a quality status based on the results of that examination, requires some understanding of the peculiarities of sampling.

Most members of the public will have a general understanding of 'random' and 'randomness', but where QC sampling is involved it is essential that the personnel involved in obtaining the sample are fully aware of its QC significance.

A sample 'should' represent all the items or parameters included in the population under examination. Taking a random sample requires the following.

1 Broad coverage of all the batch.
2 No concentration of the sample according to:

- beginning or end of the machine run etc.
- time of manufacture (i.e. not specific on-the-hour plans since these could coincide with natural peaks or troughs in the production cycle)
- speed of manufacture (i.e. not every 100th, 200th, 300th component, etc., since this could also match a production cycle)
- any repetitive predetermined pattern, since this could also coincide with a production cycle.

3 No sampling bias or selection of the items according to any natural senses, i.e. visual, aural, etc.
4 The batch quality should be unchanged on completion of the sampling routine (i.e. sampling a batch should neither improve nor reduce its overall quality standard).

To achieve this, the sampler must firmly understand that random sampling requires that each component has an equal opportunity or chance of being included in the sample. To use a legal comparison, honest, impartial and representative sampling should, like justice, be blindfolded to the peculiarities or characteristics of the item under test.

Table 4.3 gives an example of an ideal but unlikely series of samples, taken from a batch of known proportion defectives (10% bad).

To the non-QC qualified operator, this possibly represents the ideal and hoped for consistently true representation between batch and sample (every sample). In reality, faults randomly distributed in a batch could not perpetually produce the same number/percentage of faults in a sample, since 'chance' decides otherwise (but obviously if enough 'random' samples were taken, the long-term average would eventually equal the batch defect level).

It is at this stage of the consideration of 'sampling' that probability can be introduced to show why samples vary and how it is possible to calculate the likelihood (or probability) of finding a number of defectives in any sample taken from a batch.

This calculation assumes randomness of defects in the batch, and no sampling bias, and uses the binomial distribution to determine the probability levels (the detailed explanation of this distribution, as well as the Poisson distribution, is given later).

Assume: that batch N = 5,000
   that sample n = 100
   that proportion defective p = 10% = 0.10
   that proportion good q = 90% = 0.90

Then, according to the binomial distribution, the probability of finding 1 defective or 2 defectives or 3 defectives, etc. can be obtained from the expanded terms of $(q + p)^n$, i.e.

probability of 0 defectives = $q^n = 0.90^{100} = 0.00003$

probability of 1 defective = $nq^{n-1}p = 100 \times 0.90^{99} \times 0.10 = 0.0003$

$$\text{probability of 2 defectives} = \frac{n(n-1)q^{n-2}p^2}{2!} = \frac{100 \times 99 \times 0.90^{98} \times 0.10^2}{2}$$

$$= 0.0016$$

$$\text{probability of 3 defectives} = \frac{n(n-1)(n-2)q^{n-3}p^3}{3!}$$

$$= \frac{100 \times 99 \times 98 \times 0.90^{97} \times 0.10^3}{3 \times 2} = 0.0059$$

Table 4.3 Ideal series of samples

	Batch	Sample 1	Sample 2	Sample 3
Size	5,000	100	100	100
Quality	90% good	90 good items	90 good items	90 good items
	10% bad	10 bad items	10 bad items	10 bad items

The values for 4, 5 defectives etc. are: 0.016, 0.034, 0.060, 0.089, 0.11, 0.13, 0.13, 0.12, 0.099, 0.064 . . .

These values can be plotted as a graph to show the probability distribution for this sample plan (Figure 4.2). This graph shows that the probability distribution peaks with a defect level of around 10 defective, but the figures reveal that there is a very similar probability of finding 9 defectives, 10 defectives and 11 defectives.

With this insight into the mechanism of sample plans, we should not be surprised in the earlier example that samples of 100 items, taken from a batch of 5,000, where the 'known' defect level is 10, will not always produce just 10 defectives.

The graph reveals one other useful point: if we sum the total probabilities of 0 defectives through to 10 defectives inclusive (using the probability addition law), we obtain a figure of 0.583. By this calculation we can now say that there is a 58.3% probability that a sample taken from the test population would reveal ≤10 defectives. This is the type of calculation on which the recognised sampling tables for inspection by attributes are based, and which is covered a little later.

At this point it is worth reviewing the options available in assessing batch quality.

Not to take a sample

With a batch of unknown quality (e.g. a new supplier or new production unit), the decision not to take a sample does not realistically arise. However, where the supplier or source is known through long-term experience and probably supplier audits, it can be practical to accept a batch on certification release but with the precaution of an identity unit check.

For strict batch statistical quality confidence this option is very rarely considered, but it does have its economic benefits. (Note that the FDA, through the Code of Federal Regulations (CFR), makes no allowance for acceptance on certificate.)

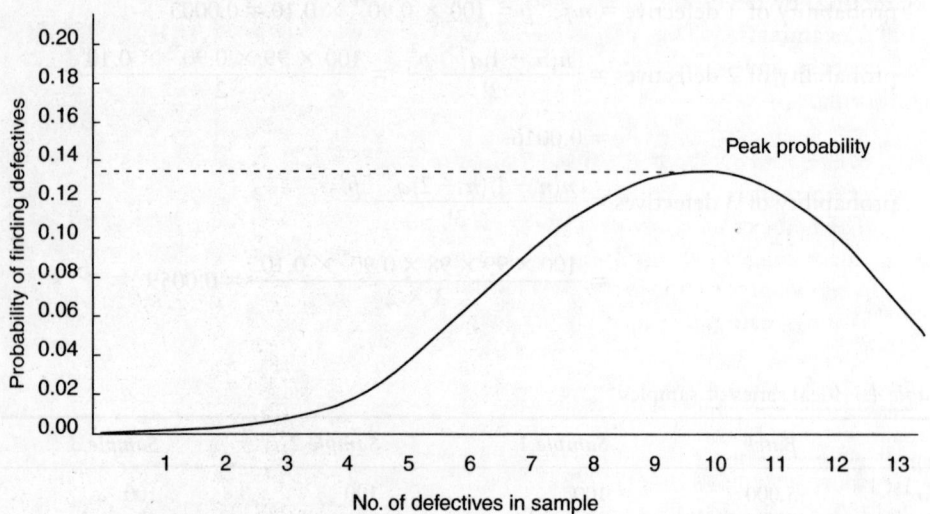

Figure 4.2 Probability distribution for sample plan (defectives)

To take a sample

Having decided to take a sample, the type of sample falls into just four categories, as follows.

A spot sample

By this means a batch of many units is released based on the examination of one or two units. This routine does not afford a reliable quality check or allow any precise understanding of the variability of the batch. Its use should be restricted to identity (see above), for example where a supplier manufactures glass containers, a spot check of one unit or one collated group of units could establish that the delivery consists of amber screw neck containers and not a white flint screw neck design.

Fixed percentage/number

It is not uncommon to find historical sampling routines based on the use of a fixed number or percentage of units (Table 4.4). However, it is without argument that decisions can be misleading when coupled to a simple mathematical calculation of quality, e.g. in the earlier example of a 5,000 batch size with a known defect level of 10%. From our previous consideration of this example it is obvious that sampling results can and will vary and should be related to a probability calculation for confidence.

A second important inefficiency of a fixed percentage plan is that as batch sizes increase, what starts as a simple examination of a small number of items can become excessively large and expensive in time and effort for very little appreciable gain in confidence of the result.

100% sampling examination

Sampling, by definition, cannot really be encompassed by a check which involves a 100% examination. This level of inspection is therefore usually disregarded for reasons of expense and/or impracticality, although there are some exceptions, such as the following.

1   Where historical records show that a problem routinely exists at the point of manufacture, it is sometimes feasible to employ 100% in line checking for that defect. The best example of this is in the glass industry where certain dimensions are routinely gauged, and deviations automatically rejected, or during ampoule filling when all production is checked for particulates.
2   During customer receipt checks on reel-fed labels, automatic counting equipment

Table 4.4 Sampling routine based on fixed number of units

Sample	Results	Interpretation
1st 100	10 defectives	Batch is 10% defective
2nd 100	11 defectives	Batch is 11% defective, i.e. worse than 'known' quality
3rd 100	9 defectives	Batch is 9% defective, i.e. better than 'known' quality

can be combined with electronic code readers to ensure count reconciliation as well as register and identity.

This type of examination is additional to normal statistical checks and can usually be equated with near 100% confidence (assuming the check has been properly validated).

Random statistical sampling

The QC of packaging components for the pharmaceutical industry requires an understanding of the technology of the supplier industry, and uses as a tool multiple sciences and technologies, e.g.

1   chemistry – glass neutrality, plastics analysis
2   engineering – limits and fit gauges.

Statistics, as employed in packaging QC, must be viewed as a further tool to be used where necessary and practical. Before use, consideration must be given to the source of supply, the method of manufacture/assembly, whether multiple components are blended into specific patterns and whether random sampling will identify the variability of each component/assembly.

The main benefits of a statistical random sample include calculable levels of confidence regarding the average, medium and long-term quality standard, as well as an appreciation of the risk involved in the quality decision on any one batch.

It must be stressed that statistical sampling is not infallible and in particular can never reliably detect 'rogue' pockets of excessive variability, since its confidence relies on faults being randomly distributed throughout the batch under examination. This is not always the case, since in any batch process isolated 'rogue' defects can occur which may escape the defect detection system operated by supplier or customer.

To minimise this risk, customers must work with and encourage suppliers to measure their process capability actively, and to carry out routine SPC. By determining the route and frequency by which defectives (and in particular rogue defectives) can occur, effective remedies can be agreed to prevent or minimise their manufacture, or to remove them at a later time.

All processes have a natural, calculable variability, with assignable causes of defects. Initial, perhaps high-intensity, sampling is necessary to determine this variability and remove the causes for the unacceptable 'rogues'. Once a process is operating on a steady state basis, normal random SPC sampling of the batch will provide supplier and customer protection.

Sample size

It must be expected that the size of the sample will vary, primarily for two reasons:

1   not all materials can justify the same QC effort
2   generally, the larger the sample size, the lower will be the sample risk (this point is covered below).

Most countries now have national sampling and inspection tables which relate batch size to sample size and, by using precalculated accept/reject figures for a range of 'preferred' AQLs, allow acceptance of a batch at 90/95% probability levels. In the USA these plans are identified as MIL-STD-105, in the UK as BS 6001 and internationally as ISO 2859.

It is recommended that any intending user of sampling plans should examine these documents closely, since they have the major advantage of being internationally accepted and practised. Procedures are very clearly explained and a knowledge of statistics is not essential to their implementation, although a clearer understanding of their derivation and scope will aid the total quality operation.

For example, a 95% probability that a batch is as good as the AQL does not exclude other probabilities that the batch is worse (for example the 10% probability level, sometimes called the lot tolerance per cent defective (LTPD) or unacceptable quality level, can be several percentage points worse than the AQL). It is the relationship of AQL to LTPD that more closely identifies the quality risk in any statistical sampling plan, and illustrates why the use of national plans as simple accept and reject figures fails to tap their full potential.

Risk is itself related to the chosen AQL and the sample size, and of course the unknown level of defectives, randomly distributed (it is hoped) in the batch. We shall consider the AQL first.

1 The AQL is the maximum percentage of defectives which for sampling purposes can be considered as the process average. With a variable quality of supplies, and over a period of many successive deliveries, the long-term average quality of accepted batches will be equal to or better than the AQL.

2 If several batches considerably worse than the AQL were supplied, the majority would be rejected.

3 It is essential that all manufactured materials have been quality assessed by the supplier. The customer's examination should therefore always start with the confidence that the material has at least 'passed' one quality examination (the procedure for which has previously been mutually agreed).

The customer's examination need not therefore be as detailed as the supplier's, but if it is, and duplicates the supplier's plan, then quality confidence in the accepted batches must be considerably enhanced. For example, the multiplication law of statistical probabilities shows that if there is a 1/10 probability of a batch significantly worse than the AQL being released by an inspection, then if two independent examinations are correctly carried out the probability of release is reduced to:

$$1/10 \times 1/10 = 1/100$$

If we now combine these points, in a comparison of some simple sampling plans, where the batch size is ignored and the AQL is considered to be constant, then it is clear that sampling risk is directly dependent on sample size (Table 4.5). (The theoretical plans used show that, depending on the acceptance of 'special risks', a batch of 20,000 items could be inspected against a 4% AQL with a single sample of from 13 items to 315 items.)

Two points are apparent in this comparison:

Table 4.5 Relationship of sampling risks and sample size

Sample size	AQL	Decision number		Defect level at:	
		Accept	Reject	95% probability of acceptance	10% probability of acceptance
13	4%	1	2	2.73	29.9
20	4%	2	3	4.09	26.6
32	4%	3	4	4.26	20.9
50	4%	5	6	5.23	21.0
80	4%	7	8	4.98	14.7
125	4%	10	11	4.94	12.3
200	4%	14	15	4.62	10.1
300	4%	21	22	4.73	8.95

1 the AQL is never actually 4% at the 95% probability level (since we can only operate with whole number accept/reject figures)
2 as the sample size increases, there is a correspondingly reduced level of defectives potentially acceptable at the 10% probability level.

This can be generalised as:

• small sample = high risk potential
• large sample = low risk potential.

This sample size versus risk dependency is covered in detail below.

One further point in dealing with the size of sample is the choice between single, double and multiple samples. Plans have been produced which allow comparison between these options at the same AQL, and using the same example as above (i.e. a batch of 20,000, AQL 4%) (Table 4.6).

Table 4.6 Comparison of single, double and multiple samples

Type of sample	Sample size	Decision number		Total sample
		Accept	Reject	
Single	50	5	6	50
Double	1st sample 32	2	5	64
	2nd sample 32	6	7	
Multiple*	1st Sample 13*	–	4	91
	2nd Sample 13	1	5	
	3rd Sample 13	2	6	
	4th Sample 13	3	7	
	5th Sample 13	5	8	
	6th Sample 13	7	9	
	7th Sample 13	9	10	

* This sample size does not allow acceptance of the batch, but does allow rejection if 4 or more defectives are found.

Reasons for choosing multiple samples

The obvious first reason for choosing a double or multiple sample plan (and possibly the only real reason) is the opportunity to take a smaller initial sample, i.e. the ability to make a status decision using a smaller sample than if a single plan were used. This reduction in the QC effort is only achieved when the status decision can be made on the first 1 or 2 samples; when a further sample is necessary, the advantage is lost.

The main requirements for double/multiple sampling can therefore be detailed as follows.

1   There must be high confidence that the routine quality standard of the items is high, and can be passed on the preliminary samples. This is often the case with in-company manufacture, or where suppliers have proven/validated and audited QC systems.
2   That the unit cost of the item is high and, perhaps, the test is destructive.

Distributions and operating characteristics

It has previously been stated that the use of national sampling plans does not require a detailed knowledge of statistics, but in practice a working understanding of their derivation will aid the user. All sampling plans are derived from either the binomial distribution or the Poisson distribution, by calculating either:

1   the probability x of finding 1, 2, 3, etc. defectives in a sample (n), where the level of defectives (p) in the batch is known or postulated, or
2   the number of defectives (y) in a batch when the sample size (n) is known and the probability of success is stipulated (e.g. as 95%).

The binomial distribution

This distribution is based on the expansion of the simple equation:

$$(q + p)^n = 1$$

(i.e. the total probabilities). If we use QC terms, then
p = the known proportion of defective items
q = the known proportion of acceptable items
n = the sample size.

Using a simple example, say of a sample of 2 items, the expansion gives us these terms:

$$(q + p)^2 = q^2 + qp + pq + p^2$$
$$= q^2 + 2qp + p^2$$

The individual terms of this expansion are the probability values for 0 defectives, 1 defective and 2 defectives, i.e.

129

q^2 = probability of 0 defectives

$2qp$ = probability of 1 defective

p^2 = probability of 2 defectives

→ The total probability of ≤2 defectives = 1

Extending this example into the full distribution, we obtain:

$$(q + p)^n = q^n + nq^{n-1}p + \frac{n(n - 1)q^{n-2}p^2}{2!} + \frac{n(n - 1)(n - 2)q^{n-3}}{3!} \ldots p^n$$

               0 def. 1 def.   2 def.   3 def. n def.

This distribution is now in a format which can be used in a QC environment, for example a typical QC sample (n) is 50 components, and a not untypical defect level (p) in a batch is 1%. (The non-defect level (q) is therefore 99%.)

We can then substitute these figures into the binomial:

$$(q + p)^n = (0.99 + 0.01)^{50}$$

and expanding this equation gives

$$p(0 \text{ def.}) = q^n = 0.99^{50} = 0.6050 = 60.5\%$$

$$p(1 \text{ def.}) = nq^{n-1}p = 50 \times 0.99^{49} \times 0.01 = 0.3056 = 30.56\%$$

$$p(2 \text{ def.}) = \frac{n(n-1)q^{n-1}p^2}{2!} = \frac{50 \times 49 \times 0.99^{48} \times 0.01^2}{2!} = 0.0756 = 7.56\%$$

These individual values are not always useful, but if we pose the normal QC question of what probability of acceptance is attached to the above example, when the sample acceptance number is say 1 or 2, we can use the addition law, i.e.:

(a) $p(0 \text{ def.}) + p(1 \text{ def.}) = 0.6050 + 0.3056$

$$= 0.9106$$

Probability of accepting on ≤ 1 def. = 91.06%

(b) $p(0 \text{ def.}) + p(1 \text{ def.}) + p(2 \text{ defs}) = 0.6050 + 0.3056 + 0.0756$

$$= 0.9862$$

Probability of accepting on ≤2 defs = 98.62%

The Poisson distribution

This distribution approximates the binomial, and is used as an alternative when:

- the sample is large, $n \to \infty$ (i.e. >50)
- the level of defective (p) is small (i.e. <0.1)
- the form of the distribution used by QC is

$$1 = e^{-m} + me^{-m} + \frac{m^2 e^{-m}}{2!} + \frac{m^3 e^{-m}}{3!} + \frac{m^4 e^{-m}}{4!} \cdots$$

The individual terms of this expansion are the probability value for 0 defectives, 1 defective, 2 defectives, etc.

e^{-m} = probability of 0 defectives

me^{-m} = probability of 1 defective

$\dfrac{m^2 e^{-m}}{2!}$ = probability of 2 defectives

$\dfrac{m^3 e^{-m}}{3!}$ = probability of 3 defectives

By using the same example as for the binomial distribution, we can make the comparison:

$n = 50$

$p = 0.01$

m = mean number of defectives expected in sample

$m = np$

$m = 0.5$

$p(0 \text{ def.}) = e^{-m} = e^{-0.5} = 0.6065 = 60.65\%$

$p(1 \text{ def.}) = me^{-m} = 0.5 \times e^{-0.5} = 0.3033 = 30.33\%$

$p(2 \text{ defs}) = \dfrac{m^2 e^{-m}}{2!} = \dfrac{0.5^2 \times e^{-0.5}}{2} = 0.0758 = 7.58\%$

and similarly:

$p(0 \text{ def.}) + p(1 \text{ def.}) = 0.6065 + 0.3033$
$$= 0.9098$$

probability of accepting on ≤ 1 def. $= 90.98\%$

$p(0 \text{ def.}) + p(1 \text{ def.}) + p(2 \text{ defs}) = 0.6065 + 0.3033 + 0.0758$
$$= 0.9856$$

probability of accepting on ≤ 2 defs = 98.56%

It can therefore be shown that the two distributions do provide good comparisons, and using the above examples it is not difficult to calculate one's own individual plans, perhaps to meet specific requirements or more realistically just for experience of the construction of documented plans.

It is worth stressing that the AQL is simply the defect percentage level which defines the 95% probability of acceptance. From the example it is obvious that there are other probabilities which can be calculated and, if graphed, provide the operating characteristic (OC) of that sampling plan, i.e.

sample size (n) = 50

acceptance number (a) = 2

proportion defective (p) = 1%, 2%, 3%, 4%, 5% etc. (since we cannot be certain of batch variability)

If we now use the binomial distribution $(q + p)^n$ for each level of defectives, i.e. by expanding

(a) $(0.99 + 0.01)^{50}$
(b) $(0.98 + 0.02)^{50}$
(c) $(0.97 + 0.03)^{50}$
(d) $(0.96 + 0.04)^{50}$
(e) $(0.95 + 0.05)^{50}$, etc.

1   $(0.99 + 0.01)^{50}$ gives p (≤ 2 def.) = 98.62% (see above)
2   $(0.98 + 0.02)^{50}$ gives the following terms:

$$p(0 \text{ def.}) = 0.98^{50} = 0.3642 = 36.42\%$$

$$p(1 \text{ def.}) = 50 \times 0.98^{49} \times 0.02 = 0.3716 = 37.16\%$$

$$p(2 \text{ defs}) = \frac{50 \times 49 \times 0.98^{48} \times 0.02^2}{2!} = 0.1858 = 18.58\%$$

$$p(0 \text{ def.}) + p(1 \text{ def.}) + p(2 \text{ defs}) = 0.3642 + 0.3716 + 0.1858 = 0.9216 = 92.16\%$$

By the same method, the probability for ≤ 2 defectives can be calculated for batches containing 3%, 4%, 5%, etc. defectives (Table 4.7). These probability values can now be graphed as shown in Figure 4.3.

Several comments can be made from a consideration of the OC shown in Figure 4.3.

1   All sampling plans have an OC in which no matter how low the defect level is at the theoretical AQL, there will be a risk of accepting a batch with a considerably higher level of defectives.
2   The sampling plan cannot be adequately defined by reference to just one point on the curve (i.e. the AQL), but two points will define the plan.
3   The second point usually chosen to define the plan is the 10% probability (risk) of

Table 4.7 Probabilities of ≤2 defectives for batches containing various percentages of defectives

No. of defectives	Probability of finding up to 2 defectives									
	1%	2%	3%	4%	5%	6%	7%	8%	10%	20%
0	0.6050	0.3642	0.2181	0.1299	0.0769	0.0453	0.0266	0.0155	0.0052	0.0000
1	0.3056	0.3716	0.3372	0.2706	0.2025	0.1447	0.0999	0.0672	0.0286	0.0002
2	0.0756	0.1858	0.2555	0.2762	0.2611	0.2262	0.1843	0.1433	0.0779	0.0013
Total probability of ≤2 defectives	0.9862	0.9216	0.8108	0.6767	0.5405	0.4162	0.3108	0.226	0.1117	0.0015

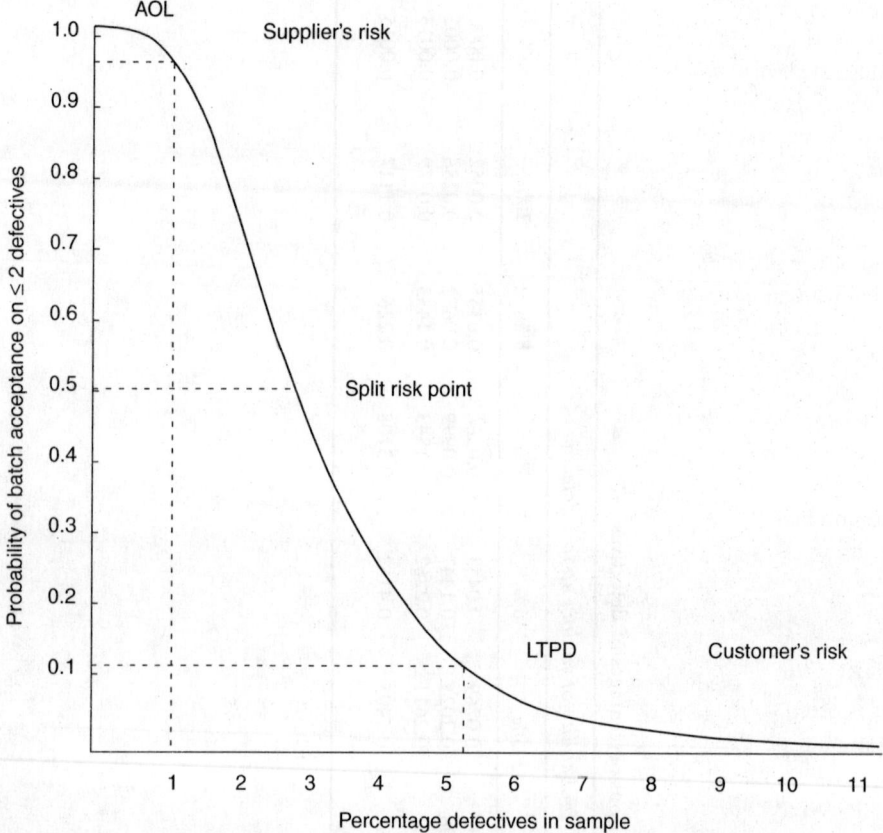

Figure 4.3 Probability of ≤2 defectives for various percentage of defectives

acceptance, and as previously mentioned is termed the *lot tolerance per cent defec-tive (LTPD) or the unacceptable quality level (UQL)*.

4   At the AQL of 95% probability of acceptance, there is a 5% probability (i.e. 100%–95%) of a batch being rejected although it is as good as or even better than the AQL. This 5% probability value is referred to as the supplier's risk.

5   Similarly, the LTPD of 10% probability of acceptance is sometimes referred to as the customer's risk.

6   The mid-point of the OC curve, or the 50% probability level, is sometimes known as the split risk point, since there is an even chance of batch acceptance or rejection.

Comparison of OC curves

All sampling plans have OC curves, and any consideration of a scheme for sampling inspection should begin with an examination of the curve (see MIL-STD-105, or BS 6001). The ambition in examining the curves is to obtain the smallest sample size that provides the greatest confidence of batch compliance with the required quality, i.e. reducing the degree to which the batch may be different from the chosen AQL.

However, it has to be recognised that small samples must equate with a greater chance of accepting a batch significantly worse than the AQL. Larger samples, because they have steeper OC curves, will conversely have a lower chance of accepting a batch significantly worse than the AQL.

In general, very small samples should only be used with a high/lax AQL, and large samples when the AQL is very low/tight.

Supplier evaluation

The supplier plays a key role in the chain of quality events that concludes with the sale of the ultimate final product. This point is sometimes overlooked or consideration and implementation left too late to utilise fully all the potential advantages that can be gained by the correct choice of supplier.

Any realistic QC function must therefore have a policy of supplier evaluation which will ensure that the capability of the supplier matches the requirements of the customer. This is all that can be requested of a supplier, but while assessing the capability it is essential that the customer is equally thorough in stipulating the quality requirements.

Supplier evaluation can usually be subdivided into three categories: new project with existing supplier, new supplier, and new project with new supplier.

New project with existing supplier

This is often the easiest evaluation to monitor since it operates with a full project team and quality objectives can be co-ordinated into the complete design requirements. It is also founded on long-term commercial relationships where the company history will exist to support the actual quality of performance.

A new supplier

This can be more complicated, since it will rely on the assessment of a company's potential ability, separate from the actual context of historical performance. Ideally any new supplier should be certificated to a national or international quality standard (e.g. ISO 9000), with an already audited and proven quality system. (During the 1990s many UK packaging companies have been independently certificated to the Pharmaceutical Supplier Codes of Practice, which are linked to ISO 9002.)

To obtain a realistic assessment, the method and detail of the purchaser's evaluation of a new supplier must be formalised, and the results documented. The opportunity must be taken to view the supplier under normal operating conditions, with the involvement of the relevant technical staff. Systems of working routines must be made available and the operation of quality systems defined. The supplier company should explain its organisation (line/functional disposition), its personnel training policy, and its philosophy and commitment to quality.

The results of the evaluation must be made known to the supplier, and the opportunity presented for comment (to resolve differences, to extend the evaluation or to discontinue the evaluation).

New project with a new supplier

This category will naturally involve a combination of the previous two and, to a great extent, the quality evaluation should parallel the design project team which could itself possibly be involved in the development programme with a research subdivision separate from the manufacturing plant.

Care must be taken with a new innovative company which may initially lack in-depth quality systems, and it may be necessary to help introduce quality procedures compatible with the quality demands. This would be far easier than trying to teach innovative design concepts.

The intention under this title must be to design quality into the component, and to ensure that conformance is achievable.

In general, the evaluation of a supplier will fall into just three categories:

- the supplier's manufacturing capability
- the supplier's quality capability
- the customer's quality requirements.

The supplier's manufacturing capability

The supplier must invite an unconditional tour of its plant, or, at least, of the part that involves or impinges on fulfilling the contract.

This will cover areas of design and development, the production support facility (the tool room for manufacture, refurbishing of moulds, dies, etc.), the manufacturing plant (all the multiphases of the operation including machining, moulding, printing, assembly, packaging, warehousing, distribution, etc.).

Details of normal GMP (perhaps specific to that particular industry) should be highlighted, such as machine layout and space; floor and wall conditions; segregation and separation of material in storage, work or awaiting use; level of lighting; material and work identification; quarantine areas; etc.

Quality capability

The size of the quality organisation and the extent of documented procedures will vary according to the size of company. Independent of size there should be an appreciation that quality systems must be formalised to ensure material consistency. Each manufactured batch must be subjected to the same control, ideally involving pre-running start-up checks, in-process SPC checks and pre-delivery conformance checking.

It is for these reasons that all companies should possess a quality manual which contains the formal policy on company quality. This should be produced by the quality department but have chief executive authorisation. Specific quality procedures should be included in a quality plan, which can be presented as either one complete plan containing a sub-chapter for individual components/component ranges, or a separate plan for each and every individual component/component range.

The assessment of the company's quality capability should review the quality policy, and establish the following.

1   The role, responsibilities and training of staff delegated with the quality function (in both production and QC).

2   The person named as responsible for quality, his or her status and to whom he or she reports.

3   The inspection facilities and equipment must be suitable for the control of manufacture, and able to meet the contract quality specification, i.e. main laboratory and/or line testing areas, measuring equipment, component function testing equipment, sample storage, calibration and validation procedures.

4   Quality procedures must detail the type and route of sampling, inspecting and testing, which will include:

- raw materials and manufactured products
- the means for quarantine segregation of defectives, their status identification and the mechanism for sorting and resubmission to QC
- the action on finding defectives
- the means of disposal of defectives
- the production/QC action to remedy the cause of defectives.

5   The degree and type of production-based line inspection, and its relationship to the QC operation. Ideally line inspection should be based on SPC and involve an element of continuous improvement to remove defect causes.

6   The manufacturing process documentation for stipulating the type and amount of materials required per batch; the machines/moulds etc. required for producing the product; the specification details/drawing; the degree of process checking; first-off checks; etc.

7   The documentation system for recording all results obtained by QC (of raw materials and manufactured materials).

8   The means of storing batch data, its accessibility to supplier and customer, and duration of retention.

9   The system for incorporating special customer requirements into production operations, e.g. certificate, special packaging, labelling.

10   The company GMP system covering work practices throughout the plant and warehouse, e.g. in-company audits, line clean down procedures, material identification and segregation, quarantine areas, general traceability.

11   The company system for routine training of operators involved in the manufacturing process.

12   The system for regular review of:

- specification and procedures
- control equipment calibration (in production and QC)
- subcontractor or suppliers
- customer's quality contract
- internal quality systems.

The customer's quality requirements

To be competitive in terms of specification and quality, a modern supplier must have a thorough understanding of its own process capability, its quality ability and its market position. The evaluation must therefore work to the strength of the supplier, by relating that ability to the customer's quality requirements. To that extent, the customer must ensure that its component specifications are complete, that its quality procedures are comprehensive and realistic, and then classify all the details to the supplier's satisfaction. At that point it may be necessary for the customer to use its quality expertise to aid the supplier in improving its quality systems (see above).

Any doubts about the supplier's total ability to meet specific requirements must be resolved before commencing production (machine trials should be utilised to remove doubts, as well as to acquire confidence for either party).

The intention of the evaluation is to ensure that the supplier can control its manufacturing operation and meet agreed standards. It is therefore in the interests of both parties that sufficient time is taken to form the basis for a good long-term commercial relationship.

On completion of the successful examination, the supplier must agree the final component quality procedure since this is an integral part of the commercial contract.

Customer–supplier working relationship

The customer and supplier form the opposite ends of the same commercial chain. To be successful, both must contribute:

1   the supplier must achieve specified standards and service
2   the customer must accept the commercial cost of specified standards.

The arrangements must start with an open evaluation and, through agreement on realistic quality standards confirmed by results on successive deliveries, achieve a steady working relationship.

A review of the quality standards can be initiated by both parties, either because the standards are too low (usually by the customer when problems are occurring in manufacture or market) or because the standards are too high (usually if the supplier is suffering excessive wastage or process downtime).

The quality standard should be automatically reviewed after several consignments or 6–12 months, whichever is more realistic. This review allows performance of supplier and in-use customer data to be incorporated into a more fully validated standard. The longer term ambition of supplier and customer must be to achieve complete inter-company quality trust (evidenced by supply on certificate).

Quality control of material, to be effective, must be close to the point of manufacture. Hence the emphasis on the supplier controlling its process while the material is being produced, backed-up by separate batch testing. The delivery that reaches the customer and is then found to be defective has far-reaching implications on product scheduling, market supply and, eventually, customer confidence.

It is therefore self-evident, as well as cost-effective, that supplier and customer should concentrate most of the QC effort at the supplier's production line, for example by the supplier using strict in-process controls backed-up by a single, large sample, while the customer employs double, smaller samples. The supplier, not the customer, must be responsible for the quality of delivered components.

This system of 'commercial' QC trust should lead to the customer expending more effort in aiding/improving the supplier's quality system(through regular quality audits), and less on routine conformance testing. The supplier has to be aware that a substandard delivery, unknowingly accepted for use, can have serious implications for the customer's production efficiency, but more critical consequences on patient efficacy.

Manufacture and qualification controls

Once a delivery has been received by the purchasing company, and assessed for specification compliance, it is held in a quarantine warehouse awaiting manufacturing use.

The systems required for in-house manufacture are developed as part of the product launch product team, and within the overall time scale. The manufacturing brief will encompass a variety of parameters depending on the type of product and the scale of the manufacturing launch.

Objectives will have to be rationally established, and will probably include:

1 the equipment specification
2 the environmental specification (sterile or non-sterile area, temperature/humidity controlled, etc.)
3 the raw material specification
4 the packaging components specification
5 prestocking for materials and components
6 standard operating procedures
7 staff training (including training in SPC techniques associated with the new process)
8 operator process controls
9 finished product qualification controls.

All these prime activities, and many others, will need in-depth assessment and resolution (usually within a qualification and validation programme) before production can commence, but once production is initiated, confirmation of compliance with the finished product specification depends on the last two activities.

In the modern organisation it is difficult to separate production-operated SPC from QC-operated finished product controls. They must complement one another within the following broad definitions.

1 *Statistical process controls:* manufacturing procedures designed to ensure that process operators 'self-check' their production output (to record results, maintain process variation within established limits, correct the causes of ongoing deviations, detect trends and minimise wastage).
2 *Finished product control:* QC procedures, separate from production operations, to ensure that released product complies with agreed standards (which can be company-based or nationally/internationally imposed specifications).

It must be emphasised that transfer of the 'research product' to the 'manufacturing division' cannot occur in an information vacuum, divorced from the background information and experience of the project team. In many companies it is common for several full-scale 'development' batches to be produced in the manufacturing facility before complete hand-over to production.

This phase-in period allows for better co-ordination of the development technology into the production technology of the detailed product manual. It maintains the skills and expertise of the project team through the difficult learning cycle of the production operators. It enhances GMP and consolidates the process controls necessary to ensure production efficiency combined with 'making it right first time' policies.

Process controls

The degree and type of process controls will vary from company to company and from product to product. Some new products (such as a pharmaceutical drug) may require complicated and new blending/homogenising operations, but then be presented in a standard tablet form. In this example process controls would include routine checks for tablet weight, thickness, hardness and possibly friability and dissolution.

If the process were a large volume liquid filling line, then in-process controls would include measurement of fill levels/weight and, if a screw closure, the release torque.

The following are equally important as determining the type of test to carry out.

1 How many items to check.
2 How frequently the tests should be carried out.
3 At what point of the manufacture the sample should be taken (e.g. checks on label presentation should also be made after cartoning of the container, to avoid over-looking label damage caused by carton insertion).
4 The action to be taken if items are found to deviate from specification. This is the key point and comes from the correlation of defect causes with efforts leading to continuous improvement and the avoidance/prevention of defectives. Answers to these questions can often be found from experience with products of a similar nature (for example, although a liquid filling line may be new, the cap-tightening equipment may be identical to machinery in another part of the plant. Records will show equipment capability and tests can be duplicated).

If, however, the actual filling line is to a new design, fill level testing procedures can only be obtained from first principles, as follows.

1 What is the desired product specification?
2 What is the equipment manufacturer's recommendation? (All manufacturers carry out detailed 'qualification' trials, although not always with exactly the same liquid characteristics.)
3 Carry out detailed trials at the manufacturer to establish consistency standards before the equipment is shipped to the purchaser's plant. Standards will need to be contractual.
4 Once installed in the purchaser's plant, the first three 'development' batches should be used to carry out in-depth process capability trials (with the manufacturer's engineering representative possibly in attendance). The process capability trial is the best opportunity to establish not only the capability of the equipment, but also the in-process checking necessary to ensure batch consistency. The trial will require multi-comparison data:

- frequent but small sample sizes, taken throughout the batch and repeated on later batches
- less frequent but larger samples, covering all filling heads, throughout several batches as above
- repeat testing following batch change-overs from one pack size (of fill) to another, to establish variability induced by engineering adjustment and changes.

The statistical analysis of this data will determine the sample size and frequency of later routine checking by indicating:

- mean fill and range (including standard deviation)
- long- and short-term machine cycling variability
- head-to-head variability
- fill drift (since it is well known that level of fill can drift as the machine 'warms up/settles down' and can require an initial operator adjustment)
- stop/start variability (it is recognised that stop/start interruptions to a process can introduce excessive process variability).

The trials should deliberately investigate the mode for variations and failure route (care must be taken that trial-induced variations in the product are not released for consumer retail unless extensively checked). For example, failure/variation in a vacuum filling line can be caused by loss of vacuum, the result of seal damage from abrasion with the bottle rims. In a piston/cylinder operation, density variations in the product (requiring strict analytical control) are a principal source of fill weight variation.

Although it is not unusual for equipment to cause excessive variations occasionally, defects can often be related to maintenance faults (e.g. seals not replaced at specified times, volumetric adjustment controls not secured after adjustment). One of the most important process checks is at the start of the batch, particularly after a change-over from a different fill quantity or after a maintenance period. This start-up check is the best opportunity to find the gross error and to ensure that all filling heads are set correctly.

Provided that process capability trials have shown process consistency, with only nominal head-to-head variations, only small sample sizes are needed to maintain process control.

Statistical data can be employed to construct control charts (Shewart charts) which provide action limits and warning limits for values of mean and standard deviation. Charts can be used for measurement of variability (size, volume, hardness, etc.) or attributes (good/bad or acceptable/rejectable). Values calculated from routine samples are plotted onto the relevant chart, and provided the results fall within the acceptance area, manufacture can continue until the next sample is called for.

SPC charts have proved their value over many years and no longer need justification or a detailed explanation. They allow for the normal expected process variability, e.g. action can follow a failure at 99.8% probability (1/1,000), with a warning at 95% probability (1/40). They allow easy operator understanding of results, without which data can be misconstrued leading to excessive operator-induced variability (under the impression that the process is out of control).

Where certain process characteristics are important, it is sometimes feasible to incorporate automatic in-process checking of 100% of production. This can remove the risk of low-frequency faults escaping detection and provides virtual 100% quality confidence, as follows.

1 Automatic in-line weight checking programmed with calculated net values of the container weight distribution (provided this is very small relative to the net fill standard). Similar statistical systems exist for the weight-checking of samples, and these can be programmed to indicate whether the fill process needs an increase or decrease adjustment.

2 Automatic code reading and missing label detector. Process control results must be recorded, since the records can be invaluable for later analysis. They will allow immediate action over gross deviations:

- to quarantine current production and re-examine product from the time of the previous acceptance results
- to accumulate daily data for medium-term assessment of line efficiency/wastage levels
- to act as a warning that a deviation is developing which could eventually cause specification failure
- to show long-term process drift indicative of machine wear requiring planned maintenance
- to provide historical data to support customer feedback
- as a means for 'continuous improvement', where causes of deviations are examined and reviewed continually giving an improving quality capability.

One last responsibility after the transfer of a new process/product into the production operation is to institute a review of production records after a set time period or number of batches. This review can be used to consolidate existing limits and test procedures, or to introduce modified or new routines. It should include data from market reports and any customer reactions (good or bad).

The intention of GMP is firstly to design systems, facilities and procedures so as to avoid failure, and secondly to detect at the earliest opportunity process drift that can lead to failure and thereby avoid the manufacture of failures. GMP is dictated by the company need to ensure product constancy within the specifications and to maximise efficiency. For good GMP, process operators must be in control of the production operation and this requires predetermined and relevant process control checks.

Finished product control

Before development of modern QA principles and QC technology, finished product control was the main (and perhaps only) preoccupation of the QC department. Finished products were often sampled at the end of the process and, after inspection, classed as acceptable or not acceptable. Following this decision, it was expected that the 'surprise news' of a quality problem would be investigated and remedial action introduced.

No company can be expected to survive in a competitive market if quality assessments are divorced in time from manufacture. It is for this reason that pharmaceutical manufacturers must believe in production-operated in-process checks where the process operators have the responsibility to self-check. These checks will be complementary to the independent (and legally required) QC assessment.

The finished product control will be based on the finished product specification and will detail the tests, sample size and frequency necessary to ensure compliance. As with the inspection of bought-in components, testing procedures will include details extracted from national and international standards (pharmacopoeias, military standards, etc.). They will however have one major advantage over systems designed to vet bought-in materials, i.e. the higher confidence synonymous with in-house manufacture.

QA/QC will have been involved in the project phase which developed and introduced the new process/product. They will have participated in devising the 'manufacturing specifications' used to produce the product, in particular the in-process production checking. They will have ensured that bought-in materials meet the specification and that all items (components, facilities and process) have been validated in a process capability trial.

With these advantages, the finished product control can be implemented during, or at the end of, the batch manufacturing process, and will include a thorough assessment of the regular documented results of the in-process production checking. (Note that the production in-process checking will normally be at a higher frequency than the QC check, although perhaps not always to the same depth or detail.)

The QC control inspection can therefore justify the economical use of double or multiple sampling techniques (these depend on high confidence of passing on the initial sample(s), otherwise they become uneconomic of sampling effort if further samples are required).

As with in-process production checking, finished product control can employ statistical techniques and control charts or can be derived from national sampling procedures such as MIL-STD 414 (sampling, procedures and tables for inspection by variables for per cent defectives). These sampling procedures are very similar to and complement the sampling, procedures and tables for inspection by attributes (e.g. MIL-STD 105E) and can be used in a similar manner.

The finished product control will be a standard procedure covering primary and secondary pack characteristics such as the following.

1   Primary characteristics:

- weight/volume of fill
- tablet count
- integrity of pack
- efficiency of closure
- functionality of pack assembly.

2   Secondary characteristics:

- presentation of pack
- label details
- carton details
- batch data (lot and expiry).

In general, its format will be similar to that for component inspection.

Validation as part of packaging quality

Validation, in the European Guide *The Rules Governing Medicinal Products in the European Community Volume IV*, is defined as 'Action of proving, in accordance with the principles of good manufacturing practice, that any procedure, process equipment, material, activity or system actually leads to the expected results'.

From this definition it is obvious that packaging components come within the scope of validation (via the 'material' route). In the context of the earlier review of quality of design and quality of conformance, it may seem that the validation concept does not offer a great deal of additional confidence. However, this would ignore the recent history of validation and its expansion into qualification.

While validation has a relatively short technical history, in practice it has largely been directed at aseptic processing (autoclaves and media fill vials, etc.). In recent years validation has been progressively expanded, firstly to cover all manufacturing, then computer systems, analytical methodology and more recently into packaging processes. Coincident with this, validation has itself evolved into qualification, with defined parts:

- SQ (specification qualification, i.e. equipment specified against key requirements)
- PDQ (pre-delivery qualification, i.e. optimised assessment at supplier)
- IQ (installation qualification, i.e. inventory, services, function check)
- OQ (operational qualification, i.e. dynamic assessment against specification, under production conditions)
- PQ (performance qualification, i.e. technical review of first batches).

As was common with validation, qualification can be as broad as an entirely new line, or focused on a new or modified sub-part, e.g. a new capper in a filling line. No matter how large, the important aspect is to ensure that the assessment covers all the possible interactions between constituent parts of the process (i.e. input and outputs), the materials being used and the operation of the process (i.e. operators).

For example, a company which experienced a customer complaint involving a large glass fragment in an aseptically filled powder vial introduced procedural preventive measures but concluded that the issue required automated vision inspection equipment. Once the corrective equipment was identified, a validation master plan detailed the key qualification elements for hardware, software, defect detection system, infeed/outfeed links, but also the specification requirements of the component and component quality, e.g:

1 the specification – supplier, component dimensions, glass type, surface design, etc.
2 the vial quality – particulates, cracks, surface marks, contamination, etc.

Details needed defining with the supplier and the trial components needed to be assessed prior to the trial to document the quality datum, since the whole performance assessment would be based on the components 'as used'. During the trial using laboratory produced 'defectives', false positive/spurious rejects were qualified and assessed in order to determine the true quality performance of the unit. At the conclusion, the unit was certificated in the context of:

1   the inspection unit
2   the process
3   the environment
4   the operational procedure
5   the trained operators
6   the specified components
7   the re-validation schedule.

It is worth stressing that future changes to the process (e.g. a new component supplier or component design) could degrade the operational performance and take it out of 'certification'. Any change must therefore lead to a review, an outcome of which could be re-validation/re-qualification.

A further example of how validation is having an effect on component quality is where regulatory authorities impose new requirements. These are naturally intended to support or expand GMP, and must be viewed positively, but they can create additional quality demands.

The FDA recently confirmed that market feedback showed that mislabelling recalls were not associated with packaging processes with on-line bar code readers. This has led to the relaxation of the need for full component reconciliation, but indirectly upgraded the technical demands on validating bar code readers.

To put this into context, when bar code readers were just one part of an integrated quality system (e.g. supplier count verification, QC count checks on incoming deliveries, line receipt checks, line cleandown checks and reconciliation), only the function of the bar code readers needed to be the focus of attention. As a stand-alone system, full validation/qualification becomes a necessity and takes the issue away from the line and onto technical support (i.e. QA). Just as with the earlier vision inspection equipment, qualification is not just of the bar code reader and the detection performance, but also of the component quality, e.g.

1   the specification – supplier, component dimensions, surface type and finish, colour, print design/coverage, code design, etc.
2   the component quality – colour and surface variation, text location (related to size variation), etc.

Final certification of the unit must relate to specified components and the supplier, with changes, as pointed out earlier, requiring review and possible revalidation.

Validation is not therefore an entirely new requirement for packaging components, but purely an extension of the original 'fitness for purpose' and the desire to ensure that all constituent parts (material and *matériel*) are not only as specified, but also function together as specified, before material is used in a production process.

What is possibly new is the interest of regulatory authorities in the combination of packaging component and process validation, which directly increases the need for a fully professional and interested component dossier covering:

•   the specification
•   the quality standard
•   supplier audit

- QC tests
- line and material/process validations
- change history.

This total approach to the integration of quality takes suppliers and users close to a performance guarantee that materials and processes will perform as specified.

Conclusion

It is difficult to write a concluding summary without incurring the risk of paraphrasing the salient features of the main text or simply repeating verbatim. However, product quality, as a topic to manufacturer and lay person alike, cannot be repeated too frequently since it is one of the critical factors that:

- directly affect consumer appreciation
- are directly controllable by the manufacturer or producer
- are cost-effective aids to production efficiency when properly devised and implemented.

All products have a quality horizon. While some are intentionally low, others are intentionally high. This is no different in the pharmaceutical industry, where the 'product' must be considered to be the drug and pack and both will warrant equal quality considerations. Emphasis might vary from company to company or from industry to industry, but whatever the product standard it is essential for the manufacturer to know its market sector and whether quality objectives are being achieved at the right market cost.

Manufacturing costs are important and are always undergoing scrutiny on the basis of reducing costs to improve efficiency. Costs cannot be divorced from quality, but it is wrong to consider that high quality automatically implies high costs, or conversely that low quality means low costs. In many companies the true 'quality costs' (as opposed to the straightforward cost of QC) are often unknown, and lost in departmental or divisional budgets, e.g. the costs of

- line waste or scrap
- line inefficiency or low running speeds
- line downtime
- defect investigation
- customer complaints
- customer replacement products
- company public relations following up complaints (and cost of 'low' image).

The correct product quality is achieved not by luck or chance but by the consistent application of quality principles to the design of the product, the inclusion of these principles within the GMP of the manufacturing operation, the relevance of the design specification and quality standards, and the follow-up investigation of consumer acceptance/feedback after launch.

Appreciation of the need for real quality standards must therefore be one of the considerations during the conceptual studies by the product research department of the large multinational companies and by a market research assessment of the potential market slot. It requires an assessment of the market the product is intended to satisfy, followed by the incorporation of these market requirements into the first 'paper' designs.

The initial development phase of the design will primarily involve detailed investigation and liaison between the research and marketing organisation. However, as the design concept 'hardens' and consideration is given to eventual launch, a close relationship is needed with the technical specialists of the manufacturing division (engineering, purchasing, product scheduling, QC, production, etc.).

Control of the multitechnical requirements of these different functions, together with those of suppliers and sub-suppliers, cannot be left to the whims of an *ad hoc* committee, but must be the responsibility of a co-ordinating team. This team (sometimes termed a product launch project team) is ideally composed of delegates from the above specialist functions, and is charged with the responsibility for guiding the new product through the manufacturing operation to its satisfactory launch into the market.

This team will be required to operate at different intensity levels and to differing time scales, i.e. the occasional moderate pressure, but long-term involvement of the research/development group in conjunction with the more intense, short-term brief of the manufacturing division. These different time scales will have to be contained within a critical path network (CPN) once a launch 'window' has been selected, in order to avoid a launch-restricting bottleneck.

Within the CPN different factors will be investigated and actioned, e.g.:

1   research finalisation of the viable design and product specification via in-house assessments, market trials varying from one-off test examples to pre-production trials
2   manufacturing finalisation of

- choice of manufacturing equipment, process speeds, throughputs
- production schedules
- stocking of raw materials, components, etc.
- training schedules
- standard operating procedures
- quality standards for raw materials, components, and intermediate/finished products.
- qualification validation of the process.

These last few points are perhaps the most important in the whole design for quality, since validation provides full objective confirmation that the whole process is fully integrated to achieve the quality specification.

While validation is the final company challenge of the design capability, validation documentation is often the first point of challenge by regulatory inspectors, looking for proof that quality requirements have been built into the design and process.

From the inspectorates' viewpoint, however, quality documentation is critical for all the key stages before and during manufacture. In the event of complaints or referrals from the market or regulatory inspectorates, it is archived batch and test documentation that must provide 'traceability' to the quality conformance history of:

1 the component (in-house and at the supplier)
2 the materials (in-house and at the supplier)
3 the manufacturing process
4 batch and material testing
5 standard operating procedures
6 staff training
7 manufacturing and support equipment maintenance, calibration and validation.

Through unique reference identification of materials, components, products, processes, trials, evaluations, etc., traceability is comprehensively built into the total pharmaceutical process.

It may seem that only immediately prior to commencing the production phase will the word 'quality' be commonly documented, and here in the context of QC objectives of measurements, procedures and standards. In practice, quality principles are consciously and subconsciously being viewed, assessed and re-assessed during the earliest product investigations.

As stated previously, marketing must consciously decide the market in which the new product will compete. This will have involved in-market assessments and possibly laboratory studies of competitive product and national standards that govern sale, use and distribution.

Research studies will cross-evaluate the 'home' product design against the best of the competition and disregard characteristics which do not exhibit significant advantages. The definitive pharmaceutical product must be subjected to governmental approval using data obtained from laboratory and market evaluations, i.e.:

1 clinical trials – where the test product is clinically assessed for efficacy
2 presentation trials – where the product–pack presentation is tested, initially using 'one-off' or pre-production samples for

- shelf-life expectation
- shelf-life stability
- user acceptability.

Results will invariably be subjected to statistical evaluation before the company decision to proceed is taken, or acceptance by the government's licensing authority. They must therefore be capable of withstanding independent scrutiny.

The disciplines necessary to ensure registration of a product require the efficient research establishment to follow highly detailed routines of GLP. These routines reproduce in the laboratory environment the procedures, disciplines and systems comparable with the manufacturing operation. They have proved important to industrial research in maintaining consistency of manufacturing standards and product reproducibility.

The inspectorate of most national health organisations devotes equal investigations time to the QC operations and to the manufacturing process. This has been reflected in the corresponding attention paid by the legislature to the control of practices by research and clinical evaluation laboratories. It is essential that in the design stage of new product, the importance of the supplier's effect on finished product quality is not overlooked. Most modern products are the sum of many different parts and processes, all of which should be equally under control.

Customer and supplier have to agree the raw material/component specification and the associated quality standard. The supplier must be encouraged to operate a system of manufacturing controls to ensure that not only is the material produced in the right quantity and at the right cost, but also to the agreed quality. These manufacturing controls, while perhaps being simpler than those in a pharmaceutical company, should be sufficient to guarantee that standards are achieved.

The launch of a new product, through the manufacturing operation, should be attended by a deliberate but temporary 'overkill of controls'. The intention must be to measure the quality of the product as it progresses from one operation to the next as well as to establish other performance parameters such as:

- line speeds
- downtime
- wastage
- operation efficiency

As the learning curve is extended for each of these, production efficiency improves while quality is maintained. With this intention, the first batches of a new product (usually three to five) should be under a development jurisdiction to confirm transfer of the design requirements into production conformance (this is often termed performance qualification). Specialist departments other than QC will also be present (training, engineering, O&M, etc.) to ensure the relevance of procedures, systems and performance.

The intention of the quality specialist is not only to confirm the correctness of the quality standards but to ensure that quality monitoring is effective in detecting deviations at the earliest opportunity. Close monitoring by production, through process controls or through quality control checks, detects process drift before the manufacture of defectives and minimises the risk of rejected product.

The quality system should not be satisfied with the mere release of a conforming batch of product, but should also assess the market response in comparison with the original batch results. Reaction from the market can be invaluable in detecting (and correcting) a minor deviation or trend before it becomes a major complaint. For that reason market opinions should be positively sought rather than passively awaited.

A predetermined time after the launch of the product, or after a specified number of batches, specifications and quality standards should automatically be reviewed to confirm relevance. (This initial review should be the beginning of regular updating and assessment of procedures, specifications and standards.)

To conclude this chapter, quality systems of quality-conscious pharmaceutical organisations can be divided into two categories and summarised as follows.

1   QA (the activities and functions concerned with the attainment of quality). This can take into account the establishment of GLP in the laboratory environment (of research as well as QC), as well as GMP in the production environment. It is concerned with the manufacturing facilities, together with the systems, procedures and disciplines that guarantee that manufacture is right first time. It is equally concerned with the operation of the internal quality assessment systems, which should include efficient self-checking by production of the production process as well as the independent measurement of quality conformance by QC.

2 QC (the function responsible for the maintenance of product quality to the agreed standard). Standards must be documented to show the company's requirements for the consumer (individual, group and/or national regulatory) combined with the economic and efficient utilisation of resources.

QC specialists, or *aficionados*, sometimes engage in technical arguments with specialists from other disciplines over whether QC is primarily concerned with compliance with specification or with suitability for purpose. Consideration of the option of suitability for purpose is sometimes an emotional issue when non-specification/conforming product is quarantined pending detailed investigation. In this scenario the first objective priority of the QC inspector must be to determine defect causes and prevent manufacture of further defectives, in conjunction with assessing the degree of non-conformance to the specification.

As stressed repeatedly above, the setting of a specification or standard must be a realistic technical study which includes all criteria that could affect suitability for purpose. Hence failure to meet the specification must automatically imply non-suitability for purpose (exceptional occasions can occur which necessitate rewriting the specifications).

There is therefore no reason why, provided that:

1 product design encompasses basic quality principles
2 the manufacturing process is correctly chosen and operates to strict GMP
3 specifications and standards are correctly set and implemented

the successful conclusion of the manufacture of a new product should not be summarised by the QA philosophy: 'it came to pass'.

Technical references

BS 6001: 1996, *Guide for the selection of an acceptance sampling system, scheme or plan for inspection of discrete items in lots.*
Part 1: 1999, *Sampling Schemes indexed by acceptance quality limits AQL for lot by lot inspection.*
Part 2: 1993, *Specification for sampling plans indexed by LQ for isolated inspection.*
Part 3: 1993, *Specification for skip lot procedure.*
Part 4: 1994, *Specification for segregated sampling plans.*
Part 0: 1996, *Inspection by BS 6001 attribute sampling system.*
MIL STD-205 E, Military Standard 205 E, *Sampling procedures and tables for inspection by attributes.*
MIL STD-414, Military Standard 414, *Sampling procedures and tables for inspection for product defectives.*
BS 7782: 1994, *Control charts: general guide and introduction.*
BS 7785: 1994, *Shewart Control Charts.*
BS EN ISO 9001: 1994, *Quality systems – model for quality assurance in design, development, production, installation and servicing.*
BS EN ISO 9002: 1994, *Quality systems – model for quality assurance in production, installation and servicing.*

Pharmaceutical Supplier Code of Practice (obtained via Institute of Quality Assurance, London.) (i) *The manufacture of printed materials for use in the packaging and labelling of medicinal products (document reference P00021). (ii) The manufacture of medicinal product contact packaging materials (document reference P00022).*

The Orange Guide, *Rules and guidance for pharmaceutical manufacturers and distributors* 1997 (London: The Stationery Office).

Code of Federal Regulations, CFR 21 Parts 200 to 299, Part 210 – *Current good manufacturing practice in manufacturing, processing, packing or holding of drugs; general*. Part 211 – *Current good manufacturing practice for finished pharmaceuticals*.

Rules Governing Medicinal Products in the European Community, Volume IV, *Good manufacturing practice for medicinal products*.

United States Pharmacopoeia and The National Formulary, USP 23/NF 18.

5

PAPER- AND BOARD-BASED PACKAGING MATERIALS AND THEIR USE IN PACK SECURITY SYSTEMS

I. H. Hall

Introduction and history

In this chapter, packaging materials based on 'cellulose' or natural fibres will be discussed. They provide a major contribution to the packaging of pharmaceuticals, the size and nature of which can readily be overlooked since the number of applications is far more diverse and more paper and board is used than glass, metal or plastics.

The history of paper-making in particular is long, and the earliest recorded British mention is in the thirteenth century. It has always used forms of cellulose fibre, but began to use wood pulp in the mid-nineteenth century, which has continued gradually to replace the older materials, so that 98%+ of the papers and boards made today are from the wood pulp route.

Boards (in the case of pharmaceuticals, lined folding box boards) were introduced in the mid-nineteenth century, as hand-made constructions to help protect and transport products. Only at the end of the nineteenth century were machines invented to produce what we would now know as cartons.

Corrugated boards are a fairly recent introduction, starting in the early 1870s and becoming widely commercially available in the late 1890s. From then on there has been a continuous development, both where corrugated board is used and in the technical production processes of developing better, stronger and more hazard-resistant boards.

Papers and boards are used in the following pharmaceutical packaging applications (the list may not be comprehensive):

- labels and leaflets
- wrapping materials
- bags and sacks
- collapsible and rigid cartons and boxes
- shipping and transit outers, both corrugated and solid
- gummed tape
- fitments for cases
- composite tubes and drums
- moulded pulpboard containers
- paper liners, linings and laminations.

Being based on 'natural' fibres, i.e. cellulose, potentially from a wide range of sources, paper and board are seen as renewable resources as distinct from petroleum- and metal-based resources. However, in some circumstances the energy required for conversion of the natural fibres into packaging materials may be more than that required for non-renewable sources in a competitive form. This is part of the debate on environmental/ecological factors which is exercising the minds of the packaging profession, and will be discussed as we go through the chapter in relation to the use of recycled material in paper and board.

There is a major problem with 'natural' products. They are not as consistent as synthetic products, therefore anything made from a natural material cannot be guaranteed to be exactly the same all the time, i.e. they usually need wider tolerances than, for example, glass, metal or plastics. Its easy to see why. Living organisms grow with a large number of factors influencing that growth: availability of nutrients, light conditions, damage to seedlings by animals, local environment, difference in age of each tree, etc.

Sources of cellulose fibre

Although trees are the major source of wood pulp, other cellulosic fibres such as cotton, flax, bamboo, esparto, jute, hemp, straws, bagass (from sugar cane), grass, rags and sisal have been used in the manufacture of papers and some of them for boards. The quality of the fibre varies according to the source, with certain hardwoods being excluded on the grounds of cost or undesirable constituents. Softwoods such as spruce, fir, pine and eucalyptus are usually commercially preferred, as they are grown in colder climates where they are arguably the best use for the land. In the past 20 to 30 years the 'farming' of softwood forests has developed into an environmentally friendly industry, under the term 'silviculture'.

The basis of all paper and board is 'pulp', which is in fact refined cellulose $(C_6H_{10}O_5)_n$, where n is between 800 and 1500. The crude extracted cellulose is made up of three parts, as follows.

1 Holocellulose – this is 70–80% of the wood. It is the whole water-insoluble carbohydrate fraction comprising:

- alpha-cellulose, which is insoluble in strong caustic soda
- hemi-cellulose, which is soluble in dilute caustic soda
- beta-cellulose, which is reprecipitated by dilute acid
- gamma-cellulose, which is the remainder of the cellulose fraction.

There is in fact no single compound holocellulose, since the structures and crystallinity of the cellulose fibres vary with the source of the wood. This is part of the reason for the variation in properties of pulps.

2 Lignin – this varies between 17% and 30% of the bulk and is an amorphous phenylpropane polymer which is found intimately associated with the holocellulose. It is not a fibrous material and therefore is of no value in the pulping process.

3 Extractives, which form between 3% and 8% of the bulk, are mainly other carbohydrates, soluble mineral salts, resins, fats and tannins which may be washed out with water.

The individual fibres of cellulose are very strong and of varying lengths, e.g. esparto grass 1.5 mm, coniferous wood 3.5 mm and broadleaf wood 1.2 mm, and those that are preferentially used for paper and board are between about 1 and 4 mm in length.

The manufacturing process

To manufacture paper or board there are two basic processes: pulping, then machine conversion into paper or board.

Pulping

The treatment of the fibres (pulp) is the major influence on the properties and costs of the paper or board produced. The objective in pulping is to 'tease' out undamaged fibres from the mass of the wood, so that these fibres can be reworked into the smooth paper/board required.

There are three major processes which reduce raw material, i.e. any of the cellulose-containing materials mentioned above, to 'pulp':

1 mechanical pulping
2 chemical pulping
3 semi-chemical or combination pulping.

For practical purposes only wood pulp will be considered. The wood pulp is supplied from the two most popular sources which are the managed softwood forests, mentioned above, and 'recycled' fibres, which will be covered later.

Most label papers are chemical pulp, with additives, only. Most box boards are layers of mechanical or semi-chemical pulps with chemical pulps on the face and sometimes the back facings. Corrugated will probably, today, be nearly all recycled material, whereas unbleached semi-chem would have been used in the past for the corrugated medium. Any Kraft facing paper will probably still be 80–90% virgin Kraft pulp in make-up.

Bleaching

If this is required it is achieved by using either hydrogen peroxide or chlorine (or a hypochlorite) dissolved in water to remove the coloured residues that are in the cellulose fibres. It is usual to bleach only the chemical pulp made from the sulphite or soda processes, as these are grades probably used for white paper and the white plies of board.

Beating and refining

Beating is the batch process where the pulp suspension is recycled through a specially designed vessel which shortens the fibres and softens (plasticises) them (Figure 5.1). Refining is a continuous process whereby the pulp suspension is pumped between a static outer housing and a tapering rotor (Figure 5.2). Figure 5.3 shows the properties of paper/board influenced by beating.

154

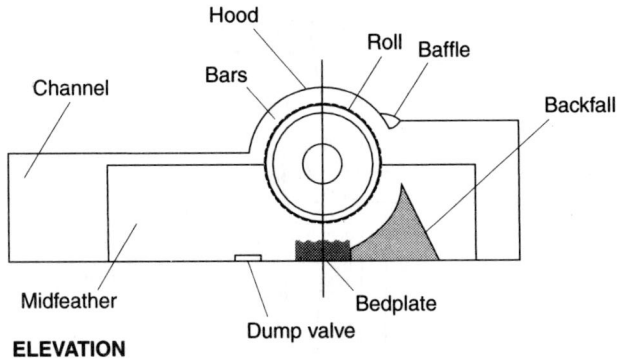

ELEVATION

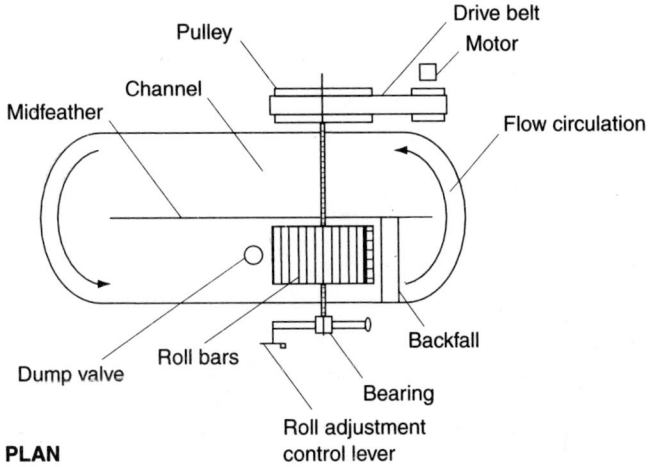

PLAN

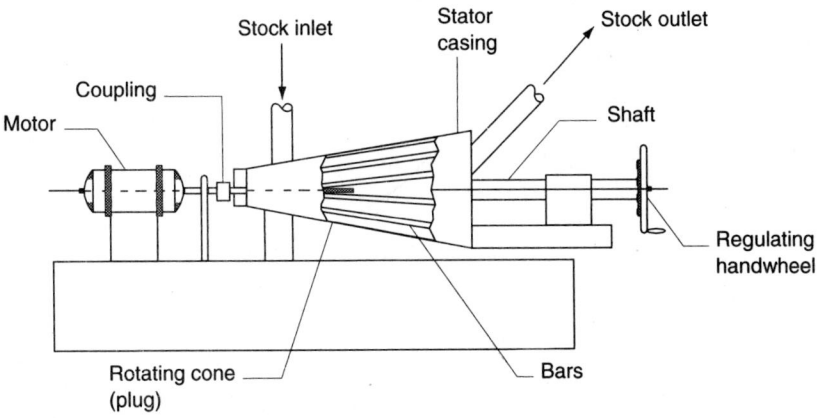

Figure 5.1 Beating

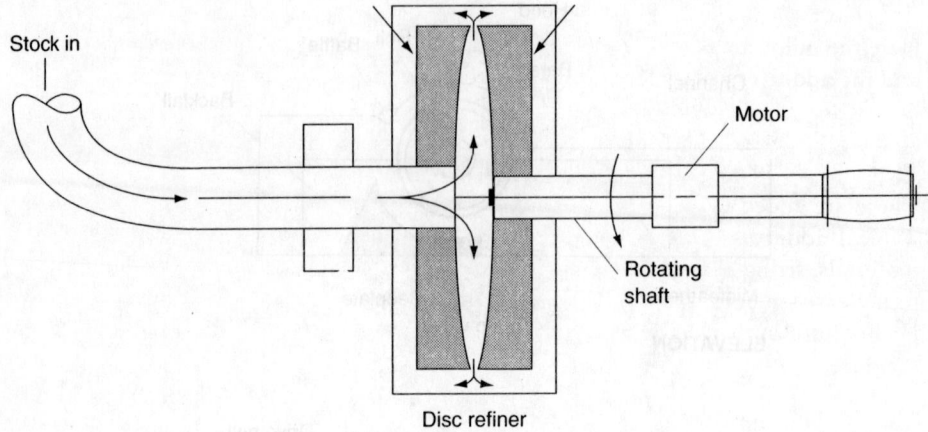

Figure 5.2 Refining

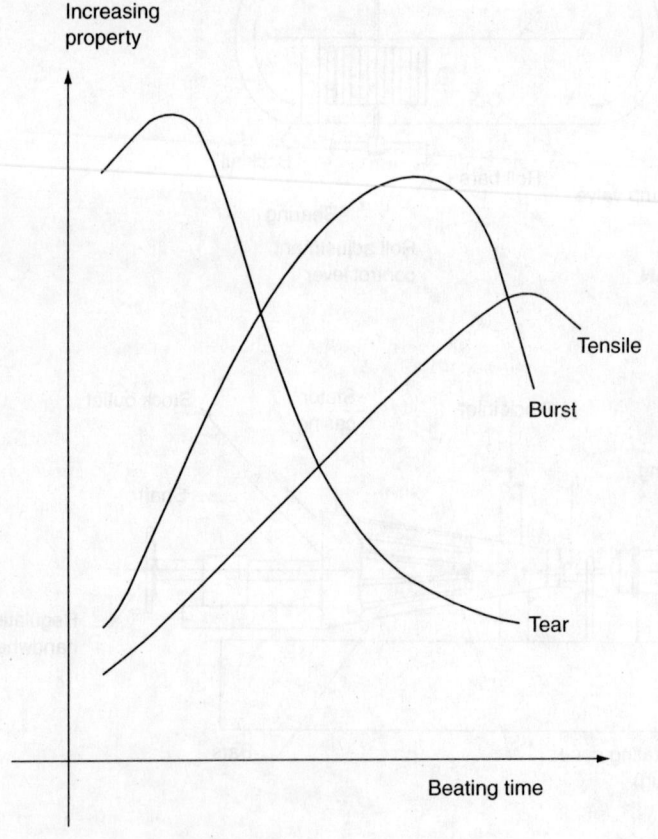

Figure 5.3 Effect of beating on strength

Mixer stage

Here the pulps are stirred vigorously in a hydropulper with copious amounts of water and the additives are added to make the final mixture.

Additives

These are added to the beaten or refined pulp to produce the final form of the paper. Typical additives are loadings and fillers (to improve opacity/brightness), colouring materials, sizing agents which reduce the penetration of water and inks, binding agents to increase strength, gums, antifoam agents, wet strength resins and optical brightening agents (OBAs). It is at this stage that the pH of the paper can be adjusted to make it 'acid free'.

Machine conversion into paper

Fourdrinier system

This is the most popular system still used today, even though the basic system was invented in the early nineteenth century (Figure 5.4). The machine starts at the 'wet end' (1–4) and finishes at the 'dry end' (5–9), thus:

1   a stuff chest
2   a breast box or head box
3   a slice
4   Fourdrinier wire with vacuum boxes
5   presses
6   driers
7   machine glaze drier
8   calender stacks
9   reeling.

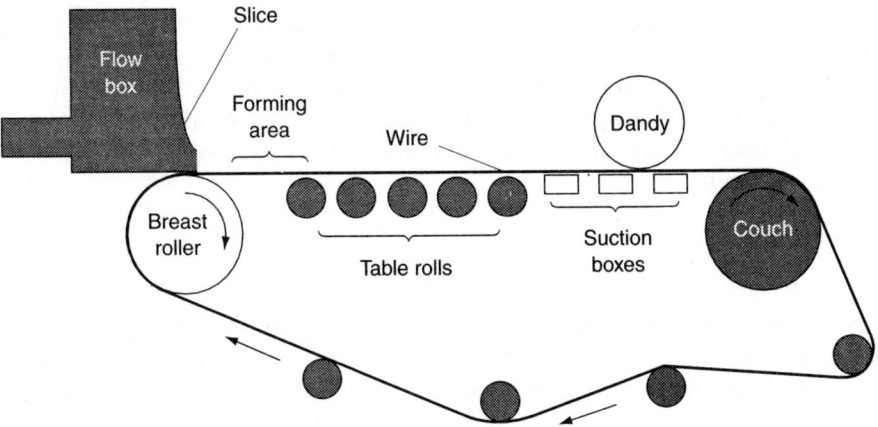

Figure 5.4 A Fourdrinier system

Pulp, including all the additives needed for a particular paper, in suspension is pumped into the stuff chest then let down into the 'head box' which sits over a continuously fast moving fine 'wire' (nowadays usually nylon) mesh, i.e. the Fourdrinier wire.

The suspension (99% water) is fed onto the wire mesh through the variable 'slice' in the bottom of the head box. (The aperture of the slice and the speed of the wire mesh control some of the physical properties of the paper, i.e. caliper.) The water from the suspension drains away and then is pulled through the wire by a vacuum, leaving a mass of solids on the wire. The movement of the wire induces the fibres to align themselves preferentially in the machine direction (MD), producing the 'grain' of machine-made papers, although a cross-directional oscillation is built into the machine to try to minimise the orientation of the fibres.

Towards the end of the wire the water content is below 85%. The material leaving the 'wire' is called the 'felt'. This 'felt' is pressed through speed-synchronised cold rollers (the presses) to reduce the water content to 65–70%. This is followed by the drying section, which is a series of steam-heated cylinders over which the felt winds its way with alternate sides being dried.

Sizing or coating is carried out about two-thirds of the way through the drying section. A machine-glazed (MG) finish is applied towards the end of the drying section, by a very large diameter steam-heated highly polished roller.

The paper is then taken up the calender stacks which are stacks of rollers that press onto the alternate sides of the paper. Only the bottom roller of the calender stack is driven; all the other rollers burnish the paper by slippage.

The paper has by now been dried down to 3–4% water content. It is then conditioned to 7–10% water so that the paper is no longer brittle, prior to reeling. The reels are stored on end on skillets under covered conditions, until needed for reel slitting and/or sheeting.

Papers in use in the pharmaceutical industry vary from about 40 g/m^2 substance up to about 175 g/m^2.

Finishing processes

These consist of additional treatments which are carried out on the material after the paper-making process. Surface sizing may, for example, be performed by applying a solution of gelatin, together with other chemicals, to the paper. This improves water resistance and printing properties, and is called 'tub-sizing'. Coating suspensions, e.g. containing china clay, may also be applied to the surface by spraying, air knife or rotating brush methods.

Other surface treatments

These processes include coatings (Figure 5.5), impregnations and laminations which are mainly aimed at reducing moisture, gas, permeation, etc. or for creating a heat-sealing capability. Typical examples include both dry and wet waxing processes.

Paper may also be solvent or aqueous coated, e.g. PVdC, emulsions, varnishes, lacquers, or laminated to plastics by adhesion or direct extrusion or to foils by adhesion, all to form laminates. These laminates containing paper are dealt with in Chapter 9.

METERING BAR

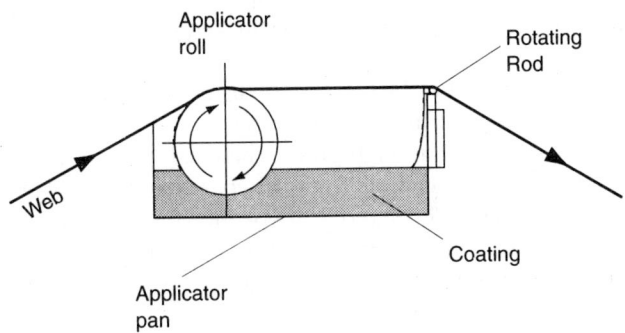

AIR KNIFE

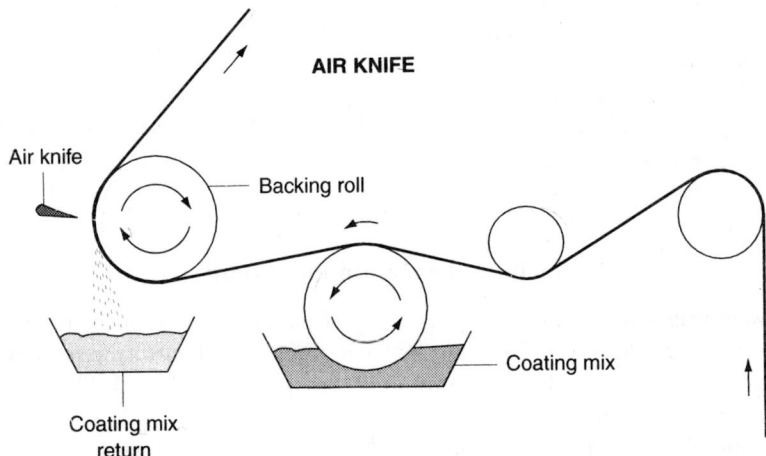

BLADE

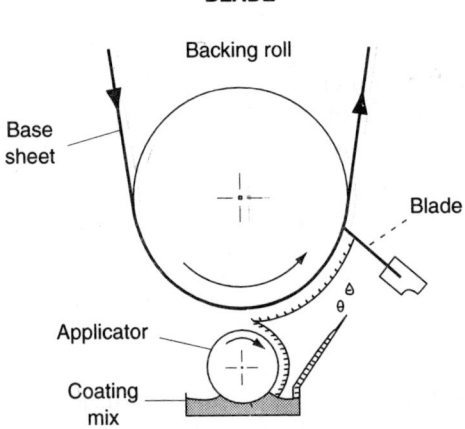

Figure 5.5 Coating methods

All surface treatments are used either to enhance the 'printability' of the paper or to modify and 'improve' the characteristics of the paper.

The more common types of paper used in pharmaceutical packaging are as follows.

1   'Kraft' paper used as an outer facing for corrugated board, solid board, spirally wound kegs and fibreboard drums.
2   Uncoated paper, usually from high-grade chemical pulp source, used in thin calipers for small labels and leaflets. One-side coated and MG papers are used for the heavier weighted labelling material. Two-side coated lightweight papers are used for leaflets. Glassine paper is super-calendered greaseproof paper. Greaseproof paper relies on the closing-up of the pores between the fibres achieved by beating the fibres for a very long time.
3   White wood-free paper for laminates is usually one-side coated paper that has been super-calendered to make the outside (coated) surface less permeable.
4   So-called test liners in two grades are made entirely from recycled material. Used for internal liners in corrugated board production and as both liners for corrugated fitments.
5   Vegetable parchment paper is made by a process of treating the absorbent paper with sulphuric acid, which enhances the wet strength of the paper. This is the most water-resistant paper of all. It is usually used for 'dressing' packs. It has good resistance to fats and greases.

Machine conversion into board

In many ways this is very similar to the making of paper, except that the multi-ply production systems are more suitable than the basic single wire Fourdrinier system. Board covers rigid and folding boxboards, solid and corrugated fibreboard, fibre drums and components of composite containers.

One of the different types of machine used at present for making board is the vat or cylinder machine. The machine starts at the 'wet end' (1–4) and finishes at the 'dry end' (5–9) just like the Fourdrinier machine:

1   pulp preparation
2   make-up tanks with different pulps
3   vats with a constant level of pulp
4   vacuum applied cylinders in vats
5   presses
6   dryers
7   machine glaze drier
8   calender stacks
9   reeling

Figure 5.6 shows a vat system.

Twin wire machines are Fourdrinier-type processes which are drained between the two forming fabrics or wires in a horizontal plane. There are also multiwire Fourdrinier types of machine in operation today. Figure 5.7 shows a twin wire system.

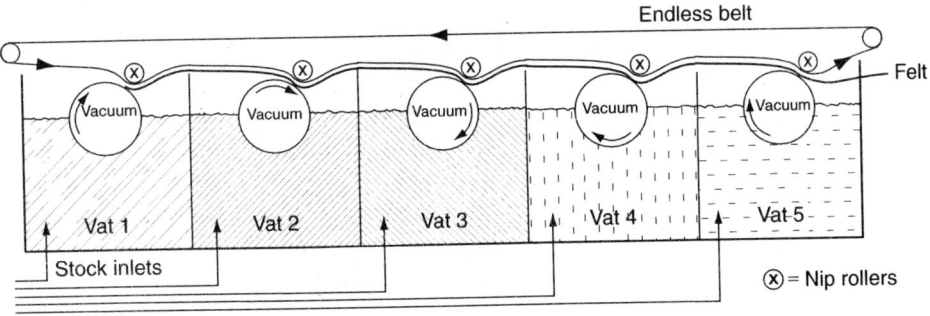

Figure 5.6 A vat system

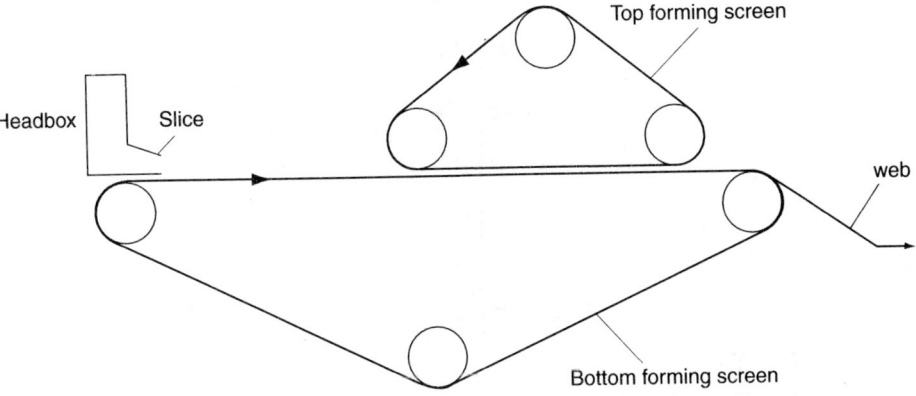

Figure 5.7 A twin wire system

Vertiform machines are twin wire machines arranged vertically. Figure 5.8 shows a vertiform system.

The inverform process is that in which the slurry is forced between two wires. Figure 5.9 shows an inverform system.

Common types of board in use

Millboard

This can be made on a single cylinder or vat machine, where a moist web of thick paper is built up in plies and then milled between heavy rollers.

Chipboards

These use post-industrial waste (PIW) and some post-consumer waste (PCW) in their middle plies. They can be faced with better quality facing materials and may or may not have a quality backing used for low-grade small boxes and cartons.

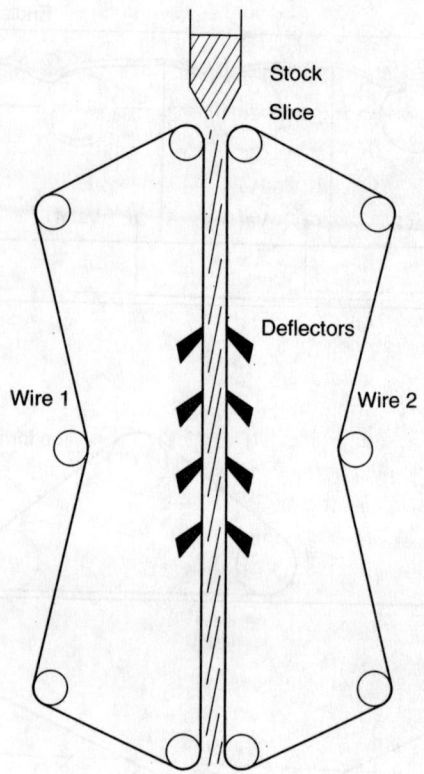

Figure 5.8 A vertiform system

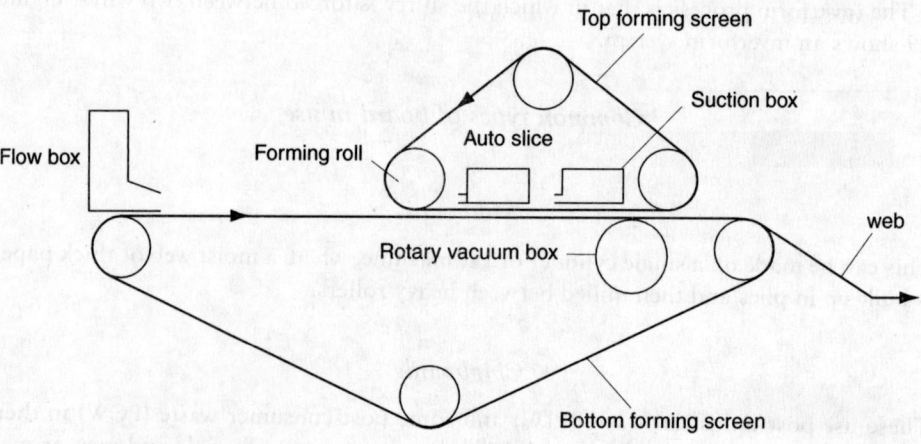

Figure 5.9 An inverform system

Box boards and coated box boards

VIRGIN PULP USED

Figure 5.10 shows a white lined folding boxboard in section. High-grade mechanical pulp is usually used for the centre plies of the board, with high-grade bleached sulphite pulp in front and behind the core plies. On the face 'printing' side of the sulphite pulp there is a base coating and finally a clay/size coating (up to 20–25 g/m^2).

'RECYCLED' BOARD

Figure 5.11 shows a typical high-quality recycled board structure. Typical 400 µm grade plies from printside inwards consist of: 28 g/m^2 clay coating; topliner 47 g/m^2 bleached virgin sulphite pulp; under-liner 69 g/m^2 unprinted recycled newspaper pulp; main body up to six plies of general recycled pulp adding up to 134 g/m^2 of mostly PIW waste; back-liner 22 g/m^2 bleached virgin sulphite pulp. This means that the average percentage of recycled fibre is about 75% by fibre weight and 68% of total board weight, including coatings. Most recycling mills will claim to be to be well inside *any* current or proposed limits on any part of effluent control.

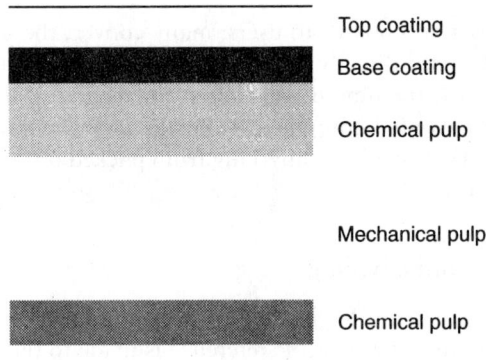

Top coating
Base coating
Chemical pulp

Mechanical pulp

Chemical pulp

Figure 5.10 A white lined folding boxboard in section

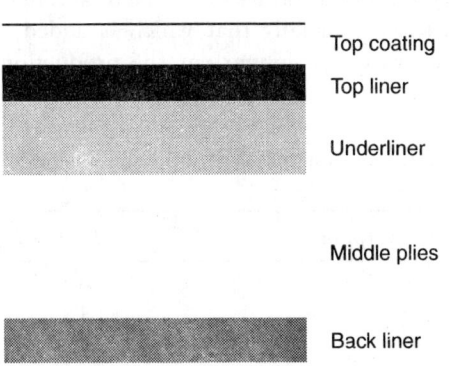

Top coating
Top liner
Underliner

Middle plies

Back liner

Figure 5.11 A typical high-quality recycled board structure

It is also claimed that the bacterial count in the finished recycled board (which is obviously variable) compares with virgin board. For polybichlorinated phenols (PBCs) the claim is <1 ppm against a limit of 2 ppm specified for the contact of greasy foodstuffs. See Table 5.1 for contamination levels.

Strawboards (lined or unlined)

Used for some rigid boxes, e.g. solid board enema boxes where the slight odour and high chlorine content are of little importance. Fibre is provided by straw and is made on a conventional board machine. Lining is achieved by pasting paper, of the desired type, to one or both sides on a continuous process machine. It is quite rigid, but has limited use in pharmaceuticals because of the slight odour.

Paper and board merchandising

Usually the larger paper and board mills do not sell their final 'jumbo' reels direct to printers or converters. They sell them to merchants who store the reels of the many specifications of paper and board available (in controlled conditions) and market the papers and boards to the printers and converters. These jumbo reels can vary from 1 to 4 m wide and be up to 2 km long.

All paper merchants market the papers and boards to users; many convert the paper or board into a form in which it can be used directly. The latter type of merchant has substantial quantities of machinery to slit the jumbo reels down for reel-fed printing equipment or slit, sheet and pack for sheet-fed equipment. The slit reels are usually delivered on end to the printer, but the sheets could be anything from packed on special skillets to wrapped in Kraft paper parcels.

Labels and labelling

The following discussion covers the requirements for labelling with paper onto various types of packaging material used in this industry. Specific reference is made to the four main types of paper labels, i.e. plain with adhesive added, pregummed, heat sensitive and pressure sensitive.

Printing can be basically divided between information which is 'fixed' and information which is 'variable'. Variable information is usually that which is added either immediately prior to the production line process or as part of the production line process (see below).

Table 5.1 Contamination data (mean values) based on samples taken and tested by the University of Graz (Austria) in 1992

Heavy metal	Virgin fibre (ppm)	Recycled (ppm)
Cadmium	0.3	0.2
Arsenic	5.45	4.2
Lead	7.6	10.6
Mercury	0.15	0.14
Chromium	0.8	4.1

Label systems are also found in combination with leaflets, of which the Denny Bros FIX-A-FORM system is an example (PEEL 'N' RESEAL from Harlands, INSEAL from Instance, MULTIPEEL and DOUBLE-DRI are others).

A dictionary definition of a label is 'a slip of paper, cardboard, metal, etc. for attaching to an object and bearing its name, destination, description, etc.'. A label may therefore be made of any material and may be attached to its parent item or pack by any means, e.g. tying, stapling, nailing, adhesion. Decoration or wording may be achieved by any printing process (depending on the material), i.e. embossing, debossing, letterpress, flexographic, offset litho, gravure, screen, dry offset, etc.

Labels are, if anything, increasing in importance as carriers of more and more information about the product, e.g.:

- product identity
- corporate image and sales appeal
- pack contents and ingredients (in ever more detail)
- legal and moral warnings
- bar codes (of both the retail and security variety)
- security (increasingly a problem in manufacture, retail, distribution and transportation)
- identity and address of manufacturer (and marketing company)
- instructions/warnings for use
- information on handling, disposal, destination, hazardous goods, etc.
- promotional information.

This list is not exclusive, but is a guide to the pieces of information which one part or another of the packaging chain could be required to affix to a product, not forgetting the warehousing and transportation systems. The amount of information is more likely to increase than to decrease, due to consumer demand for more and more relevant information on what they buy:

- more awareness of health and safety issues
- better inventory control needed, therefore more bar coding to carry more easily automatically retrievable information
- more environmental pressure
- more legislation by the UK and the EU
- more security, either as devices or preventive.

Will it be necessary to design packs where the information will dominate the design parameters? This is already a reality in some limited areas of packaging, e.g. leaflets on small parenteral antibiotic packs! More importance is now placed on eye appeal with the creation of consumer preference for the product, particularly in the case of OTC medicines. However, less ornate and more functional forms of labelling must not be ignored, i.e. identifying features for parcels, cases, crates, etc. and as seals to show when a product has been tampered with.

Labels may be used in addition to the main pack decoration (special offers, price tags, etc.) and, as in the case of certain materials, for instance glass, are the most economical means of applying printed detail. (Ceramic printing has limited applications to reusable glass containers.)

As this chapter is concerned only with paper label material, the foils, foil laminates and plastics are not considered.

Label fundamentals

When working with labels and the designs thereof, the prime responsibility of the packaging specialist is to look after the technical side, i.e. paper, adhesive, carriers, etc. However, in order to perform that function correctly the fundamentals of decoration need to be understood. (This chapter does not deal specifically with the printing processes: see Chapter 16.)

1   A good design – prominent brand image.
2   Well printed, full use of colour: note that a single printing on a coloured surface gives a two coloured label at the cost of one printing. The method of printing is important as the best overall effect is what matters, allied with the best price. For example, do not use gravure printing on short run labels for outer cases.
3   Best paper for the purpose, i.e. white, tinted, coloured, coated, substance (most label papers between 60 and 110 g/m^2), etc.
4   Features that may be critical for machine application:

- direction of grain
- dimensional tolerances – frequently dependent on the method of paper cutting (punching or guillotining)
- paper substance/caliper
- absorbency (Cobb test) – water absorbency
- porosity – vacuum pick-up is used on many labelling machines
- method of storage and handling, i.e. top and bottom card stiffeners, wrap around banded (not rubber bands), restrict number per bundle (say 500s) for block cut labels
- shape – artistic value, radiused or square corners
- size of area (and tolerances) to which label is being applied.

5   Surface finish (also critical to (4) above):

- varnished (roller coated, plate varnished – varnish type (water varnish, spirit varnish), coating weight)
- high melt varnish – critical for heat sealing areas or export markets
- nitrocellulose or PVdC coating systems
- laminated to other materials – PVC, PP, cellulose acetate, etc.

Note that any external coating (varnishes etc., solid print, bands of print) can have a direct effect on the 'curl' of the paper, which is liable to occur when the paper is wetted or dried. This is because inks and varnishes 'stiffen' the paper in both the machine direction and the cross direction. Coatings may vary from matt to high gloss.

6   Print requirements:

- colour standards – target plus light/dark tolerances (e.g. Pantone)
- rub resistance, fade resistance, odour level (see Chapter 16)

- product resistance
- ink thickness.

7   Suitable adhesive (mechanical or specific) – dependent on the surface to which the label is being applied. Note the importance of tack, setting time, polarity (polar or non-polar) of materials.
8   Cut or roll form (i.e. singles or rolls).

The fact that paper has fibres oriented mainly in one direction, i.e. 'grain' or 'machine direction' and 'cross direction', plus the fact that it consists of hygroscopic vegetable fibres, frequently has a strong influence on the labelling process. The application of an aqueous based adhesive to a paper label causes a swelling of the fibres. This change in dimension is greater in the cross-grain direction, hence the paper curls around or parallel to the machine direction. This 'curl' is away from the wetted area and may be accentuated if the outer surface is covered by a less moisture sensitive covering: varnish, printing ink, etc. Any labelling process which involves the application of water must recognise 'curl' as a distinct problem which can be reduced to a minimum by consideration of a number of factors, i.e. label shape, size, grain direction, adhesive (solid to water content, tack), method of application, speed of application, etc.

Label 'curl' also occurs when paper is heated and moisture is 'lost'. In addition to the relationship grain direction has with moisture (this applies to both loss and gain), two other factors associated with it are as follows.

1   Tear strength – this is lower along the grain; note difference on edge appearance when paper is torn in both directions (at right angles to each other). Tear along the cross-grain direction shows a more fibrous (feathered) edge.
2   Rigidity or stiffness – paper bends more easily in the cross direction. Another test for grain: cut two strips of paper 0.5 inches × 6 inches at right angles from the same sheet. The length which shows the greatest bend has grain parallel to the 0.5 inch measurement.

Grain can also be detected by a Mullen burst test (and tensile strength) – see 'Paper and board testing' below.

Types of paper labels

As indicated above there are basically four types of paper labels, as follows.

1   Plain paper – applied after the addition of an adhesive.
2   Pregummed paper – where the label is applied after wetting with water. The paper is pre-coated with dextrine or gum arabic using single to treble coatings.
3   Heat sensitive labels – applied after the activation of a thermoplastic coating by the use of heat. Two types of thermoplastic resin exist:

- instant type – activation is a factor of heat, pressure, time; sets immediately the source of heat is removed
- delayed action type – activation by heat, pressure, time but once activated, adhesive remains tacky.

4   Pressure sensitive or self-adhesive – applied by the application of pressure. Paper is pre-coated with a permanently tacky adhesive which is attached to a separate backing paper (which has an easy release coating on it).

In addition to the above, there are shrink-and-stretch plastic sleeving and pressure sensitive plastic labels. These two are not dealt with here, but they are making considerable headway in pharmaceutical labelling at the present time.

The above labelling methods are listed in ascending order of cost; using for example a label printed in two colours, size 90 × 63 mm, prices quoted in Table 5.2 are per 1,000 labels delivered, based on orders of 100,000 and 10,000 using 1991 prices.

Plain paper labels plus suitable adhesive

The thin film of adhesive applied costs only a few pence per 1,000 labels, plus labour costs. Plain paper is most widely used for glass, but can be applied to metal, particularly in the form of a complete wrap around label. Application can be by hand, semiautomatic or fully automatic methods. Speeds of 1,000 or more per minute can be achieved. Pharmaceutical labelling usually ranges from 10 to 300 per minute.

Hand application

This routine is not covered in detail here, but application speeds can reach as high as 400–600 units per operator hour.

Semi-automatic labelling

In this operation the machine selects, glues and applies the label but the item to which it is applied is placed into position by hand. Labels may be picked up by vacuum or the adhesive. Higher tack is necessary than that used for hand labelling. Speeds range from 25 to 60 per minute, i.e. 3,600 per hour maximum.

Fully automatic labelling

The item is positioned and labelled automatically. This requires even more critical limits in terms of setting-up, material and adhesive tolerances. Change over time or adjustments also take longer. Speeds can range from 3,500 to 60,000 per hour.

Table 5.2 Costs of labelling methods (1991 prices)

Type of label	Order-size		Approximate ratio (plain paper = 1)
	100,000	10,000	
Plain paper	£6.00	£13.00	1
Pregummed paper	£8.00	£18.50	1.3
Thermoplastic coated	£9.00	£20.00	1.5
Self-adhesive	£12.50	£26.00	2.0

Adhesives

The type of adhesive used depends on the surface of the item to be labelled. The adhesive must provide an adequate bond between the label and container. Labelling of paper-based materials (unless specially treated) and glass usually presents little difficulty. Tinplate, although slightly more difficult, can involve problems of corrosion unless special corrosion inhibitors are incorporated into the adhesive. Labelling to plastic surfaces requires the use of specialised adhesives which may be based on latex or synthetic resins, e.g. polyvinyl acetate (PVA). In certain instances pre-treatment of the plastic (in common with printing) with flaming or corona discharge can aid adhesion.

Dextrine is the most widely used adhesive involving different levels of solid content. For instance, a low solid content is used for hand labelling since low tack (after initial placement it may be slid into position) and a long setting time are necessary. On mechanical labelling, particularly where the label is picked up by the adhesive, a high tack plus quick set is important. In addition, the adhesive must be non-threading and non-foaming. The addition of borax increases tack and setting speeds.

Problems of curl

Although this has already been mentioned, it is always a factor to consider when any label is applied by a wetting adhesive. Both printing inks and coatings tend to reduce the moisture absorbency of a paper and thereby increase any curl (which is always parallel to the grain direction). If the amount of water used in an adhesive can be kept to a minimum, curl will be reduced. Using a thin film of adhesive is also effective. When labelling a round container there is a choice between a complete wrap around (probably leaving a varnish-free area on the under lap) and using, say, three-quarter wrap with a gap. It should be recorded that many containers (particularly injection moulded plastic) have a natural taper which may cause problems of alignment.

It is normal to have the grain direction parallel to the base of the label, but there are occasions where this does not apply, i.e. some labels on circular containers.

Pregummed labels

Paper is pre-coated with dextrine or gum arabic. As only water is required to activate the adhesive, the labels are clean to apply and a complete labelling operation can be carried out by one operator. They are ideally suited to small runs or intermittent production, such as parcel labels. They provide good adhesion to paper, board, glass, but as the range of adhesive types is very limited, they lack flexibility in terms of adhering to a wide range of surfaces.

Pregummed labels are difficult to apply if large, due to problems of creasing. They also have a high tack and therefore cannot be adjusted readily once on the item to which they are being applied.

Heat sensitive or thermoplastic adhesive-based labels activated by heat

As indicated above, two types are in use: instant tack and delayed tack. Both are based on synthetic resins; the former has to have heat and pressure applied to affect the transfer but sets immediately the source heat is removed. The latter is usually activated to tacky state after which it can be affixed to any item without a heat source. However, most frequently the heating operation plus pressure of application are applied simultaneously. The tacky state remains for some time after the source of heat is removed.

As heat sensitive labels do not rely on conventional gums or water as a wetting agent they will adhere to a wider range of materials including metals, plastics, and varnished, coated and printed surfaces. However there is one criterion that is very important in storage of thermoplastic materials either as flat sheet prior to printing or as labels after printing. All heated areas (pipes, radiators, overhead heaters) must be avoided; also high stacking pressures, both of which can cause partial activation and/or blocking. Care also has to be taken in the selection of printing inks and varnishes, as certain volatile constituents of these decorative materials will also cause activation and blocking.

As the delayed action resin takes up a permanent set very slowly, the grain direction (shrinkage after heating) will cause curl to occur. In certain circumstances this can be greater than the adhesive forces so the label may lift, particularly if the radius to which it is applied is tight. For this reason labels should be produced with the grain parallel to the axis of curvature of the container to which they are applied.

During activation, temperatures above 100°C are used, causing drying-out of the paper and shrinkage. Labels return to normal after exposure to the atmosphere, but on larger sizes (say 100 cm^2) there is a tendency towards creasing and blistering. Activation by steam can partially overcome these problems provided the outer (printed) surface is not waterproof.

Instant tack labels

There are a few well-known makes on the British market. They may be applied by hand (hot plate), semi-automatically or automatically. Machinery is similar in price to conventional gluing/labelling machines but those with more sophisticated heating systems can be more expensive. The machines involve far less cleaning time and generally get less 'gummed up'.

Instant tack labels find special usage on seals, pleated overwraps, various header labels (cellulose films must be heat sealable variety). They are not used for bottle or can labelling.

Delayed action labels

These are more versatile than the instant tack type, particularly in their application to bottles, tinplate, plastics, coated or laminated surfaces. Speeds of around 600 per minute can be achieved.

Both instant tack and delayed action labels are more costly than the conventional paper – adhesive labelling. Selected advantages may offset the cost increase, i.e.:

1   virtually no cleaning down, no wastage of adhesive
2   shorter setting-up time
3   adhesion to a wider range of surfaces
4   less affected by powder contamination or varying ambient atmospheric conditions (humidity and temperature)
5   provide a high standard of cleanliness – no labour for wiping down.

Thermoplastic adhesive labels generally find a special usage and are now meeting increasing competition from self-adhesive or pressure sensitive labels.

Pressure sensitive labels (created by RS Avery 1935)

It is preferable to call these pressure sensitive labels, rather than self-adhesive, as both the pre-gummed and heat sensitive labels can be thought of as self-adhesive.

They consist of a suitable label paper coated on the reverse side with a permanently tacky adhesive which is in contact with a backing paper that protects it prior to use. The backing paper is coated with a special release coating which permits the label to be removed easily. Labels may be provided in reel or sheet form; both can have the label 'laid on', i.e. the non-printed area has been cut and removed. Sheet label forms also exist as split top type – both printed and non-printed area is present but printed area is 'split' away so that it can be removed. Split back type has the backing paper split or cut so that it can be removed. (Applies to larger sizes.)

Numerous papers, usually of the single face coated types, are now available with a wide range of pressure sensitive adhesives. These adhesives may be:

- *temporary* – can be easily removed from the item onto which it has been placed
- semi-permanent – difficult to remove
- permanent – virtually impossible to remove without a fibre tear.

Pressure sensitive labels are removed from the backing paper and then applied by pressure. Ideally they should be removed by turning the backing paper over a right angle so that the label comes off straight. If some labels are peeled off (backwards) a curl is induced, which in the less permanent form may result in a peel back or lifting from the item to which it is applied. Figure 5.12 shows the structure of a pressure sensitive label.

Self-adhesive labels normally have the following type of structure (layers):

- facing material   (90 μm)
- key coating adhesive   (12 μm)
- silicone release backing (50 μm)

giving a total thickness of 150 μm (0.006 inches).

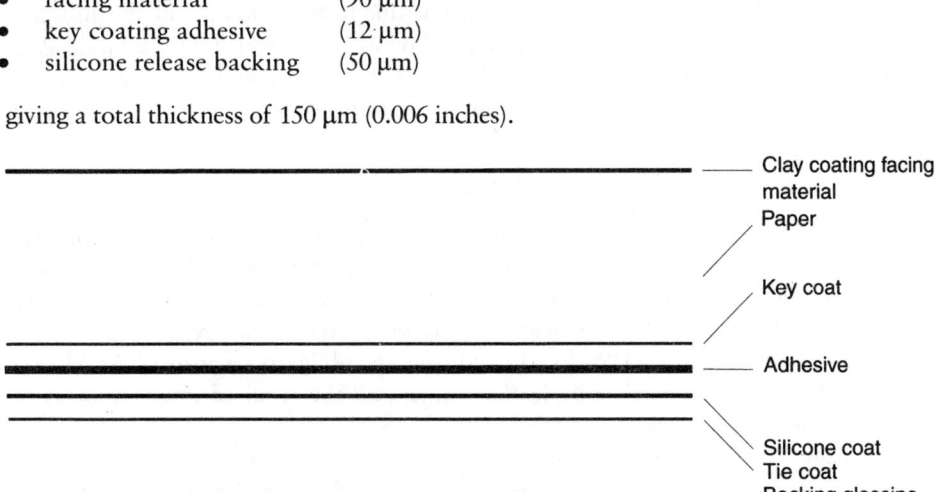

Clay coating facing material
Paper
Key coat
Adhesive
Silicone coat
Tie coat
Backing glassine carrier

Figure 5.12 Structure of a pressure sensitive label

The silicone release usually has a coating weight of approx. 0.5 g/m². Die cut accuracy is usually ± 5 μm.

Self-adhesive labels can be applied to most materials: wood, plastic, metal, glass, paper and board. As the adhesives are resin-based (plasticised thermoplastics), migration problems can occur when they are applied to certain plastics (PVC, LDPE, etc.). Adhesive systems for pressure sensitive labels include latex and acrylic bases and adhesives which may be applied as a hot melt, or via a solvent, emulsion or dispersion base. Water-based adhesives are currently increasing in use.

Until recently the printing processes have tended to be limited, i.e. flexographic, rotary letterpress (four colours), with gravure (occasionally). The labels are produced in accurate register on the backing paper – on reel-fed machines, printing, punching and removal of trim are carried out as a continuous operation (platens are also used.)

Labelling can be carried out by hand, semi-automatically or fully automatically. In all instances accurate positioning is essential as the label cannot be slid into position. Machine speeds of 800 per minute are attainable. The cost of pressure sensitive labels is higher (than that of all other forms).

Reel-fed labels offer one huge advantage in security – they dramatically reduce the risk of admixture, which is particularly important in the case of pharmaceuticals.

Applying labels to tight radii still may give butterflying (edge lift) with certain label types and styles. Improvements can be achieved either by an adhesive change or using a paper of a lower substance weight (i.e. replace 90 g/m² with 65 g/m²), or by reducing the stiffness of the printed face by reducing the amount of ink used, ceasing to use a varnish or using a lighter coat weight paper.

Modern adhesives for self-adhesive labels include acrylic, polyethylene combinations. There is a distinct move away from solvent-based adhesives (for ecological reasons) to water-based dispersion/emulsion systems.

Adhesion can be normally checked by a press-down test, followed by removal after 3 s, 6 h, 24 h. Bond normally improves with time due to the cold flow of the adhesive. Long-term adhesion may use a test involving 7 days at 70°C, which gives an indication of any change over 12 months. Be certain that 70°C is well below the degradation temperature of the adhesive, otherwise the results are spurious.

Leaflets

Leaflets have loomed large in the minds of packaging people in the industry in the past few years, primarily with the implementation (from 2 January 1994) of the relevant parts of the European Community Directive 92/27/EC, which brings together requirements for labelling and package leaflets into one directive by repealing parts of Directives 65/65/EEC and 75/319/EEC. In addition, the obligatory nature of Article 3 of Directive 89/341/EEC on packaging leaflets (unless *all* the required information is on the pack or label) is confirmed and reinforced.

Paper leaflets can be found broadly as one of four types, as follows.

1   *Cut sheet*. Usually printed both sides, delivered as blocks of cut sheet and folded on the cartoning machine. The restrictions on block cut papers are also relevant, i.e. they should be backed and fronted with band bound card.

2   *Reel-fed*. Like reel-fed labels, but with no backing paper. They are both guillotined and folded on the cartoning machine. Claimed to be more secure than all other types of leaflet.

3   *Pre-folded*. Are delivered as bundles (these need to be 'broad banded', *not* with elastic bands round them) or contained in plastic cartridges and fed via a hopper system direct to the cartoning machine,

4   *Combined label/leaflet*. Delivered as a thick pressure sensitive label (either reel-fed or block cut), containing a fold-out portion which is the leaflet itself. Applied as one would apply a pressure sensitive label. These have now been around for a number of years. As far as can be ascertained, at least six patents have been taken out in this field. Recently there has been more use of multi-ply construction of these types of label, often using dissimilar materials with rather specialist adhesive systems. Probably the best known are Fix-a-Form from Denny, Peel 'n' Reseal booklet labels, Multipeel, a peel off promotional leaflet or sticker, Dri-peel, Incore and the Double-Dri system. Leaflets use high-opacity (80% + EEL) lightweight ($40-70$ g/m^2) coated or uncoated papers.

In order to maximise the smooth production of these thin (lightweight) papers, the following facts about paper should be borne in mind when designing the leaflet.

1   *Grain direction*. The grain of paper has been mentioned several times already, but with lightweight papers it becomes once again a critical feature, as the papers are both thinner and weaker than label paper or board.

2   *Stiffness*. Paper is nearly twice as stiff in the machine direction as it is in the cross direction. The degree of stiffness is related to the caliper (substance), so that the thinner the paper, the lower is the stiffness, to the extent that the stiffness factor is proportional to the cube of thickness. Arising from this is a basic recommendation that the thinner the paper the more advantageous it is to print in the machine direction because of its greater stiffness.

The other parameter of lightweight paper to be considered is the porosity of the chosen paper. This is because many cartoning machines use a vacuum type of pick-up for the leaflet no matter in what form it may be presented to the cartoning machine. Even so-called reel-fed leaflets have to be cut, picked and moved through folding plates up to the insertion point into the carton. For this reason both specification of paper porosity to air and pick tests (to keep down the amount of lint or dust) are sensible.

The other point to take into account is the 'conditioning' of the lightweight papers prior to printing and folding. This just means that the paper should be kept, as far as practical, in optimum storage conditions.

All leaflets, though folded tightly for insertion, have inherent problems of ink 'show through', particularly with ink colour solid blocks, e.g. photos or pictures. Security bar code reading can be a severe problem on the thinner papers. The amount of copy required on all types of leaflets has increased dramatically over the past ten years, so much so that packs have had to be devised to accommodate very large leaflets (A3); this has created its own cartoning machine design problems.

Folding or collapsible cartons

These difficult to handle, temperamental objects in white lined folding boxboard are popular in the industry because they are good at their job, which is to contain, protect and distinguish the product from *all* others in an economical manner. They are sometimes known as 'secondary' packaging.

Ethical products should either have a print free area or a printed area which does not contain vital or legally required information which would be covered or obliterated when the pharmacist's label giving information for the patient is applied. The standard size for this label is 70 mm × 40 mm, or 70 mm × 35 mm.

Choice of design

When choosing a carton design the following points should be noted and fully discussed with a printer used to dealing with pharmaceutical products and with the necessary levels of hygiene control, QC, and inspection.

1 *Style* – This could be from a catalogue of carton designs, e.g. that of the European Carton Makers Association (ECMA). This includes the method of flap retention in its style parameters, e.g. lock slit, friction fit, claw lock, crash lock, envelope lock. Are dust flaps required? Is reverse tuck or aeroplane tuck wanted? Figure 5.13 shows a typical reverse tuck twin lock slit carton.

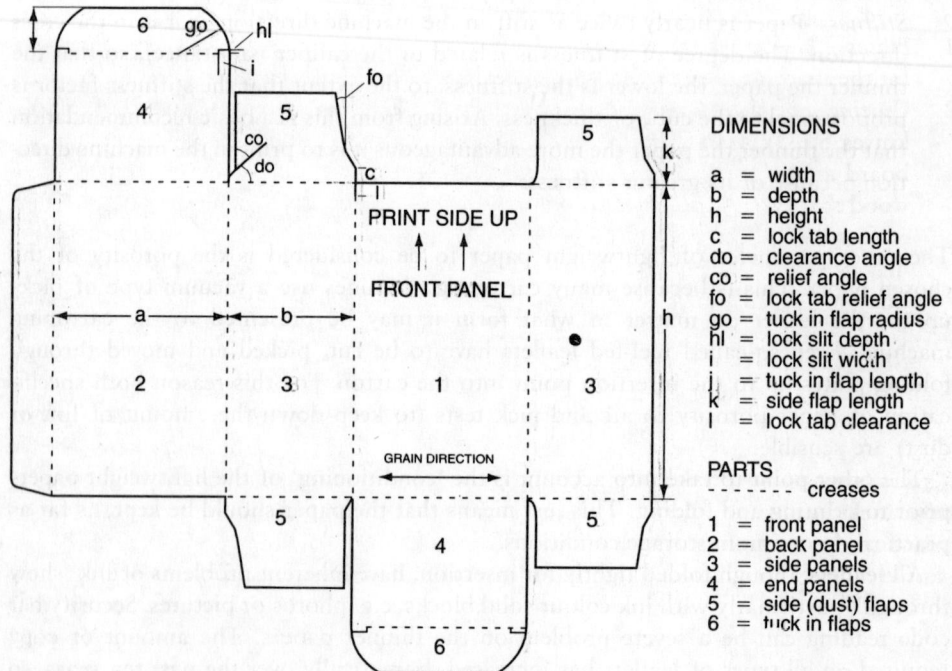

DIMENSIONS

a = width
b = depth
h = height
c = lock tab length
do = clearance angle
co = relief angle
fo = lock tab relief angle
go = tuck in flap radius
hl = lock slit depth
i = lock slit width
j = tuck in flap length
k = side flap length
l = lock tab clearance

PARTS

------- creases

1 = front panel
2 = back panel
3 = side panels
4 = end panels
5 = side (dust) flaps
6 = tuck in flaps

Figure 5.13 ECMA 2120 style carton with twin lock slit flaps

2   *Type of board* – This has been discussed above. Each of the types of board mentioned comes in various calipers ranging from about 200 µm up to around 700 µm.
This will depend to a large extent on what is going to be put into the carton, allied with
the size. Board surface facing materials need to be decided, as these will affect the type
of printing chosen and may affect the creasing and subsequent carton erection.

3   *Layout* – It is usual to have the top opening flap opening away from the opener,
with the 'glue flap' around the back of the carton, placed so that it interferes as little as possible with the overprinting operation.

4   *Size* – This has been mentioned above. Only make the carton big enough to contain the contents and allow enough clearance for machine operation.

5   *Graphics* – Understand what graphics are needed and the limitations of each of the
printing processes you are likely to use. One colour is easier and cheaper to print
than four colour process.

6   *Quantity to be produced* – If only running a few hundred cartons of one particular type, then choose the process with the cheapest plates and shortest make ready:
that will be the cheapest, e.g. one colour flexographic or letterpress printing. At the
other end of the scale, if you wish to produce four colour process printing with
screens and tones and produce them by the tens of millions then either offset litho
or gravure printing is the choice.

7   *Method of printing* – Usually using offset litho, flexography, letterpress or gravure.
May include hot die, stamping, foil blocking, embossing, debossing.

Origination

1   *Plates* – Need to be made from the artwork, one per colour specifically designed
for the machine on which it is going to be used.

2   *Cutting and creasing formes* – These are the cutting (sharp) and creasing (blunt)
knives fitted into a sheet of thick plywood so as to cut the flat printed sheet of
board and press in the creases needed to form up the carton. Each sheet of plywood that carries the knives is called a forme. The knives are surrounded by strips
of foam rubber, to prevent them from tearing the board. Opposite to this sheet is a
'negative' sheet of plywood called the 'counter'. On this there is a mandrel of hard
material for the sharp knives to cut against.

3   *Cost of origination* – This entails looking to the best way of minimising the costs
of artwork, plates, printing processes, sheet, sizes, formes and counters, etc.

Make ready

This is 'simply' the preparation of the printing machine to make it ready for production, including the selection of the board sheet size and which way the grain of the
board in the finished carton will run. The figures, drawings of cartons and artwork
should all indicate in which direction the grain is to run.

Printing

May be printed on flat sheet or from reels. May use either a four colour process system
(cyan, magenta, yellow and black), or a multi-colour system. As indicated above,

almost any printing process can be (and is) used. The most common methods of printing today are all sheet fed, mainly using letterpress and offset litho.

Cutting and creasing

The basic purpose is to stamp in the crease lines, at the same time cutting out the outline of the carton. The prime reason for creasing the carton blank is to define the shape of the carton panels and allow it to fold without distortion. This is achieved by using sharp cutting and blunt creasing 'rules' (either flat bed or rotary). The sheets of preprinted board are fed into what looks like an ordinary small printing press, located over the counter and the forme comes down with some force, cutting and creasing that single sheet.

Stripping

This is the removal of unrequired waste surrounding the printed cut and creased flat carton blanks on the sheet. It is still quite often a hand-based operation.

Pre-folding and gluing

Cartons are usually supplied in a collapsed state, with a glued side seam and two of the folds already made. Folding/gluing is done at high speed and it is necessary for the adhesives used to have a high tack, since freshly folded creases are quite resilient. At this stage, crease quality is very important, since unduly stiff creases will resist gluing.

Following gluing the carton is usually compressed to a flat state where it already exhibits some degree of 'crease set'. To minimise this it is frequently advisable to open the carton through 90° to 180° momentarily to literally break the crease, reduce possible crease set and generally assist final erection. This process is termed pre-folding. (Tests that it is sensible to know about and use during a carton design sequence are covered below.)

Packaging and identification

The cartons should be loosely bundled together, stacked on their edges into strong corrugated box. It is detrimental to stack them 'flat' as the weight of cartons above will inhibit the pre-break (or natural springiness of the carton), making automatic handling an impossibility. The looseness is for similar reasons to prevent having problems with cartons. The case should be securely sealed and identified in the manner prescribed by the specification, with at least the security code (item code, part number), customer, batch/lot, a QC pass stamp/mark and a description.

Carton erection and filling

The action of mechanically erecting, inserting primary pack, insertion of leaflet, then the closing of the carton is another world in which technical expertise may be required. The criteria on which the form of carton filling will be decided include, quantity per batch/lot/order, size and weight of the goods to be cartoned, cartonboard caliper, design of closure flaps, and what else, apart from the primary container, has to be inserted.

Hand cartoning

Basically any carton style, with any form of goods, of any caliper board, with any of the closure flap designs (lock slit, friction fit, claw lock, crash lock, envelope lock), with any number of leaflets or measures or droppers etc. can be used in hand cartoning.

Semi-automatic

This is usually a machine where the carton is erected, the bottom closed and the top opening presented to the operator who drops in the goods and any accessories. It would be expected for this type of machine to have an overprinting unit of some type built into the cartoning machine.

Quantity per batch/lot/order needs to be greater than the time needed to change the machine from one size of pack to another, which could be from 30 min to 3 h. Works at a speed of 40–60 items per minute with two to four operators. The size and weight of the goods to be cartoned have some relevance, as large heavy objects (2 l Winchesters of liquid) will need to run more slowly than, say, 5 ml bottles.

The cartonboard caliper, particularly the consistency, is more critical than for hand cartoning as it affects the 'pre-break' of the carton and once a machine is set to open pre-break there is little tolerance for variation. The faster and more sophisticated machines need tight tolerances.

The following designs of closure flaps, lock slit, friction fit, claw lock, envelope lock and glued flaps can be made to work on an appropriate semi-automatic machine. One would recommend for simplicity that attention be paid when using claw locks and envelope locks, ensuring that they are really necessary before introducing them, as they are not the easiest carton closures to handle.

Note that cartons can have different locks on each end, e.g. lock slit at the bottom and friction fit at the top, or (more usually) envelope lock base seal with friction, lock slit, claw or glued flaps at the top.

Automatic

There are two basic types of machine – intermittent motion and continuous motion. The intermittent is the smaller, slower and cheaper, usually with a blade opening action for the carton pre-break, so that it is likely to accept a lower quality of carton than the really high-speed machines. The continuous motion machines tend to be much larger, faster and more expensive and, being much faster with vacuum pick-up of the carton for a 'knock' pre-break, are much more sensitive to the quality of the carton presented.

Automatic cartoning should only be used when the quantity per batch/lot/order is large enough to keep the machine running for more time than it is down on change-over.

The size and weight of the goods to be cartoned is something of a limiting factor, as our 2 l Winchester would probably not be candidate, but a 300 ml bottle certainly would be run automatically. Speeds range from 60 to 350 per minute, with machine prices rising to match the speed. The design of closure flaps is probably practically limited to lock slit, friction fit and glued flaps. This again is in the interests of speed. What else, apart from the goods, has to be inserted may create a problem. Leaflets can be inserted, as can probably one other accessory, but for more than this specialist machines have to be designed to do the job.

Rigid boxes

These are still occasionally used e.g. rigid nested fibreboard boxes for ampoules, but nowadays any paper-board near parenteral products is viewed critically, due to the fibre load from the board itself contaminating the local atmosphere.

Rigid boxes need similar stages to folding cartons see 'Choice of design', 'Origination' and 'Make Ready' above. Printing, if necessary (but usually labelled with a pregummed label, which might act as a tamper-evident seal as well), is usually applied as a pre-printed liner after the rigid box has been formed. Hence the further stages are:

1 selection of board, board size and cutting to size on a cutter/scorer machine, e.g. one of the chipboards
2 corner cutting – removing the corners so that the box can be erected
3 corner staying – adding gummed paper to each corner to make the erected box rigid
4 quad staying – an alternative to (3)
5 paper slotting – printed or plain covering
6 QC to specification
7 packaging and identification.

Rigid boxes are normally hand packed.

Overprinting

This is sometimes known as 'batch coding' as well as the more popular term, over-printing. This has become a necessary evil in the modern world. All overprinting (this may include off-line methods as well) is used to add variable data as late in the production cycle as possible, i.e. batch/lot numbers, manufacture and expiry dates, price blocks for the Middle East in particular and registration numbers for many other places. If these problems are approached by the method of using fixed copy for a large area of the world allied with a fairly sophisticated overprinting system, one can save the cost of the system in inventory savings alone.

The overprinting of 'variable' information as late as possible in the label application and carton closing processes gives the production company a high degree of flexibility to allow for unforecasted emergency information to be added. This copy is normally added to the printed label or carton either just prior to the packaging operation or during the operation itself. As with all printed copy, the print must be indelible, legible and not fade during the shelf life of the product under normal usage conditions. It is usual to overprint in black and occasionally red. *Note* that red is traditionally used for warnings or poison markings, so check carefully before using.

Overprinting is usually carried out with one or other of the following printing processes: hot foil stamping, flexographic, letterpress, tampon, thermal printing, and stamp debossing.

Some of the information required may be in the form of bar codes. This has stimulated the European Pressure Sensitive Manufacturers Association (EPMSA) in line with the Article Numbering Association (ANA) EAN guidelines, to produce a standard for bar code overprinting on pressure sensitive labels. EAN bar codes can now be successfully printed onto labels using flexographics, or thermal transfer printing.

Contact printing techniques

Contact printing is the more traditional type of printing in the industry.

1 *Letterpress* – the traditional slugs of type in either lead/antimony alloy or hardened steel letters. Usually locked up (set) in a chase (holder), or using a 'baselock' type of system where the type has a foot which slips into a holder and can be locked by a spring clip, being inked each pass and 'kissing' the substrate to deposit the ink. Can be used on most substrates, but is best on paper and board which is not too shiny. Cast coated papers and boards give problems.

2 *Debossing* – the same as letterpress except that no ink is involved and the characters are pressed quite hard into the substrate. Used occasionally for paper, but more normally for blister and strip packs. This method is likely to generate complaints, due to the difficulty of reading it clearly.

3 *Hot foil* – again similar to letterpress, but the ink is carried as a solid on a PET carrier and is stuck to the substrate by the type face using a combination of heat, pressure and time. This means that it is probably not as quick as letterpress or debossing. This system can now be operated by a clip-in rotary flickwheel typeholder, which means that information can be changed very quickly.

4 *Thermal transfer* printing is the selective heating (computer-controlled) and cooling of small elements in a print-head which can be used to impress a one-use thermal ribbon onto the substrate surface. Resolutions of up to 12 dots per mm can be achieved.

5 *Flexographic* – here the characters are formed on a flexible 'plate' of rubber or plastic. The characters pick up ink (probably thinner than letterpress ink) and transfer it to the surface of the label or carton. Can be made to run quite quickly. There is today a cheap rubber-type 'baselock' system on offer, primarily designed for the Third World.

6 *Offset litho* – this technique has occasionally been used in the past by using a special paper plate that can be photocopied and uses the properties of oil and water separation. Usually used only for fairly large labels.

7 *Impact dot matrix* – where a block of 'needles', usually nine but sometimes more, are electronically selected to strike forward onto a typewriter type of ribbon, thereby placing the ink from the ribbon onto the substrate.

Non-contact printing techniques

These are more modern types such as ink jet (solvent-based and hot plastic based) and laser.

Ink jet

These printers come in two types:

1 Drop-on-demand printers have an array of nozzles which fire a drop of ink when commanded by their computer control. Can use either a solvent-based ink or a solid base which is melted and ejected by the print-head.
2 Continuous flow works by using piezo electric crystal to generate an ultrasonic beam to disturb the flow of ink by producing uniform sized droplets. These are then electrostatically charged under computer control. The charged droplets are deflected to a catching mechanism and the neutral ones pass onto the substrate forming the image.

Toner-based laser

A computer-controlled laser beam forms an image on a charged photosensitive drum. A carbon toner is applied and adheres to the charged areas, developing the image which is then transferred to the substrate and fixed with heat and pressure. Text, graphics and bar codes can all be produced this way.

Ion deposition printers are used in similar circumstances, but their method of operation is different. A latent image is formed on a dielectric cylinder which is directly imaged by a projection of ions. Development is by a toner adhering to the charged areas and simultaneously transferred and fixed to the substrate under pressure.

It is predicted that on short-run label production/overprinting there will be increases in use of non-impact printing, especially thermal, thermal transfer and laser technologies. Ink jet coding design with small characters is also expanding into pharmaceuticals.

On-line or off-line printing?

In all overprinting operations the economics of the situation must be addressed, e.g. on-line or off-line.

On-line overprinting has the advantage of being directly under the control of the person in charge of the operation, but has the disadvantage that if there is a problem with the overprinting operation the production line halts. Off-line overprinting has the advantages of not directly holding up production if it has problems, and having staff that are usually better trained and specialist in printing. The disadvantages are that generally extra overprinted components have to be supplied to compensate for potential packaging line problems, and the overprinting operation can sometimes become a bottleneck.

A capability for in-house design in overprinting and printing in production is discussed referring to EPiSYS or the MAP80 systems of in-house label design and printing (as often currently used in clinical trials packaging).

Reel-to-reel laser printers are seen as part of the answer to low-volume orders needing variable information, along with the success of the EPiSYS technology. These laser printers will probably have an expanded use in the not too distant future to encompass primary pack labels, when the development of better and more light-fast colour printing is achieved. More recently both Indigo and Xeikon have introduced 'digital' in-house printing systems.

Solid and corrugated boards for casing

Too little attention is usually paid to this important area of packaging. If the transit packaging is poorly designed then the product will not reach the market in usable condition. This automatically puts up costs and leads to intense customer dissatisfaction. There are several types and structures of boards for casing.

Solid fibreboard

This is two to six layers of recycled paperboard which is treated with an adhesive between the layers and press-laminated together. The outside layer can be of 'Kraft' paper to improve the strength and help better resist water and water vapour. It has good crush-resistant and anti-puncture properties.

It is usually specified as just the thickness of the board, 0.95 to 2.9 mm (340 to 700 g/m^2 with 60 to 125 g/m^2 of Kraft). It may be printed by flexography or letterpress or ink jet.

Corrugated fibreboard

Popularly known as just 'corrugated', this is the most popular form of outer protection used in the industry today. It comprises one or more sheets of fluted (corrugated) paper secured by an adhesive to two or more liners. The paper used for the 'corrugations' is made up of recycled paper, e.g. semi-chem chipboard or 'strawboard', 25–75% straw with various quantities of waste-based pulp added. As the corrugated layer is impregnated with a stiffening agent (usually starch or synthetic vinyls) during the corrugating process, the relative strengths of the three types of recycled paper are not too different. Usually printed by flexography or ink jet, which can weaken the board.

Note that pre-printed sheets may also be employed using offset or gravure printing techniques. With a pre-printed outer liner, care has to be taken in the print design and layout so that when a case is made the print corresponds to the case shape, i.e. is kept in register on the cutters. Figure 5.14 shows a corrugator. There are various types of corrugated fibreboard:

1   single wall, i.e. one sheet of fluted paper between two liners (Figure 5.15 shows single wall corrugated)
2   double wall, i.e. two sheets of corrugated paper between three liners (Figure 5.16 shows double wall corrugated)
3   triple wall, sometimes known as Triwall (trade name), i.e. three sheets of fluted paper between four liners (Figure 5.17 shows triple wall corrugated).

Flutings are described as A, B, C, E and micro flutes. This describes the depth of the fluting (see Table 5.3).

Abbreviations commonly used for describing the structure of boards are:

- K, Kraft liner
- BK, bleached Kraft liner
- T, test liner

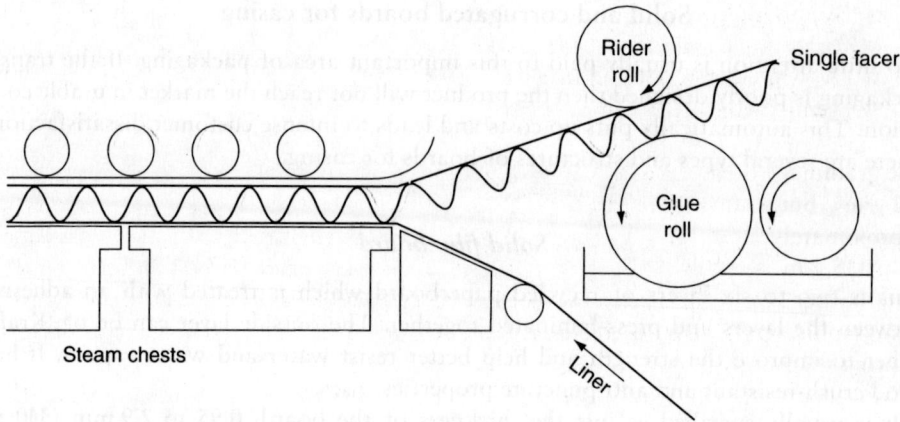

Figure 5.14 A corrugator

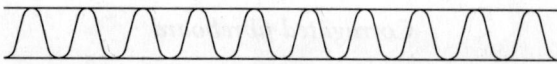

Figure 5.15 Single wall corrugated fibreboard

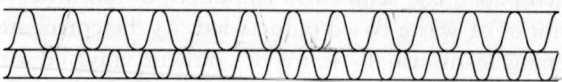

Figure 5.16 Double wall corrugated fibreboard

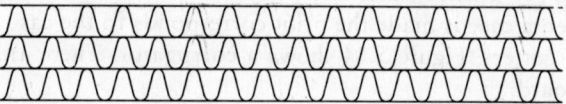

Figure 5.17 Triple wall corrugated fibreboard

Table 5.3 Flutings in corrugated fibreboard

Flute form	Approx. height of corrugations (mm)	Approx. corrugations/m	Case wall corrugations
A flute	4.5–4.7	105–125	Triple
B flute	2.1–2.9	150–185	Single and double
C flute	3.5–3.7	120–145	Single, double and triple
E flute	1.1–1.4	290–320	Single
F flute	1.0–1.2	340–390	Single
Micro flute	0.9–1.0	400–440	Single

- C, chipboard liner
- MK, mottled Kraft liner
- WTK, white-topped Kraft liner
- SC, semi-chemically prepared board.

The grammage (substance) of the corrugated fluting would normally be expected to be 112 g/m^2, but 125, 150 and 175 g/m^2 can be found in use. The liners should be of approximately equal grammage so that the corrugated board is balanced; anything from 115 g/m^2 right up to 400 g/m^2 has been used. It is usual to use Kraft liner, with its better water resistance and smoother surface, as the outside liner. To print (usually flexographically) the corrugated board, the smoother the liner, the better the quality of printing that results.

'Test' liner (pulped waste-based paper) is usually used both as the inner liner and for fitments. The centre liner(s) in double or triple walled containers could be semi-chem, chipboard or test liner according to the properties required.

There is no single industry-wide way of describing a corrugated case wall, but below are examples of those recommended in BS 1133 section 7.5.

- 150K/C/150T – single wall case with C flute 112 g/m^2 with an outer liner of 150 g/m^2 Kraft paper and an inner liner of 150 g/m^2 test paper.
- 150K/B/150SC/C/150T – double wall case with B flute outside C flute, both with substance of 112 g/m^2, with 150 g/m^2 Kraft outer liner, 150 g/m^2 semi-chem middle liner and 150 g/m^2 test inner liner. Note that this system assumes a 112 g/m^2 corrugated layer, so that if a 150 g/m^2 corrugated layer is really needed then this must be specified to the supplier.

Use of corrugated boards in distribution

Manufacture of corrugated and solid-board cases

The flat sheets of board (solid or corrugated) are fed into machines which produce the cases. These may consist of:

1. a slotter creaser
2. a printer slotter
3. folder/gluer (or stitcher or stapler)
4. rotary or flat bed die cutters (including waste stripping).

Any decoration is usually done flexographically and currently uses solvent-based inks to improve drying. Delivery is usually of made-up cases in the flat, stacked onto pallets and either stretchwrapped or banded.

Collation and casing of packs

In packaging, a carton may or may not be chosen as the prime container. If it is not chosen then a number of containers may be held together in a tray, or containers on their own, both held together with some form of film wrap, e.g. shrinkwrap. Product in a carton must be arranged so that the longest side of the carton is vertical, as this is the way to use the maximum strength of the carton.

Structure of cases and design parameters

Cases should be designed to the FEFCO, sometimes called the International Fibreboard Case Code (IFFC), system. This is an international system which has codified the various designs of cases into a simple book of basic designs. Figure 5.18 shows FEFCO case designs.

At this point it is sensible to include fitments, either solid or corrugated, into the equation. Fitments are also described in the FEFCO book, and are used to provide added strength and protection to the casing system by:

1   thickening the walls of the case
2   thickening the top and base of the case
3   being added as nests to prevent collisions between products in the case
4   preventing movement of the product
5   increasing the puncture resistance of the case.

Fitments are usually made of entirely waste-based materials.

In order to optimise the strength/cost balance an understanding of the way cases behave under load is vital. In helping to determine this optimisation, tests and estimates of the various parameters surrounding cases must be considered. Probably one of the most useful tests performed is the edge crush test.

Edge crush test (ECT)

This is defined in ASTM 2808 and BS6036 and TAPPI 811 and is a useful way of estimating the way a particular board will react under standard conditions. From the ECT, box compression ratios (BCRs) can be calculated for any case, thus:

$$BCR = 17.7 \times ECT1.06 \times d0.85 \times (L + B)0.31$$

where ECT is in kN/m, d is the board thickness (mm), L is the length of the case (mm) and B is the breadth of the case (mm).

When one is designing a case, a useful piece of knowledge is that in general each 1 g substance of fluting is as strong as 2 g substance of liner. Cases may be held together at the 'manufacturer's join' by:

- stitching the join together – abbreviation 'S'
- gluing the joint together – abbreviation 'G'
- taping the joint together – abbreviation 'T'.

Factors affecting design

Determine whether the product is going to be single, double or higher stacked on pallets, as this will create the need to increase the strength of the board accordingly.

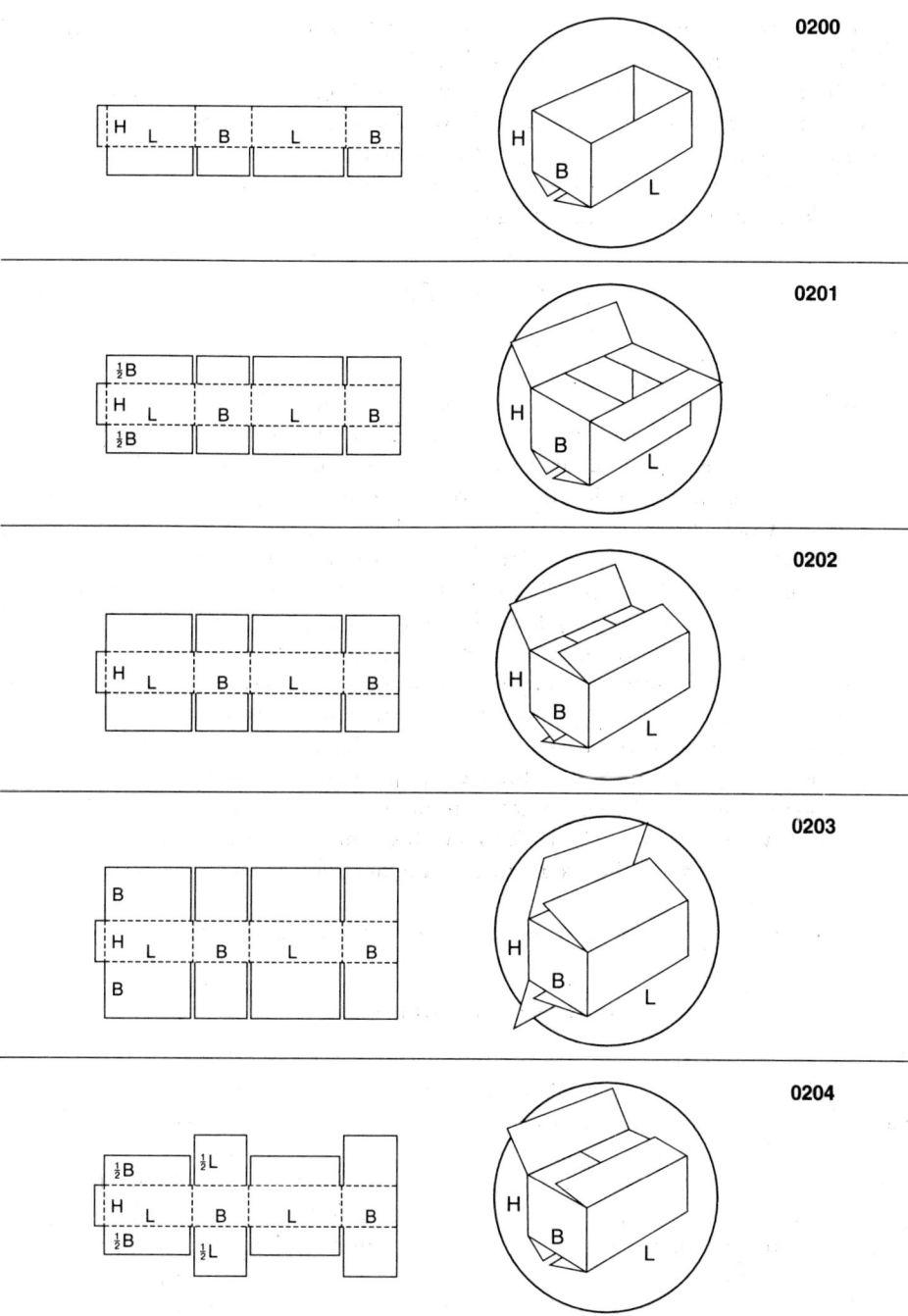

Figure 5.18 FEFCO case designs

Note the design of pallet being used, as the gaps between the deck boards may be too wide for the case size, letting case edges 'dive' down between the boards. Note also the pallet 'footprint' in any option used for multi-stacking pallets. Ensure that cases are stacked with their vertical walls directly above each other as this is the best way to carry load from above. Know the weight of the product to be carried per case. There are weight limits in various parts of the world. The author's personal experience suggests about 12 kg as the maximum case weight.

Closing of cases

This is carried out by one of five methods.

1   Gluing, either hot melt or cold adhesive. This would only be used on cases where the inner flaps of the case protected the product, e.g. FEFCO 0204 design.
2   Large staples can be used, but they puncture the liners of the outside corrugation and can let in water to the corrugations; nevertheless they form a secure closure and are widely used.
3   Water-based adhesive tape, where the adhesive is activated by wetting and this soaks into the outer liner of the case forming a strong closure, provided the relative humidity remains reasonably low. Not recommended for tropical markets where the high humidity makes paper taping a security risk.
4   Pressure sensitive adhesive tape, probably the most used today. At least 50 mm down leg of tape is needed to form a positive bond with the surface of the liner and there needs to be a substantial overlap of tape over the join of the outer flaps. For this reason 50 mm or 2 inch tape is the most popular. Clear tape pressure sensitive adhesives are susceptible to UV light degradation. It therefore makes sense to incorporate UV blocking agent either into the plastic material or into the adhesive itself.
5   Interlocking flaps may be used, but they are not considered to be a secure form of case closing.
6   Specific hot melts are used for very hot and very cold climates.

Environmental issues

All vegetative materials undergo respiration and transpiration, thereby making a major contribution to the atmospheric balance in which we live. Since trees are a major land-based part of this balance, forest destruction is a concern. There is also a linkage to global warming.

In addition to the management of the forest, great strides have been taken to salvage *all* waste wood, bark, chippings, sawdust and waste pulp so that it can be turned into fuel for the upkeep of the paper mill itself. Rain forest hardwoods make very weak, poor paper or board and are not used. The use of chlorine-based products for the bleaching process has virtually died out in Scandinavia, but remains in some other parts of the world.

Some questions are posed in the next few paragraphs. There are probably no right answers, but many opinions and certainly many more questions.

The impact of the use of paper and board has to be seen in the context of what we would do without it. One could print directly onto containers all the information discussed above for labels and leaflets. One might suspect that massive warehouses would need to be built in order to contain all the printed variables on the prime containers, and this would be a doubtful benefit to the environment.

The prime containers in warehousing and distribution could be protected with plastic boxes or in wooden crates, which could be made returnable and therefore reusable. This would entail the problem of retrieving the containers, cleaning (thereby creating effluent), re-marking them and putting them into the cycle.

The trite answer is to do a life cycle analysis for each material used, theoretically from 'the cradle to the grave'. That is all very well, but where is the cradle and where is the grave? It has been suggested that with materials tied into the 'carbon cycle' there is no cradle and there is no grave. What has to be done is to make the best analysis possible taking account of as many factors as are known!

Paper- and board-based containers

Fibreboard kegs and drums

Fibreboard kegs can be used for solid bulk drug, bulk tablet, or bulk excipient containment and transport. These are made up of multiple plies of test or Kraft liner board, convolutedly wound on a mandrel and bonded with sodium silicate adhesive between the plies. There may be an LDPE or other inside liner and the exterior may also be varnished. The base could be of either metal or plain thick board, the latter waterproofed by dipping into paraffin wax.

There may also be a galvanised mild steel base chimb bonding a board base to the wall. The lid may be of the slip-over type, in which case there is no need to protect the top of the keg, or of the push-in type, where a top mild steel chimb is added to the wall of the keg to carry the lid. This latter type of lid, made of either metal or plastic, will usually have some more sophisticated closure, e.g. lever lock.

Paper and composite open mouth sacks

These may be used for bulk excipients where there is no risk to or from the environment, e.g. chalk. They comprise two to six plies of sack Kraft types of paper, with possibly LDPE coated or metallised paper or one ply of LDPE in the case of composite sacks. The sacks may or may not have a gusset. They will all be either stitched or glued at the base and usually stitched to close the open mouth.

Composite containers

These can be used as tubes for protection or for small powder drums of 100–200 g. They are made by spirally or convolutedly winding the various plies in turn around a mandrel (similar to kegs), bound together with suitable adhesives. The materials are basically grades of paper or light board but may contain PE, aluminium and fine calendered coated decorated paper as an outside layer.

They are usually closed with metal (tinplate) or plastic bases, with closures of similar materials which may also contain dosing devices.

Paper liners, linings and laminations containing paper

Papers of various grades are used as liners inside bags made of another material. Glassine has been used as linings for the inside of plastic, metal or fibreboard kegs, where there has been a suspected problem with the compatibility of the drug and bulk container.

Paper is used extensively in laminations where it is bonded, usually by heat and/or adhesive, to other films, notably plastics and aluminium, e.g. LDPE/adhesive/aluminium/adhesive/calendered paper. This type of lamination can be used for form fill and seal work, e.g. sachet packs of deliquescent powders.

Cellulose films

The coated film is usually used as an overwrap, has been used for strip packaging when metallised, but has lost popularity in recent years with the better barrier and stronger olefin-based films becoming more available, cheaper and with 'tailored' properties. Cellulose acetate (CA), cellulose nitrate (CN), cellulose acetate propionate (CAP) and cellulose acetate butyrate (CAB) may all be found in use. The poor tear resistance, once the tear has started, does not help their case. Also, the most popular method of using cellulose films is deadfold wrapping holding down the envelope corners by heat dabbing which bonds the coating. This method has proved not to be tamper-evident.

Paper and board testing

All uses are related to the function requirements which are necessarily linked to the material properties and characteristics. Details of material tests for paper, board, cartons and corrugated are given in Appendices 5.1–5.4.

Pharmaceutical product and pack security

To cover this subject fully product issues are reviewed independently and in the context of their contribution to overall security made by 'paper'-based materials and printing.

Paper and board as security features may seem a little far from reality to the uninitiated, but seals, tapes, labels and cartons can all be utilised as devices to ensure the security of your product. The security issues will be dealt with in two ways: first the really criminal issues, i.e. tampering and counterfeiting in particular; second the security of ensuring that the correct copy gets onto the correct paper material, onto the correct substrate containing the correct pharmaceutical product.

The security environment in pharmaceuticals

There is massive fraud or illegal activity in the sale of all goods worldwide. Figures quoted in 1993 indicate that up to 5% of world trade or $80 bn per annum is involved, and this is rising each time fresh estimates are released. Pharmaceuticals are not exempt from these problems ($200 m per annum estimated), despite having theoretically tighter systems of manufacture, storage and distribution due to governmental licensing of products, storage, and distribution, thereby authorising sale by wholesalers and dispensing by pharmacists. Here it must be pointed out that this refers largely to Europe, the USA and Japan. Procedures may not be as tight in developing countries, despite government controls and licences.

The illegal, fraudulent and unauthorised practices can be placed into eight broad categories:

1   product copying
2   product substitution
3   'pass off' or counterfeit packaging to support (1), (2) and (7)
4   adulteration or tampering
5   'shrinkage'
6   illegal parallel trading
7   'poaching' of territories by agents
8   invention of 'new' products.

Some of the examples which follow will fall into more than one category, e.g. how does one substitute something in a pack without tampering with it? Two further points should be considered that will affect the way in which companies react:

- producer liability legislation
- the legal need to track hazardous materials comprehensively

Product copying

This category of illegal activity attempts to copy the physical appearance of the pharmaceutical formulation without going to the massive expense of setting up all the legally necessary control systems, thereby producing something similar but cheaper and probably of much lower quality. The copy could be in either original packaging or 'pass off' packaging. Copies that have been seen have either contained impure amounts of drug substance or no active ingredient whatsoever.

The dangers of these copies are:

- impure active ingredient – uncontrolled effects on patient
- no active ingredient – no therapeutic effect for the patient and overall loss of confidence by patients and the medical profession
- impure or incorrect excipient substances – as above (note that deaths have been recorded where, in the Third World, 'glycol' was added to a product to extend the volume).

Product substitution

The substitution of one product by another, 'dressed up' to look like a more expensive product, e.g.

1   the labelling of a low-cost antibiotic as a much more modern and potent antibiotic
2   refilling or recycling vials using even non-sterile products
3   one company's counterfeit product in a second company's reused packaging.

The great danger inherent in this type of activity is that the substitute is probably cheaper, older and a lot less potent than the original, consequently the patient may not react in the way the health professional intended. The result here may not be fatal, but at the minimum a loss of confidence in the original product by the health professionals.

'Pass off' or conterfeit packaging

The term 'pass off' is the correct one in English law, since 'counterfeiting' is theoretically used only for offences concerned with currencies. However, 'counterfeiting'is the term usually used.

In the past few years some remarkable copies of packaging materials have temporarily fooled packaging experts. At the other end of the scale there have been many poor copies that would cause one to wonder how anyone could be so easily fooled.

Any of the examples quoted in 'Product copying' and 'Product substitution' above can be taken, plus out-of-date material or factory rejects 'obtained' and recycled with fresh packaging and different manufacture and expiry dates.

The danger in date-expired materials is that pharmaceutical products are given very strictly controlled shelf lives. Past the end of the shelf life there is *no* guarantee that the degeneration products produced will not be harmful to a patient. If the 'obtained' materials were factory rejects, then they had been considered by the factory QC system as not within the specification necessary for administration to patients.

Adulteration or tampering

Adulteration is the deliberate contamination of a product for extortion or for some other malicious intent, e.g. personal revenge. The two best known examples in the pharmaceutical industry are the 'Tylenol' affair in 1982 and the 'Sudafed' affair in 1991, both in the USA.

In both of these cases OTC pharmaceutical preparations, analgesics contained in capsules, were contaminated with a cyanide salt and deaths resulted. In the author's opinion, making packs fully tamper-evident is one of the hurdles that the industry has to tackle. Many companies have decided to add additional tamper-evidence, but it can be argued that there is still a long way to go. Experience to date suggests that adulteration appears to be more prevalent in the more sophisticated markets whereas tampering, in its widest sense, is worldwide.

Shrinkage

This describes the loss of goods through pilferage in production, storage, distribution or even disappearance from hospital and pharmacy stores. This is more prevalent than might be thought. Even lorry-loads of goods have been known to disappear.

The only real answer, at present, is the rigorous 'policing' of all parts of the manufacturing, storage and distribution areas. The pharmaceutical industry tries very hard to reconcile all input materials, be they drug substances, excipients, drug delivery systems or packaging materials. Some companies and countries claim that their control systems are so good that 'it cannot happen here'. Despite very rigorous systems and controls, materials still 'disappear', especially if there is money to be made! Human ingenuity knows no bounds.

Illegal parallel trading

All parallel trading of pharmaceuticals inside the European Union is legal, provided that the following three conditions are fulfilled:

1   the product is registered and approved in the receiving market
2   the manufacturer is fully licensed to manufacture the drug in the country of origin
3   the importer in the country of sale is registered and licensed to handle pharmaceuticals.

The reasoning behind parallel trading is that of the 'free market' and that the best (i.e. lowest) prices can be obtained for any particular pharmaceutical presentation. Having worked in the industry for 36 years, there is one point the author has learnt – Ministries of Health actually control all the prices.

Over the past several years parallel trading has increased into the high-priced countries (e.g. Holland, Germany) from countries where the prices are lower (e.g. Greece, Belgium and Spain). Included in this trading have been products that are pass offs.

There is also the problem of illegal imports from both within the EU and non-EU areas. Illegal imports from within the EU usually do not comply with the three conditions above. In the UK the levels of control exercised by the DoH inspectorate have recently been revised, to try to combat illegal parallel imports.

Poaching of territories by agents

This is what might be termed a contractual offence between a manufacturer, an agent (who is contracted for specific markets) and the regulatory authorities in those markets. In many ways it is similar (if not identical) to the illegal parallel trading mentioned previously.

Inventing 'new' products

Human ingenuity in making money is nowhere more evident than where illegal operators have 'invented' a new product for the company, e.g. a well-known dermatological product name from an international company was used for a soap in certain markets and allegedly sold quite well.

There are two dangers here. First, the patient is paying good money for a product that has little or no therapeutic effect, and in certain cases might be exactly the wrong thing for the consumer's complaint. Second, the reputation of the company involved can suffer.

Two major factors which influence the reactions of pharmaceutical companies to the eight problems discussed above will now be considered.

Producer liability

There is a growing need for companies to be able to trace and authenticate their products so that claims arising from customer complaints and product performance liabilities, in particular, are proved. The probable nightmare scenario to a pharmaceutical company is where deaths are reported in the international media and attributed to its product – and it cannot 'prove' conclusively that the product was not its own but a 'pass off'. To the best of the author's knowledge this has not happened yet.

Most pharmaceutical companies are taking responsible counter-measures to avoid this dramatic situation.

Tracking of hazardous materials

There is a legal obligation to be capable of tracing hazardous goods, i.e. those classified under the UN hazardous goods scheme. It may not be appreciated that a number of pharmaceutical products are UN certified. Pharmaceutical companies can trace any 'batch or lot' of product up to the time it leaves their immediate control. There are techniques of 'trace back' used to investigate product complaints. Each company tries to reconcile 100% all materials, e.g. raw materials, drug substances, excipients and packaging materials, during all stages of progress through the company. It also holds records of the sources of all those materials, and today most of these sources are regularly audited.

Parameters needed for the design of a pharmaceutical security package

In this section only the solutions that encompass the use of cellulose-based materials in their make-up will be covered.

Project objectives

First, project objectives must be clear through an analysis of the problem(s) appertaining to the product(s). Do not proceed blindly into a strategy which does not suit the situation. The final objective will be to prevent, or at least minimise, product copying, substitution, etc. at a realistic cost. There are only two options:

1   do nothing and hope that the problem is solved by the forces of law and order
2   protect the product with the most cost-effective systems to minimise the problem. The totally criminal-resistant pack may never be achieved, but building in a number of layers of protection increases the chances of the criminal making a detectable error, or giving up the attempt and going to try it out on someone else's pack.

As stated earlier, one should carefully analyse the problem before deciding which of the above eight problem categories one intends to protect against.

1   Is more than one protective system needed?

2   Are the correct reasons for introduction being considered?
3   Is protection against more than one type of activity being considered?

Some of the issues – the vulnerability of packs and the concerns of the industry – are discussed below.

The issues involved in the initial evaluation of what, if any, actions should be taken are probably the most demanding. They must not be taken in isolation but supported by the company management. An approach to consider is the effects of an illegal action and the follow-up company action, e.g. is the incident fully understood? Have the reasons for the illegal incident really been analysed? Has the company the expertise to examine the problem and think the way the criminal thought?

Probably the hardest decision that has to be made is the need for public announcement. Is it worth taking the risk of losing public and professional confidence in the product, or is it better to rely on their understanding that what is happening is not the fault of the company and that the company is making considerable efforts to rectify the situation?

Which systems are considered to protect the goods? This will largely rest on what illegal activities have happened to the goods, the markets involved, and the type of packaging. Is an overt or covert feature to be used to protect the goods? Whatever overt measures are taken, an eye must be kept on public education because without it, vast numbers of inspectors might have to be employed to achieve the same level of inspection and coverage.

Have all the avenues of supply with reference to security considerations been examined, for example, security of printed materials supplies and suppliers and the movement of security packaging (and indeed ordinary genuine packaging) materials between the supplier and the final assembly workplace?

Vulnerability of the packaging system could include the following.

1   Product 'look alikes' can be easy to produce using conventional printing processes. The average label and carton used in pharmaceuticals are quite easy to reproduce well enough to fool both the pharmacist and the patient, even though they may not mislead the expert.
2   There is a very long period between drug patent and market approval, during which information and graphics can leak from a company. It is not unknown for the illegal route of pharmaceutical supply to outstrip the legal route into certain markets.
3   There are different prices in different markets, with more likelihood of illegal parallel trading and the introduction of 'pass offs'.
4   The multiple supply chains used by pharmaceutical companies can be bewildering, sometimes leading to the genuine product landing up in a market for which it is not intended.
5   No tamper-evident systems are employed on packs. This omission is gross negligence on the part of the company, since a degree of tamper-evidence can be provided very easily and cheaply, e.g. tamper-evident fragile paper labels. Anti-counterfeiting systems should, as has already been said, only be used after long, detailed and very careful consideration of the problems.

The concerns of the pharmaceutical manufacturer could include the following.

1 · That patient safety is of paramount importance. The biggest risk is to the patient and all else should be a secondary consideration. The pharmaceutical company exists to supply safe, secure, therapeutic treatments to its customers. Any break or interference in the chain can only result in the final consumer, the patient, receiving inferior product with results ranging from loss of money for a placebo product look alike to serious health complications if a parenteral product is compromised.

2 Either of the above could cause a loss of confidence to the health professionals and the public, with the most serious effect on the economics of a company. Loss of confidence by anybody means loss of prescriptions, therefore loss of business. This could feasibly occur even though the product itself was OK, if the mass media were given a story of a drug being substituted. This does not have to be true, and the company can probably prove to the authorities that the product is not affected, but the medical professionals and the general public will be difficult to convince that the product is safe if anti-tampering and anti-counterfeiting measures have not been taken.

3 The product liability laws are such that if the company cannot prove that the goods that were bought/prescribed/taken by a patient are not its own, then the company is liable. How much easier to prove that the goods were not the company's if there are security features which are not to be encountered on an illegal pack.

4 There is a great fear of going public when one of these types of problem arises in the industry. When faced with this problem certain companies have introduced packaging measures, gone public and advertised the overt counter-measures to the health professionals. The net result was a rise in sales for 8–10 months after the event.

5 The fear of loss of revenue is always present in these cases. Facing up to the security problem and being proactive might in the short term cost money, but in the long term will protect the company revenue – look on it as insurance!

Key features

1 It is suggested that a 'horses for courses' approach be adopted, i.e. look at each problem individually and decide on the best answer. With cellulose-based materials the following might be considered: specialist inks (UV, photochromic, thermochromic), holograms, special prints, clever multicolour designs, watermarks, chemically marked paper and board, etc. Any of them could be appropriate, depending on the circumstances of the problem.

2 This is why clearly defining the problems and what is to be achieved is critical, so that any counter-measure designer is in a better position to defend the product. If the company doesn't have an expert in this field, there are consultants who will help identify problems.

3 What is wanted: authentication or deterrent, or both? This decision will change the way to approach the design.

4 This goes back to covert or overt features, depending on the answer to (3) above.

5 Assess whether there should be a single feature on one product pack or continuous throughout the product range, even though it may only be one or two product presentations that are being targeted.

The produced anti-criminal device must then have the following characteristics.

- Very difficult to counterfeit. While this may be obvious, some pharmaceutical products are like currency in some parts of the features world. Hence consider if currency without anti-criminal features built in would be accepted. The answer will be *no*!
- A device which needs no specific marketing monitoring i.e. self-policing after public education.
- An obvious deterrent to put off the criminal.
- The ability to maintain public confidence, through a form of label/seal with a distinctive secure print on it, advertised wherever advertising is allowed in order to get the public to check the goods on receipt.
- Relatively easy to introduce, for speed is of the essence. If the company is seen to be taking steps to protect its customers, then those customers will probably react favourably.

Which deterrent?

1 It is important to treat security as security features and not to be drawn into treating them as promotional. There may be a promotional angle that the marketing department can employ, but security of the system is paramount.
2 Simple design can be easily reproduced particularly with the advent of the colour photocopier. Review the design and include features that change when photocopied.
3 All markets will need consideration for both literate and illiterate patients, i.e. a company logo may not be a good idea as it might mean little to the end user.
4 Ensure that a secure supplier is chosen for the designs that are being considered. Although obvious it is often missed.
5 The format must be carefully chosen as it must fit in or onto production lines efficiently and securely. All staff must understand what is happening and how important is the (particularly) overt device. It may not be necessary to tell them about covert devices, as the less said about them outside the security circle the better.

Other considerations

1 The issue of public education will only apply to overt devices. Educate the health professionals first and rely on them and legitimate publicity to ensure that if the security device is not on the pack then questions are raised immediately. Speed is important, as the trail of the criminal will go cold very quickly.
2 The total security throughout all the supply, manufacture, and distribution chain

has been mentioned before. It has been known for a counterfeit supply of goods to be sold in original packaging material. If the counterfeiter can counterfeit goods he can do the same with individual company's purchase orders. Build in checks throughout the system, particularly the habit of making personal contact with people in the supply chain to check that orders received are genuine.

3   There are other controls, e.g. governments, patents, discarded production equipment. Ensure that the government being dealt with doesn't 'leak' any security secrets. Use patents whenever possible to protect packs. Ensure that on disposal of production or packaging equipment there are no tools, change parts or packaging materials belonging to the company that go with the old machines. It has been known for the criminals to get hold of them and reproduce counterfeit packs.

4   It is essential that a series of controlled changes of security feature be devised to keep ahead of the criminal. Change small features of the design, keeping accurate records of when and what was changed. This means that the company can take account of the latest in technology and keep the criminal guessing as to what might be done next.

Deterrent design and use

The type of deterrent

Is it to be label, a specially designed sealed carton or perhaps watermarked paper or board, chemically marked paper or board security inks, holograms etc.? In a large proportion of the potential methods of protection you will need to ensure that the device, print, etc. actually 'permanently adheres' to the substrate.

The substrates

The substrates could be any of the following:

1   cartonboard – what surface is to be used (cast coated, clay coated, uncoated)?
2   label materials – what paper surface (cast coated, clay coated, uncoated)?
3   cellulose films – with or without surface coatings?

The primary pack could also be glass, metal or plastic needing a security label, carton or overwrap.

The adhesion system

It is vitally important that the adhesion between the security system and the final substrate cannot be breached by any means without leaving conclusive 'easy to see' evidence. It is no use using a hot melt adhesive, which can be reheated and allows either a label to be removed and a 'pass off' put on or a sealed carton to be opened. More harm than good may be done with such a system.

Tests must be performed so that one can be satisfied that the above criterion is fulfilled all the time, throughout the distribution and storage chain, worldwide if necessary.

Additional items to be considered when designing security systems

1   The surface exposed to the public: This must be robust enough to withstand the scuffing and vibration of a normal pack in transit and use by the medical service. If overt it must have a bright clear image to attract the public.
2   Production systems of transferring the system to the final pack: Again this may seem obvious, but check carefully the feasibility of the laydown of final design onto the final pack. Also make sure that there is equipment to do the job economically and accurately. The design must have a high degree of accuracy and design procedures which cover the entire system of design production, including all aspects of producing and applying the design to the final pack.

The evaluation for end use must be thorough and realistic, e.g. fragile papers for seals might not apply well on machines and fracture in transit, yet be easy to open. The post-addition of additional security system packaging processes, e.g. overwrapping with securely marked or designed cellophane incorporating a tear band, can also be practical.

Costs

1   There are project and evaluation costs (non-recoverable).
2   Possible research costs into an adhesive, carriers and substrates to be considered.
3   The implementation and education costs to introduce a total security system (setting up and training everyone from designer to supplier and company staff).
4   The cost of educating health professionals and the public if the system is to be monitored effectively.
5   Audits of supply distribution system are needed to check system integrity.
6   Costs of additional material needed for the job.
7   Additional capital needed for machines.
8   Possibly additional staff to monitor and work in key areas.

What the project must achieve is total security of production, public education (particularly health professionals), security of supply chain, effective monitoring and keeping features updated.

Security in the packaging operations

The second form of security to be addressed is the one of ensuring that the printed word, as laid down by the competent authority, is securely translated onto label, leaflet or carton by whatever means, and affixed/placed on or around the correct drug container.

Although simple in principle, the industry gets it wrong time after time. Both the FDA and the MCA state that the single most common cause of a product recall is a mistake in 'labelling' or identification, commonly known as a 'mix-up'. A breach of internal security has been devised to prevent such a mix-up happening. Detailed below are some recommendations on the best way to approach the problem when handling labels, leaflets and cartons.

There must be an integrated approach to the problem. Putting a bar code reader on a packaging line doesn't address the problem: it is an important addition to the system, but not the whole answer. Some additional points that might assist in the discrimination of one piece of printed material from another are as follows.

1 Distinction in colour layout and shape, especially when manual inspections are the norm.
2 Critical information should be in one colour, to minimise problems should one plate in the printing process cease to function.
3 Use ISO 9000 registered suppliers especially those used to dealing with pharmaceutical printing. Codes of practice are issued by the Pharmaceutical Quality Group of the Institute of Quality Assurance and linked to ISO 9002, specifically aimed at printing suppliers to the industry.
4 In-house systems, e.g. warehousing, should be set up in such a way as to minimise the risk of mix-ups, e.g. using discrete lidded storage bins.
5 All machines, packaging areas, printed material transport systems, etc. should be specifically designed to facilitate clearance of all the 'current' set of printed material.
6 Formally document all the checks that are carried out, ensure that the person checking has been trained and knows what to look for, knows what to do when a mix-up occurs and knows that the success of the system depends on their ability. Note: The results of checks must be recorded.
7 Increase the number of security safe positive accepting electronic/mechanical machines. Be careful in choice of systems and never forget that an integrated system that cannot be bypassed ensures the best security for your company.

The next few paragraphs work through the procedures for designing, approving, printing, supplying and using a label (but the same principles apply to all printed materials).

First, the copy must be written by a competent person, fulfilling copy guidelines laid down by the various regulatory authorities. This approved copy is then laid down as artwork which meet the demands of the pharmacy label/leaflet regulations, regulatory authority, company corporate identity and the container label design (size) which is best suited to the container and application system.

Note that the adhesive performance requires validation on the substrate being used, beyond the shelf life of the product and in the extremes of storage and use conditions predicted for the markets that are to be supplied with that particular label/adhesive/container application. A label that does not remain on its container is a security risk! The problem of adhesion failure occurs in cartons with the 'glue flap' being a vulnerable point, due to inefficient gluing on the folder/gluer, or the wrong adhesive being used.

When the artwork is completed it must be authorised for use by the originator, regulatory affairs, marketing, quality assurance and packaging to ensure that all the parameters are in accordance with requirements. The completed colour separated artwork should be sent, by the purchasing department, along with the remainder of the label specification, to an audited authorised printer.

The printer should be used to dealing with pharmaceuticals and have been audited to ISO 9002. This will ensure that all the correct procedures for line checking, physical separation, printing plate separation, line, make-ready, records, absence of gang printing etc. are in place and followed. Some companies call this GMP at suppliers. Colour proofs of each colour to be used should be returned for checking prior to the actual print run.

The artwork must include a unique part number (or item code) as the basis of identification, security and reference, which will change for every change to the printed component (however small). This identification is the key to all security traceability. This code may be represented by either alpha-numeric human readable characters or an associated bar code. This requires the capability for automatically reading either the bar code or the part number using suitable equipment on the printer's press and on packaging lines. The printed part number and/or the bar code should be unique and verified on the printed component artwork, in as many colours as the reading system is capable of reading to ensure that all the printing is there on the label.

If the printer is equipped to read either type of code then ensure that all labels are read, not just one line of codes on an unslit label reel, for example. This last reading should take place as the final act of inspection just prior to the labels being securely wrapped and sealed into their transit packaging ready for dispatch.

There are options to sample and test each delivery of labels or, through confidence in the printer, accept a 'certificate of conformance' and only randomly sample occasional deliveries. Labels, once delivered and accepted, should be stored in individual, segregated and secure closed bins, one bin per part number. They should be issued on a 'first in first out' (FIFO) system.

When quantities of the label are requisitioned against the packaging documentation, (based on the packaging specification) they should first be visually identified, counted and code checked (preferably by machine reading) and then signed off by the authorised store issuer. The materials are then securely held away from the packaging line area, awaiting use.

If the overprinting of LOT, BATCH, or EXP, etc. is to be carried out away from the packaging line then a similar separate loop of the checking procedure must be written and used.

When the order is ready to be packaged on a production line it must be preceded by a formal line clearance procedure and the material then carefully visually checked for accuracy of part numbers and accuracy of quantity.

The printed packaging material should be kept away from the packaging line machinery while the bar code reader or vision system code is set from an independent source of information, e.g. the pack specification or the works order document. The printed packaging material itself must not be used to set the checking equipment as this is a known GMP risk. With the advent of computer integrated lines it is possible to download the bar codes or number directly to the reading system, leaving the packaging line personnel the task of only aligning the reading heads.

The system of code reading must be challenged at regular intervals by feeding slightly wrong codes to it and confirming that they are not accepted. It is advisable for automatic systems on packaging lines to be 'positive accept'. This means that the line/machine will reject everything unless a positive accept signal is received from the sensor, which then 'opens' to 'pass' the package.

The parts of the packaging line between stations (open conveyer) should be covered so that the goods once passed through the automatic checks cannot, as far as is practical, be handled by operators again. This is because it has been reported that up to 70% of product mix-ups and adulteration in the whole British industry are caused with the supply company deliberately bypassing systems.

A mix-up leading to a recall means at least a loss of reputation through adverse publicity in pharmaceutical journals, loss of revenue, cost of collecting the recall and stock replacement and loss of confidence in the company.

Bar coding

This is an essential form of printing nowadays, usually in two forms for two totally different reasons as detailed below.

Non-security bar codes

These codes are used every day in the UK on the supermarket checkouts, and an extended version of them is used to control movements of goods in warehouses. They are being applied in the pharmaceutical industry, both on OTCs and, less obviously, on POM classified medicines. The OTCs are sometimes sold by the large supermarket chains, and therefore have been brought under the same rules and regulations as all other fast-moving consumer goods.

EAN (UPC) codes

These codes are 'market' codes designed to be used at point of sale, so that the inventory can be kept up to date to the minute. They are made up of thirteen numeric characters all with a meaning. Note that there are some eight character codes, discussed below.

The first two EAN codes denote the country of issue of the number, e.g. UK for the number 50. The last or thirteenth number is a 'check character' calculated to modulo 10, which completes the code, confirming that the code is genuine and has conformed to the number structure. The remaining ten are split into two groups of five. The first five is the number assigned by the Article Numbering Association (ANA) to the purchaser of the sequence of numbers, e.g. 50 99999 00001?. The 99999 is specific to company 'X' and no other company or supplier can use it without permission of the owner. The next group of five is the number that the owner assigns to the specific product name and size, e.g. in 50 99999 00001? the 00001 could describe a bottle of 50 Cureall tablets, 100 mg.

So the code tells us that it is UK issued, the code is owned by company 'X', the product is a bottle of 50 Cureall tablets, 100 mg.

To return to the last character, i.e. the check character, at modulo 10 it would work out as 9 so the full code reads 50 99999 00001 9, and thirteen meaningful characters.

Difficulties in printing these codes in a readable form resulted in a complicated series of specifications written by the ANA. These specifications have been somewhat modified in the light of improved readers, but if codes are to be read efficiently, follow the ANA guidelines.

To optimise the contrasts between the bars and spaces, it is preferable to print black onto a white surface. Print gain is a term used by printers to quantify the amount by which the printed bar is bigger than the plate used. Different printing processes and machines have different gains, so leave control to the professional printer to obtain the code films to the correct gain.

A normal 100% magnification EAN 13 code is exactly 37.29 mm long and 26.26 mm high. These dimensions include the quiet zones around the bars themselves. The magnification has been reduced successfully to 80%, and the height can be reduced or 'truncated' 16 mm overall.

There is an EAN 8 code. These are certain numbers in the code sequence in which the zeros can be ignored, giving only eight digits, thereby reducing the code width to 26.73 mm overall. The same rules on reduction and truncation apply.

Warehousing codes, e.g. EAN 128 or traded unit outer codes

This is a system of extending the basic EAN code to 'add on' data to the basic code, e.g. bar coded batch code and/or expiry date. In order to achieve this, 'addition identifiers' (AIs) are used to delineate where the additional part of the code begins and ends. This code is much larger than the primary EAN code, e.g. 123 mm long by a minimum of 27 mm high. As it would usually be printed onto cases or trays or tray or case labels, there is more space in which to accommodate the code. Figure 5.19 shows an EAN 128 code.

Interleaf two of five (ITF) codes

An alternative to the EAN 128 is an ITF code. This is a bar symbology which allows numeric characters only (i.e. 0–9 inclusive) to be portrayed as a series of thick and thin bars and spaces. Using our EAN number we have to add a zero to the front of it, making it a fourteen numeric code. The overall size of this code is 159.828 mm across (remember this is totally inclusive of all the margins) and 48.1 mm high. Figure 5.20 shows an ITF codes. Again, supplementary information can be added to this code.

(01) 05412345678908 (15) 921231

Figure 5.19 An EAN bar code (not to size)

050   00144 01570   5

Figure 5.20 An ITF bar code (not to size)

Other codes

Interleaf 3 of 9 or code 39 has been used, particularly in some European markets, as a means of helping to control the reimbursement of drug costs, by electronic reading means, to the patient. It is similar in structure to ITF, but allows the full alphanumeric range of characters to be used.

The Health Industry Business Communications Council (HIBCC) code was originally developed in the USA to establish its own codification structure for the full range of health sectors, but has come to be used mainly within the US hospital system. In the UK, HIBCC is also called the Health Industry Bar Code Convention by the Article Numbering Association (ANA), and also the Health Industry Business Code Council. In the Netherlands it is known as the Health Industry Bar Code (HIBC). The code is composed of five elements:

1   1st character '+' denotes HIBCC
2   2nd to 5th characters denote the manufacturer or proprietor of the product at international level – 'E' as the second character denotes Europe
3   6th to 18th characters (variable in number) identify the product (could contain an EAN code)
4   19th character denotes the level of packaging, e.g. unit of sale, pallet, case
5   check character in a maximum of the 20th position calculated at modulo 43.

The code can be represented in any of the following standard bar formats: code 39, code 16K, code 49, and code 128.

Other codes coming onto the market are answering the problem of more and more information being required by the warehousing, wholesale and retail pharmaceuticals trade. It may soon be possible by using an individual bar code to be able to trace at least every batch of product right down the chain to individual patients.

Security codes

These are usually called 'Pharmacodes'. This is a misnomer, as the term 'Pharmacode' belongs as a trade mark to one company only. They are in the form of thick and thin bars of dark print on a light background. The thick and thin bars are of specified dimensions and give the effective signal of '1' and '0' respectively when moved past a scanning head. The 1s and 0s are then compared with a pre-loaded code and the result passes or fails.

The pre-loaded code can be entered in one of two ways. It can be loaded as a number, e.g. 112. This is then set by the decoder as 110001, i.e. to read thick, thick, thin, thin, thin, thick. The other method is to set the code directly by pressing usually the thick bars on one side of a decoder and the thin on the other side. Whichever method is used, the information for the code reader must be obtained from a controlled source, e.g. pack specification or works order.

The purpose of the code is to provide an affordable easy machine-readable form of the item code (part number) and prevent mix-ups at any point in the system. The mechanism by which this is achieved is by the code moving past a combined light source and sensor. The reflected light generates a peak voltage over a short time for a thin bar and about times three for a thick bar. In order to prevent mis-rejects the contrast between the background and the bars must be as great as possible. The background should always be white, but there are many problems with white: shine, uncoated paper, print show-through, etc. This means that the ground voltage (that voltage from which the spike is measured) might *not* be zero volts. Figure 5.21 shows high ground voltage.

Ground voltages up to as high as 0.9 V have been experienced. The reason for this is that the light source is constant (over a short period, even though it might decay in value over months). If it is calibrated to zero volts on the whitest source available, e.g. standard white tile, calcium carbonate block, any white darker or less reflective will not register zero volts but a positive value as the conditions controlling the detector must remain the same for the duration of the testing period, i.e. the production run. Again if the contrast between the bars and the background is poor, there is a greater chance of a misread.

There are a number of competing systems on the market, all doing approximately the same job and being successful provided all the systems governing the running of these bar codes are themselves secure.

The advent of vision verification systems is now competing with bar codes in the security field. These systems read the preprinted part number and either compare it with a pre-loaded independently obtained code or the whole system can be fully computerised and the reader told what component to expect and read as it passes.

Conclusions

This chapter has covered one of the oldest yet most useful of pharmaceutical packaging materials which has survived the onslaught of plastics and, being biodegradable, has considerably contributed to the store of natural materials that can be used for product protection. The chapter has also included sections on security, since papers (in

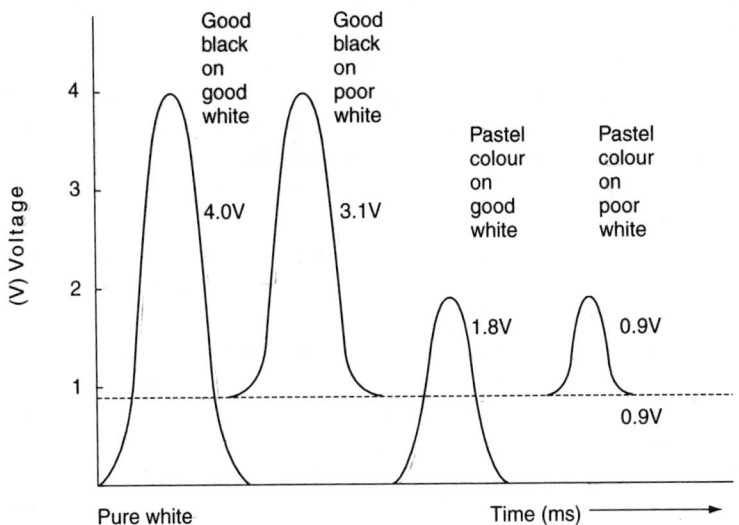

Figure 5.21 High ground voltage

particular) are frequently involved to assist security, a key example being the printing of bar codes – both for security and for efficient stock control and movement tracing.

The objective of the chapter is to provide a reasonably detailed amount of information on this very important and varied group of packaging materials, widely used in the pharmaceutical industry.

The best known applications of paper and board are labels, leaflets, folding boxboard cartons and corrugated cases. Without these, packaging or products would be more expensive and difficult. Please also note some of the 'rarer' or more hidden uses of cellulose, e.g. cellulose film, layers in laminates.

The major problem discussed in this chapter is not in the technologies of cellulose materials but in the question of security. Companies can be made less competitive by non-adherence to security rules. The two major areas are mix-ups in the production, delivery and use of labels, leaflets and cartons and the more modern phenomenon of passing off counterfeit drugs.

The future is bright for cellulosic materials, due to the more detailed requirements needed for information – particularly the expanded EU leaflet requirements.

On the environmental front, the success of Scandinavia (in particular) in managing its forests in an eco-friendly manner and cutting pollution of the environment during the manufacture of paper and board has countered many of the environmental objections to the paper- and board-making industries. Trees, grasses, etc. are renewable and as such preferable, where they are an economic alternative to petroleum-based materials.

In short, paper board and other cellulosic materials have a major future in this industry.

Appendix 5.1: Testing of paper and board

It is fundamental to a good understanding of paper and board that the testing regimes that can be used and the specific tests and the reasons for using those tests are appreciated.

The reason for testing is to gain information, thereby ascertaining the acceptability of the test piece in comparison with a specification. That specification should be drawn up so that if all results pass, the material is fit for the purpose that it is intended to fulfil. All tests must be relevant to the use of the material, and must be understood by all the parties involved. This need has led to a series of standard tests: British BSI, ASTM, etc.

Testing conditions have also to be defined, as paper and board are very susceptible to humidity and temperature changes. It is therefore essential that the test pieces for paper and board are in fact 'conditioned' so that the tests can be carried out under 'standard' conditions, thereby giving fair comparisons. Those conditions usually quoted are:

- temperature – $23\,°C \pm 1\,°C$ (BS 3431 and ISO 187)
- relative humidity – $50\% \pm 2\%$ (BS 3431 and ISO 187).

Note that there is one major exception to this rule – moisture content of the material. How to test is simple. Just follow carefully and accurately the standard test methods. Note also that test pieces should be cut accurately for tests where dimensions are critical. If one is using specific test instruments it must be ensured that the instrument is properly set and calibrated (if necessary) prior to the commencement of a test.

The reporting of results should include at least the following data:

1　The test method used, e.g. Grammage BS 3432:1980 (always specify the date of the method, as the BS and all the other standards are routinely updated)
2　the instrument used (its reference no.)
3　the test conditions
4　the size of the test piece, where relevant
5　the number of replicate tests per sample
6　the units used – this is very important, as a number of different units are used in reporting (both the SI and Imperial systems are in use together)
7　any other facts relevant to the test piece, e.g. discoloration of a white test piece on moisture content testing.

Appendix 5.2: General tests for paper and board

1　Sample conditioning of paper and board: BS EN 20187; 1993, ISO/R187 1990. This is the way to condition any test piece prior to testing by the appropriate BS method.
2　Pre-test procedures for paper and board. BS 3430:1986 (91) ISO 186 (1985) sets out the methods of obtaining a representative sample of the paper or board for testing in order to ensure that an average can be taken and compared with the original specification.
3　Moisture content of paper and board is measured according to BS 343:1986 (91) ISO 287 (1985). All papers and boards can be covered, i.e. all calipers of paper, chipboard, pasteboard, folding boxboard, solid and corrugated fibreboards provided there are no substances that will escape at the temperature specified for the test.
4　Folding endurance: ISO 5626:1993 describes four methods, i.e. Köhler Molin, Lhomary, MIT and Schopper. These various instruments fold the test piece back and forth through a specified angle until rupture occurs. Applies to all forms of paper and board, but there may be different instruments for different boards.
5　Density of paper and board: BS 4370:1973–1991. These are methods of test for rigid cellular materials. There are fourteen different test methods for aspects of the physical properties – dimensions, apparent density, compression strength, dimensional stability, cross-breaking strength, shear strength, shear modulus, thermal conditioning, water vapour transmission, tensile strength, friability and coefficient of linear thermal expansion.
6　Methods for determining air permeability: BS 6538:1985 (95) ISO 5636 (1984). Permeability is the mean airflow through unit area under unit pressure difference in unit time, under specified conditions, expressed in $\mu m\ Pa^{-1}\ s^{-1}$. Beware as there are several types of instruments that can be used and the results may be quoted as, for example Bendtsen. Note that this is only a valid test in what is termed the 'medium air permeance range'. This is important when you are using lightweight uncoated papers on machines that have a vacuum pick-up system.

7   Methods of test for the assessment of odour for packaging materials used for food-stuffs: BS 3755:1964 (71) This particular test has been deleted from the latest lists of the BSI.

8   Grammage or substance: BS 3432:1980 (90) ISO 536. The weight of material per unit area of the sample, usually confined to papers and boards, excluding the man-ufactured corrugated sheet but including the component parts of the corrugated sheet. Units are usually g/m^2.

9   Paper caliper BS EN 20534 1993 ISO 534 1988. Single sheet thickness between one surface and the other. Measure over a specified area and under a specific static load by means of a high precision dead-weight micrometer.

10 Tensile strength, both wet and dry: BS 4415:1992 ISO 1924 (1992). The maximum tensile force per unit width that a paper or board will withstand before breaking. The stretch at break is the measured elongation at the moment of rupture of a test piece, when tested under specific conditions.

11 Tear strength either across or along the grain: BS EN 21974 1994 ISO 1974, 1990. The mean force required to continue the tearing of an initial cut in a single sheet of paper and four torn together through a fixed distance using a pendulum to apply the tearing force. The work done in tearing the test piece is measured by the loss of potential energy of the pendulum. This obviously can be done either across or along the grain. The scale is calibrated to indicate the average force.

12 Burst strength, both wet and dry: BS 3137:1972 (95) ISO 2758, 2754, 3689. The maximum uniformly distributed pressure, applied at right angles to the surface, that a test piece of paper and board will stand under the conditions of the test.
The test piece is placed into contact with a circular diaphragm, the test piece being clamped around the periphery, but free in the centre to bulge with the diaphragm. Hydraulic pressure is applied to the diaphragm, bulging it until the test piece bursts. This denotes the general strength of the test piece.

13 Puncture resistance: BS 4812:1972 (93) ISO 3036. A triangular pyramid puncture head is attached to a pendulum. It is released to swing onto a test piece. The energy required to force the puncture head right through the piece, i.e. to make the initial puncture and to tear and bend open the test piece, is measured.

14 Stiffness of thick papers and boards: BS 3748:1992 ISO 2493 1992. This is the degree of resistance offered by a paper or board when it is bent under specified conditions.

15 Ply bond of boards: TAPPI 403. This test ensures that the various plies of a multi-ply board have bonded together enough to ensure that they will perform satisfactorily in service. This test applies not to boards that use an adhesive as the bonding agent, e.g. pasteboard, but to those in which the plies are joined by heat and pressure only.

16 Creasability of boards: BS 4818:1993 described the method of determining the creasing quality of cartonboard within the range of 300–1000 μm. This is important to the packaging line, since if the creases are not correct and do not assist the carton erection, the cartoning machine will not function correctly.

17 Cobb test: BS EN 20535 1991 ISO 535 1991 for water absorbency. This measures the mass of water absorbed by 1 m^2 of the test piece in a specified time under a head of 1 cm of water. It is determined by weighing before and after exposure to the water, and usually quoted in g/m^2.

18 Rub resistance: BS 3110:1959 (94). This is the resistance of a printed test piece to withstand rubbing against either another similar printed test piece or against a plain test specimen. The objective is to see that the ink/print has cured and will not scuff or smear in service.

19 Pick test: BS 6225:1982 (95) ISO 3782, 3783; also called the IGT test (Instituut Voor-Grafische Technical TNO Amsterdam). It is a small printing unit which allows one to print a small strip of paper under controlled conditions. A specified amount of a special oil is added to the printing system and printed onto the test piece. The surface is then examined for signs of disruption (otherwise known as 'pick' in the trade). Results are correlated from a time calibration table. It is essential that the paper surface does not pick when printed, as pick means that some of the deposited ink may be lost from the surface, and in extreme cases the paper surface may start 'dusting'. This means that the sizes and binding agents are not working and the fines of the fillers and opacifiers are loose on the paper surface.

20 pH, chloride or sulphate by BS 2924:1992 Parts 1–4, ISO 6588, 6587, 9898, 9197 or DEF STD 81–1. These factors are tested on a aqueous extract of the test piece. The acidity or alkalinity (pH) can help the life of the paper or board, as the natural pulp is slightly acidic and goes dusty and powdery in 50–70 years. Most papers today are neutral. Sulphates should be >20 mg/kg of sample and chlorides can vary with the cleaning processes of the pulp. The conductivity of the test piece can be also be determined in the aqueous extracts.

21 Roughness/smoothness: BS 4420:1990 (95) ISO 8791 (Bendtsen) or BS 6563:1985 (90) (Parker Printsurf). This is a measure of the extent to which a paper or board surface deviates from a plane and involves the depth, width and number of departures from that plane. This is very important for the 'printability' of the paper.

22 Brightness to BS 4432:1980 Parts 1–4 (95) ISO 2469, 2470, 2471. This is the reflectance factor measured at the effective wavelength of 457 nm with a reflectometer having specified BS characteristics. Note again that this might be quoted with a manufacturers name behind it, e.g. Technibrit.

23 Opacity to BS 4432:1980 Parts 1 and 2 (95) ISO 3688. This is the ratio, expressed as a percentage, of the luminous reflectance factor of a single sheet of the paper with a black backing to the intrinsic luminous reflectance factor of a layer, or pad, of the same paper which is thick enough to be opaque.

24 Dennison wax test. This is an older test that was largely replaced by the IGT test, but is still used by some older paper and board mills. It consists of a series of specialised waxes, which are heated to a specified temperature, placed on the paper surface, left to cool, then removed. The wax formula 'picks' dust and debris from the surface, and the wax formula number that shows the picking indicates the degree of ink viscosity (or stickiness) that the particular paper will tolerate without risk to the print.

25 Wet burst strength: BS 2922 (PT1):1985 (95) ISO 3689. This is used for determining the wet bursting strength of any paper or board following immersion in water.

26 Wet tensile strength: BS 2922 (PT2):1984 (95) ISO 3781. This is a method of determining the wet tensile strength of any paper or board after immersion in water.

27 Ash in paper and board: BS 3631:1984 (94) ISO 2144. This is a method of determining the ash content (i.e. the inorganic matter left after controlled combustion) in paper and board. The method is suitable for most loading materials and coating pigments.

28 Detection and estimation of nitrogenous agents in paper: BS 4497:1969 (93). This standard describes the problems involved with the nitrogenous treating agents for paper and gives qualitative and quantitative methods for use with certain agents used in paper treatment. It applies only to substances that have a strong affinity for acid dyes.

29 Ink absorbency: BS 4574:1970 (91). This gives recommendations for the determination of the ink absorbency of paper and board by K & N ink. Applies to both paper and boards to be printed by the litho gravure or letterpress process.

Appendix 5.3: Specific tests for cartons

1 Compression to BS 4826 (PT3):1986 ISO 2234. This standard lists three methods which can be used to assess the strength of the erected package, thereby estimating the degree of protection that it confers on the contents. This is particularly useful for products with no inherent strength in one plane or another, e.g. strip packs.

2 Carton opening force. The method that is often used is to hold the flat carton, as delivered, by its creases between thumb and first finger and press. The carton should spring open into the 'square' position without a need for unreasonable force. If the carton does not spring open, or buckles in on itself, then it is reasonable to assume that those particular cartons will cause problems on any cartoning machine. This can be measured by instrumentation.

3 Coefficient of friction: BS 2782 (PT2):1983 method 824A or ASTM D1894. Both the static and kinetic coefficients of friction are determined by sliding the specimen over itself under specific test conditions. As discussed earlier, the finish of board can differ dramatically. Compare a corrugated case with a test liner and with a Kraft liner, or a cast coated or varnished carton with an uncoated carton. Where machines are involved there could be problems with different coefficients of friction, since friction is used as part of the control on carton and corrugated case erecting machines.

4 Crease stiffness: BS 6965:1988 (94). Also called the crease recovery test. This involves testing a carton board piece and folding it through 90°. It will then try to recover its former position when the bending force is removed. The increase or decrease in the inherent board stiffness after folding is measured. As with all tests involving forces, the test should be performed both along and across the grain.

5 Joint shear strength: BS 5350 Part C5 1990. This is a method of testing the glued lap seam on the side of a carton for strength of the adhesive, using a tensile testing machine. This quantity is important in ensuring that the correct adhesive for the cartonboard finish has been used, and in the right quantity. Another problem that frequently occurs is skewed lap seams. This means that the carton is out of true, and will not erect on a machine.

Appendix 5.4: Specific tests for corrugated

1   Flat crush resistance test for corrugated board: BS EN23035:1994 ISO 3055 1982. This only applies to single wall and single faced corrugated. Test pieces are placed perpendicular to the paper surface between two platens, which move together until the fluting collapses. Measure the maximum force obtained.

2   Edge crush test for corrugated board: BS 6063:1992 ISO 4097. A rectangular test piece of corrugated FBB is placed between the platens of a crush tester with the fluting perpendicular to the platens. Compress until failure, measuring the maximum force. Useful in assessing stacking strength

3   Ring crush test (corrugated): TAPPI T818 1987. A compressive force is exerted on a specimen, held in a ring form in a special jig and placed between two platens of a compression machine. The upper platen approaches the lower platen at a uniform speed, until the specimen collapses. This correlates with the edgewise compression strength of the paperboard or fluted medium.

4   Flat crush of corrugating medium (Concora test): BS EN:ISO 7263 1995. Paper is fluted by passing between heated rollers and then formed as a single faced corrugated board using a pressure sensitive tape as the liner. A crushing force, perpendicular to plane of the paper, is applied and measured at the point in time the paper crushes.

5   The specific apparatus and detailed procedures for the measurement of corrugated board caliper are contained in BS 4817:1972 (93) ISO 3034. This obviously differs from the other methods already described in that the corrugations could be crushed when using calipers or any other form of measuring equipment.

6

GLASS CONTAINERS

D. A. Dean

Introduction

Glass is believed to have been first discovered around 3000 BC in the East Mediterranean. It has been established that hollow glassware existed in Egypt around 1500 BC and was made by the sand core method. A core or clay was attached to the end of a metal rod then coated either by dipping into molten glass or by winding threads of molten glass around it. The vessel was then reheated and made smooth by marvering, i.e. rolling on a flat surface. Even in those ancient times such containers were used for ointments, perfumes and cosmetics, but due to the restricted availability they were only used by the extremely rich. The sand core method was supplemented by the pressing of bowl shapes, until true glass blowing was invented in the first century BC. Early glass blowers were the Egyptians, Syrians and Jews based at Sidon. With the emigration of Syrians and Jews, glassworks gradually became established throughout Europe. Thus as glass expanded, so did its use for pharmaceuticals.

Glass has served the pharmaceutical and cosmetic industries as an effective container for many centuries, and particularly during the past 100 years. Some 40 years ago, with the advent of plastic containers, glass was virtually condemned as an obsolete material and a rapid decline in its use was forecast by the plastics salespersons. Since then in an expanding packaging era both glass and plastic have enjoyed a period of increasing usage, at first in direct competition with one another, but now reaching a state of association and union (in the form of plastic-coated glass bottles and glass composite packs). Also, glass would not have become such a universal container for pharmaceuticals had the plastic closure not been available.

In 1969 approximately 14% of blown glass containers were supplied to the pharmaceutical and toiletry industries (9.2% and 5% respectively); in 1971 this reduced to 11% (7.3% and 3.5% respectively), in spite of an increase in total production. The major users were the food, beverage, beer and spirit industries. Although the use of glass again dropped in the late 1980s, this trend generally reversed in the early 1990s. Part of this is attributed to the popularity of bottle banks and the belief by the general public that glass is a more 'friendly' material. In the same period, coatings on glass have improved the colour range options and general strength, coupled to further light weighting.

The fact that glass has been so successful for such a long period reflects not only the fact that it was discovered before other materials but also that it still meets most of the requirements of a modern packaging material. Glass is economical, can be handled at high speeds on production lines, is inert (thus giving excellent product–pack compatibility), and provides good product presentation (clarity, sparkle, design) and good product protection. Early limitations in the use of glass were associated with the production process and difficulties in finding a fully satisfactory closure system.

Glass could be defined as the original plastic material in that it closely resembles a thermoplastic. It is softened by heat, capable of being fashioned in a mould, and can be reheated and remoulded into another shape many times with little deterioration. However, glass is inorganic in origin, whereas plastics are organic.

Both the earlier glasses and today's major usage are based on soda glass, which is a product of the fusion of sand, soda ash and limestone, hence the name soda or alkali glass.

Early uses of glass included the preservation of food. In 1805 Nicholas Appert in France showed that heat would preserve foods by arresting their natural tendency to spoil. For this he recommended glass containers closed with long corks. Usage was, however, restricted due to poor processing techniques and the variability of closures. In 1858 an American, John Landis Mason, invented a screw-topped jar which was subsequently used by housewives. Domestic food-preserving jars are frequently known as Mason jars. The cost of the closure and method of handling did not make fuller commercial usage worth while. Louis Pasteur in the 1860s explained the spoilage of foodstuffs by micro-organisms, how they could be destroyed by heat and the product preserved by the use of air-tight containers. He too used glass containers, but also had problems with the closures.

One of the first bottle-making machines, invented in 1882 by Phillip Arbogart, was based on a press and blow technique. With the development of further ideas at the beginning of the twentieth century, improved closures soon appeared. The roll-on closure was invented in 1923 and the pry-off cap in 1926. However, the cork reigned supreme for many years in both waxed and unwaxed forms. Ground glass stoppers were also very popular at one time, each bottle bearing its own stopper which had been individually ground into the neck, thus assuring a good fit. The medicine bottle, as such, probably first came into regular use as a narrow-necked glass vial for liquids.

Bottles for general use became known by their shape, i.e. rounds, ovals, panels, hexagonals and flats. Others bore special names such as Winchesters, corbyns, ampoules, vials, Mexicans and carboys.

Composition of glass and types

The exact structure of glass is not clearly known. It can be formed by mixing together various inorganic substances which on heating give a homogeneous molten mass. On cooling this does not arrange itself into crystal pattern but becomes a super-cooled liquid in which ultimately the state of flow has ceased to exist. When most liquids cool, the transition from a liquid to a solid state occurs abruptly at a specific temperature with the simultaneous evolution of heat. This freezing process depends on the formulation of crystal nuclei. However, certain liquids increase in viscosity with cooling and this hinders the formation of nuclei. Since, in the case of glass, nuclei are not formed, it remains in a super-cooled state until a solid state is reached. The properties may be varied according to the raw materials used. Sand, which is the main ingredient and consists mostly of silicon dioxide, requires very high melting temperatures (1700°C+). If certain fluxing agents such as soda ash (sodium carbonate) are added, the melting temperature reduces to around 800°C but the resulting substance, widely known as water glass (Na_2SiO_3), is soluble in water. If a stabiliser such as limestone ($CaCO_3$) is added, conventional (insoluble) glass is obtained. Normal alkali glass is basically fifteen parts sand, five parts soda ash and four parts limestone – the mixture being heated to about 1500°C. At this temperature the three ingredients gradually react. To help melting, cullet or broken glass (of the same type) is added to the basic raw materials. Early glasses had a green tinge due to the presence of iron. Today virtually colourless glass is produced by using decolourisers such as selenium or cobalt oxide. For each 10% of cullet added, energy (heat) can be reduced by approximately 2.5%.

Compared to plastics, glass additives cover fewer purposes, i.e. colourants, opacifiers, decolourisers, modifiers, and stabilisers. Certain additional technical ingredients may be employed, e.g. alumina to improve durability. Coloured glass may be obtained by solution (glass acts as a solvent for certain oxides) or by colloidal dispersion: the following are examples.

- *Amber:* May vary from light yellowish to deep reddish brown. Obtained by the addition of carbon and sulphur or iron and manganese dioxide.
- *Yellow:* Compounds of cadmium and sulphur.
- *Blue:* Various shades of blue, cobalt oxide or occasionally copper (cupric) oxide.
- *Green:* A range of greens can be achieved by varying additions of iron oxide, manganese dioxide and chromium dioxide. Actinic green is the name usually given for glass of a bright emerald green which absorbs the ultraviolet wavelength of light.
- *Opal:* Involves fluorides or phosphates.

Although most glasses are coloured in the main melt, it is possible to add the colourisers as a frit at the feeder conditioning stage prior to extrusion as gobs into the glass blowing unit. This obviously gives greater flexibility in allowing additional colours to be produced, but the resultant cullet frequently cannot be reused (coloured cullet can only be used to produce containers of the same or similar colour). Normally a glass furnace has an expected life of 8–10 years and will run most economically on one colour. Frequent changes from one colour to another can obviously cause lengthy and costly downtime – for this reason unusual colours made by a continuous batch process will be more costly to produce.

Three types of furnace are in use: regenerative, recuperative and unit melters. The last, while cheaper to install and easier to maintain, with shorter downtime on colour changes, is more expensive on fuel. Regenerative furnaces are in the majority.

Several types of container glass are generally recognised:

- type I – neutral, a boro-silicate type glass
- type II – soda glass with a surface treatment
- type III – soda glass of limited alkalinity
- NP – soda glass (non-parenteral usage) or European type IV.

Colourless white flint soda glass has the following composition range: silica (SiO_2)

59–75%, calcium oxide (CaO) 5–12%, sodium oxide (Na_2O) 12–17%, alumina (Al_2O_3) 0.5–3.0%, and possibly small quantities of ferric oxide, titanium dioxide, potassium and magnesium oxide.

Type I glass

Neutral or borosilicate type glass has the following composition range: silica (SiO_2) 66–72% alumina (Al_2O_3) 4–10%, sodium oxide (Na_2O) or potassium oxide (K_2O) 7–10%, boric oxide (B_2O_3) 9–11%, calcium oxide (CaO) 1–5%, barium oxide (BaO) 0–3.0%, and possibly small quantities of magnesium oxide, ferric oxide and titanium dioxide.

These types of glass require a higher working temperature, have a narrower working range and hence are more difficult to process (1700–1750 °C). Borosilicate glasses with high boric oxide contents (over 12%) show reduced chemical resistance, and are more prone to atmospheric weathering. Type I surface treated glass is also available with certain smaller tubular containers.

Type II glass

This is a soda glass which has had the surface treated, usually by a process of sulphating or sulphuring. In the former a pellet of ammonium sulphate is dropped into each bottle before it passes passes through a heated tunnel known as the lehr. This then sublimes and coats the inside of the glass. Sulphuring usually involves sulphur dioxide being injected into the container while it is within the lehr. Evidence suggests that the ammonium sulphate process confers better resistance than sulphuring.

In all these treatments the excess surface alkalinity is neutralised by forming a coating of sodium sulphate which is soluble in water. All treated containers must therefore be washed prior to use in order to remove the soluble coating which shows a 'bloom'.

Other surface treatments

Various surface treatments are now in use for improving surface lubricity, reducing damage by impact, or giving additional decorative effects.

Surface lubricity can be improved by the use of silicone coatings (it also assists drainage from the container) and hot/cold end treatments. The latter operate at the beginning (hot end) and the end of the lehr (cold end) and can involve titanium dioxide, tin tetrachloride at the hot end and waxes, waxes in combination with polyethylene, oleic acid, polyethylene glycol, stearates, etc., at the cold end. Currently tin tetrachloride is the most popular hot end treatment being applied from bottom up or neck downwards, with the latter being more likely to give some internal contamination. These coatings generally provide greater slip in their role as lubricity coatings.

Other inorganic and organic treatments are available. In one Japanese process, surface sodium ions are replaced by surface potassium ions in the molecular structure of the glass. Organic coatings include various polymers – surlyn, polyurethene, etc., – or the direct application of plastic sleeves as shrink or stretch wraps (PVC, PP, PET, LLDPE, etc.) at the glass manufacturing site. All these processes can reduce surface damage and maintain bottle strength and/or be used to add decorative designs, colour, etc. It should be noted that coatings cannot fully replace either poor glass distributions or bad design. A more recent inorganic coating involves silica. A special finish coating is required where an induction sealed diaphragm is to be employed.

Selective coating to improve the image of glass seems assured. By such techniques and good design, Japan has already produced cylindrical containers of half the weight and twice the strength of those previously available, but at a relatively high cost.

Properties

Glass shows a high degree of chemical inertness in that hydrofluoric acid is the only substance which appreciably attacks it. Instances of surface attack which can lead to the detachment of 'flakes' are few. This can occur with type I, alkali or treated glass either after autoclaving or on long-term storage in contact with certain inorganic alkali salts such as sodium citrate, tartrate, phosphate or saline solutions. Alkali glass, as indicated by its name, can give up alkali to aqueous solutions and can therefore affect either suspended or dissolved substances. For instance, the amount of sodium extracted from 100 cm^2 of glass varies according to temperature, i.e. 5 mg extracted after approx. 6 months at 20°C or 120°C for approx. 1 h. Some of the factors which influence the degree of chemical attack on glass are:

1   chemical composition of the glass
2   temperature of attacking agent
3   time in contact
4   previous history (e.g. weathered glass is more prone to attack).

Salts of sodium, potassium, calcium and magnesium can be extracted in small quantities – usually ppm (this passes EU extractive tests with reference to food contact).

In certain instances the use of neutral glass becomes essential – ordinary insulin was quoted as a prime example where pH control is critical. Neutral glass is far more resistant to chemical attack. Treated neutral glass is also available.

Glass is completely impermeable to all gases, solutions and solvents. It has a high degree of transparency when clear but can, in either amber or selected green shades, offer good resistance to the passage of UV light. Amber glass will show the greater absorbance of IR rays (see USP XXIII)

Soda glass has a density of 2.5 and borosilicate glass 2.25. Hence it is lighter than most metals. Its rigidity and ability to withstand top weight (i.e. stacking) is particularly good. The same rigidity and strength make it capable of withstanding internal as well as external pressures. Heat resistance and a high melting point make it a material suitable for both moist and dry sterilisation. Borosilicate glasses are particularly good against thermal shock. Soda glass is quite suitable for hot filling operations providing attention is paid to design, container size and the temperature difference (see thermal shock testing, pp. 231, 260) (coefficient of thermal expansion is three times greater for soda glass than for borosilicate glass).

The smoothness of a glass surface makes cleaning easy and generally restricts surface damaging, scratching or bruising to an acceptable level. The weakness of glass relates to the fact that a glass is only as strong as its skin. Surface damage (usually traced to minute fissures) can cause significant reduction in its strength which is readily

a Semi-automatic

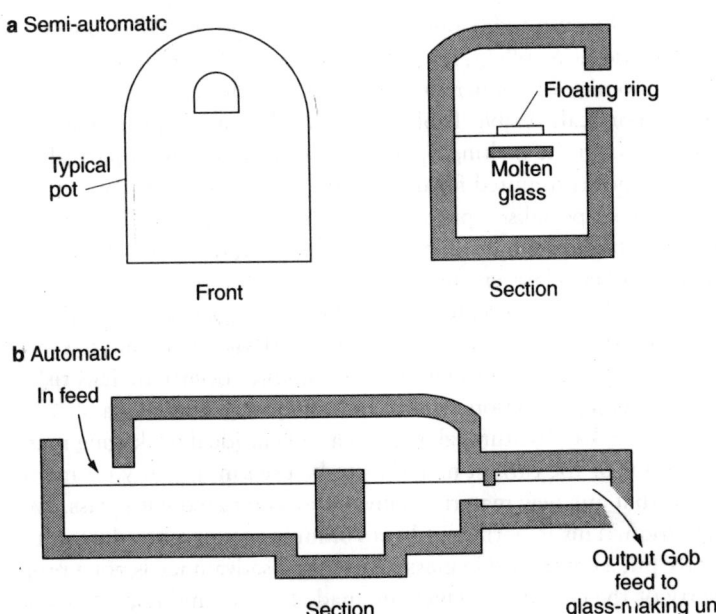

Front   Section

b Automatic

Figure 6.1 Melting tanks

shown by internal pressure testing. Strength based on bursting tests on new, delivered and used bottles have shown a ratio of 7:4:3 – i.e. a steady reduction. Glass-to-glass contact or glass in contact with harder materials must therefore be minimised. If the surface of a glass can be increased in lubricity or slip, then impact damage can be reduced and its strength maintained by the use of the coatings previously mentioned. Glass is basically a strong material (20 × steel) but it ends up with approx. 1% of its original theoretical strength. Glass is strong in compression but weaker in tension.

Glass also presents low microbiological risk both as delivered and after storage. Glass is therefore a rigid, inert container which will generally withstand the rigours of handling, filling, closuring and use, and if required for reuse can be easily recleaned. Its weight and stability with the right designs enables extremely high-speed processing through a plant (speeds in excess of 1000/min are achieved in the food industry). In terms of basic cost of raw materials, soda glass is relatively cheap but the energy processing cost (1500°C) is high when compared with the competitive plastics. In total energy (i.e. the energy needed to collect and convert the raw materials to a finished product), glass is favourable in comparison to other materials. However, the cost of setting up a glass blow moulding facility is very high (£30 million plus). Glass containers need an extra process known as annealing – the container is reheated to dull red heat and then cooled under controlled conditions in a lehr, whereby 'setting' strains are minimised. Annealing temperatures are around 560°C for soda glass and 580°C for borosilicate glass. Strains basically arise when the inner and outer surfaces of glass cool at different rates and the hotter surface is in compression and the colder surface in tension.

Providing a satisfactory closure rarely presents a problem if conventional practices are followed. Pourability is generally good and special screw-threaded finishes with pourer lips are available, but these add to bottle and cap costs.

With any packaging material in use today one must also consider its effect on life in terms of disposability, pollution, recycling, etc. and the possible drain on natural resources. Although the economics of total reuse present some difficulties, the partial recovery of glass remains economically viable. Broken glass (of the same type) or cullet, as it is known, considerably assists in the melting operation and is an essential part of the manufacturing process. Glass not committed for direct reuse or recycling can be satisfactorily used for land fill or other specialised purposes. At this point the obvious hazard associated with glass must be emphasised. It can be easily shattered, fractured and broken by sharp impacts, and the broken glass creates severe hazards for people or animals. Although this hazard has generally been accepted, one still has to recognise that a splinter of glass found in a product must be considered an extremely serious complaint, irrespective of how the product is likely to be used or how the glass splinter occurred. This risk is ever-present even if every apparent precaution is taken to avoid it (e.g. coated glass).

Apart from its weight and breakage feature, glass rates as a near ideal packaging material. This fact, plus it being one of the earliest materials to be used in quantity for manufacturing containers, means that any new material is invariably compared with glass, even when not in direct competition. This is borne out by a common testing procedure in the pharmaceutical industry to 'put a control on in glass'. Another disadvantage is not a property of glass but a property of the containers which are made from it, and relates to storage. Glass containers store air and are generally more expensive than most competitive materials for warehousing. Whereas plastic containers can be made immediately prior to filling or consecutively by a form fill seal process, this type of operation is virtually impossible with glass due to the cost and the type of manufacturing processes employed.

One final feature which has caused comment is the weight of glass containers. Thus there have been consistent efforts over the past 25 years to 'light' or 'right' weight most containers. This has been achieved by combinations of design, the processing machinery, and computer-aided design and manufacture (CAD/CAM). However, not all designs can be reduced in weight and in more angular shapes this is neither practical nor critical. In fact the solid feel of the pack may be an asset. Glass is, as indicated earlier, a strong material which is readily weakened by surface damage. The advent of the extremely thin walled container with a plastic covering or skin shows that a marriage has been achieved between two apparently competitive materials.

Manufacturing processes

Glass containers can be fabricated by certain basic processes:

1 blown glassware based on either press and blow or blow and blow principles
2 tubular glassware – a tube of glass is first produced and subsequently cut and shaped (after reheating) by a separate process
3 pressed glassware – rarely used for packaging containers.

Blown glass

This can be produced on automatic or semi-automatic equipment or can be handmade. Manual blowing of containers is still used on a limited scale for specialised ware, and is not covered here.

Few bottles are now made by the semi-automatic process but it is used for limited quantities of specialised ware. As it employs a basic team of three or four persons, the work is very labour-intensive with a low output speed. A pot furnace supplies the molten glass and each team is fed by a 'gatherer' who is highly skilled at lifting out the right amount of glass (gob) on a metal gathering iron. This glass is allowed to gravity feed from the iron into a parison mould, the glass gob being cut with metal shears. The parison is blown to shape and then transferred to a finishing mould where it is blown into the final design. It is then taken to a lehr for annealing. Semi-automatically made containers cannot be fully light weighted. The process is otherwise similar to that used in a fully automatic blow and blow process. The cost for semi-autoware can be five to ten times greater than a similar bottle made by the fully automatic process. Automatic glass making machines are supplied from a tank furnace. These usually have a capacity of up to 300 t (1 day's processing) and are continuously supplied with the mixed ingredients at the infeed/melting end and deliver accurately sheared gobs to the glass blowing machine at the other end (see Figure 6.1).

In the blow and blow process the gob is dropped into an open blank or parison mould. The neck is formed by top blow and then the parison or blank is blown from the base (Figure 6.2). The blank shape supported by the transfer ring is then transferred to the finishing mould where it is blown into the final shape. This blow and blow process is the major process employed – usually with IS (i.e. independent or individual section) machinery. Other machines include Roirant R7, S10 and Lynch 44. IS machines may have 4, 5, 6, 8, 10 or 12 stations. For small containers double, triple or quadruple gobbing may be employed. The last can give speeds of over 400 containers per minute.

Alternatively a press and blow process may be used for wide-mouthed (and now certain narrow-necked) containers. The first stage is a gob feed into a mould which is followed by a plunger descending or ascending to form both the neck finish (at end) and the parison shape. As in the blow and blow process, the blank is then transferred to a finishing mould where it is blown into the final shape (Figure 6.3).

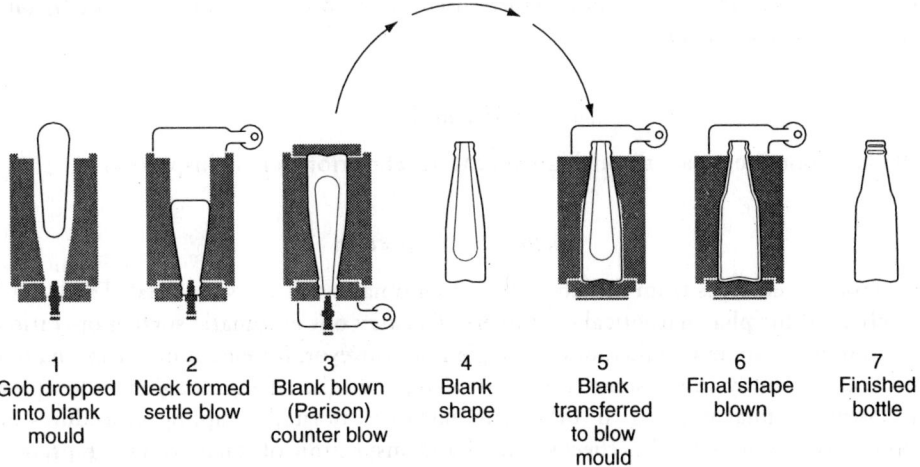

1	2	3	4	5	6	7
Gob dropped into blank mould	Neck formed settle blow	Blank blown (Parison) counter blow	Blank shape	Blank transferred to blow mould	Final shape blown	Finished bottle

Figure 6.2 The blow and blow process (bottles)

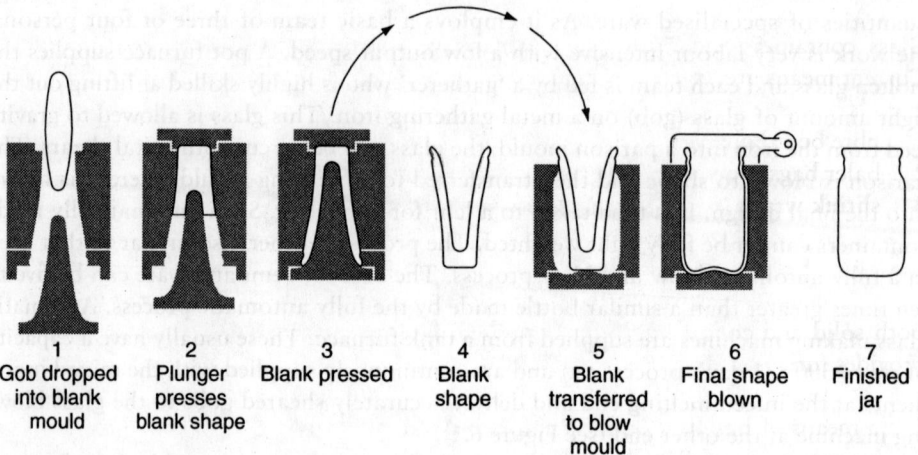

Figure 6.3 The press and blow process (jars)

Press and blow processes have recently found new applications for narrow-necked containers resulting in up to 25% further light weighting on cylindrical containers, i.e. pharmaceutical 100 ml cylindrical rounds (90+ g reduced to less than 70 g).

Pressed glassware involves only the first stage of the above process, the final shape being achieved by one pressing of the glass which is entrapped and shaped between the mould walls and the plunger. All automatic glass producing processes operate around the clock, for approximately 360 days per year.

Borosilicate type glasses are more difficult to produce on conventional glass making equipment (than soda glass), because they are inherently tougher and have both a high working temperature and a narrowed working temperature range, hence production rates are lower with higher rejection levels. This further increases the container cost as base material is already higher than soda glass, and is the main reason why larger neutral glass containers are not more widely used. Treated glass containers (type II) form an economical substitute.

Annealing

All glass containers pass through an annealing lehr prior to final inspection.

Sorting and inspection

As glassware emerges from the lehr, hand or automatic sorting is required. The latter is widely used for pharmaceutical containers. To carry out automatic sorting operations the containers are marshalled onto a single line conveyor, for electronic or mechanical checking for body dimensions, bore, visual damage (i.e. using imaging techniques), etc., prior to final packing. In other circumstances normal sampling procedures are applied for laboratory QC checks, plus hand inspection of each container prior to packing. The sorting area is usually screened from the dirtier manufacturing process, and is under positive air pressure in order to assist cleanliness.

Outer packaging

Glass containers were supplied for many years in open returnable wooden crates. Current means are:

1 fibre board outers
2 baler bags (now in limited use)
3 shrink wraps (palletised).

Fibreboard outers/baler bags/shrunk wraps

Both solid and corrugated board are used, but the latter is more common. An outer provides for:

1 a means of handling, identification and transportation
2 storage of empty bottles and maintaining them in a clean state
3 protection against journey hazards
4 suitable unloading onto a production line.

For handling and stacking, a brick shape giving a ratio of $3:1.5:1$ is ideal. H tape or single strip sealing is usually applied to the top case flaps to exclude dirt and dust. The base flaps are less firmly closed, as it is often necessary to deposit the containers at the beginning of a production line by opening the base flaps. The bottles are usually inverted in the outers.

However, fibreboard has been criticised because of loose fibres. Baler bags received favourable publicity a few years ago but found rather limited use against the more competitive shrink wrapping systems. Shrink wraps as sleeves or overwraps may be used around complete pallet loads or small unit quantities. In the case of wrapped pallet loads the bottles may be separated with layer pads. On smaller quantities, bottles may be trayed or left without additional support (i.e. direct shrink wrap). Again the pallet may have a full shrink wrap to give added security and protection, and this is now the preferred method of packing.

Tubular glassware

'Cane' for tubular glassware may be made by one of two processes – Danner and Vello. Danner was the earlier process but is not detailed here, since it has been largely replaced by the faster Vello system. Both can produce 'cane' in soda or neutral glass.

Vello process

Glass flows from a forehearth into a bowl or reservoir in which a hollow bell-shaped mandrel rotates in a ring which allows the glass to flow via the annular space to give a continuously emerging tube. Blowing air is fed via the end of the bell where there is a hollow tip. The dimensions of the tubing are controlled by the glass temperature, the rate of draw, the clearance between the bell and the ring, rate of draw-off, and the pressure of the blowing air.

During the process the tubing is gauged, classified for use, and cut into lengths. In subsequent production the tubing may be used in a horizontal or vertical plane. The latter is currently more popular.

Containers are made by flame cutting the tube to length, flaming and shaping each end. The containers are subsequently annealed.

Due to these processes producing greater control on the side wall thickness, tubular glass containers can be made with very thin sections and of a much lighter weight than blown glass ware. Ampoules, vials, cartridge tubes and prefilled syringes all indicate the capabilities of the tubular process. In their initial use ampoules were followed by vials, originally for oral products (tablets) and then for multidose injections (Figure 6.4).

More recently glass disposable and prefilled syringes, mix-o-vials, etc. have extended the use of tubular glass. In general neutral glass is more widely used. This can be twice the price of soda glass but annealing is less critical, although still essential.

The physical cutting of tubular glass gives rise to glass particles, which also occur when any type of glass ampoule is opened. In the case of glass particle contamination in containers made from tubular glass there are various methods for reduction or elimination, i.e. high-pressure air blowing, high-pressure water washing, each with or without ultrasonics, and heating to dull red heat (during annealing) to fuse the glass fragments to the walls of the container.

Tubular glass containers are made in neutral type I, surface treated type I glass, soda glass, etc., and may also be siliconised as a separate process after manufacture. Surface treated type I glass is occasionally necessary in smaller containers, where now and then a sample fails the neutral glass test.

Design and decoration

The design of any container involves two basic considerations – aesthetic appeal and functional efficiency. With an established type of product, designs either follow tradition or endeavour to break from it in the hope that a new association can be created. Size impression frequently dictates design limitations such as a big looker, bigger than x approach. So often the requirements of appeal and functional efficiency are conflicting in the extreme: Functional efficiency can be applied to many aspects, i.e. delivery to factory, production line (stability, handling speed), closuring, packing, warehousing, and finally stability at point of sale and consumer convenience. If taken to the extreme, the basic alternatives appear to be round or square sectioned containers, the former for general ease of handling and strength and the latter for the maximising of space. The compromise is a square or rectangular bottle with well radiused edges, an in sweep at the base, and an even taper from the body to the neck finish, e.g. a modern rectangular tablet bottle. The relative strength of various shapes is of the following order: circular 10, oval 5, square with radiused corners 2.5, square with sharp corners 1. Thinning, which may occur in a square-cornered container, is indicated in Figure 6.5.

From these general observations one can identify basic guidelines.

As glass is weakened by surface damage, designs which lead to point to point contact (Figure 6.6) are particularly susceptible to damage if handled on conveyor belts. If the areas of contact can be spread over greater areas there is less risk of damage (Figure 6.7). Designs must also aim at providing a uniform wall section and avoiding

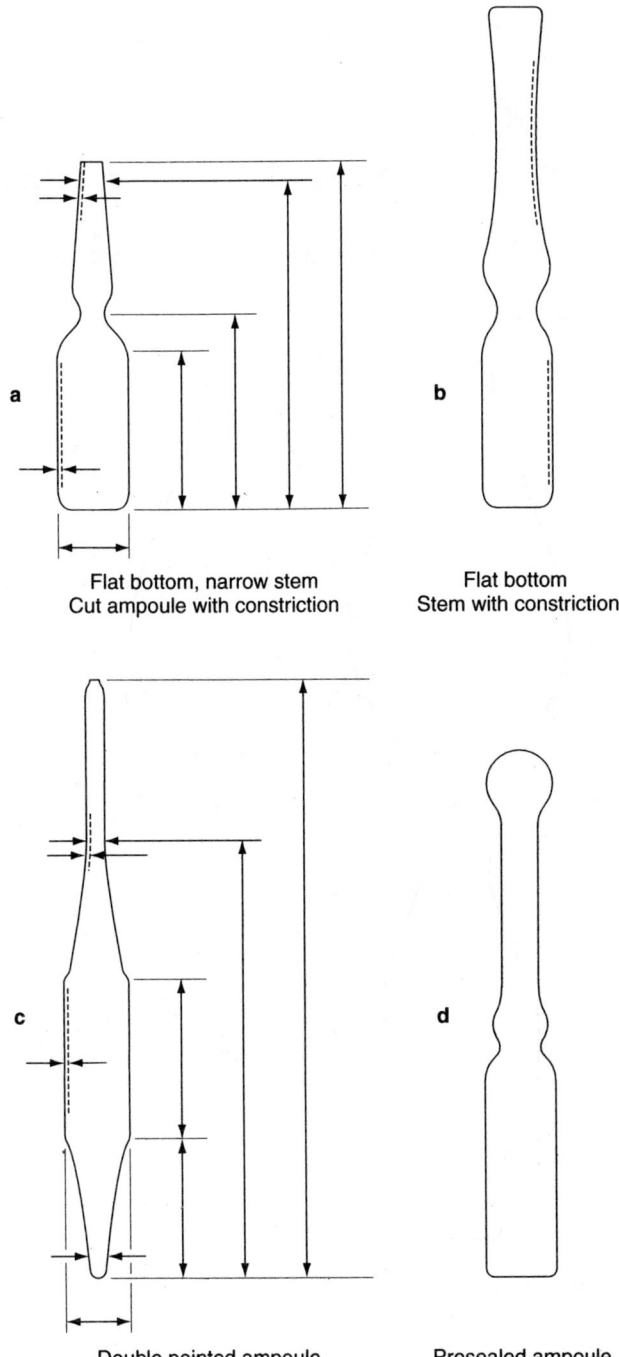

a — Flat bottom, narrow stem
Cut ampoule with constriction

b — Flat bottom
Stem with constriction

c — Double pointed ampoule

d — Presealed ampoule

Figure 6.4 Ampoules

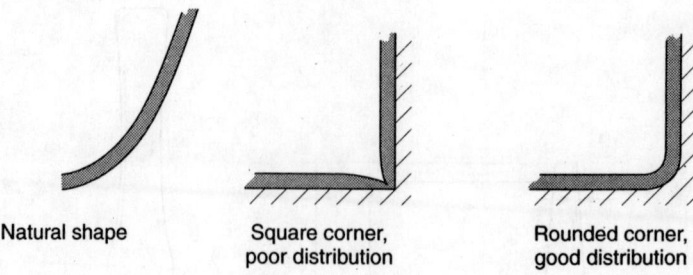

Natural shape   Square corner,   Rounded corner,
poor distribution   good distribution

Figure 6.5 Glass distribution

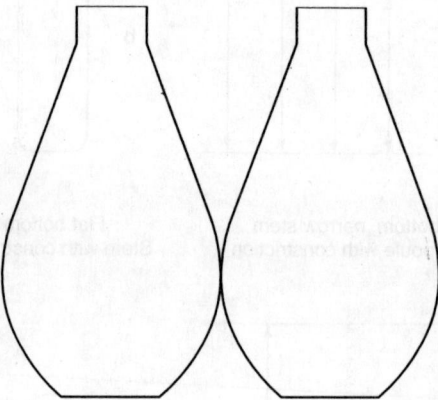

Figure 6.6 Avoid point to point contact

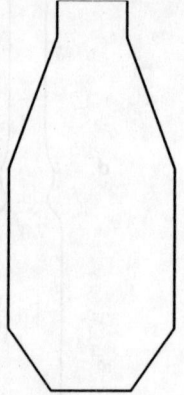

Figure 6.7 Good contact area

thick and thin areas which offer points of weakness in use and areas of extra strain through cooling differentials. Even distribution depends on the design of both the final shape and the parison mould.

Square sections should be avoided whenever possible. This can be achieved by consideration of a suitable radius – see Figure 6.5. At the base of the bottle one has to reach a compromise between maximum stability (a broad wide base with near square edges) or optimum glass distribution with a 'drawn in foot' which naturally reduces the total base area.

Stippling of the base is useful in improving base grip, masking mould scars and improving the strength of the container. Damage to individual stipples does not normally lead to surface weakening as the strength (and surface which may be weakened by damage) lies in the plane at the base of the stipples. Similarly, the neck of the bottle should avoid sharp changes in direction, preferably utilising gradual slopes and incorporating adequate radii.

The ability for a neck to accept a vertical load is shown in Figure 6.8. High stacking strength is a recognised feature with glass.

Large flat surfaces should be avoided as these tend to sink during the cooling of the glass and may give rise to labelling and capacity problems. A large radius should therefore be used, as exemplified by Figure 6.9.

A bottle must be designed to be removed from or clear the mould. This can be illustrated by taking a bottle of rectangular section as shown in Figure 6.10. It is apparent that the mould fouls the edges A and B as it opens. In this case the bottle manufacturer

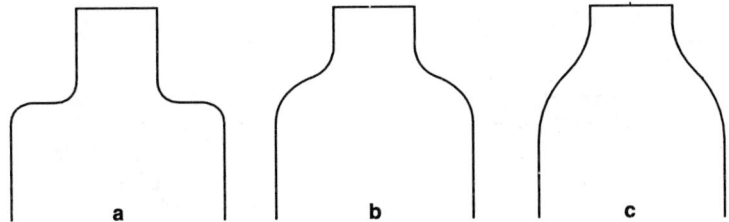

a   **b**   **c**

Figure 6.8 Neck/shoulder design: capable of accepting vertical load of (a) 500 lb/in^2, (b) 4,000 lb/in^2, (c) 10,000 lb/in^2

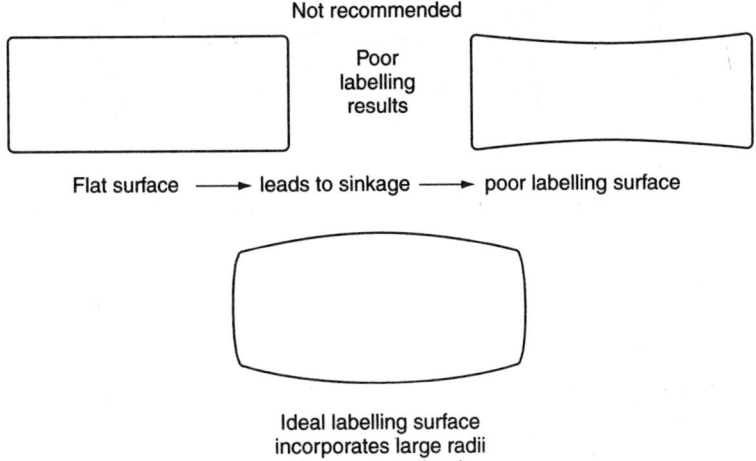

Not recommended

Poor labelling results

Flat surface ⟶ leads to sinkage ⟶ poor labelling surface

Ideal labelling surface
incorporates large radii
(converse surface)

Figure 6.9 Labelling surfaces

will arrange the mould as shown in (c), where the part lines are diagonally across the bottle. While this would produce a satisfactory bottle, it is better avoided as adjacent parts of the mould are not symmetrical, and can lead to uneven mould wear. This problem could be overcome with the rectangular shape by radiusing the ends of the bottle as shown in (d) where a symmetrical mould can be used.

In a more complicated bottle as in Figure 6.11, neither a diagonal part line nor an asymmetrical shape is avoidable.

Embossing of a bottle, such as that employed on intravenous solution containers, can induce stretch lines, but the correct use of radii can minimise the problem (which tends to be visual rather than a point of mechanical weakness). The height of the embossing should be kept at a minimum – usually around 0.4–0.75 mm. This feature of the bottle clearing the mould can easily be overlooked and however good a design is, it fails if the bottle cannot be made! Bottles may also have debossed areas, e.g. to take a hanging harness.

Examples of improving a design are given in Figure 6.12, which shows an old and an updated Winchester. Not only has strength been increased and light weighting

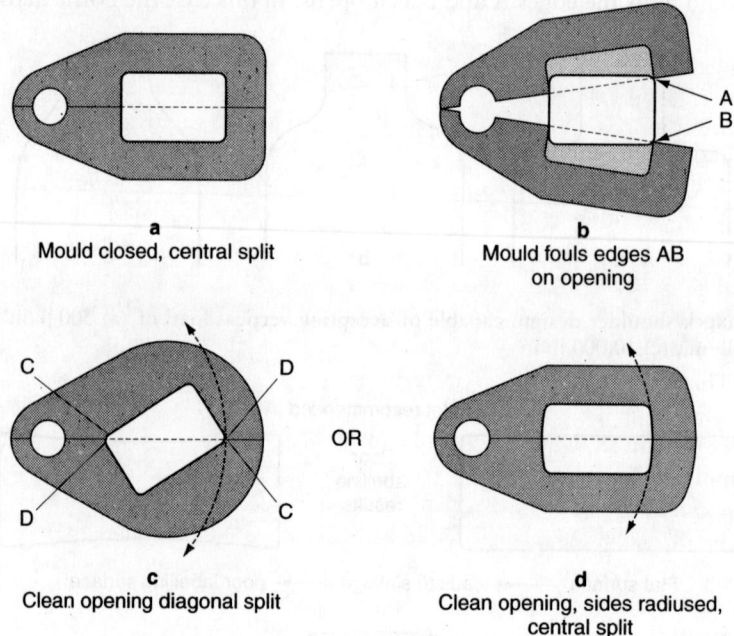

a
Mould closed, central split

b
Mould fouls edges AB
on opening

OR

c
Clean opening diagonal split

d
Clean opening, sides radiused,
central split

Figure 6.10 Design of bottle to clear a mould

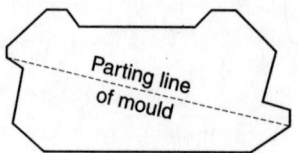

Figure 6.11 Asymmetrical design: diagonal split essential

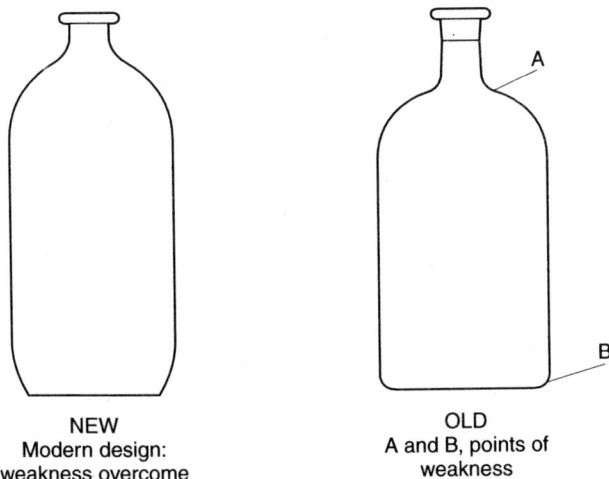

NEW
Modern design:
weakness overcome

OLD
A and B, points of
weakness

Figure 6.12 Design improvements

achieved, but pourability has been improved (by lessening the risk of air entrapment when tilted).

Panels inevitably cause glass distribution problems, and Figure 6.13 indicates steps taken to modernise a typical panelled pharmaceutical bottle.

A   Original bottle – note angular base, long narrow neck.
B   Improved shoulder – wider and stronger neck section.
C   Removal of panel: maintain parallel sides, draw in base–neck. Design now follows total shape better, front panel convex – eliminates sinkage risk and makes for better labelling. Finally bottle weight reduced and glass distribution maintained – stronger bottle. This final bottle also offers advantages in faster filling and better pouring..

Toilet bottles give more scope for the imagination, but the same rules of good practice should be applied when possible. Occasionally, rules may have to be relaxed as in many instances special shapes are said to be 'essential' and light weighting and high-speed filling may be of less importance. While a square edge is still not good practice, this may be disguised by a double radius. A bevel may be improved by superimposing a series of fine flutes (see Figure 6.14).

It is frequently necessary to design a family series, and as a general rule a 25% increase of the original shape in height, depth and width will double the capacity. One final trick with any design is to turn it upside down – it may look much better that way (Figure 6.15). The use of CAD/CAM and computer technology generally is now widely applied to glass design, thus providing a faster service and improved design. 3D models can also be screened.

It should be noted that like plastic, glass has a shrinkage factor – usually 0.3% (which is less than for plastics). Moulds are therefore slightly larger than the item produced.

Insufficient study of the design related to the mould can lead to bottle distortion

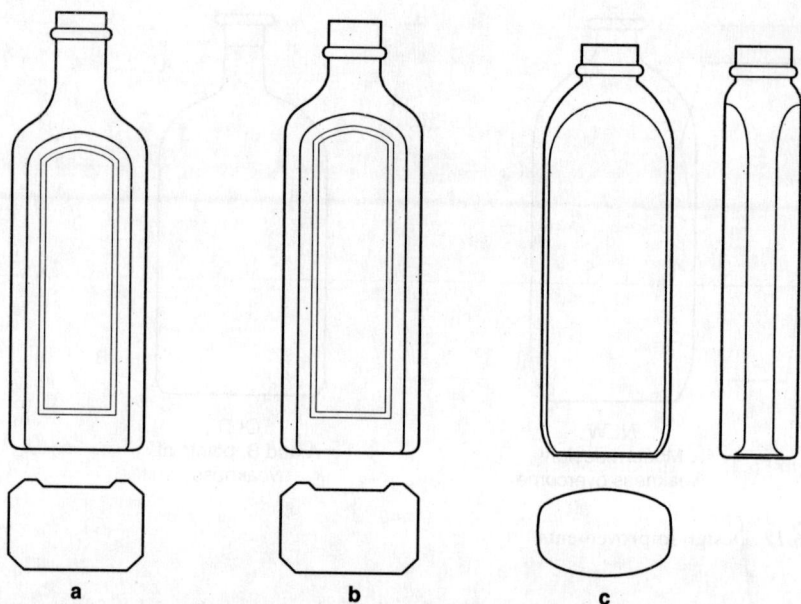

Figure 6.13 Design improvements

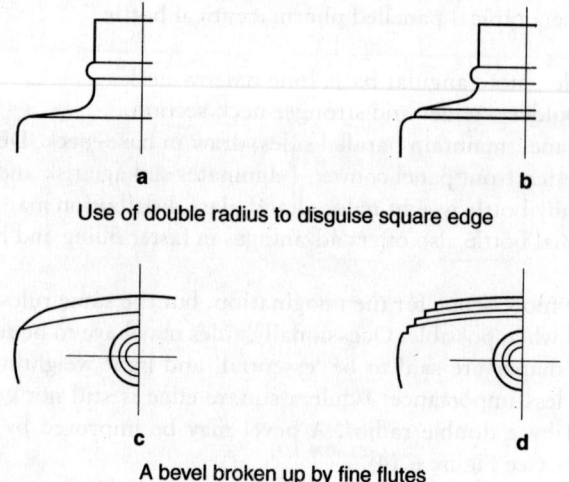

Use of double radius to disguise square edge

A bevel broken up by fine flutes

Figure 6.14 Design improvements

while it is still at the 'red' heat stage. This aspect must be considered a function of the glass manufacturer and the mould maker.

Lastly, designs cannot be separated from closures – the total effect therefore must be a major consideration (Figure 6.16).

To evaluate the functional aspect of design one should first outline various points which require consideration. These may be listed as follows.

226

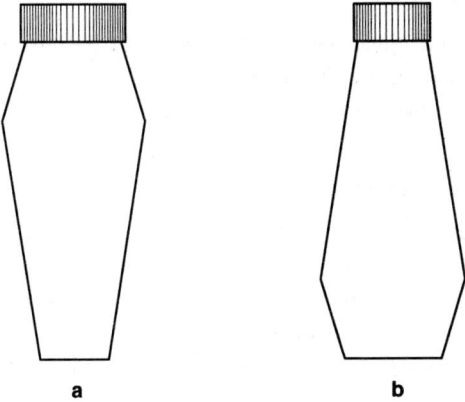

Figure 6.15 Design impression

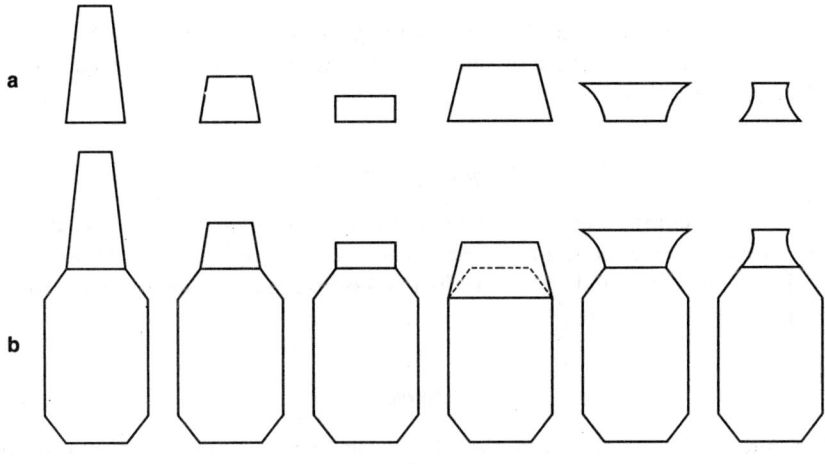

A design consists of a bottle with a cap

Figure 6.16 (a) Closure shapes; (b) closure plus bottle

Production line handling

This comprises unscrambling, cleaning, filling, capping, labelling, etc. For instance, the air blowing of containers with square shoulders and narrow necks may present difficulties, and figure eight shapes create swirl patterns.

Filling speeds relate to both the container shape and the neck diameter. If conveyor feeding is likely to lead to excessive surface impacts then alternative methods of feeding may become essential, e.g. worm or screw feed (scroll). Capping speed and efficiency depend on gripping the container, the design of the neck finish and the design of the closure.

Labelling also depends on holding the container, the shape of the label, the evenness of the surface to which it is applied and the type of labelling process. A convex surface is preferred to a flat or concave surface. Excessive fall away can lead to creased labels.

Strength

This depends on design, glass weight, and glass distribution. A badly designed container can lead to excessive weighting to reduce the zones of thin areas. Note that strength bears a relationship to handling, processing and stacking.

Consumer convenience

Does it rest comfortably in the hand? Are the hands likely to be wet, as they frequently are in the bathroom and kitchen? Can the cap be easily removed? Can it then be poured without changing the grip? Does it pour well? Can pouring be controlled? Where will the container be stored? (If in a bathroom, then good stability is essential.) A bottle which falls over is a danger to the user and may damage the bath or sink onto which it falls.

Display stability

Are there restrictions on display height or arrangements? Is it necessary for the pack to be self-stacking, i.e. for the base of one container to fit neatly into the top of the closure of the container beneath it?

Display potential

What is the pack competing with? What is the predominant issue – size impression, stability, confidence in handling by salesman or user(!) or appearance? How important is the label area compared with product visibility? Can a decorative process be employed rather than labelling?

Reuse

This may refer to a reclosable pack after use by the user, or multi-trip. Can it readily be rewashed, both internally, and externally, and can the label(s) be removed?

Capacity

This may be based on product sold by weight, volume, or number. Container capacity is a critical feature bearing relationships with product filling speed, the declared contents and headspace (vacuity or ullage). The ullage (airspace above product) must be adequate to allow for the thermal expansion of the product. This is particularly important with alcohol-based products in narrow necked containers. The capacity usually relates to either a brimful capacity or a defined fill point.

There is also the visual aspect of the point of fill which may, in certain designs, lead to the appearance of a low fill. Powder or granular products which settle require consideration at the design stage, the settling effect being exaggerated in narrow containers or containers with long narrow necks. Container capacity tolerances increase with size, e.g. 30 ± 0.5 ml and 650 ± 12.5 ml.

Costs

Bottle mould costs are likely to be of the order of £3,000 ($4,500) per mould set (i.e. around £30,000 for a ten-station IS machine).

Recyclability

All glass is recyclable, but borosilicate or soda glass must be segregated. In addition to the above functional issues it is essential that a designer receives a full marketing brief before commencing a design, covering:

- full knowledge of the product – nature, how, when, where it is used, etc.
- full knowledge of the market – is it new, what is the competition, where will it be sold?
- the content requirement (see Capacity above)
- full knowledge of any price or production restrictions which may be applied
- knowledge of the distribution system to be employed
- knowledge of legislation.

Added to this are the aesthetic issues of design, frequently requested as being better than or different from a particular product. A container should ultimately provide an economical basis for a balance between presentation, identification, protection and convenience. Models of new designs for bottles, closures, etc. can be produced either in wood or opaque or clear plastic, bearing in mind that a clear plastic model frequently looks better than the final glass bottle.

Design protection – registration and patents

Depending on legal aspects bottle shapes can be design registered but not patented unless they involve specialised features such as new innovations involving closures.

Legislation

In the USA the regulatory body for legislation associated with drug and cosmetic products is the FDA. The Food Additives Amendment to the Federal Food, Drug and Cosmetic Act places a requirement on the manufacturer to submit data on packaging materials and components to the FDA prior to marketing of pharmaceutical (and food) products. The same applies for pharmaceuticals under EU legislation. Submission for clearance of product/pack must include data on all packaging material constituents (i.e. glass type) and adequate toxicological studies to prove these constituents innocuous if not previously cleared (e.g. with plastics).

The Fair Packaging and Labelling Act 1966 also has widespread impact and is regulated by the FDA for drug and cosmetic products. The Act not only legislates against deceptive package (usually associated with packaging design and construction) but also details minimum label area size and a minimum size (height) of letters. Exemptions are included for small drug, cosmetic and toiletry containers. Additional legislation on ethical or prescription drugs is given in Section 507 (e) (i) of the Food, Drug and Cosmetic

Act. OTC drug products must prominently carry the established or proprietary name on the principal panel and must also carry a statement on the general pharmacological category.

In the UK legislation is similar to the USA involving various Acts of Parliament, e.g. Trade Description Act, Food Labelling Act, Weights and Measures Act. The last is covered by the 'Model State Packaging and Labelling Regulation' first adopted in 1952 within the USA.

One other Act, the Poison Prevention Packaging Act 1970, is now having wide influence on child-resistant safety packaging and is dealt with separately in Chapter 11.

Glass has been cleared by the FDA for a wide range of products. Closures present few difficulties.

Decoration

Certain decorative processes other than the more conventional labelling may be used. Some of the most brilliant effects may be achieved by ceramic printing. This is a screen process which applies pigments and powdered glass in a carrier of waxes or oils. After application the ink is 'fired' on by passing through a lehr at 900–1100°C, whereby the carriers are burnt away and the pigment–glass mixture melts and becomes affixed to the container. The result is a near permanent decoration which will withstand heat, cold, abrasion, etc. The texture can be high gloss, matt, satin, or rough.

Another process is the Thermo-Cal system in which ceramic decalcomanias are released from a carrying paper on to a preheated container and then fired.

Organic coatings and inks have been developed which will adhere to glass at lower temperatures, i.e. 450–500°C. These organics could be more economical than ceramics and offer a wide range of colours but are less scuff-resistant. Inorganic metallic oxide coatings may also be employed, particularly for coloured iridescence (i.e. Spectrasheen – Owen, Illinois).

Although the decorative processes apply certain restrictions (particularly half tones), the overall possibilities are gradually extending when cost is not a prime factor. In addition to paper labelling and those mentioned above are plastic labels, or tapes, close fitting sleeves (shrink or stretch) or cards, plastic fitments and plastisol dip coatings (as used for aerosols). Thus a glass pack may reach its final objective by a combination with other materials such as paper and plastic or decorative processes. New coating technologies (organic and inorganic) can provide both coloured and protective coatings, with the latter reducing surface damage which could weaken a container. More recent coatings have included Surlyn and SBR (styrene butadiene rubber) with polyurethane.

Quality control and quality assurance

QC or QA is essential to the maintenance of quality by the regular checking of parameters that will:

1   lower the aesthetic appearance and therefore give rise to adverse consumer reaction, loss of sales, etc.

2   reduce the functional characteristics – pouring, standing, opening, reclosing – and the protection of the product

3   increase the cost by increasing wastage and/or reducing output on the user's production line.

These parameters should be directly or indirectly covered in a specification which represents a negotiated agreement between a supplier and the using company.

QC and QA as a means of measuring and controlling quality can be applied to both the glass producer's input and output, i.e. from raw materials to finished product. They are therefore a production aid and a user's guarantee. QC must only check those parameters which are critical or essential – the unnecessary measuring of non-critical aspects only adds extra processing cost. For instance, if the burst strength of a bottle is either directly or indirectly related to its performance, then measure it – if not, it may be of interest but not of practical importance, hence do not check it.

Two fault categories are associated with quality control – variables and attributes. Variables are those faults that can be measured, usually instrumentally, i.e. dimensional measurements, burst strength, etc. Attributes are those faults which either cannot be accurately assessed (frequently associated with appearance, i.e. visual defects) or can be assessed by go–no go procedures without resorting to accurate measurements.

It must also be pointed out that the basic materials from which glass is made have to be subjected to QC in order to ensure consistency between batches of glass and the processing of the materials. As the majority of glass containers are produced in a continuous process, this aspect is particularly important, e.g. control of colour.

Modern QC is based on recognised statistical programmes. The parameters to be controlled vary with the consumer's requirements. For instance, pressurised products must have a high resistance to internal pressure, while containers to be hot filled or sterilised require good thermal shock resistance. Possible defects have first to be recognised, classified and in some cases further defined by limit samples, i.e. a sample showing a defect to the agreed degree is acceptable; beyond this point it is unacceptable and therefore a defective sample.

The importance of recognising those aspects which are critical to a container, its subsequent processing and sale is one of experience and proper consultation between manufacturers of the packaging materials, packaging machinery suppliers, the user, etc. Being an old established industry, glass reject terminology tends to be advanced and complex (see appendices).

Prior to launch, a provisional specification should be tentatively agreed and then subsequently verified in the light of actual experience. Acceptable sampling schemes are now applied by most producers working to an AQL (acceptable quality level) agreed between producer and user. The AQL defines the acceptable proportion of detectives per batch. Further goods receipt QC schemes may be applied by a user, which means that all supplies are subjected to a second QC check. Under such circumstances it is advisable that the acceptance sampling schemes are clearly defined so that agreement on acceptance and rejection is reached with the minimum of friction. Alternatively, a user may either request a batch sample from the producer or accept deliveries on warranty without further major QC checks, for example as follows.

A batch sample consists of an agreed number of units taken throughout a production run. These are sent to the user with special identifications, but without prior checking or sorting. The user then applies its normal QC checks to these samples only. This offers some advantages in that samples are received from the whole production run and the user is not faced with the sampling difficulties associated with stacked and palletised components. As all opened stock has to be resealed, this not only is labour-consuming but also unnecessarily exposes stock to additional handling and atmospheric contamination.

Buying under warranty/certificate usually implies that the supplier and user have discussed and accepted the level of QC and QA carried out by the supplier. However, as all schemes involve risk, it must be recognised that occasionally a delivery or part delivery below the agreed standards may be received. This risk may mean that faulty bottles are found when they reach the production line or that some defectives will go undetected. (Note that even a second QC check does not guarantee that a defective batch will be found.) A scheme placing total dependence on the supplier is a practical proposition but requires a high level of confidence and understanding between the two parties. This can only be achieved by an effective and continuous interchange of information thus ensuring a proper basis for each to understand and acknowledge the other's problems, requirements and limitations.

The success of obtaining consistent supplies must therefore be met by effective QA/QC schemes and specification. The main feature of a specification should include a clearly defined dimensional drawing covering profile, side elevation and plan together with glass mass, volume and finish details. The written specification will also show accepted container name, stock and/or computer code number, AQLs, including performance tests and mode of delivery. The last is particularly important as it includes the method of packing which should be designed to meet the user's handling requirements on the production line, i.e. is it designed for efficient hand or mechanical? A specimen specification is detailed in Appendix 6.3.

As part of AQLs one must understand a number of terms and their technical meanings. Individual faults must be defined as critical, major, minor, with each group being controlled to an acceptable AQL. For instance, the AQL for a critical fault is usually nil and the discovery of a critical fault will cause either a rejection of the delivery or, if found at the glass producer's, a complete resort of the batch. A single example of a critical fault would be a bird cage or bird swing (Figure 6.17) as this would risk broken glass in a container reaching a consumer. It is fair to say that instances of bird cages or bird swings are now rare.

Critical, major and minor defects may be defined as follows:

- *critical* – type of defect which renders a bottle unsuitable for use and frequently implies a risk of personal injury; AQL usually 0
- *major* – defects which reduce usability or saleability; AQL usually 0.65–1.5
- *minor* – other defects, undesirable but accepted to a certain level; AQL usually 4.0–6.5.

The figures given are typical ones, which can vary according to the product.

QC sampling

Acceptance sampling schemes are based on the Dodge and Romig tables, Military standard 105E or BS 6001. Single or double sampling may be employed.

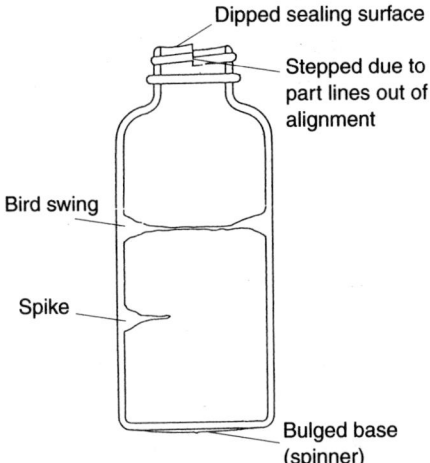

Dipped sealing surface

Stepped due to part lines out of alignment

Bird swing

Spike

Bulged base (spinner)

Figure 6.17 Bottle defects

Tolerances – no manufacturer of glass containers produces bottles with identical physical characteristics, therefore recognised tolerances are part of any manufacturing process. The probability for the chosen tolerances is usually 0.998, thus 998 containers out of every 1000 should be within the specified tolerances. Some tolerances are inter-related, i.e. capacity, glass mass, and dimensions. If certain dimensions are particularly critical to a production line, pregauging may be carried out by either the glass manufacturer or the user on its production line prior to filling.

Dimensions may be measured automatically by either gauges or instruments. Typical gauges are shown in Figure 6.18 and are detailed in Appendix 6.1. Glass defect terminology is given in Appendix 6.2. Appendix 6.3 gives a typical bottle specification.

Bottles and production lines

Glass bottles offer advantages on weight, stability, and rigidity on production lines. Most designs can be handled on normal conveyor systems. Where the design gives a high centre of gravity, has limited contact points (for impact damage), is asymmetrical or an unusual shape it may be necessary to create a specially designed production line, or resort to individual handling (i.e. use of pucks).

Unscrambling tables must be designed to limit impact and rubbing of surfaces which weaken the glass by surface damage. Similar care must be taken with manual handling. Many lines feed via star wheels, which must be correctly shaped, positioned and sized to accept the bottle at the right point with the full tolerances of the specification.

Glass bottles may contain a variety of products, liquids, solids or gases (aerosols). The mode of filling therefore depends on the item being filled. However, prior to filling a container must be clean. Years ago all containers were washed, but other than sterile products and treated glass most bottles are usually inverted and air blown. To be effective air blowing must use dry oil-free air and have proper facilities for controlled removal of blown out debris (i.e. by vacuum).

233

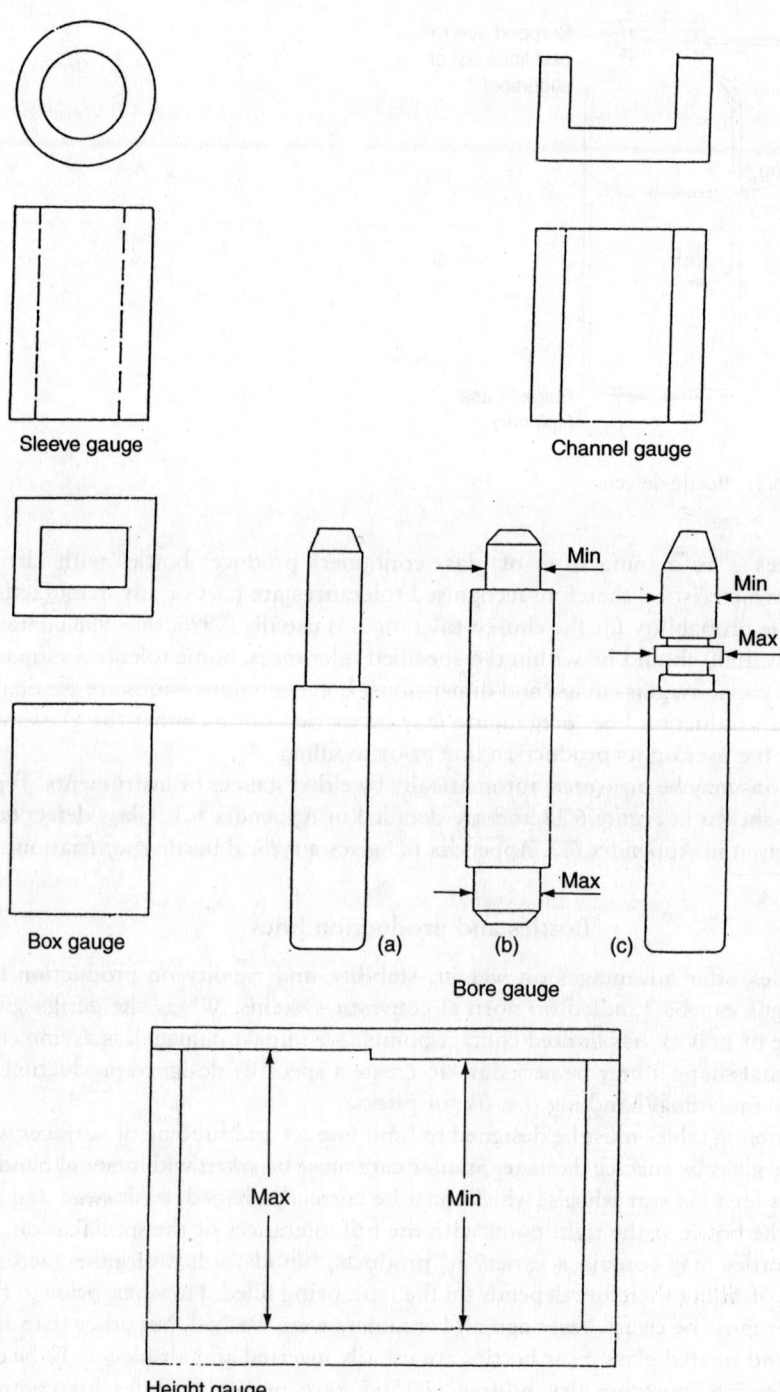

Sleeve gauge

Channel gauge

Box gauge

Bore gauge

(a)   (b)   (c)

Min
Min
Max
Max

Height gauge

Max   Min

Figure 6.18 Gauge types

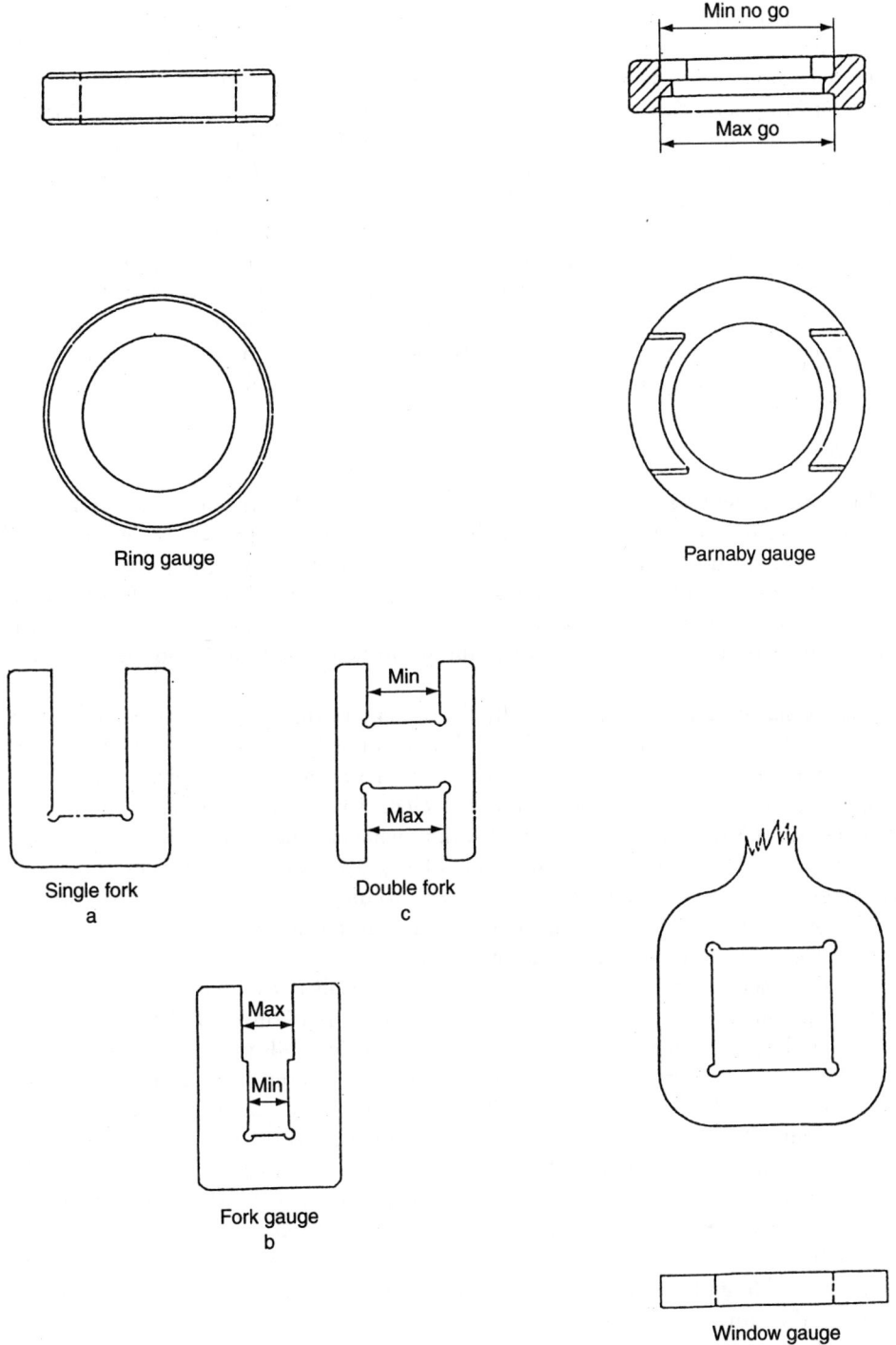

Min no go

Max go

Ring gauge

Parnaby gauge

Single fork
a

Min

Max

Double fork
c

Max

Min

Fork gauge
b

Window gauge

Figure 6.18 Gauge types (cont.)

Tests under controlled conditions have shown that the cleanliness of blown bottles can be equal to or better than that of traditionally washed bottles in terms of both fibres and bacterial count. One reason for this is the fact that bottle washing is not usually carried out in line with the filling operation, but usually a few days previously. The accumulated stock therefore has a further chance to collect dirt and bacteriological contamination unless stored under special clean conditions. When bottles exit the lehr they are sterile due to the high temperature of the process. If these receive the minimum handling under relatively clean conditions and are then either packed in fully sealed fibreboard cartons or effectively closed with shrink wraps, a low level of microbiological and dirt/dust contamination is preserved. This may seem obvious now but one must remember that traditional open wooden crates were stored under poor conditions, frequently in the open, and encouraged dirt, dust, condensation and surface corrosion. Full washing was then essential. Type II and treated neutral glass must always be washed to remove the soluble surface film of sodium sulphate.

Filling

Filling speeds depend not only on the item and quantity being filled but invariably on the aperture of the container. Although wider mouthed containers are easier to fill, an effective closure is slightly more difficult to achieve. Some comparison between types of closure and container diameter are given later. Items to be filled include liquids of varying viscosities, solid items – tablets, capsules, powders, etc. – and gas-containing products such as aerosols. Filling can be carried out by count, volume or weight.

Count may be achieved electronically (breaking a beam of light) or mechanically by counting devices such as slat, revolving disc, column fillers, or lever trip. Volumetric fillers may be the piston principle coupled with non-returnable valves whereby the product is drawn into a cylinder and then ejected via a filling nozzle. Alternatively, gravimetric volume fillers may be employed in which cylinders are filled to brimful or to a defined fill level (with overflow), then a base valve opens and empties under gravity, or gravity with positive pressure assistance. Volumetric filling can also be combined with a weight feed whereby the greater part is delivered by volume with a trickle feed weight top-up to give the final requirement.

An auger screw for powders or very viscous materials is another means of volumetric filling and relies on a number of whole turns or part turns of the screw. Weight fillers can be based on a bulk weighing plus a trickle feed fill-up.

Filling to a predetermined distance either from the container base or from the container sealing surface can be employed for both liquids and powders. Vacuum or negative pressure filling is widely used. Two tubes, a filling and vacuum tube, pass through a resilient disc which makes a seal with the container sealing surface. The vacuum tube determines the height of fill by acting as an overflow system, which can be taken off in a vacuum trap. The vacuum filling system may be assisted by pressure. With liquids which froth, a tendency aggravated by vacuum, the containers may be filled by positioning the filling tube at the base of the container and then raising it to the final point of fill at the same rate as the product is delivered.

By whatever means a fill is achieved the critical factors are cleanliness of fill, accuracy and guarantee of declared content with a minimum overage. For particularly viscous liquid products or under special circumstances, hot fills may be used. Hot fills are useful where a partial vacuum is required in the closed pack.

Placing inserts into glass bottles, e.g. pouring devices or plugs usually made of LD polyethylene, may call for a more accurate bore control than is provided by normal commercial processes. In the pharmaceutical industry, cotton wool in tablet packs, if not pre-dried, can add moisture to the product and small strands which bridge the sealing surface can act as a wick (wicking).

With a moisture sensitive product, moisture pick by this means can be quite rapid. Alternative materials to wool are either plastic shapes or plugs of expanded polystyrene, polyethylene or polyurethane foams. Closures can also be obtained which incorporate spring extensions. Such closures may have chambers which hold desiccants. Transit tests (vibration/drops) would be advised to check whether space fillers are necessary.

Closuring

It is not long since the stoppered or corked bottles were the basic containers for both the pharmaceutical and the toiletry trade. Although these still exist, their use rapidly declined with the advent of the screw-necked container. In more recent years glass has used wadless closures which started as screw versions but can now be applied and removed by other means: plug, twist-off, lever-off, etc. In these forms the flexibility of certain plastics have been utilised to provide both the resistance and the resilience required of a closure. Although press in/over closures can be applied at a higher speed than screw caps, tolerances for bottle neck and closure have to be tighter.

Screw finishes follow recognised standards for shallow, medium deep and deep finishes, etc. All must ensure adequate thread engagement between cap and bottle so that an even pressure is applied over the entire sealing surface – if the closure is wadded or flowed in, this can be checked by the 'wad' impression. If less than $\frac{3}{4}$ of a turn of thread of engagement occurs (possible on a standard shallow finish by a combination of low start of thread on the bottle, over-thick wad, and high thread run-out in the cap) then the cap is likely to tilt and make an unsatisfactory seal. Screw finishes use two basic types of closure – prethreaded (metal or plastic) or rolled on (metal or plastic). Prethreaded closures usually rely on the torque being applied by the spinning action of the cap-holding chuck. Some machines' application torque can be read directly from a gauge, but more usually closures are checked on a separate instrument and recorded as unscrewing torques. As there is a tendency for unscrewing torques to have a time–temperature relationship, checks should follow an agreed schedule.

Although loose closures or low torques obviously run a leakage risk, high torques contain other dangers such as distortion of the closure and customer removal difficulty. Excessive torque can cause cold flow loosening of thermoplastic closures and the doming of metal and plastic caps. If the former is then knocked or flattened (stacking), a low torque can result. Softer metals can also flow or distort (e.g. aluminium alloys) if subjected to excessive forces.

Rolled-on caps can offer some advantages on torque control provided that the bottles, caps and wads are of a good commercial standard. The procedure of applying top pressure to ensure a good seal with the wad and then rolling on a thread to retain the seal offers very effective sealing. However, as the metal employed is an aluminium alloy which is considerably softer than tinplate, the thread must be well formed on both the bottle and the cap, or the threads will over-ride when the closure is replaced and retightened.

The principle of applying top pressure and then affixing it in that position while the wad is compressed is also used on most vial closures, where an overcap is subsequently locked under a bead by either clinching or rolling. Rubber discs or plugs provide the resilient and resistant part of the closure. From a range of natural and synthetic rubbers, properties can be varied in terms of moisture and gas permeation, chemical resistance, etc. and acceptability for irradiation or autoclaving. The industry has yet to discover a replacement for rubber in one essential property for injectable products, i.e. the ability of a needle to pierce without tearing or splitting and reseal upon needle withdrawal. In spite of this advantage, rubbers present problems when they are pierced in terms of shredding or fragmentation (small rubber particles removed by friction between rubber and needle) and coring (pieces of rubber actually cut out by the needle bore – usually associated with the design of the needle point, size, bore and sharpness of the needle heel) (Figure 6.19). Rubber closures for pharmaceutical usage are briefly dealt with under 'Homogeneous liners' later in this chapter.

Whatever the type of closure used on a glass container, the sealing surface is of prime importance. It is critical that this is even and smooth with no sharp features. Mould split lines should be inconspicuous, or alternatively a seamless neck ring can be used so that the risk is completely removed. Sealing surfaces may be radial, flat, stepped, sloped, etc., as indicated in Figure 6.20. The pressure applied by either top pressure or screw torque is taken up by the wad (impression) making intimate contact with the sealing surface. Hence there is either a high pressure confined to a limited area (i.e. raised ring contact) or a lower pressure when it is spread over a greater area, as presented by a broad flat sealing surface. Torques therefore have a direct relationship with the surface area, hence as the neck size increases so increased torques are required. Similarly there is a relationship between the neck size and apparent closure efficiency, as moisture pick-up tests with a desiccant show increasing moisture gain with widening diameters (see Table 6.2, p. 253). This may mean that wider diameter finishes are not advisable for some products but since the product quantity may also increase, the gain per unit weight of product may not be significantly different.

Glass in the form of ampoules offers the apparent facility of a near-perfect primary closure in the fusion of glass. This does produce a perfect pack in terms of compatibility (assuming the product is compatible with glass), nil exchange with atmosphere, etc., but difficulty in opening together with the hazards involved lower its overall performance. It is difficult to break open an ampoule either by using a file, or snapping at a score (OPC, one point cut), or at a ceramically fired-in ring, without spicules of glass arising. The presence of such spicules is undesirable, although various opinions have been expressed on the actual risks.

Bottles using wadless bore-type seals may need better quality neck finishes than conventional screw caps because bore seals exert an outward force which may cause cracks or similar imperfections to proliferate. Instances of necks 'cracking off' have been reported.

Special mention should be made of closures for IV solutions. The use of any screw closure with an inner rubber wad or plug always presents an unscrewing risk due to a watch spring effect. In addition, threading may hide a contamination due to residual

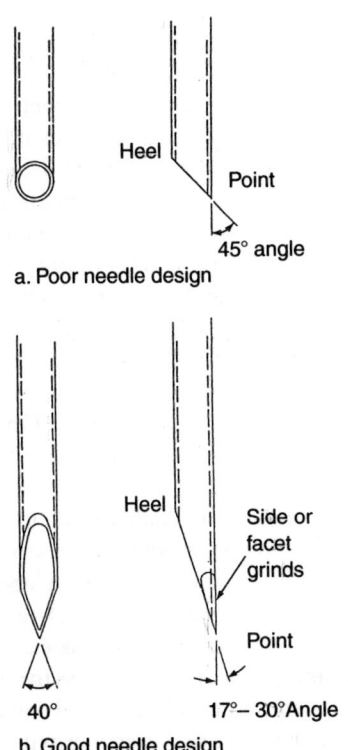

Heel

Point

45° angle

a. Poor needle design

Heel

Side or
facet
grinds

Point

40°   17°– 30° Angle

b. Good needle design

Figure 6.19 Needles for injectables

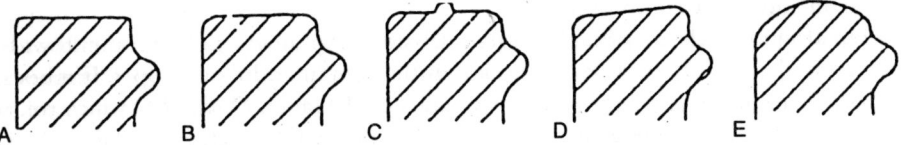

A   B   C   D   E

Figure 6.20 Sealing surfaces: (E) is preferred

cooling water. An overseal-type closure, similar to that employed for vials, appears to offer advantages (DIN Standard).

Labelling

Labels may be applied to the main body of the bottle, to the neck, or may enshroud the closure (TE). Each label must be designed for a selected bottle area allowing tolerances for the bottle, the label and the process by which it is applied. A label should be applied to areas of large radius, as several changes of radius within a limited area will cause creasing. Provided that the glass surface is free from silicones or surface lubricants, one of a number of labelling processes may be used, i.e. label plus adhesive, delayed action heat sensitive or pressure sensitive.

An additional critical aspect is product security, i.e. an insurance that the correct label is applied to the right product. Reel-fed labels offer advantages over precut or bundled labels, but even with reel-fed labels there is a tendency for a bar code (or similar coding) to be incorporated onto the label at the printing stage. This is then electronically scanned either just prior to container labelling or immediately after it. The legal requirements for pharmaceutical products are making more and more demands on the product label, i.e. identity including official name, strength, quantity, product licence, manufacturer, batch no., expiry date, etc. This is thereby increasing the difficulties associated with product security. Frequently colour is used to differentiate products and while this has advantages, colour-blind users may find problems, therefore there is no substitute for careful reading and clear and concise text. It is here that we find an obvious difference between many pharmaceutical and OTC products. Ethicals have to maintain a degree of professional confidence to pharmacists, doctors, veterinary surgeons, etc. and must therefore display this by simplicity and clarity. On the other hand, certain proprietary medicines frequently rely on both visual impact and the ability to convince the user of efficacy.

OTC products may cover all extremes in order to create some individuality. Therefore we have simplicity, such as printing of black on white or white reversed out of black, to half tone printing in up to seven colours. The reader may say that the ability to apply a label to a glass container bears no relationship to the design. In some instances this may be true, but on many occasions problems can arise from the design – even the thickness of ink can play a part. Similarly, application of a varnish to protect the ink will reduce water loss through the surface, so that when an aqueous adhesive is applied to the under side, the label will curl more rapidly. One must therefore select an adhesive of the right tack together with the proper smoothing down of the label by wiping pads or rollers. On heat sensitive labels the varnish must not contain solvents which activate or plasticise the adhesive.

As a general rule, labels with radiused corners (not for wrap around) are easier to handle on automatic equipment.

Wrap around labels are suitable for parallel-sided containers. Before committing to a wrap around label it is essential to check that the container does not taper. If it does, it is advisable to have a gap between the two ends of the label. Machinery which rolls on the label from a leading edge may give rise to an unsightly effect, as the label tends to follow a spiral if the container has a taper.

Siliconising or other surface treatments, particularly on the outside of injection vials, can lead to labelling difficulties or the label dropping off on storage. Any glass container which has received a treatment either inside or out should have an adhesive stability check. Silicones tend to creep and internal spraying could affect the outside. Silicone coatings normally do not produce any extraction hazards. Labelling problems may also arise where plastic coated glass is used.

Cartoning and outerisation

Filled glass containers may be cartoned, directly outerised or shrink wrapped. This secondary packaging must be considered in the container design as a means of providing adequate protection against mechanical hazards. Among these effects, vibration is one hazard which results in labelling scuff and damage. Round containers tend to rotate under transit vibration and all shapes tend to show some up and down movements.

Any movement can cause scuffing if the label inks are not dry or rub-resistant. The use of cheaper carton board can be a false economy if this leads to surface damage of a label. Certain protective varnishes are also abrasives – that is, once the varnish has started to rub, damage is accentuated by the abrasive nature of the varnish powder created.

Bottles can be designed to minimise label damage by the use of recessed areas. These should be sufficiently deep to allow for variations in the surface uniformity but not so deep as to cause glass distribution problems. Labels applied to bulged bottles or zones of prominence obviously run a risk of concentrated rub. Heavy containers may need to be retained in cartons with base locking flaps (200 g or more in weight).

Labels provide little in the way of light protection unless the base is thicker than normal, selectively coloured (i.e. black), or a foil ply is incorporated. Plastic sleeving (shrink or stretch) as well as coatings applied by the bottle manufacturer have been used on light weight bottles to reduce container weakening due to surface damage.

Warehousing

The stackability of finished stock is a final factory consideration prior to the evaluation of transit hazards – fortunately, glass is a strong material and can take at least part of the stacking pressures. Dangers therefore relate to the effect on the closure rather than the container. Undue pressure can be transmitted to the cap wad, thus inducing a compression set which reduces the seal efficiency. Compression and transit vibration may also increase such an effect to the point of closure failure.

Transit damage

The fragile nature of glass, from impact damage, exposes many risks during transportation with the result that a nil loss can only be insured against by overpacking. One therefore accepts that reasonable handling is expected with occasional exceptions and that there is a recognised economical level of outer packaging. This is frequently achieved by a combination of cartons, internal carton fitments and fibreboard outers with or without internal fitments. The use of shrink wraps with and without base (and top) trays or nests is growing, and brings with it new palletisation requirements. The designer of a pack for a glass bottle must consider the protection requirements. A study of the bottle design and laboratory drop tests (burst tests are also useful) should indicate weaknesses which require selective protection. Where possible, containers should be filled to the normal filling height as the air space or ullage may affect results (water hammer effect).

The degree of protection afforded by individual cartons may be varied by board type and caliper, internal fitments, or even packaging inserts. There are advantages in having single corrugated pieces with the corrugated outwards – the board then acts as a double faced liner and high spot rub between corrugations and labels is avoided. Fine fluted corrugated as used for cartons provides another bonus.

Glass and the environment

Today no chapter on any packaging material is complete without a reference to the problems it may create in terms of disposal, pollution, litter, and the four Rs: recovery, recycle, reuse and reduce (e.g. light weighting).

Glass represents approximately 5–9% of waste by weight but as it is chemically inert, does not burn, rot, putrefy or degrade, there are no direct pollution hazards. Crushed glass is beneficial to land fill and in incinerators glass containers can assist in aerating the mass and thereby improve combustion.

In various surveys glass has emerged in a strong position, particularly in terms of recycling and reclamation. Resalvaged glass is primarily being used in three ways:

1   new containers (via cullet) – a Swiss plant is using 100%
2   as Glasphalt for road surfaces (still under experimental survey)
3   as bricks and blocks and as glass wool insulation in buildings.

However, glass as litter remains a serious problem. General education together with adequate and proper disposal facilities will undoubtedly reduce this hazard, but broken glass must still cause concern. Glass, however, has advantages over most other materials as it can be readily cleaned and reused, or recycled via bottle banks as cullet. In the latter case, other than the risk of admixtures (colours and glass types) no deterioration has been reported in properties.

Special pharmaceutical containers

As one of the earliest usages of bottles and jars was for drug and cosmetic products, it is natural that many of the first specialised containers bore names which became associated with the pharmaceutical industry. Glass containers can be broadly divided into narrow-necked (including sprinkler) and wide-necked – these correspond roughly with the descriptions of bottles and jars. Many general names relate to the cross-sectional shapes, i.e. round, oval, triangular, hexagon, squares, flats and panels.

More specialised container names include the following.

1   Winchesters (UK): This term is widely used in the UK and covers a range of capacities from 0.5 fl.oz upwards, although the Winchester quart containing 80 fl oz. was the best known (see Figure 6.12). These have now transferred to metric sizes, 15 ml to 2.5 l.
2   Carboys: These usually exist in two shapes, balloon shaped of either 5 or 10 gallon capacity or a cylindrical or straight side form of 2, 3, 5 gallons. Metric 22.5 to 45 l.
3   Cylindrical rounds, Boston rounds: Conventional cylindrical bottle with near flat shoulders, 5 ml to 2 l.
4   Jars: Parallel side cylindrical containers bearing no shoulder. Used mainly for creams and ointments. May be white flint, amber or opal glass.

Tubular glass containers

Tubular glassware deserves further mention, as it finds specialised usage in the pharmaceutical industry and in many textbooks on glass, detail is confined to blown glass.

Limited use was made of tubular glass containers prior to 1917, when Charles Danner introduced the first method of continuously drawing glass tube. This discovery led to the greater use of containers made from tubular glass as these then offered certain advantages:

1   lower weight (blown glass was much thicker and therefore heavier)
2   thinner and more even wall control
3   the ability to produce a hermetically sealed pack, an ampoule (early usage)
4   an ampoule met the need for sterile (unit dose) products
5   competitiveness.

These early containers used soda glass tubing. With the further mechanisation of the shaping process in the early 1920s, ampoules which had already been produced by hand became one of the first large usages. Many of these had rounded bases. Neutral glass containers were introduced in the late 1920s and today most ampoules use neutral glass.

Ampoules

Standards exist for a range of ampoule shapes and sizes with variations on the neck and the method of opening. The ampoule can be broken at the neck restriction either by scoring or by having a ceramic point (ring or spot) baked on during the manufacture thus causing a weak point. However, ampoules breaking on a ceramic colour can cause coloured particles to fall into the product. This has led to an alternative where the ampoule is scored and then has a coloured ring above or below the score to indicate the break point. In this way the break does not occur at the coloured ring, thus avoiding 'coloured' contamination. OPC (open point cut) ampoules are often now preferred.

Ampoules are normally supplied in plastic boxes with a tray lid and band plus an inner covering to minimise the ingress of particulate contamination. Recently there has been a tendency towards the use of wide stems as this facilitates cleaning and filling at high speed. However, it makes the sealing operation slightly more difficult.

Presealed ampoules can be used without a washing process, i.e. the manufacturing process produces a sterile and relatively clean ampoule. Special equipment is required to handle these so that the vacuum retained in the sealed ampoule does not draw in glass particles when it is opened. Preheating prior to opening can 'neutralise' the vacuum by using a flamed opening method. Washing is otherwise an essential stage in the use of ampoules, and specialised machinery with various combinations of ultrasonic vibrations and jets of water, steam or air is available for this purpose from companies such as Bosch, Strunck, Neri and Bonotto.

Ampoules may be sterilised by dry heat or steam autoclaved after filling provided the product will withstand this process. On-line sterilisation often uses dry heat at over 300°C for a controlled period.

Following filling and sealing, ampoules are inspected for seal and visual contamination. The seal or leakage test was performed by immersion in a water/dye solution under vacuum. It is debatable whether the test fully detected minor cracks or capillary holes through which microbiological contamination could occur. High-voltage tests which detect through cracks are now more effective.

Contamination in the form of particulate matter or glass spicules can be viewed by either direct light or polarised light. Although a Coulter counter can provide useful data, it has not been ideal for use in regular QC type counts. The ultimate objective must be to exclude glass particles from the site of the injection.

Ampoules may be preprinted or printed after filling. Preprinted ampoules can use ceramic inks which are printed by the screen process and then fired on. Printing after filling gives greater stock flexibility but requires extra security precautions during the time when the ampoules bear no identification. Printing after filling can be done either from rubber stereos or by silkscreen. The latter can use special inks such as the latest epoxy resin-based inks which can provide an acceptable degree of permanency. Self-adhesive plastic labels are currently finding more use.

The current usage of the ampoule is virtually static. Although it was one of the first unit dose containers, it is anticipated that alternatives such as cartridge tubes and pre-filled syringes (glass or plastic) will ultimately take over a major share of the ampoule market.

Typical ampoules are shown in Figure 6.4.

Vials

Vials are parallel side containers with a flat or concave base with a variety of neck finishes. These were popular in the 1920s and 1930s, when they first used cork closures followed by the more conventional screw finishes. The majority of these are produced from soda glass, when used for tablets and capsules.

The advent of the multidose injection vial with its rubber plug and aluminium overcap increased in use with the discovery of insulin and then penicillin. Insulin made the use of neutral glass essential but when penicillin was presented as a freeze dried powder, soda glass proved reasonably satisfactory, particularly as the life of the solution was dated once the water for injection was added. Injection vials can still be obtained in either neutral or soda glass and occasionally in treated soda glass. Larger vials may be made by conventional blowing techniques as well as from tubular glass. Vial usage has recently been extended by the advent of lyophilised biologicals.

Rubber closures for injectables are outlined under 'Special closures for pharmaceutical products (sterile products)' below. Various types of rubber, plug design and over (cap) seal may be employed. A range of standard neck sizes are available (13 to 20 mm). Rubber discs or plugs can be fixed into the overseal – these are usually known as combination seals. Although offering advantages in the closuring operation (only one item to be fed instead of two), washing techniques are more complicated and there is always a contamination risk from metal particles.

Aluminium overcaps may have a perforated metal, plastic flip-off or peelable foil cover. Figure 6.21 shows typical combination and conventional seals. Vials have also been introduced for unit dose packs using either an aluminium two-piece tear-off closure with a Saran coated pulpboard liner or a peel-type seal.

Cartridge tubes, disposable syringes

The use of a glass tube with an end cap seal and movable plunger is another early use of a unit dose injectable. After many years of use in the dental trade in conjunction with a resterilisable metal syringe, further applications were found with other pharmaceutical products. Thus when plastic disposable syringes became available, glass cartridge tubes became the first obvious choice, thus leading to high-volume quantities. The next stage was to combine the cartridge tube and syringe, thus creating a glass dis-

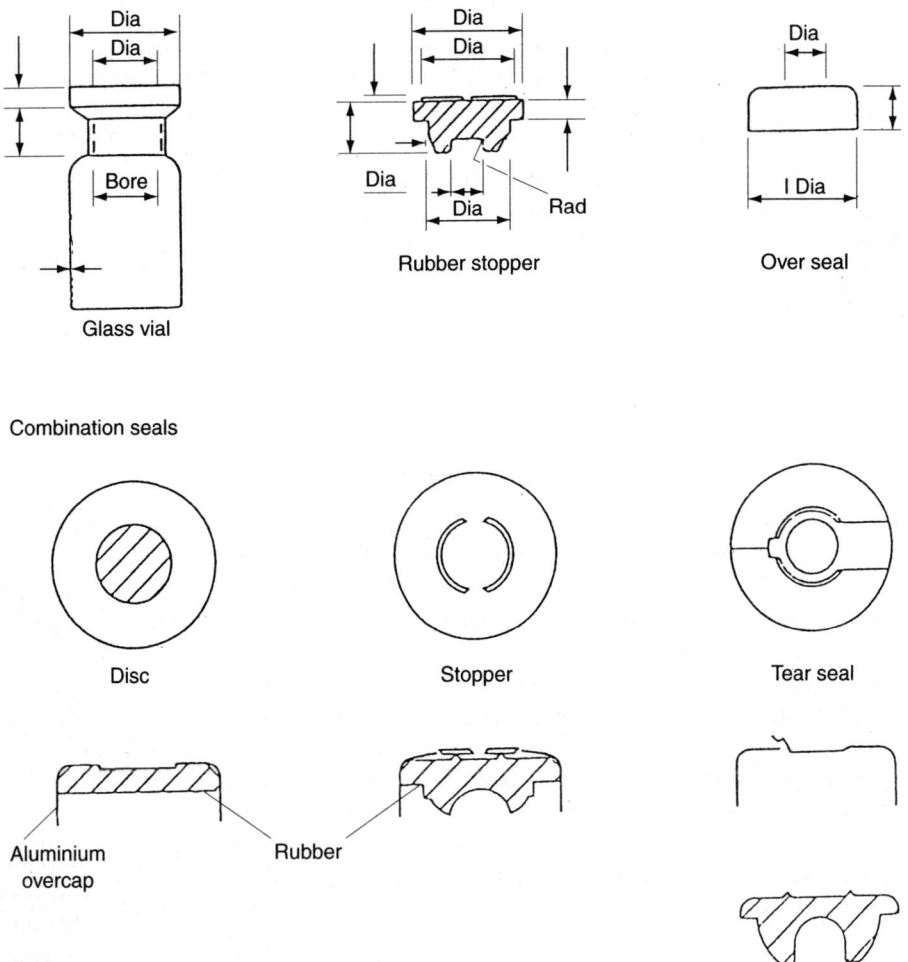

Figure 6.21 Typical combination and conventional seals

posable syringe. Syringes are also available with two compartments (bi-compartmental syringes) which allow unstable parts of a pharmaceutical formulation to be kept separate and then mixed immediately prior to use.

With packs relying on a rubber piston to effect the injection, this must both release without sticking and then move smoothly with the minimum of force. This may be assisted by including lubricants in the rubber which subsequently migrate to give a surface film, or by siliconising or coatings.

Closures for cartridge tubes are invariably based on aluminium overseals with or without a tear-off cap which are clinched or rolled on. Syringes may either have a needle mount or have a needle already fitted. Both usually employ rubber or plastic overcaps for protection and are supplied in a sterile outer pack.

Aerosols

The use of glass bottles for aerosols has received mixed comments on the risks involved. Although glass offers greater flexibility in design than cylindrical metal cans, it is essential that the breakage risk is safeguarded against either by good bottle strength/design or adequate bottle strength plus an external coating of a flexible plastic (usually PVC). Uncoated glass bottles are usually used in conjunction with low pressure aerosols (less than 25 lb/in^2 at 21°C). Coated bottles do not usually contain excessively high-pressure formulations.

Glass aerosols inevitably cost more than metal cans but offer plus features on appearance, which is highly desirable for toiletries and cosmetics.

The valves are set in an aluminium overseal (which is frequently polished and anodised or lacquered) and clinched or rolled under an external bead on the glass finish. Finishes range from 13 to 20 mm.

Future potential

What does glass offer for the future? It still serves the pharmaceutical and cosmetic industries well in offering effective, attractive packs. If it were not for the breakage risk, glass would offer the best product protection with distinct advantages relating to hygiene, inertness, zero permeation, sterilisation by heat, etc. Ultimately, a glass pack is as effective as its closure.

The percentage of glass used in pharmaceuticals reduced over the period of 1987–1991, although the overall production of glass remained static. Thus one might predict a slow decline but not a drastic drop, as glass usage is still expanding in certain parts of the world. However, under conditions of material shortage, glass is the least likely to be affected and therefore could enjoy further success.

The marriage of glass and plastic, originally started with the plastic coating of aerosols, has shown a continuing trend for the future. Coated glass, which involves very thin coatings to improve the colour range and strength, shows the greatest promise. Coatings of both organic and inorganic origins are being employed. The latest involves a thin coating of silica. From a pharmaceutical aspect the FDA acceptance of glass rarely presents problems – it therefore encourages the choice of glass as a packaging container. Surface attack and shedding, however, can be a problem, particularly in detection and identification. This can be done with a scanning electron microscope fitted with an energy dispersion analyser. X-ray fluorescence now provides a fast means of analysing glass.

Closures, caps, seals and stoppers

'A bottle can only be judged by the effectiveness of its closure.' The subject of closures, briefly discussed above, is now dealt with more fully. The specific suitability of glass as a recipient of a closuring system may be as one use or multi-use types. The latter should be easy to apply, open and effectively reclose until such time as all the product is used. This ideal may clash with the requirements of a child-resistant closure, but this is adequately covered if the word 'easy' is applied to adults and a phrase such as 'difficult to open by children' is added. With a child-resistant closure it is important that an adult finds it easy to reclose, as failure to do this defeats the very objective that one is trying to achieve. The one-use closure is widely used in the pharmaceutical industry and is in some instances specially designed to prevent reuse.

The primary objective of a closure is to effect a seal, and this is usually achieved by contact between at least two components, one which is relatively hard and resistant to pressure and the other which is soft or pliable and therefore receptive to compression (a ground glass stopper is an exception). A seal can also be made between two pliable or flexible materials, but either or both has to be supported by a rigid background or framework. In order to provide an effective seal on a ridged glass bottle, the closure must provide both resilience and product resistance. There must also be uniformity of compression so that the seal is effective over the full circumference of the container's sealing surface. In this combination glass can offer a fully hermetic seal which permits no exchange between the product and the outside atmosphere.

A seal can be secured by one or more of several basic closuring processes:

1   screw on – by thread or lug (single or multi-start)
2   crimp on or clinch on
3   roll on (in or under)
4   press on, i.e. push in or over
5   heat
6   adhesion
7   vacuum or differential pressure.

Although closures are important to all types of pack, this is particularly so with glass, where any exchange between the product and the external environment can only occur via the closure system. A glass pack therefore relies on its closure effectiveness, but it also must be remembered that function during use and ultimately disposal is also part of the overall 'fitness for purpose'.

Although a wide variety of closure systems are described in Chapter 11, those particularly important to glass are described in detail below. As closures and closure testing in general remain a weakness for many packs, no apologies are given for some overlap with Chapter 11. The two chapters contain complementary information.

Sealing materials

Prior to the invention of screw closures, corks, glass stoppers, pulpboard discs and parchment covers were the main closures. Historically, prethreaded screw closures have consisted of a threaded shell containing a wad or liner and a facing. The wad or liner may be made from cork agglomerate (gelatin or resin bonded), pulpboard, feltboard, plastic or rubber. It provides a resilient backing which receives the compression. In the case of screw closures the compression is due to the application of a controlled torque. Other closures, e.g. roll on, clinch, press on, may achieve this by the simple application of top pressure. Under the normally recommended torques, composition cork compresses by about 50% and pulpboard by approximately 20%.

The facing or liner material in direct contact with the product must be compatible with it, i.e. must not impart anything to or extract anything from the product. However, in the selection of a liner, factors in addition to compatibility must be considered, for example.

1   appearance
2   caliper – liners if too thick or too thin can reduce closuring efficiency or in certain circumstances prevent a seal being made
3   removal – should give a smooth removal without sticking or tearing; silicone coatings can sometimes be used to improve release
4   permeation – gas and vapour transmission
5   shelf life – must not deteriorate or break down
6   heat resistance – necessary when hot fills or heat sterilisation procedures are employed
7   economical – cost must be acceptable
8   function – a liner must not become distorted or fall out in use, i.e. must maintain a good fit; must continue to accept pressure or compression without bottoming
9   cleanliness, i.e. not create particles or support microbial growth.

There are two main classes of liners, namely heterogeneous and homogeneous. The former consists of a separate facing material laminated to a resilient backing; the latter consists of a single material which serves as both a facing and a backing. The main materials used are as follows.

Heterogeneous liners

1   Laminated papers – these materials are usually laminated to paper and include foils and polymers detailed in Chapter 11.
2   Coated papers

- Thermosetting resins coated onto (and into) paper are now obsolete in the UK but are still used in some parts of the world. They are not covered here.
- Thermoplastic coated papers: These include PVdC, vinyls, polyethylenes and occasionally polypropylene; more recently SiO_x and carbon coatings have been introduced.

Homogeneous liners

Cellulosic materials

Cork, feltboard, pulpboard – used widely as a wadding material, but have limited use in pharmaceuticals and toiletries without a facing.

Polymeric materials

1   Rubber: Still has limited use outside of injectable products; see Chapter 11, specifically relating to natural and synthetic rubbers. Has specialised applications for injectables.

2   Polyolefins. Polyethylene and polypropylene – some use as a separate disc or wad, but are now widely used in the form of wadless closures where the closure acts as its own wad.

3   Fluorocarbons and chlorocarbons: PTFE may be used as a separate disc for strong acids, alkalis, etc. – a very resistant material.

4   Plastic foams: Foamed polyethylene, polystyrene, polypropylene, and vinyls. These are also finding uses as a backing material, being an economical replacement for composition cork and pulpboard. While they exhibit similar advantages to flowed-in liners over the cellulosics, additional advantages are obtained in product compatibility and permeation resistance depending on the facing used. EPE is now widely used, with compression factors of 20% and 50%.

Flowed-in compounds

These are essentially a variation on the liners described above, but they are applied *in situ* as the name suggests rather than as a separate disc. They may be applied to the whole area of the cap top or at the edges or within a sunken ring. Materials used as plastisols, organosols, latexes, etc. may be based on aqueous dispersions (rubber and synthetic rubbers) or solvent solutions or dispersions of synthetics in organic solvents. Flowed-in compounds generally provide a good sealing medium but have limitations related to compatibility/migration and moisture permeation. A flowed-in compound offers the following features.

1   Can be operated on a full automatic system at high speed with the minimum of waste when applied to metal closures.

2   It is clean and dust free (cf. cellulosic-based liners).

3   The closure can frequently be rewashed and reused as it is not wetted.

However, there are disadvantages.

1   Difficult to use with certain plastic closures due to the high drying and curing temperature which is about 171°C, but retention is aided by cap design.

2   Solvent-based compounds require a special extraction plant. Residual solvents can cause problems (safety hazards).

3   Aqueous dispersions dry slowly. It is important that all traces of water are removed. There is also a possible odour hazard. These are now preferred.

4   Frequently contain migratory ingredients, or the compound may adsorb from the product. Therefore some compatibility limitations.

5   Investment in plant is high (see (2) above).

Economics of use of flowed-in liners resides in replacing a full conventional liner by a ring or restricted area of flowed-in compound. This especially applies on wide diameter closures. Most widely used are PVC and EVA plastisols.

Finally, the use of flowed in compounds is particularly significant due to supply restrictions on natural cork.

Screw closures

Screw closures based on single (continuous) or multi-start thread constitute the most widely used form of closuring. Prethreaded closures made from metal or plastic rely on achieving an adequate torque which is measured as N m or lb force inch to effect a seal. In general the unscrewing torque is 50–75% of the application torque, but variations occur according to the materials, time elapsed, temperature conditions and, in the case of thermosetting closures, humidity.

Torque control is particularly important with some thermoplastic closures which if given excessive torque will exhibit cold flow. Most countries have standards for single start screw finishes, such as the GCM1 400 series in the USA or BSI R3/2 and R4 in the UK. Progress is already being made in Europe on a series of standard finishes which will ultimately be common to the EU.

The GCM1 series includes a wide range of finishes, of which the 400 series is the most popular. Some of these are given in Table 6.1.

The tolerances of both the cap and the glass screw finish are critical in a number of areas, including the following.

Diameter – cap and bottle finish

- Clearance (e) between cap thread (E) and bottle neck wall (E)
- Clearance (t) between cap wall (T) and bottle neck thread (T)
- The minimum value of e varies from 0.004 inches (100 µm) for an 8 mm finish to 0.014 inches (350 µm) for 63 mm.
- The minimum value of t varies from 0.002 inches (50 µm) (8 mm) to 0.008 inches (200 µm) (63 mm).

These tolerances should provide adequate allowance for both bottle and closure ovalities.

The maximum clearances are equally important, as too much clearance can lead to the cap tilting or over-riding.

- The maximum value of e varies from 0.016 inches, 400 µm (8 mm) to 0.059 inches, 1.475 mm (63 mm).
- The maximum value of t varies from 0.016 inches, 400 µm (8 mm) to 0.053 inches, 1.325 mm (63 mm).

Table 6.1 Finishes of screw closures

No.	Type	Diameter (mm)	Threads per inch	Turns of thread
400	Shallow CT	38–120	8–5	1
405	Shallow CT with depressed thread	18+	8–5	1
425	Shallow CT with depressed thread	8–15		2
415	Tall CT (deep)	13–28	12–6	2
410	Medium tall	18–28	8–6	1.5
430	Tall CT four cut	18–38	8–5	1

Height – cap and bottle

For critical appraisal the external bottle height should be measured against the internal cap height with the wad fitted and an allowance made for the correct degree of wad compression. A cap should not stand proud, as this can lead to an unsightly appearance, or bottom on either the bead or the shoulder of bottle or jar.

Thread start

The thread start on both cap and bottle determines, particularly on a shallow finish, the length of thread engagement and therefore the number of turns or part turns required to tighten or release (Figure 6.22). Insufficient thread engagement can lead to cap tilt or uneven wad compression. This may also be caused by an over-thick wad.

Thread starts on plastic caps are virtually fixed by the tooling. In metal caps where the thread is rolled or formed, thread engagement can suffer due to a high thread start, a poorly defined run-out or when the thread is improperly formed (i.e. of insufficient height or depth, etc.).

However, if a bottle thread starts too high (nearer to the sealing surface) this may cause problems with plastic caps which employ a stopped rather than a run-out thread or where caps use a wad retention recess – see Figure 6.23. General metal and plastic cap drawing are shown in Figures 6.24 and 6.25. A typical glass finish is shown in Figure 6.26.

Pitch

Caps and bottles must have the same thread pitch or tpi (threads per inch). The number of threads per inch reduces as the neck diameter increases i.e.

- 8 mm finish = 15
- 63 mm finish = 5.

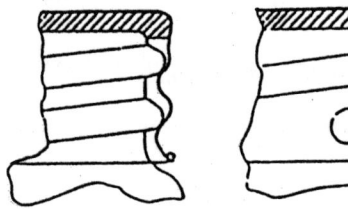

Figure 6.22 Illustration of the desirability of prolonging the thread as near to the brim as possible: 0.05 inch start (left) versus 0.1 inch start (right)

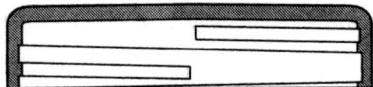

Figure 6.23 Type of plastic cap that is liable to prevent a seal: the upper end of the thread is stopped too low, and is liable to meet the top end of the thread before it is screwed home

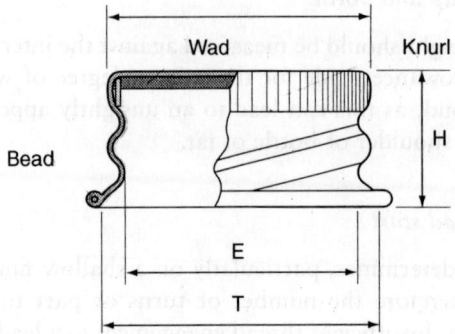

Figure 6.24 Metal screw cap

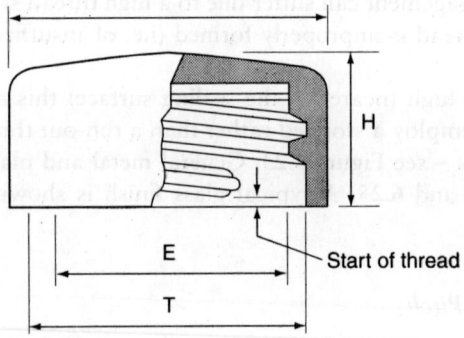

Figure 6.25 Plastic screw cap

Most glass screw finishes use a thread form based on 60° (earlier semi-round threads were employed). Metal screw caps also follow a common shape, but with plastic caps various configurations have been and still are used (see Figure 6.25).

Closuring diameter – relationship with seal efficiency

The effectiveness of a seal bears a direct relationship to the container diameter because:

1   the wider the container diameter, the more difficult it is to achieve a uniform seal-ing surface which lies in the same plane, i.e. perfectly flat
2   the wider the diameter, the greater is the seal area.

Therefore a wider diameter container must have a more resilient wad. Even with a good wad, higher moisture figures should be expected on wider diameter containers (see test data in Table 6.2). However, as larger containers hold greater amounts of product, the critical factor is the moisture gain per item or per gram of material.

For the tests documented in Table 6.2, containers contained dried calcium chloride with wadless PP caps applied to a normal torque. Although the results include some

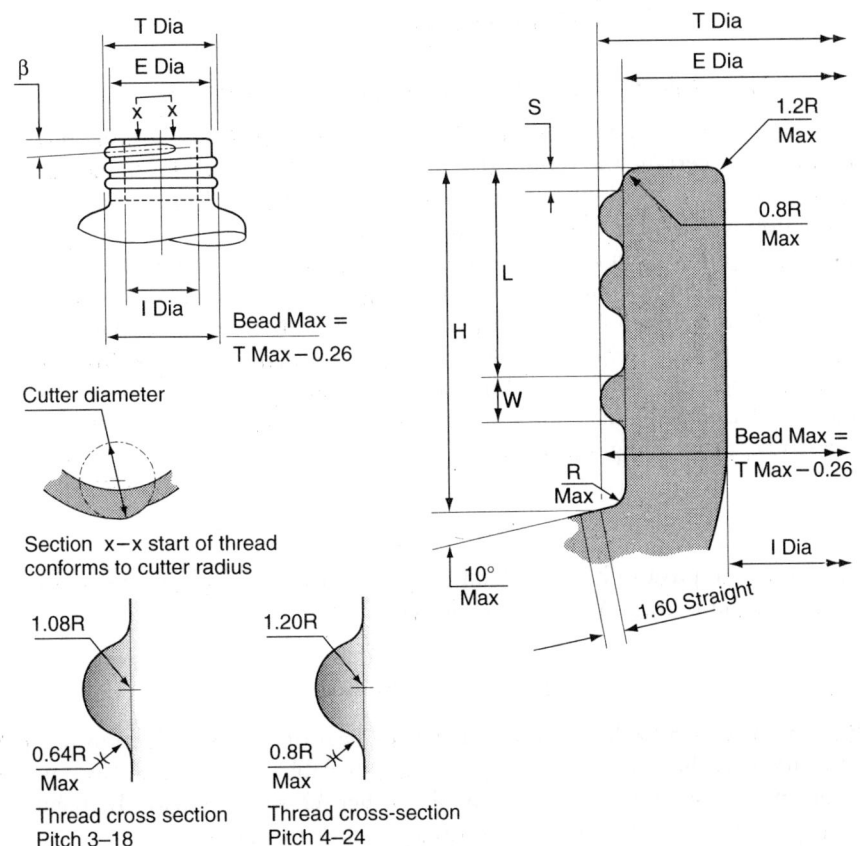

Figure 6.26 Typical drawing of bottle finish

Table 6.2 Results of moisture tests

Container	Finish	25°C 90% moisture gain (mg)			37°C 90% RH moisture gain (mg)		
		1 month	2 months	6 months	1 month	2 months	6 months
Glass 30 ml	22 mm	2	6	6	2	7	10
Glass 60 ml	24 mm	3	11	33	9	47	61
Glass 100 ml	28 mm	32	122	198	11	434	531

moisture gain due to permeation through polypropylene, a flowed-in compound lined cap gave comparable figures.

Multi-start as distinct from single start threads have two or more threads. These provide a more even pressure on the liner and require fewer turns to tighten or remove, e.g. on a four start thread, engagement is obtained in a $\frac{1}{4}$ turn. A conventional single start closure requires a minimum of $\frac{3}{4}$ turns of thread engagement to ensure that even pressure is obtained, and with less than $\frac{1}{2}$ turn of engagement a distinct tilt and/or a poor wad impression results.

Rolled-on closures are covered in Chapter 11.

Other means of closuring

Clinching, crimping, swaging, spinning or rolling

Each of these primarily applies to metal closures, although a similar action could be carried out with certain thermoplastics under the influence of heat. Basically each operation starts with the application of top pressure (like the RO seal) followed by a shaping action which locks metal under a retaining feature.

Clinch-on applies a simultaneous bending action over the total circumference of a skirt. Crimped-on applies both flutes and a bending action in the case of closures – the prime example is a crown cork closure invented by W. Painter of Baltimore in 1882. The word 'crimped' is frequently misused when 'clinched' is correct. Rolled-on and spun-on use wheels to bend in a skirt extension, thus providing a similar effect to clinching. Both clinched and spun-on metal closures are used in injection vials, IV solutions, cartridge tubes and glass aerosols.

Press-on

Press-on, push-on, push-in have gradually expanded in their applications, particularly on tablet vials and bottles. All are made of plastic.

Heat or adhesive seal

Finally, containers can be diaphragm sealed using heat (including induction sealing) or adhesive either as the sole closuring means (i.e. peelable tops for unit dose preparations) or in conjunction with any of the other closures previously mentioned. Diaphragms can be a useful means of forming a tamper-evident seal, e.g. used in conjunction with a child-resistant closure.

Dispensing closures

A closure may serve additional purposes to its prime objective of product retention. Dispensing closures offer pouring aids, facilities for providing drops, sprays, or a measured (metered) dose. Perhaps one of the earliest dispensing uses was the dropper-pipette which locked into a retaining hole in a conventional screw cap. This is still used today, with the bulb made from either natural or synthetic rubber or silicone elastomer, and a pipette of either glass or thermoplastic material.

Bore/plug fitments can be used to improve pouring or to restrict the flow so that a drop can be dispensed. Various pump systems can be fitted to glass bottles in order that a metered volume can be delivered as a 'shot' or as a coarse or fine spray. These employ special break-up features according to the product characteristics and the spray requirements. These devices have found wide usage for nasal products and have further potential in the pharmaceutical field. Captive closures can also incorporate a tear ring, thus creating a tamper-evident closure. These are invariably a wadless type of closure which can make its seal on any of three areas on the glass finish:

1   internal, cone or valve type seal – seals on either the lead-in edge or the sides of
     the bore
2   land or top seal – seal is made on the container sealing surface
3   external seal – seals on the edge or sides of the outer container wall.

Any combination of the above can be employed (see Figure 6.27).

   While pharmaceuticals have many closures in common with other groups of products, certain closuring systems are unique to pharmaceuticals. These are dealt with
below.

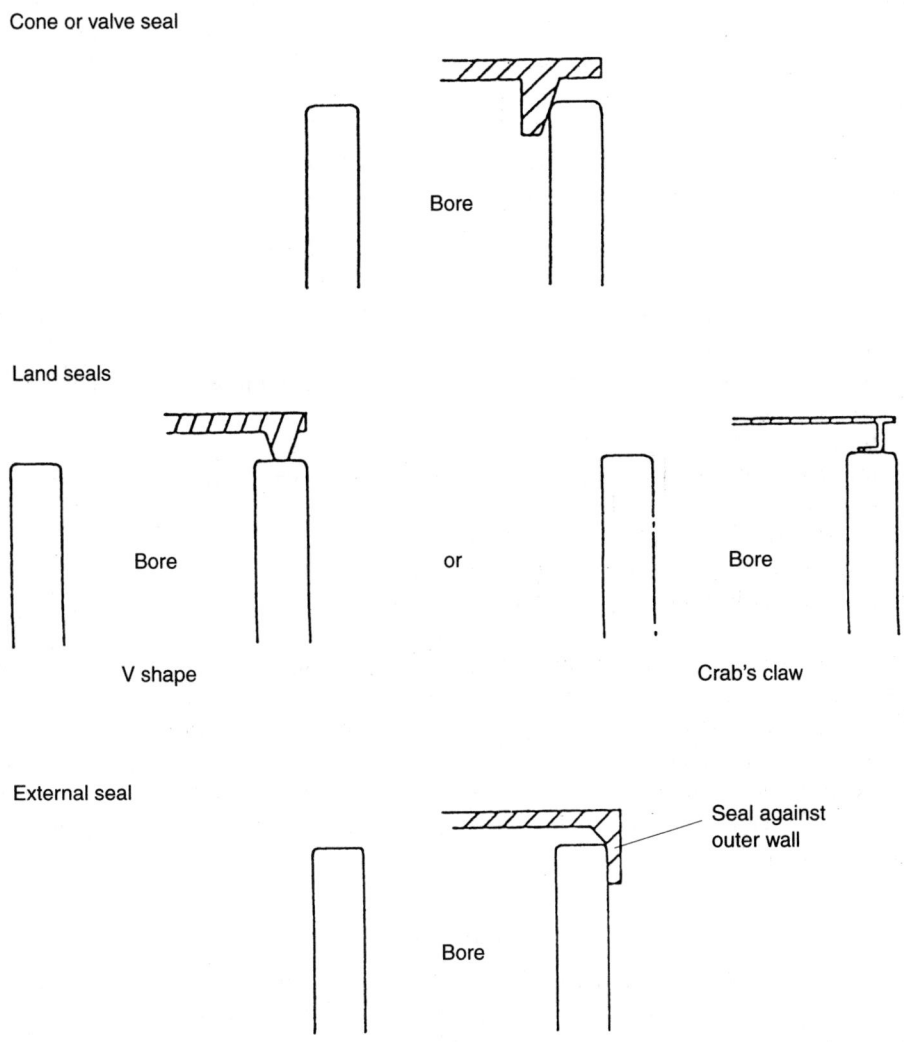

Figure 6.27 Types of seal

Special closures for pharmaceutical products (sterile products)

Fusion of glass – ampoules

Although ampoules have already been mentioned as an example of a near-perfect closure, all closuring systems require some means of checking their effectiveness. The basis for testing the seal of ampoules was immersion in a solution containing a dye and applying a vacuum (vacuum dye test). This is now being superseded by electrical conductivity testing, or capacitance testing (Eisei, Densok, etc.).

Intravenous solutions, multidose vials

The majority of sterile products rely on the use of a rubber closure (synthetic or natural) which is held in position by some form of overcap. The latter may be a metal screw cap or seal which is clinched or rolled under a bead. The rubber may be a disc or a plug and be applied either as a combination seal (the disc or plug is pre-fitted in a metal seal) or as separate components.

A closure for an injectable product has to fulfil the following requirements, which are additional to or more critical than the requirements for other closures.

1   It must make an air-tight seal and maintain sterility (i.e. not admit any micro-organisms).
2   It must be compatible with the product – not extracting or absorbing from the product or imparting anything to it.
3   It must be clean or capable of being cleaned to minimise possible particulate contamination.
4   It must be pierceable by a wide range of needle sizes and needle types, without leaking, splitting or shedding fragments by either friction (i.e. fragmentation) or coring.
5   It must reseal when needle is removed.
6   It must be capable of sterilisation at least once or twice by autoclaving. Gaseous or gamma sterilisation may be other possibilities.

Rubber meets most of these requirements, but so far no plastic material has been found as a substitute. The nearest alternative is a silicone rubber which is expensive, has a relatively high water vapour permeability and readily absorbs preservatives.

The range of rubber materials includes natural and synthetic-based materials. Special designs of rubber (e.g. castellated) are available for lyophilised/freeze dried products. Surfaces may be coated, e.g. with PTFE or Parylene, to reduce any extractability risks.

Summary

Closures are important to all packs, but particularly so with glass, where any exchange between the product and the external environment can only occur via the closure system. The total effectiveness of a glass pack is therefore reliant on its closure. However, function during use and ultimately disposal are also part of the overall fitness for purpose.

Appendix 6.1: Gauges

Gauges form an essential tool in the checking of glass containers. The main types are as follows (Figure 6.18).

1   Ring gauge – usually separate minimum and maximum gauges.
2   Parnaby gauge.
3   Single and double fork gauges:

- single fork – separate maximum and minimum
- single fork – with both maximum and minimum
- double fork – shaped like a letter H, covers maximum and minimum gauges.

4   Window gauge – usually for square or rectangular containers.
5   Channel gauge.
6   Box gauge.
7   Sleeve gauge.
8   Bore gauge:

- single
- minimum and maximum on separate ends
- minimum and maximum on same end.

9   Height gauge.
10 Verticality gauge.

It is important that gauges be correctly positioned during use – this usually means holding the gauge in a plane at 90° to the dimension being measured. If the gauge is tilted it can give an incorrect result.

Appendix 6.2: Glass terminology, test procedures and gauges

The fact that glass is a long-established packaging material has led to the gradual development of testing procedures and terminology.

Glass terminology

Figure 6.28 gives the basic terminology which is expanded in the text. A bottle consists of a finish or neck ring, a neck, shoulder, body and bottom or base. The finish varies according to the closure requirements. The bead, which is also known as the transfer ring (it supports the bottle when it is transferred from the parison to the finishing mould), may either be prominent, i.e. remain visible below the closure, or be concealed, i.e. covered when the closure is applied. The sealing surface may either be seamless (obtained by using a 'thimble' in the mould) or seamed. In the latter mould part lines are visible on the sealing surface.

The neck and shoulder may exist as two definable shapes or in certain circumstances may converge whereby they are virtually one (i.e. ill-defined).

The concave base is frequently known as the punt, and may be well defined as in certain wine bottles.

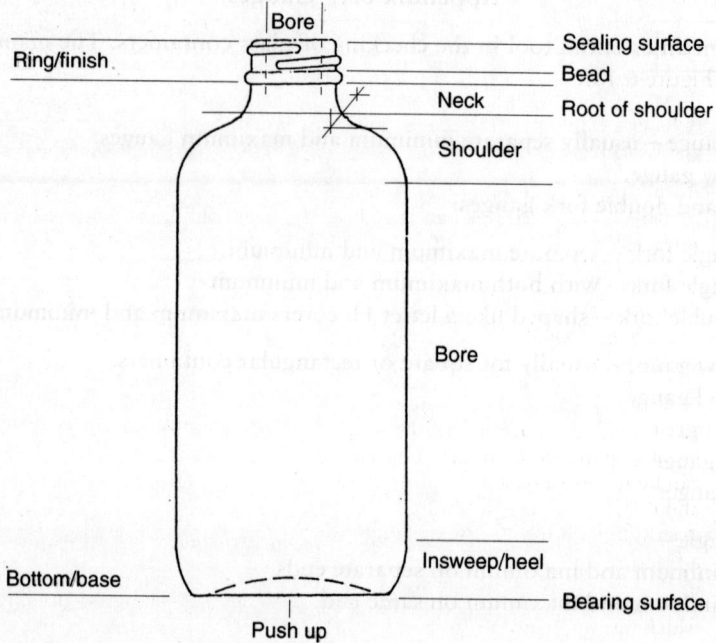

Figure 6.28 General terminology (glass bottle)

Glass defect terminology

As with many established industries, terminology can vary from company to company. Efforts have therefore been made to standardise certain terms. The list in Table 6.3 serves only to introduce the subject – a fuller list may be obtained from glass manufacturers or manufacturing federations.

Terms not involving fractures or cracks

1 Ring

- Bulged ring: profile bulged out of shape though not necessarily out of specification.
- Bent ring: a ring which is tilted to one side.
- Dipped ring: a severe dip or depression in the sealing surface.

2 Neck and shoulder

- Bent neck: a neck which is tilted.

3 Body defects

- Sunk: where the body is sunk inwards.
- Bulged: where the body has bulged outwards.
- Uneven distribution: varying thickness of bottle wall.
- Corrugated: undulating surface.

Table 6.3 Terms involving fracture or cracks

Defect	Description	Example
Split*	A fracture normally exceeding 6 mm in length which penetrates into the glass surface.	Split ring – a vertical split extending from sealing surface. Split body – in any direction in the body.
Check	A fracture normally less than 6 mm in length which penetrates into the glass surface.	Checked ring – anywhere on ring. Checked body – anywhere on body.
Crizzle	A surface 'fracture' of any length which does not penetrate into the glass to any appreciable extent. It reflects light in a similar way to checks and splits.	Crizzled sealing surface. Crizzled ring – elsewhere on ring than sealing surface.
Tear	A fissure as opposed to a fracture. Can be of any length or width. Allows a piece of paper to be inserted into it, i.e. can be felt as opposed to splits, checks and crizzles, which can rarely be felt – usually does not reflect light in the way a fracture does.	Tear under ring – usually occurs horizontally and directly under ring. Body and bottom tears – any orientation in body or bottom.
Chips	Distinct loss of a fragment of glass, which has not caused it to break.	Chipped sealing surface, chipped ring, body, bottom, etc.
Broken	Where a piece of glass has broken away from the main body or is so fractured that it will break away.	

* Splits can often lead to bottle failure and are therefore more important than checks or crizzles.

4   Bottom

- Wedged bottom: glass is thicker at one side than the other; unsightly but not thin enough for rejection.

5   Thin corner: wedged bottom with a thin corner which warrants rejection.
6   Rocky bottom: rocks from one side to the other.
7   Spinner: will spin freely due to central bulge.

The third group above covers general defects, for example the following.

- Bird swing: see Figure 6.17 – a thread of glass extends between two internal points in either neck or body.
- Stuck: lump of glass annealed to outside of container.
- Stones: refactory or batch inclusions in the glass.
- Seed: small bubbles in glass.
- Blisters: large bubbles in body of glass.
- Skin blisters: a soft surface blister which can be broken
- Hair or air line: a faint single line in glass surface.
- Wrinkle or washboard: a wrinkle or series of horizontal marks, one above another like a washboard.

- Spike: a projection, usually sharp, on inside of container.
- Glass inside: a piece of glass annealed to inside of container.
- Bloom: a hazy deposit or film, soluble in water, as found with type II glass.
- Weathered: a white surface deposit, not soluble in water.

Other defects refer to specific areas, e.g. thin shoulder, thin body, thin bottom. In each of these the area is too thin for safety.

These are only some of the many possible defects and faults (see Figure 6.17).

Specifications or dimensional defects can generally be detailed as over maximum or under minimum. Some categories may be further divided: under minimum bore, tight bore (slightly below minimum); choked bore, well below minimum. Typical AQLs for critical, major and minor defects are detailed in Appendix 6.3.

The following are examples of performance tests applied to glass containers.

Thermal shock test

The samples are placed in an upright position in a tray which is immersed into hot water for a given time, then transferred to a cold water bath. Temperatures of both baths are closely controlled. Samples are examined before and after the tests for outside surface cracks or breakage. The amount of thermal shock a bottle will withstand depends on its size, design and glass distribution. Small bottles will probably withstand a temperature differential of 60–80 °C, and 1 pint bottles 30–40 °C. A typical test uses a 45 °C temperature difference, hot to cold.

Internal bursting pressure test

The most common instrument is the American Glass Research increment pressure tester. The test bottle is filled with water and then placed inside the test chamber. A sealing head is applied and the internal pressure automatically raised by a series of increments.

Each increment is held for a set time. The bottle can either be checked to a preselected pressure level or the test continued until the container finally bursts.

Annealing test

The sample is examined by polarised light in either a polariscope or a strain viewer. The strain pattern is compared against standard strain discs or limit samples. Normal annealed glassware shows limited strain patterns usually with colours of red/blue – greater intensities of strain are indicated by colours ranging from white/orange through red/purple to green, yellow and white. Both extremes indicate strain due to either tension or compression. The interpretation of strain is frequently one of experience. When a glass bottle leaves a mould the outside tends to cool more rapidly than the inside, leaving the inner surface under a state of tension. This strain is normalised in the lehr, where the whole container is raised to dull red heat and then cooled slowly.

Vertical load test

The bottle is placed between a fixed platform and a hydraulic ramp platform which is gradually raised so that a vertical load is applied. The load is registered on a pressure gauge.

Leakage tests

These may be based on product tests, vacuum tests, feeler gauge tests, or newer special tests as given in Chapter 11.

Autoclaving

The ability of a filled or empty container to withstand autoclaving may be checked. It should be noted that when large numbers of glass containers are autoclaved some occasional breakages can be expected. Those that break are assumed to be substandard containers with certain defects such as surface damage which are difficult to detect by prior inspection. Autoclaving may be used to test the possibility of extractives from the glass surface. As a general rule 60 min at 121° C is considered equivalent to a shelf life of half to one year.

Limit tests for alkalinity or chemical resistance

These are employed to check the alkalinity extractives. The pharmacopoeial tests may be based upon surface extraction tests (i.e. type II surface treated glass) or crushed glass where the glass composition is checked (type I neutral glass).

Appendix 6.3: Packaging material specification

STANDARD NAME: BOTTLE GLASS AMBER RECTANGULAR TABLET 30 ML	**DATE:** **CODE REF:**

SUPERSEDES SPECIFICATION:	**CODE:**	**DATED:**	**NEW DESIGN:**
REASON FOR REVISION:			

GENERAL DESCRIPTION:	As above (new design) fitted BS 28R3 neck finish. Rectangular cross-section with rounded ends and sloping shoulders, seamless sealing surface
MATERIAL DESCRIPTION:	Soda lime silica glass amber
CONSTRUCTION (PROCESS):	Blow and blow
SIZE/CAPACITY:	35.0 ml +/− 1.9 ml at fill point Fill point 19.0 mm from sealing surface
DRAWING NUMBER:	(with tolerances for weight and dimensions)
DECORATION:	Plain
SPECIAL TESTS:	See glass manual
ACCEPTABLE QUALITY LEVELS:	Critical 0.0% Major 2.5% ALSO SEE NOTES ON REVERSE Minor 6.5%

MODE OF PACKING FOR DELIVERY

To be packed in good quality cartons with taped upper flaps and stitched base flaps to exclude dirt and debris. All cartons to be correctly identified.

AUTHORISATION:	
SUPPLIER:	**DATE:**
RECEIVING COMPANY:	**DATE:**

Notes

1. Where company has approved buying samples for goods, any orders for goods of the same description subsequently placed by the company shall, unless otherwise indicated, be deemed to be placed on the basis of such buying samples as well as on the description and/or specification, and in all such cases the goods shall conform both to such buying samples and the description and/or specification.

2. The supplier shall effect no physical or chemical change to the product or its method of manufacture without the prior agreements in writing of the company.

3. The company reserves the right to revise or amend the specification after formal notification to the supplier.

4. Sampling, inspection and classification of defectives is conducted strictly in accordance to .... (the AQLs for this are shown overleaf).

5. Visual defect classifications

CRITICAL

Defects which are likely to result in hazardous conditions for potential users or packing operatives.

MAJOR

a) Defects which are likely to materially reduce the usability of the container or end product.
b) Defects which are likely to result in the product not meeting the required standard.

MINOR

Defects which are not likely to materially affect the usability but are a departure from normal commercial standards.

AUTHORISATION:	
SUPPLIER:	DATE:
RECEIVING COMPANY:	DATE:

References

1. Moody, B., *Packaging in Glass*, Hutchinson Benham, London.
2. Pfaender, H.G., *Schott Guide to Glass*, Chapman & Hall, London.

7

PLASTICS – AN INTRODUCTION

D. A. Dean

Historical background

The wider acceptance of plastics as a basic packaging material took a positive step forward in the early 1950s, with the entry of polyethylene into full commercial use. Until that time the use of plastic in packaging had been mainly limited to certain thermosetting resins used for closures and a few containers (for menthol cones, shaving sticks, etc.). Reference to the history of plastics indicates that the knowledge of plastics was much further advanced in those early times than most packaging people would expect. Even today this state of affairs can still exist. Although specific substances, now recognised under the term plastics, can be identified as far back as the early nineteenth century, the name 'plastics' did not come into general use until the mid-1920s. These early plastic discoveries were generally scientific in nature without any insight into the possible applications. Phenol formaldehyde, for example, although a chemical entity in 1840, was not exploited until around 1916 when it became synonymous with the word 'Bakelite'. Nitrocellulose, which subsequently became known as 'celluloid', was also discovered in the nineteenth century and was exploited far more quickly. It became one of the first commercially accepted plastics when produced by the Hyatt Brothers in the USA around 1870. Celluloid subsequently found use for numerous household articles (brush backs, mirror holders, trays, etc.).

The objectives of this chapter are to provide a basic knowledge of plastic materials, their characteristics which are likely to appertain to pharmaceuticals and the processes by which they are converted into packaging materials.

What are plastics?

Plastics may be defined as any group of substances, of natural or synthetic origins, consisting chiefly of polymers of high molecular weight, that can be moulded into a shape or form by heat and pressure. They usually consist of large molecules of organic materials which are based on certain building block molecules referred to as monomers. When these monomers, which are relatively small molecules, undergo a process known as polymerisation, a plastic or long chain polymer is produced. This process of polymerisation may involve various chemicals which assist the process, such as accelerators, initiators, solvents and catalysts, and as a result are present to some small degree in the plastic produced. These, if found in the plastic after polymerisation, are generally known as process residues. Plastics may also incorporate processing aids (usually added to assist a process) and additives which modify the plastic chemically or physically in some way. Polymers can broadly be divided into two categories: thermosetting plastics and thermoplastics. Certain plastics may involve high pressure (LDPE) or low pressure (LLDPE, HDPE) processes.

Polymerisation

Plastics are basically produced by the process of polymerisation, which may be either addition or condensation polymerisation (see below)

Structure

Three structures are found – linear, linear branched, and cross-linked.

Linear

Linear polymer chains arise where the monomers join together in long chains with few or a limited number of side chains. These chains may, however, be in a twisted and tangled formation giving an amorphous type polymer or in a more orderly layout to give a crystalline structure. When the chains are made from a single (identical) repeating unit, a homopolymer is produced. If there are two separate (different) repeating units (monomers), a copolymer is formed with either a random or a block structure.

Random: A+A+B+A+B+A+A+A etc

Block: A+A+A+B+A+A+A+B etc

Branched

These are again long chain type polymers with far more side chain branches. These usually occur randomly, producing a more open structure which will be reflected in certain physical and physical–chemical properties. Under selected conditions the repeating unit B may be 'grafted' onto the linear chain A. This formation is called a 'graft copolymer', i.e.

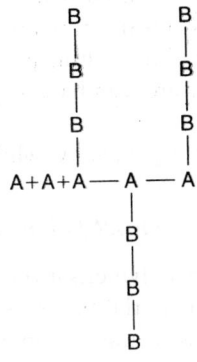

Cross-linked

Cross-linkage consists of joints between chains which occur in three dimensions. Cross-linkage usually again is reflected in physical properties, increasing, for example, polymer rigidity. In general, thermoplastic materials have linear and branched chains whereas thermosets are cross-linked.

Most polymers exhibit stereoisomerism, hence may appear in three forms:

- atactic, a random arrangement of the unsymmetrical groups
- isotactic, a structure where all groups are lined on the same side of the backbone chain
- syndiotactic, a structure where the placement of each group alternates on either side of the backbone chain.

Reference to the amorphous or crystalline nature of plastic has already been made. Crystallinity is supported by a regular chain structure whereas amorphous materials are irregular. Few polymers are, however, 100% crystalline or amorphous; frequently 'crystallite' or 'spherulite' areas of crystallinity are found in an amorphous background. Stretching a polymer by orientation increases the degree of molecular alignment, particularly with amorphous materials. Crystalline materials usually melt before a polymer degrades, hence have a melting point (T_m).

The presence of crystalline materials has a strong influence on their properties, e.g. polymer chains pack more tightly together, hence have a higher density, as shown by LDPE (60–65% crystalline), HDPE (90–95% crystalline), with densities of, say, 0.915 and 0.965 respectively.

General properties

Amorphous materials give good clarity, transparency, hardness with possible brittleness, are usually more permeable to gases and moisture and are less inert. Crystalline materials are opaque or translucent, more flexible, with low permeability to gases and moisture and are more inert.

Amorphous materials can be found as hard glassy plastics (polystyrene) or can be soft, flexible and rubbery (polyisoprene). This means that there is a temperature range where an amorphous material is in a glassy state and above which it is rubbery. This temperature is known as the glass-transition temperature T_g. However, a truly amorphous material cannot have a crystalline melting point (T_m). Crystalline materials (usually an amorphous–crystalline mixture) can have a T_g – in the case of polyethylene this is around −85°C.

For a specific grade of polyester, T_m is 267°C while T_g is 69°C.

Thermoset polymers

These are polymers produced by a polymerisation process involving a curing or vulcanisation stage during which the material becomes 'set' to a permanent state by heat and pressure. Further heating leads to the decomposition of the plastic. Thermosets usually contain additional fillers and reinforcing agents to obtain the best properties. Examples of thermoset resins include phenolics, melamine, urea, alkyds, expoxies, certain polyesters and polyurethanes, and are predominantly cross-linked polymers. Typical packaging applications include closures, small cases (as one time used for menthol cones), protective lacquers and enamels (as applied internally and externally to metal containers) and a range of adhesive systems. Thermosetting contact materials, such as lacquers, will probably receive more attention in the future. This will involve more effective compatibility studies and the use of the newer surface analysis techniques.

Thermoplastics

Thermoplastics are heat softening materials which can be repeatedly heated, made mobile and then reset to a solid state by cooling. Under conditions of fabrication these materials can be moulded (shaped in a mould) by temperature and pressure. Examples of thermoplastics are more numerous than thermosets, e.g. polyethylene, polyvinylchloride, polystyrene, polypropylene, nylon, polyester, polyvinylidene chloride, polycarbonate. Thermoplastics may be further divided into homopolymers which involve one type of monomer, e.g. ethylene polymerised to polyethylene, and co-polymers, terpolymers, etc., which involve two or more monomers of different chemical substances. Polymerisation producing thermoplastics and thermoset materials usually follows two basic chemical mechanisms, i.e. condensation and addition polymerisation.

Condensation polymerisation (step reaction polymerisation), is where monomers combine with the loss of some smaller molecules in the process, e.g. water:

$$C_6H_5OH + HCHO \longrightarrow C_6H_5CHO + H_2O$$
$$\text{phenol} + \text{formaldehyde} \longrightarrow \text{phenol formaldehyde} + \text{water}$$

Addition polymerisation (chain reaction polymerisation) consists of simple addition

$$CH_2 = CH_2 \longrightarrow CH_2 - CH_2 - \left[CH_2 - CH_2 \right]_x$$
$$\text{ethylene} \qquad\qquad \text{polyethylene}$$

without the elimination of any smaller molecules, e.g.

where x is a large number, up to tens of thousands.

The polymer molecules may occur as long unbranched straight chains (linear polymers), branched chains, or a three-dimensional lattice work where the branches link the main chains together (i.e. cross-linked polymers). Properties of plastic vary according to their form of molecular structure. Materials may also be amorphous or crystalline, where the latter are generally less permeable. The degree of crystallinity is usually established by X-ray diffraction studies.

From here on this chapter expands the properties of various plastics, the means by which certain physical and chemical characteristics can be identified and quantified, together with the constituents which may be 'found' in a plastic. The converting processes may contribute other factors relevant to the selection and clearance of a plastic pack. The chapter concludes by reference to sterilisation methods and references. (The next chapter places particular emphasis on the 'clearance of a plastic pack', and should be read in conjunction with this section.)

It could or perhaps should be concluded from this background that the majority of pharmaceutical products could, with the rapidly expanding technology of today, be packed in one of the plastics available. In the ultimate choice the question may not be what is the ideal plastic to choose but what is the best combination of materials. This may include several layers of different plastics (e.g. coextrusions), laminations, coated plastics, or a low-cost material enclosed in one or more 'overwraps'.

Currently the greater part of usage lies with the economic five. These consist of the polyethylenes, polypropylenes, polyvinylchlorides and polystyrenes, all at similar prices per tonne, and polyester, which although nearly double the price of the other four offers special properties, usually in thinner sections etc.

The main thermosetting and thermoplastic materials are now briefly described.

Thermosets

Urea formaldehyde (UF)

UF is made by the condensation polymerisation of urea and formaldehyde. Although it has been widely used for closures (mainly in pastel shades), use is now in decline due to wadless thermoplastic systems. Density 1.47–1.52.

Phenol formaldehyde (originally Bakelite) (PF)

PF is made by the condensation polymerisation of phenol and formaldehyde. Due to the volatile and toxic/irritant nature of formaldehyde, this is usually 'fixed' with ammonia giving hexamine. Polymerisation of hexamine and phenol not only produces phenol formaldehyde but may release residues of phenol, formaldehyde or ammonia. In certain cases some residues may remain in the moulding and be released into the product. As with UF, PF is mainly used for closures but due to the fact that the material is naturally dark, it is used for dark or deep colours. PF is generally more resistant to heat and moisture than UF. Both UF and PF are used with a range of fillers, e.g. wood flour, synthetic fibre. Density 1.25–1.45. General pharmaceutical applications have now reduced.

Melamine formaldehyde (MF)

Although offering better resistance to water and heat, it is considerably more expensive than UF and PF and has found few packaging applications.

Epoxy resins (epoxides)

Epoxy resins are polymers offering higher performance than most other thermosets. Their main packaging applications are for protective lacquers.

Polyurethanes (PURs)

Thermosetting polyurethanes are used as adhesives and to a limited extent as coatings or lacquers. They can be found as esters and ethers.

Polyesters

Polyester thermosetting resins, which are made by the polymerisation of dibasic acids with poly-functional alcohols, find uses in chemical storage tanks and chemical piping rather than any direct pharmaceutical applications. Polyester thermosets offer high general strength, particularly when reinforced with glass fibre (GRP), excellent dimensional stability and good temperature resistance for temperatures up to 200°C. Recently metal tube enamels have used polyester-based resins.

Thermoset resins are normally moulded by compression, compression transfer or, more recently, injection moulding. Two-part resin systems are used for adhesives, coatings and lacquers. Pharmaceutical applications include closures (reducing), adhesives in laminations, protective lacquers, and enamels.

Thermoplastics

The five most economical plastics are the polyethylenes (ultra low, low, linear low, medium and high density), polypropylenes (homopolymer and copolymer), polyesters, polystyrenes and polyvinylchlorides (unplasticised and plasticised) and as a result these are the materials most widely used by the pharmaceutical industry. Polyethylene and polypropylene may also be grouped under 'olefins'. The list of plastics which follows is given alphabetically rather than in any order of use.

Acrylonitrile butadiene styrene (ABS)

ABS is composed of acrylonitrile, butadiene rubber and styrene and is therefore part of the styrene group. Styrene, basically a glossy, rigid, brittle material, becomes tougher and more flexible with the addition of the other constituents. ABS produces a high-gloss finish which is particularly useful for injection moulded parts for devices and similar ancillary components. The acrylonitrile monomer was under a toxicity cloud following tests which established possible carcinogenic relationships. The primary danger is related to the polymerisation manufacturing plants, and steps have been taken to reduce significantly the free monomer level. Acrylonitrile levels of less than 0.1 ppm are now generally considered acceptable and safe.

Acetal polyoxymethylene (POM) (Delrin, Kemetal – trade names)

Acetals are obtained from the polymerisation of formaldehyde, and this is basically an engineering plastic with high stiffness, tensile strength and good fatigue endurance. Usage usually lies with devices, aerosol valves and similar engineering components. Being a polymerisation of formaldehyde, residues may have to be checked if grades and moulding conditions are not correctly selected. Copolymers are also available. The density of POM is approximately 1.41. POM is less hygroscopic than most nylons and provided it is correctly stored, it does not need pre-drying.

The acrylics

Polymethylmethacrylate (PMMA), found under the trade names of Perspex, Plexiglas, Lucite, etc., is one of the better known polymers in the acrylic group. PMMA is hard, rigid, with good clarity (92% light transmission equivalent to glass), good weather resistance and good dimensional stability. In common with polystyrene, PMMA will surface craze in contact with certain chemicals. PMMA has a density of 1.18. Acrylates are being increasingly used in adhesive systems and are found as a major constituent in heat sealants and in self-adhesive bases. PMMA has also found wide usage in hard contact lenses.

The cellulosics

This group incorporates some of the earliest discovered plastics, which are detailed individually below.

Cellulose acetate (CA)

Cellulose acetate is a clear but highly permeable plastic made by a similar type of process as used for regenerated cellulose. Cotton fibres are acetylated using glacial acetic acid and acetic anhydride, with sulphuric acid as a catalyst, to give cellulose triacetate which is then hydrolysed. The precipitated acetate is dissolved in a solvent, plasticised and made into a film by either solvent casting or slot die extrusion. Dimethyl phthalate may be added as a typical plasticiser. Cellulose acetate has a relatively high permeability to gases and moisture. It is therefore used as a film which 'breathes', especially when highly plasticised. It also has high clarity, good resistance to oils and can be moulded by most conventional processes including thermoforming.

Cellulose propionate (CAP) and cellulose acetate butyrate (CAB)

Both CAP and CAB have superior properties to plain acetate, particularly with reference to toughness and impact strength. Their main uses are as engineering plastics and occasionally for pharmaceutical devices and administration aids. Hard, gas-permeable contact lenses may be made from CAB.

Regenerated cellulose group

Regenerated cellulose is included under plastics although it is a derivative of wood pulp, which is first reacted with sodium hydroxide and then dissolved in carbon disulphide. After maturing, it is converted into a film or sheet by slot extrusion into an acid bath, followed by washing to remove the acid, and then dried. Most cellulose films contain an humectant such as glycerol or ethylene glycol which reacts to humidity changes. Various coatings are applied to confer heat sealability and resistance to moisture permeation. The coatings include nitrocellulose, polyvinylidene chloride, polyethylene, etc. Uncoated regenerated cellulose film is very hygroscopic, highly permeable to water and has poor dimensional stability. It is otherwise a strong, flexible, transparent film with good grease resistance. Coated films are mainly used as transparent overwraps, strip packs and as an outer ply in laminations. Trade names such as Cellophane and Rayophane are widely used.

Cellulose nitrate or nitrocellulose (celluloid or xylonite)

This is made by the reaction of strong nitric acid with cellulose. Today it is mainly used as a coating to provide heatsealing with general barrier properties. It seals at a lower temperature than polyvinylidene chloride, but for the same coating weight offers a considerably inferior barrier. It is highly flammable.

Ethylene-based polymers

Ethylene-vinyl acetate (EVA)

EVA is a copolymer of ethylene and vinyl acetate which can have certain properties changed according to the proportion of each monomer. EVAs are soft, flexible compounds with high elongation and high impact strength even down to low temperatures. They are widely used in conjunction with LDPE and PP to increase flexibility and as an aid to heatsealing. EVA is also the basis for certain hot melts and is used as a compound lining in closures.

Ethylene vinyl alcohol copolymer (EVAL or EVOH)

EVOH is now widely offered as an extrusion ply for coextruded laminations, where it provides a good bond, acting as a good carrier for other plies and is increasingly popular as an excellent oxygen barrier. It has to be protected from moisture absorption since this significantly lowers its otherwise excellent barrier properties.

Ethylene acid copolymers

Ethylene acid polymer is obtained by the copolymerisation of ethylene with either acrylic or methacrylic acid. These copolymers are somewhat similar to LDPE and are found as ethylene acrylic acid (EAA) and ethylene methacrylic acid (EMA). Both are used in various packaging applications, i.e. flexible packaging, adhesive laminating, hot melts, and heat seal coatings.

Ethylene-ethyl acrylate (EEA)

Ethylene-ethyl acrylate copolymers can produce very tough flexible materials and can vary from very rubbering low temperature melting products to polyethylene-like materials. EEA is used as a hot melt adhesive, for disposable gloves, tubing and sheeting.

The fluoroplastics

The fluoroplastics are a relatively pricey group which are generally more inert than most other plastics.

Polytetrafluoroethylene (PTFE)

PTFE (trade name Teflon, Fluon etc.) is probably the most well known of the fluoro-plastics. It is, however, a relatively difficult material to process. The polymer is linear, with a very high molecular weight, a high density (2.2) and a high melting point (327°C).

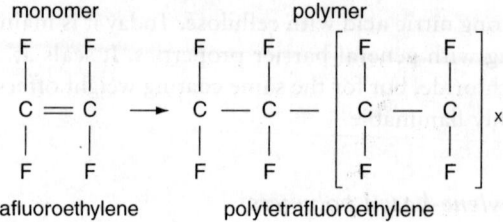

It is used as a coating for heat sealing jaws, as a low friction surface and as 'inert' coating for rubber stoppers.

Polymonochlorotrifluoroethylene (PCTFE) (trade name Aclar)

PCTFE is one of the most inert plastics, with the lowest permeability of all plastics to moisture. It has, however, higher permeabilities to O_2, N_2 and CO_2 than PVdC. The basic monomer, chlorofluoroethylene C_2ClF_3, has certain toxic properties. It is about the most expensive plastic (over £25,000 per tonne) and has so far only been used in packaging as a thin layer (laminated to PVC) for blister packing. Three types are in use: 22A, 33C and 88A. The first is usually used at 37 μm (on PVC) with a WVP figure of around 0.030 g/100 in^2/24 h at 38°C 90% RH. These all are copolymers. 33C is lower in cost because of higher yields but is far more difficult to form. 33C is used laminated to PVC at 18.75 μm and 50 μm; moisture permeation for 33C compared with earlier figure for 22A is 0.030 g and 0.015 g respectively for 38°C 90% RH, i.e. it has a similar permeability to 22A at approximately half the thickness. New homopolymers R_x 160, ultR$_x$ 2000 and 3000, SupR$_x$ 900 offer certain advantages over the copolymers, including lower costs.

Fluorinated ethylene propylene (FEP)

Has similar properties to PTFE but processes more easily. It has a crystalline melting point around 290°C.

Ethylene tetrafluoroethylene (ETFE)

This does not have the same wide temperature range as PTFE, but is easier to mould.

Ionomers (trade name Surlyn)

This group is relatively new to plastics, being available since around 1965. Ionomers are so named because of the presence of ionised carboxyl groups which provide a cross-linking effect on the molecular chain and are based on metallic salts of ethylene/methacrylic acid copolymers. The physical properties are somewhat similar to

LDPE, with a lower melting point (around 70–80°C) and a relatively broad heat sealing range. Surlyn is therefore used as a heat sealing ply since it seals well in the presence of both powders and liquids (i.e. contaminated seals). It can therefore be sealed at higher speeds and with greater security than most other heat sealants. It is more expensive than low density polyethylene, but as a heat seal ply it can be effectively used at approximately two-thirds the thickness of polyethylene (LDPE). Ionomers have excellent abrasion resistance and good resistance to puncture and impact. The side chain metals include Ca, Zn, Mg.

Liquid crystal polymers (LCPs)

LCPs are a group of aromatic copolyester polymers with high physical performance properties, high levels of inertness, low flammability with excellent high temperature resistance. Use for pharmaceuticals is predicted, possibly blended with PE or PET.

Methylpentene (TPX) polymers (ICI) – poly(4-methylpentene-1)

TPX is another relatively new plastic which was commercialised in 1968. It is an olefin-based resin with the lowest density of the plastics (0.83) but a high melting point of 240°C, which makes it a high-temperature-resistant plastic. Methylpentene can be a crystal clear or an opaque plastic. It is highly permeable to moisture and gases.

Nitrile or acrylonitrile polymers

Copolymers with a high acrylonitrile content (trade names Barex (Vistron) and Lopac (Monsanto)) have interesting properties. With a specific gravity of 1.15 these resins are glass clear, offer excellent impact resistance even at low temperatures, have good rigidity and offer high barrier to gases, especially oxygen and carbon dioxide. For instance, their oxygen transmission is approximately eight times better than PVC, 250 times better than HDPE and 300 times better than PP. Water transmission rates are higher than for PVC, e.g.

HDPE (1): PP (1.2): PVC (7.5): Barex (12.5): Styrene (40).

The material therefore readily absorbs moisture and must be effectively dried prior to moulding, otherwise a hazy or milky appearance may result. Polyacrylonitriles have a relatively low heat distortion temperature (around 75°C), hence they have limitations for products requiring a hot fill. The material is suitable for thermoforming operations but its relatively high moisture permeation is likely to restrict ultimate usage. The presence of acrylonitrile residues also placed the material under a cloud with the FDA, but use is now accepted provided acrylonitrile monomer does not exceed 0.1 ppm. Nitrile copolymers are usually copolymerised with methyl acrylate together with small quantities of butadiene/acrylonitrile rubbers.

The nylons (polyamides) (PA)

Nylon is the general name for the polyamide polymers. They cover a range of types, i.e. type 6, type 6:6, type 6:10, type 11 and type 12. The broad properties of the polyamides include low friction (good bearing properties), toughness, high fatigue resistance, high impact resistance, and good solvent resistance to aromatic hydrocarbons. Nylons 6 and 6:6, because of their lower price, tend to be the most used but have the highest absorption of moisture which tends to act as a plasticiser. The polymers are formed by a condensation reaction between amine groups and carboxylic acid groups to give an acid–basic type linkage known as amides. The nylons are classified by the number of carbon atoms in the diamine, followed by the number of carbon atoms in the diacid or by just the number of carbon atoms in the polymer chain (reference the monomer molecule).

The reaction acid + amine or diamine + diacid can be expressed as follows:

$$R-\overset{\displaystyle OH}{\underset{\displaystyle O}{C}} + R_1-NH_2 \longrightarrow \left[R-\overset{\displaystyle H}{\underset{\displaystyle O}{C-N}}-R_1 \right]_x + H_2O$$

acid + amine   nylon

Diamine nylons

          amine monomer   + acid monomer
Nylon 6:6 = hexamethylene diamine (6) + adipic acid (6)
Nylon 6:10 = hexamethylene diamine (6) + sebacic acid (10)
          (number of carbon atoms in brackets)

The above are therefore copolymers. The homopolymer nylons are made from the following:

    nylon 6 = amino caproic acid (6)
    nylon 11 = amino undecanoic acid (11)
    nylon 12 = amino dodecanoic acid (12)

Nylons have relatively high melting points and can be steam autoclaved. Nylons can be injection moulded, blow moulded or made into sheet or film, and have a density range of 1.14–1.16. Multi-ply materials are employed for their oxygen barrier properties.

Polyamide–imide (PAI)

Polyamide–imide represents another group of high-temperature engineering polymers, with good dimensional stability, impact and chemical resistance.

Polyaryletherketone

This is a relatively new crystalline plastic with a high melting point of 334°C. It has good abrasion resistance, with good chemical and solvent resistance.

Polybutylene (PB) and polyisobutylene (PIB)

Polybutylene is another new member of the polyolefin group, being similar to polyethylene but exhibiting better tensile strength. It is frequently used blended with polyethylene or polypropylene to modify the properties of films, i.e. to give a controllable peelable seal, and a good future as copolymers is predicted.

Polycarbonate (PC)

Polycarbonate is a copolymer of bisphenol A and phosgene or diphenyl carbonate. It is a transparent highly crystalline polymer with good mechanical properties, e.g. high impact strength plus high temperature resistance and fairly low moisture absorption. It is, however, attacked by alkalis and aromatic hydrocarbons. Certain reactions are similar to stress cracking. PC has a density of 1.2 with a moulding shrinkage of 0.5%. Permeation to moisture, however, is only fair. Growth in the medical area, particularly in coextrusion film applications, is predicted.

The polyolefins

The olefin group covers the following (density is shown on the right):

- ultra and very low density polyethylene   0.89–0.915
- low density polyethylene (LDPE)   0.91–0.925
  (and linear low density) (LLDPE)   0.915–0.930
- medium density polyethylene (MDPE)   0.926–0.940
- high density polyethylene (HDPE)   0.940–0.965
- polypropylene (homopolymer/copolymer) (PP)   0.900–0.910

There are also ultra high molecular weight grades of HDPE.

Low density polyethylene (LDPE)

Low density polyethylene material has branched chains and limited crystallinity, which lead to an open structure and the low density. It is particularly soft and flexible, transparent to translucent, has good impact resistance and relatively low melting points, which give good heat sealability. Most LDPEs are made by a high pressure polymerisation process starting from ethylene gas. The proportion of crystallinity to amorphous is around 3:2 (i.e. 60–65% crystalline). Recently new linear polyethylene copolymers of 0.89–0.91 (ultra or very low densities) have been developed. Special antioxidant free grades are available for pharmaceutical applications.

Medium density polyethylene (MDPE)

As density increases, materials change in both physical and chemical properties, becoming more rigid, less impact-resistant, less translucent, stronger, less flexible with an increase in melt temperature. There is also a continuing improvement in moisture and gas permeability, chemical and oil resistance, absorbency to chemicals (e.g. preservatives), etc. There is a reduction in branching and an increase in crystallinity.

High density polyethylene (HDPE)

HDPE is the most crystalline material (around 95%) and virtually free of branching and as a result has the best chemical properties, i.e. best resistance and lowest permeabilities. It is also a relatively rigid, tough material with the lowest clarity. Extra high molecular weight (HMW and UHMW) grades find specialised uses, i.e. 25 l containers and larger, due to high shock resistance and good inertness.

HDPE exists as both a homopolymer and a copolymer with higher ethylene olefins. The latter offers properties which lie between low and high density, with typical densities of 0.945–0.950. Copolymers have found wide usage for extrusion blow, injection blow and injection moulding. They are, however, generally classified under HDPE. Virtually all high density polyethylenes contain an antioxidant.

Polyethylenes generally have a high coefficient of thermal expansion and suffer increasing vulnerability towards environmental stress cracking (ESC). LDPE when under stress in contact with certain chemicals, categorised as stress cracking agents, can lead to stress cracking. These agents include detergents, wetting agents, certain hydrocarbons, volatile oils, soaps, etc. Shrinkage is high with the polyethylenes, e.g. 1.5–2.0% (LDPE). The likely variables associated with the polyethylene are chain length, antioxidant, regrind, catalytic residues, filler, antistatics, lubricants, and slip additives. Tyvek (trade name) is a spun bonded fibrous sheet of HDPE with controlled porosity which has found many pharmaceutical/hospital applications for sterile components and instruments. The fluoride treatment of HDPE is widely used to further improve its resistance to organic chemicals (e.g. solvents).

Linear low density polyethylene (LLDPE)

LLDPE is a relatively new material in terms of commercial exploitation which is receiving enormous interest, particularly as a film material where it is replacing many conventional LDPE applications. Some of the more commercially viable applications lie outside the pharmaceutical industry. There is, however, every indication that LLDPE will also find pharmaceutical usages. More immediate applications are seen with extruded film, with long-term usage in other areas where grades are already available for injection moulding, rotational moulding and cast film. LLDPE is being used for plastic tubes and as a heat seal ply where it provides high seal strength. The main advantage of LLDPE is that it can be made at lower gauges while having similar physical strength to LDPE. It is made by a low-pressure Zieglar-Natta catalytic process.

LLDPEs are usually referred to as comonomers and copolymers, where mixtures of higher olefins, butene, hexene, octene, etc. are used. Mixtures of LDPE, MDPE, HDPE, and ethylene vinyl acetate, etc. are fighting the introduction of LLDPE. LLDPE can be produced in grades which have good clarity.

Expanded low density polyethylene (EPE)

Expanded low density polyethylene is found as either a cross-linked foam or a non-cross-linked foam, with significant developments being initiated in Japan. It has been offered as a replacement moulding material for closure wadding either with or without an additional facing. When used as a wadding material, densities can be varied to give different levels of compression.

Polypropylene (PP)

Polypropylene is somewhat similar to HDPE in general properties. It exists as a homopolymer and a copolymer with ethylene and other hydrocarbons. It can also be blended with polyisobutylene. PP is one of the lowest density plastics, translucent to natural milky white with a highly crystalline structure. PP homopolymer has poor low-temperature resistance but this has largely been overcome by copolymerisation with ethylene.

Copolymerisation with ethylene increases clarity and improves impact strength, particularly at low temperatures, while still providing good resistance to chemicals, abrasion and good barrier properties to water vapour transmission. PP made by certain polymerisation routes may contain trace mineral or solvent materials, i.e. up to 300 ppm, which can be detected by smelling supplies of material in a bulk state. Grades with low levels of odour are now available and hence preferable for pharmaceutical products. Most PPs contain an antioxidant at 0.005% to 0.01%. Although PP shows better mould shrinkage than PE, it is still fairly high at approximately 2%. High temperatures and contact with copper can lead to rapid degradation. PP has high flexural strength, as demonstrated by integral hinge mouldings. When orientated, clear grades of PP can be achieved.

Polystyrene (PS or GPPS, general purpose polystyrene)

The monomer has chemical similarity to propylene in that the methyl (CH_3) groups are replaced by benzene rings. It is a clear rigid hard material with good tensile strength but is one of the more brittle plastics when dropped or flexed. PS is reasonably resistant to mineral oils, water and alkalis but soluble in hydrocarbon solvents, hence it can be solvent welded (plastic model kits). Polystyrene is fairly permeable to moisture and is not generally a suitable packaging material for pharmaceutical products. To improve the brittle characteristic, materials are frequently impact modified with rubber polymers, polybutadiene and styrene butadiene (SBR) by either blending or graft polymerisation. As a result the material shows lower rigidity, hardness, clarity, chemical resistance and higher permeability. These materials are identified as HIPS (high impact PS) or TPS (toughened PS). Styrene can also be copolymerised with acrylonitrile (SAN) and acrylonitrile and butadiene (ABS). Polystyrene is widely used as foam or expanded material (open or closed cell), mainly in either a cushioning or a thermal insulation role.

Polystyrene can be polymerised by foam processes, mass polymerisation, solution polymerisation, suspension polymerisation and emulsion polymerisation. Each contributes to the final characteristics of the plastics and the likely residues. A limit for styrene monomer may be imposed. Styrene can be readily analysed down to a 0.01% level. Polystyrene exhibits low shrinkage, hence is an excellent moulding material.

Styrene acrylonitrile (SAN)

This copolymer offers better resistance, improved impact strength and heat distortion over GP polystyrene. It is basically an engineering rather than a pharmaceutical plastic (e.g. devices).

Styrene-maleic anhydride (SMA)

SMA exists as copolymers and terpolymers with ABS. It is mainly used as an engineering plastic.

The polysulphones

Polysulphone

Polysulphone is another high-performance engineering plastic which has excellent mechanical properties up to 165°C. It has very good resistance to acids, alkalis, oils, greases and detergents, but is attacked by solvents such as ketones, aromatic hydrocarbon solvents and halogenated solvents. Certain polysulphones need annealing, rather like glass.

Polyethersulphone

Basically similar to the above but with superior creep resistance at elevated temperatures, a higher heat distortion temperature and slightly better mechanical properties. Polyacrylsulphone is another engineering plastic.

The vinyl polymers

This group covers polyvinyl chloride (PVC), polyvinylidene chloride (PVdC), polyvinyl acetate and polyvinyl alcohol, each of which has packaging applications.

Polyvinylchloride (PVC)

PVC may be formed by the polymerisation of vinyl chloride emulsion under pressure, using a peroxide catalyst. Polyvinyl chloride is found as UPVC (unplasticised PVC), plasticised PVC or as an impact modified PVC.

$$CH_2 = CH \longrightarrow -CH_2 - CH - \left[CH_2 - CH \right]_x$$
$$\qquad\quad |\qquad\qquad\qquad |\qquad\qquad\quad |$$
$$\qquad\quad Cl\qquad\qquad\qquad Cl\qquad\qquad\quad Cl$$

vinyl chloride monomer   polyvinyl chloride

Since PVCs show some deterioration or ageing under both normal or processing conditions, stabilisers are invariably added to improve stability. Rigid PVC used for blow
moulding may have its impact resistance (resistance to drop tests) improved by incorporating an impact modifier such as methyl methacrylate butadiene styrene (MBS) at
up to 15%. Thermoforming resins for films may also have impact modifiers (usually
vinyl acetate) added as this increases the forming speed and lowers the forming temperature. However, modifiers may reduce chemical resistance and increase permeation.

Plasticised PVC may sometimes seem a misnomer, as the plasticiser content can
occasionally be greater than the PVC. Plasticisation also reduces chemical resistance
and increases gas and moisture permeation. Typical plasticisers used include adipates,
citrates, sebacates, phosphates and phthalates, e.g. di-iso-octyl adipate, acetyl-tri-n
butylcitrate, di-octyl phthalate (DOP). Polymeric plasticisers and urethanes are also
used. Plasticised PVCs are soft and very flexible (see IV bag usage).

The various stabilising systems used for PVC include organotins, i.e. octyl thio–tin
complexes, calcium–zinc salts, barium, cadmium zinc salts, epoxidised materials, and a
newer group, the estertins.

PVCs frequently require other constituents as part of the formulation to aid processing or to modify the plastic. Typical requirements for processing include lubricants
(examples include amide wax and calcium stearate). Other impact modifiers include
ABS, MBS, and ethylene vinyl acetate.

The factors to consider when PVC is used for general pharmaceutical applications
include plasticisers, stabilisers, modifiers, monomer residues, regrind, lubricants, catalytic residues and chain length.

Polyvinylidene chloride (PVdC) (trade name Saran)

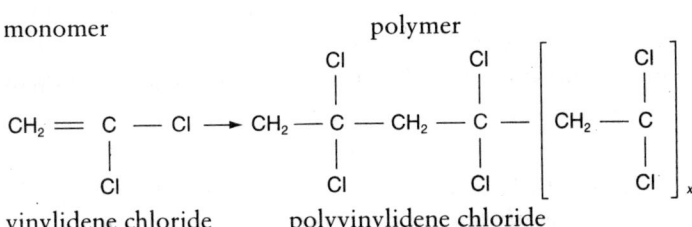

vinylidene chloride   polyvinylidene chloride

Straight polyvinylidene chloride is difficult to process, and Saran, the most widely used
material (usually as a coating), consists of a copolymer of vinyl chloride or vinyl
acetate and vinylidene chloride. These have excellent resistance to permeation by moisture and gases, very good chemical resistance plus toughness, flexibility and heat sealability. PVdC, although existing as a film, is more usually found as an aqueous
dispersion or a solvent coating. Coating weights of 4 to 180 g/m^2 are found. It normally
undergoes a maturing stage to achieve optimum barrier properties. Note that under
certain long-term storage conditions PVdC may age and discolour.

Polyvinyl acetate (PVA)

Polyvinyl acetate polymer is generally a soft, flexible and low melting polymer.
Copolymers with vinyl chloride combine the properties of the softness of PVA with the

hardness of the former. PVA and copolymers find use as an adhesive (labelling paper to metal or plastic), and a heat sensitive base.

The chemical construction of PVA is as follows:

$$
\begin{array}{ccc}
CH_2 = CH & & \left[CH_2 - CH \right. \\
| & & | \\
O \rightarrow & & O \\
| & & | \\
O = C & & O \\
| & & | \\
CH_3 & & \left. CH_3 - C = O \right]_x
\end{array}
$$

vinyl acetate   polyvinyl acetate

Polyvinyl alcohol

Polyvinyl alcohol, made by the polymerisation of vinyl alcohol, can produce a polymer which is fully water-soluble. Copolymers can also be produced with vinyl acetate. The material has excellent grease resistance and good gas barrier properties when dry. It has been used to produce water-soluble sachets.

Other vinyl plastics

Vinyl plastics also exist as plastisols, plastigels and organosols. These are usually based on PVC. A finely divided PVC powder dispersed in a plasticiser with a consistency of a cream to a thick paste is termed a plastisol. If this is thickened to a point where it will not run, then a plastigel is formed. An organosol is usually a suspension of PVC in a plasticiser with a volatile solvent which on evaporation gives a plastisol. This material is used as a dipping solution for closures and as a coating to glass (glass aerosols) and metals.

Polyesters (PET or PETP) (earlier use as Terylene (trade mark), polyethylene terephthalate)

Polyesters are formed by the interaction of acids and alcohols. The reaction is a condensation polymerisation process, producing an ester and releasing water. One of the most commonly used films (for tapes) is formed by the reaction of dimethylterephthalic acid and ethylene glycol to give polyethylene (glycol) terephthalate. PET films are particularly tough and very tear-resistant. Polyester has found wide application for 1–3 l stretch-blown containers and pharmaceutical and cosmetic/toiletry usages as small mouldings.

Copolymers also exist such as PETG, offered by Eastman Plastics. The G indicates the use of a second glycol in the polymer, i.e. 1,4-cyclohexane-dimethanol (CHDM). The resulting copolymer is an amorphous plastic which has a high degree of clarity, low haze, good resistance to acids, alkalis and many oils and excellent fragrance retention.

Polyethylene naphthalate (PEN)

PEN is a relatively recent resin based on the monomer dimethyl 2.6 naphthalate or naphthalene dicarboxylate (NDC). It is currently being commercialised as a copolymer or a blend with polyethylene terephthalate (PET), initially in order to raise the hot fill capabilities of the latter from around 75°C to 95°C or above. It is also alleged to provide improvements in moisture/gas barrier properties, give high levels of UV light exclusion and enable faster cycle times in the manufacture of bottles. PET/PEN combinations are believed to have good potential for the further replacement of glass by plastic, particularly as it is a very strong, clear material.

Rubber hydrochloride (Pliofilm – trade name)

Pliofilm was introduced by Goodyear in 1934 as the first non-cellulose transparent thermoplastic film. Until the arrival of polyethylene as a heat sealant, it was a popular heat sealing medium because of the relatively low temperature of sealing, the wide range of heat sealing temperature and the fact that a good seal could be obtained in the presence of contaminants, i.e. liquid- and powder-based products. Its use has rapidly declined, particularly in Europe, mainly because it ages fairly rapidly, becoming discoloured and increasingly brittle with time. LDPE, LLDPE and Surlyn are now utilised as heat sealing plies, particularly for pharmaceutical products.

The polyurethanes (PUR)

Polyurethanes are produced by the chemical action of di-isocyanate and polyol. The properties can be varied by the type of isocyanate used and the proportion of the two monomers. There are four main groups of classification for the thermoplastic groups of polyurethane, i.e. rigid foam, flexible foam, non-cellular and cellular polymers. Two main isocyanates used are toluene di-isocyanate (TDI) and diphenylmethane di-isocyanate (MDI). Polyurethanes have limited application in the pharmaceutical or medical industries. Polyurethane is used as an adhesive for laminations (thermosetting material). Like thermosetting polyurethane, thermoplastic polyurethanes can be found as esters and ethers.

Polyetheretherketone (PEEK) and polyetherketone (PEK)

PEEK is a newer high-performance engineering plastic. It is strong, tough, rigid, with good chemical and water resistance, withstanding temperatures of 200°C. It has high crystallinity and excellent abrasion resistance. Possible use could be anticipated for sophisticated devices. (Trade name Victrex – ICI.)

Poly(para-xylene) – Parylene (trade name)

This polymer is of interest in that extremely thin films can be deposited when the vapour is condensed onto a cooled surface. Parylene film has been shown to offer a reasonable barrier to water vapour and a good barrier to essential oils. For example, LDPE coated with a thin film of parylene has substantially increased the retention of lemon oil which would otherwise have been lost rapidly. It also withstands high temperatures of around 220°C. It is, however, an expensive plastic and has been used as a coating onto rubber.

Polyimide

The polyimide molecule consists of heterocyclic rings bracketed by aromatic rings resulting in a stable, rigid construction which will withstand temperatures up to 600°C. As a result of this high temperature, films are made by a solvent process, which also involves the final stages of a reaction. It is an expensive material.

Synthetic rubbers (thermoplastic elastomers, TPE)

Since synthetic rubbers use materials common to polymers these are now listed:

- polyisoprenes (IR)
- polybutadiene (BR)
- polychloroprenes (CR) (Neoprene) – good oil resistance
- chlorinated polyethylene elastomers (CM)
- chlorosulphonated polyethylene elastomers (CSM)
- epichlorhydrin elastomers
- acrylonitrile butadiene
- styrene–butadiene rubber (SBR)
- polyacrylates (ACM)
- nitrile rubbers (NBR) Buna N
- ethylene/acrylic elastomers
- ethylene propylene diene terpolmers (EPDM)
- ethylene/propylene copolymers (EPM)
- butyl, chlorobutyl and bromobutyl rubber
- vinyl acetate/ethylene (VAE)
- polyurethane (TPU)
- silicone elastomers – inert, expensive but highly permeable, plus fairly high absorption levels (preservatives).

Newer materials are being developed which lie between plastics and elastomers. One of these is a polyether block amide copolymer developed by ATO Chemie, Europe, called Pebax. This is a tough, highly flexible material which by changing the ratio of ether and amide can have a wide balance between hardness and flexibility. Currently this material is relatively expensive (£3,000–£5,000 per tonne).

Natural rubber (NR) and synthetic rubber usually include a wider range of constituents than plastics. A broad list of these constituents is now given, since they bear similar names to those found in plastics: accelerators, activators, anti-staining agents, antioxidants, antiozonants, anti-blocking agents, emulsifiers, chemical and heat stabilisers, odorant inhibitors, extenders, fillers and reinforcing materials, peroxide decomposers, nickel quenching agents, plasticisers and softeners, radical terminators, UV screeners, tackifiers, lubricants (mould and internal), preservatives, dispersing agents and processing aids, retarders, vulcanising and curing agents.

Silicones

Silicones, particularly silicone rubber, have plastic-like properties and are based on inorganic alternating silicon–oxygen atoms with various organic side chains. These silicon elastomers, as they are known, although relatively inert, are readily permeable to moisture, gases, absorb preservatives, etc., but have high lubricity and slow ageing properties.

Alloys and resin blends

Alloys consist of a combination of two or more polymers where each is present above the 5% level. The alloy is usually made by mixing the resins in a molten state, resulting in a miscible or immiscible material which is devoid of a chemical-type reaction. These alloys have virtually an infinite number of resin combinations, for example, ABS may be alloyed with polycarbonate, polyvinylchloride, ethylene vinyl acetate, etc.

Data sheets: information and interpretation

In spite of the availability of many standard tests on plastics, it is sometimes difficult to compare materials in terms of their characteristics, performance, equivalency, etc., by simple reference to data sheets. It is therefore perhaps more important to understand the relevance of the tests compared with what is likely to be required in the practical performance of a plastic. For instance, a test for cure is an essential QC procedure for thermosetting plastics. This can be done by sectioning the item at its thickest point, boiling it in water for 10 min followed by a check on appearance and surface hardness (a soft surface indicates incorrect cure). General tests on plastics for pharmaceutical purposes include extractive and biological tests, chemical tests and selected physical tests. The biological tests and extractive procedures cover such aspects as acute toxicity, pyrogens, chemical extractives for non-volatile matter, heavy metals, ash, pH, reducable substances, ammonia, etc. Other tests cover stress cracking, impact, print adhesion, etc.

Chemical identity tests include IR and DSC. The list below provides a brief explanation of some of the standard test procedures applied to plastics. The main British Standard involving plastics is BS 2782, which is issued as a multiplicity of parts.

Density

Ref. ASTM D792. D1505 – 68 (kg/m^3). DIN 53479. Density is a relevant factor to container weight, hence cost and yield/cost in the case of film and sheet materials.

Melt flow index (MFI)

ASTM D1238; ISO R1133; DIN 53735. MFI is the amount of plastic as measured by flow through a given orifice size under standard conditions. It is a function of the molecular weight of the material and a particularly useful factor for the characterisation of polyolefins. High melt (flow) indicates lower molecular weights and low melt (flow), high molecular weights. Measured as dg/min or g per 10 min. Increase in melt flow index is related to:

- ease of moulding (increases)
- impact strength (decreases)
- stress cracking resistance (decreases)

but does not usually affect SG, tensile strength, softening point, rigidity, solvent absorption or electrical properties.

Standard International (SI) units

With standardisation on SI units in Europe and non-standardisation in other areas of the world, knowledge of conversion between units of measurements is essential, e.g.

Length

1 inch (in) = 25.4 mm
0.001 in = 0.0254 mm

Area

1 in^2 = 6.45 cm^2
1 cm^2 = 0.155 in^2

Mass

1 lb = 0.445 kg
1 kg = 2.205 lb

Density

1 g/cm^3 = 1000 kg/m^3
= 1 mg/mm^3

Force and weight

All operate under the same units:

1 lb force (lbf)	= 4.448 newton (N)
1 N	= 0.225 lbf
1 kg force (kgf or kp)	= 9.81 N
1 N	= 0. 102 kgf
1 tonne (t)	= 1000 kg = approx. 1 ton (2,240 lb)

Stress, strength, modulus and pressure

All operate under the same units:

1 lbf/in^2 (or 1 psi)	= 0.00689 MN/m^2
1 MN/m^2	= 145 psi

1000 psi	$= 7\ MN/m^2$
1 kgf/cm^2	$= 0.0981\ MN/m^2$ and $1\ MN/m^2 = 10.2\ kgf/cm^2$
1 N/mm^2	$= 1\ MN/m^2 = 1\ MPa$

Pressure has a further unit, the bar

$1\ bar = 10^5\ N/m^2 = 0.1\ MPa$

Appearance – optical properties

Appearance of a plastic can be judged by a number of properties, i.e. gloss, or surface finish (a relationship of mould surface, moulding conditions, and material composition), haze, clarity, etc.

Gloss

ASTM 2457, ASTM D2456–65T and ASTM D523–62T measured at an angle of 45°C and expressed as a percentage (based on reflectance).

Haze and transmittance (Clarity)

D 1003–61, BS 2782 (515A). Again expressed as a percentage See-through D1746–62T (Transparency of plastic sheeting). Clarity BS 4618 Section 5.3.

Refractive index

ASTM D542.

Fastness to light

BS 1006, Fade-o-Meter ASTM G.23. The ability of a material to withstand light without discolouration (which may also indicate instability to light).

General physical properties

Prior to carrying out any comparative testing, preconditioning of the samples may be necessary. This is normally 20°C 65% RH for 15 days.

Tensile properties

Tensile testing is a widely used mechanical test from which not only tensile strength but elongation and modulus can be obtained. In the test a waisted or dumb-bell shaped sample is measured in the waisted region and then firmly gripped in machine jaws which draw away at a constant speed.

Resistance to stress and flexing

Various tests. See also folding endurance PIT 3402. The resistance to deformation is measured by a load cell connected to one of the jaws thereby producing a load–extension curve. The tensile stress applied extends the specimen so that a strain (E_1) can be equated against a change in length. The tensile strength at break is obtained by dividing the force at breaking point over the original cross-sectional area. Yield strength may be calculated from the load at which elongation continues without an additional load being applied. The ratio of stress/strain is called the elastic or Young's modulus. The value gives a clear indication of the stiffness for a set temperature. (Note that Young's modulus for polymeric materials is dependent on both temperature and speed of extension.)

Test ASTM D638; DIN 53455 (Films ASTM D–882), D1623 Tensile and elongation. Also BS 2782–326C.

- Stress at yield point – kg/mm^2 or lb/in^2 or MN/m^2.
- Elongation at yield point %.
- Resistance to flow under tensile stress – a measure of creep resistance.

Flexural properties (flexural strength)

ASTM D790, DIN 53457. Flex durability (films) see ASTM F392.

- Maximum stress kg/mm^2.
- Maximum deflection mm.
- Modulus of elasticity kg/mm^2.

All are measured over a range of temperatures.

Compression

ASTM D695 also see ASTM D-642.

- Maximum stress kg/mm^2 or lb/in^2.
- Modulus kg/mm^2 or lb/in^2.

Torsion

ASTM D1043, DIN 53447.

- Modulus of rigidity kg/mm^2.

Shear (dynamic shear modulus G)
ASTM 732, DIN 53445.

Stress (kg/mm^2)

The above may be measured against a number of factors: temperature, humidity, moisture content, etc.

Distortion and creep

Under conditions of stress most plastics will exhibit a degree of cold flow, distortion or creep depending on temperature, type and time of stress applied, and whether the moulding is restricted from movement by its surroundings. Once a moulding undergoes deformation the recovered deformation is known as elastic deformation and the permanent deformation as plastic deformation. The behaviour of a plastic material under constant tensile stress is usually estimated by creep tests. Such stress/strain behaviour as a function of time is given by isochronous stress/strain curves where tensile stress is plotted against elongation (DIN 53444). For longer periods tensile creep modulus is usually measured against loading time. Relaxation modulus as a function of loading time is described in DIN 53441.

Impact strength

Tests may be on the basic plastic or the material available as a film, sheet, component or container. One test is the Charpy notched impact strength, DIN 53453 standard. This involves either un-notched or notched samples tested against impact over a range of temperatures. The resilience is measured as kg/cm^2. The test is carried out on samples $15 \times 10 \times 2$ mm. ASTM D256 ft lb/in notch is found as the Izod notched impact test.

1   Impact breaking energy (tensile impact) ASTM D1822 ft lb/in^2.
2   Dart impact ASTM D1709A ASTM D3029 (Gardner).
3   High speed puncture test ASTM D3763.
4   Drop length to break D2436 65T.

Tear properties (tear propagation resistance)

ASTM D1922, usually known as the Elmendorf tear strength (related to test originally devised for paper and board), is carried out in the machine (MD) and cross (CD) direction of the material. Measured as kN/m. Test D689-44 also applies for films.

Torsion stiffness test

ASTM D1043.

Hardness

Hardness may be measured by several types of test:

- Rockwell hardness scale is widely used for plastics – test ASTM D785
- Shore hardness (Durometer) is another standard test – ASTM D1706
- ball indentation hardness is measured under DIN 53456.

Abrasion resistance (wear resistance)

Abrasion or resistance to abrasion is a function of the plastic, the ingredients in the plastic, the surface of the plastic, etc. Under test ASTM D1044 abrasion is related to loss in mg under standard conditions. Wear or abrasion has a relationship with the surface properties, i.e. coefficient of friction. DIN 53754E (Taber abrasion) is a similar test using a gritty material on an abrader wheel which measures wear against a number of wheel revolutions.

Coefficient of friction

D1894-63; DIN53375; BS 2782-311A, ASTM D1894-78. Here again a number of tests exist. A simple rule of thumb type procedure is an inclined plane test. This uses the plane for holding the material under test with an article or sledge (i.e. material) of a known weight. The plane is raised until the weight freely moves down the slope and the angle is measured. There are, however, a number of in-house and official variants for this type of test, i.e. dragging a sledge across a surface and measuring the resistance to movement.

Temperature and heat sensitive evaluations (thermal properties)

The procedure is to find whether a plastic converted material will distort or disfigure under a heat test, e.g. steam autoclaving, by carrying out tests on the material with and without the product present. The tests listed below, however, will give some degree of guidance.

Heat distortion temperature (or heat deflection temperature)

ASTM D648; ISO R75 measured as °C. A specimen bar is placed in a heated chamber, clamped in supports and loaded to 1856 KN/m^2 while temperature is raised 2°C every minute until the specimen bar has deflected by 0.25 cm. The apparatus used can be shared with the Vicat softening point.

Ball indentation

DIN 53456; ISO 2039 (as MPa). Measured as a constant indentation by a 5 mm steel ball under conditions of temperature, using a given (variable) load factor and a fixed time period. This is also a measure of hardness.

Melting point (T_m or crystalline melting point)

Many plastics may have an indistinct or wide melting range. ASTM D789.

Specific heat of latent fusion

ASTM C351-61. Measured as specific heat, kcal/kg/°C and latent heat of fusion, kcal/kg.

Vicat softening point

ASTM D1525, ISO 306, BS 2782 Pt 102D. A flat specimen (at least 20 mm wide × 3 mm thick) is placed in a temperature-controlled oil bath, with a flat-ended needle resting on it. The bath is raised in temperature at 50 or 120 °C per hour. When a gauge records 1 mm penetration, the temperature is recorded. The Vicat softening point should not be confused with a melting point, as it equates more closely with T_g (the glass transition temperature) with certain plastics.

Brittleness temperature

ASTM D746, i.e. how plastics stand up to low temperatures.

Thermal conductivity

DIN 52612, ASTM C177, BS 874. Measured as either, kcal/m/m^2/h/°C or BTU/ft/ft^2/h/°F
Typical examples of other materials are:

- copper: 330 (kcal/m/m^2/h/°C)
- glass: 0.6 (kcal/m/m^2/h/°C).

Plastics usually have thermal conductivities (which may be changed by added ingredients) several times lower than glass and around 1000 times lower than copper. This indicates why plastics provide excellent insulation against heat.

Heat deflection temperature (see 'Heat distortion temperature' above)

DIN 53461, D648.

Coefficient of linear expansion

ASTM D696-44 and DIN 52328 measured over a range of temperatures but calculated as expansion per °C, i.e. °C^{-1} × 10^5.
The range for most plastics is 1–20, 10^5 m/m/°C, which is higher than for most metals.

Shrinkage

Measured as a percentage, ASTM D1299. (Important for mould dimensions where allowance for shrinkage has to be made. This usually ranges from 0.5% to 5.0% depending on the plastic employed.)

Blocking (films and sheets)

ASTM D-1893.

Flammability

ASTM D635-72. Some plastics (without additives) may be self-extinguishing whereas others can be classified as non- flammable or flammable. Also classified are non-dripping and dripping. ASTM D2863, oxygen index, measured as a percentage.

Electrical properties

These do not normally have any pharmaceutical relevance unless the pharmaceuticals are part of electrical devices, hence are not discussed here.

Chemical-type evaluations

Gas permeation/gas transmission (cm³/m²/day – bar)

DIN 53380, BS 2782–514A, ASTM D1463–63, ASTM D-1484 (films). Covers both oxygen and carbon dioxide.

Water vapour permeability/transmission (g/m²/day)

DIN 53122, ASTM E-96-63T, F.372, BS 3177.

Water absorption

ASTM D570-63 equilibrium measured at 23°C or 100°C in water as a percentage or mg weight gain. Also BS 2782–43OB; DIN 53495.

Total immersion test

Weight change in 7 days.

Resistance to weak acids/weak Alkalis

ASTM D543-56T.

Resistance to strong acids/strong alkalis

ASTM D534-56T, PI-T1001.

Resistance to fats and oils

PI-T1003 (grease penetration ASTM F–119).

Environmental stress cracking (ESC)

Certain plastics suffer from a phenomenon known as environmental stress cracking, which occurs when a plastic under a physical stress is in contact with a chemical substance known as a stress cracking agent. The strain may be in-built from the moulding process or may arise from capping, plugging or top pressure (stacking pressure), etc. Stress cracking agents include most detergents, wetting agents and certain volatile oils. The preservative BKC is a mild stress cracking agent. Examples of tests to establish whether a plastic is stress crack prone include the following.

290

1   Bell telephone test: ASTM D1693-59T uses Igepal 630 at 50°C as a stress test. Results are given in hours to stress crack on a notched bent strip.
2   Pack test: known under different names including the Hedley test. Test details vary between companies and countries but generally the pack is filled, or part filled, with the product or selected commercial detergents (full concentration or a dilution) and then stored at 60–70°C for a period of 48 h to 1 week.

In the above tests plastics are likely to develop cracks if they have a tendency to suffer from ESC. Low-density polyethylenes of medium to high melt flow index are particularly prone to ESC. Moving to an LDPE of MFI less than 1.0 will normally overcome this problem.

Extractives

Simulants used for extraction procedures for foodstuffs include distilled water and aqueous solution of ethyl alcohol, or rectified olive oil. Under the EC global migration proposals, extraction is limited to either 60 ppm or 10 mg/dm^2, see EEC 90/128 plus amendments. Extraction resistance: see ASTM F-34 and USPXXIII.

Regulatory clearance

Clearance by official bodies such as the FDA, BGA (Germany), etc., on ingredients permitted to be used in plastics almost invariably relates to their use in contact with foodstuffs. Relatively few documents specifically cover pharmaceutical or medical clearance, e.g. use of PVC for blood bags, disposable syringes, etc. However, these specific clearances are slowly increasing in numbers (EP). When clearance is given for foodstuffs the recommendation states that such articles are suitable for their intended application and should not impart odour or taste to food, or yield any substance which is injurious to health. Permitted lists are currently being published for constituents which meet food grade approval.

Although clearance for use with food is a helpful check, prior to the use for a pharmaceutical purpose it remains the responsibility of the user (industry, hospital, etc.) to verify that the plastic and product are fully suitable (compatible) and safe. The EP now lists approved antioxidants for certain plastics. However, official approvals are related to human opinions which are based on the evidence available at the time when the approval was given. One should not blindly believe that such an opinion eliminates any risks and avoids the need for any additional tests.

The permeability of plastic to gases and organic substances

All plastics are to some degree permeable to atmospheric gases, i.e. nitrogen, oxygen and carbon dioxide. The first law that relates to the diffusion constant or diffusion coefficient is Fick's law, which states that the amount of gas passing perpendicularly through a unit surface against unit time is proportional to the concentration gradient, i.e.

$$q = \frac{-D\mathrm{d}c}{\mathrm{d}x}$$

where D is the diffusion constant.

The negative sign shows that diffusion occurs in the direction of the lower concentration. The second law is Henry's law, which states that the amount of gas dissolved in a given mass (of plastic) is directly proportional to the partial pressure applied by the gas. It is expressed as:

$$C = Sp$$

where C is the concentration, p is the partial pressure and S is the solubility constant of the gas in the polymer. From these two laws it can be deduced that

$$P = DS$$

where P is the permeability coefficient (sometimes called the transmission factor, permeability factor, or permeability constant).

Permeability of gases and vapours through plastic involves absorption, followed by diffusion, followed by evaporation and desorption from the other face. Permeability is greatest with amorphous plastics where diffusion occurs via the spaces between the moving mass of molecular chains. Crystalline plastics or those with crystalline regions present a greater barrier to diffusion. With thinner materials where pinholes or micropores occur, diffusion may occur via these small holes. Various other factors influence permeation, including:

1   nature of the diffusing molecule
2   nature of the plastics
3   external conditions prevailing (especially temperature).

Nature of the diffusing molecule

An example of a factor influencing the diffusing molecule is whether the gases or vapour are difficult to condense or readily condensable. With gases such as oxygen, carbon dioxide and nitrogen, which are difficult to condense and where the intermolecular forces are weak, the solubility of a permanent gas in plastic is relatively low at normal temperature, i.e. usually less than 0.2%. Where condensable vapours are involved in which the intermolecular forces are stronger, then there are two possible modes of interaction.

• Where the cohesion forces of vapour are less important than the polymer–vapour interaction in which case organic substances dissolve in or plasticise the plastic.
• Where the cohesion forces of the vapour play a larger part, and the solubility of the vapour in the plastic is relatively low. This applies to hydrophobic polymers such as LDPE and PP, and organic vapour systems which are either non-solvent or slightly solvent.

The nature of plastic

Symmetry and cohesion energy

As a general rule the permeability coefficient is low when symmetry and cohesion energy are high. For example, although LDPE and PVdC have similar degrees of symmetry, PVdC has a very high energy of cohesion and therefore has a very low diffusion coefficient. LDPE and natural rubber have similar cohesion energies but due to the lack of symmetry and the looser structure of the latter, rubber is significantly more permeable.

Proportions of amorphous and crystalline regions

The proportion of crystallinity to amorphous regions has a marked influence on both diffusion and solubility of the diffusing molecules. The coefficient of diffusion decreases as the degree of crystallinity increases. For example, PVdC is very highly crystalline, and PS is very low. In terms of permeability to water, PVdC is very low, whereas PS is very high.

Structural similarity between polymer and diffusing molecule

Another general rule is that structurally similar materials will diffuse and permeate more readily. Similarity refers to both end groups and polar moments (measured as Debye units). For example, polyvinyl alcohol is highly permeable to water but has relatively low permeability to organic vapours. PVC is the opposite, i.e. has a greater affinity to organic vapours. Polythene shows higher permeability to benzene, carbon tetrachloride, cyclohexane and hexane, the Debye units for polythene and the organics all being nil. Substances with polar moments show lesser degrees of diffusion and permeation.

Other constituents in the plastic

Plasticisers generally increase diffusion and permeation (particularly when the levels are high) for a number of reasons:

- plasticisers open up the molecules of the plastic, thus increasing their mobility
- plasticisers possess their own diffusion coefficient
- plasticisers usually have a greater affinity for the diffusing molecules.

Fillers, pigments, opacifiers, etc. may increase or decrease diffusion and permeation. This is also true of solvent residues which may increase permeation to similar organic-type solvents. Titanium dioxide usually reduces permeation; white talc and chalk as used in polypropylene will usually increase moisture permeation.

Effect of temperature

The permeability of a material generally increases with temperature, and a relationship can be derived in the form of an Arrhenuis equation:

$$P = P_0 \times (-E_p/RT)$$

where T is degrees absolute, R is the constant of a perfect gas, P_0 is a constant (the vapour pressure for infinite time), E_p is the activation energy of permention, and P is the permeability coefficient.

Gas permeation

The permeation for gases N_2, O_2, CO_2 is usually of the order of 1:4:20. Plastics with low permeabilities include polyvinylidene chloride, polyvinyl chloride, ethylene vinyl alcohol (if dry), nylon and PET.

Higher permeabilities are found with polyethylene, polypropylene and polystyrene. If, for example, an unbuffered product with a pH of around 7 is stored in LDPE the pH will ultimately shift to that of carbonic acid, i.e. pH 4.3–4.6, due to permeation of carbon dioxide.

Organic vapour permeation

Except in the case of dilute vapours, results are not always predictable. Two of the main parameters which control the rate of diffusion are the similarity of polar moments and the structural similarity of the polymer–diffusing molecule system. These may be placed in order of increasing polarity:

1   saturated aliphatic hydrocarbons
2   non-saturated aliphatic hydrocarbons
3   aromatic hydrocarbons
4   ketones
5   aldehydes
6   ethers
7   carbonic esters
8   alcohol
9   acids
10 water.

If the polarity and structural parameters are similar for two polymers then the diffusion will be related to the degree of crystallinity, i.e. HDPE, being more crystalline than LDPE, will be less permeable to organic vapours.

Constituents in plastics (residues, processing aids, additives and master batching)

Experience indicates that difficulties may occur in establishing the actual constituents in any plastic material. Certain manufacturers have at times either refused to identify constituents or only expressed a willingness to declare them to regulatory authorities. The latter compromise means that a pharmaceutical company may find itself in a difficult position, if as a result of the declaration one or more constituents are queried. Since the pharmaceutical company is legally liable for both product and pack it does seem relevant to have at least the opportunity of knowing what the plastic (or rubber, for that matter) contains. Constituents therefore may have to be quantified in terms of residues, processing aids, additives, etc. A question such as 'what are the additives?', if strictly interpreted, does not necessarily ask for the other two to be identified. Additives, which are basically constituents added to modify or change the characteristics of a polymer, can be itemised under a series of headings, for example:

- plasticisers/plasticiser extenders
- fillers, extenders, reinforcing agents
- lubricants
- stabilisers
- UV absorbers
- slip additives/anti-slip additives
- anti-blocking agents
- colourants – pigments and dyes
- antioxidants
- internal release agents
- inhibitors (mould and/or bacteria inhibitors or chemical inhibitors)
- nucleating or clarifying agents
- toughening agents – impact modifiers
- flame-retarding agents, e.g. opacifiers, whitening agents, antioxidants, biodegradable materials.

Although the number of additives used in any single plastic is likely to be low (most fall between zero and four), the list in total is fairly formidable. Several questions arise: are any of the constituents toxic or irritant, and are they extractable or simply removable from the surface of the plastic by abrasion? It should be noted that any additive which derives its effect from being present at the surface of the material may be physically removed by an abrasive action. Certain processing aids also operate at the material surface (lubricants, mould release agents, etc.). Interaction between product ingredients and plastic constituents, followed by extraction, is another, although remote, possibility. As additives are incorporated to obtain or enhance certain features considered desirable for the use of that plastic, they will be discussed in greater detail.

Plasticisers

Plasticisers improve the flow properties of a material, increase softness and flexibility, and are found mainly in polyvinyl chloride (plasticised PVC) and the cellulosics. Occasionally the word may be misused (i.e. when the general word 'additives' should be used). There is therefore sometimes a belief that all plastics may contain migrating ingredients, hence the question most frequently asked is 'what plasticisers do they contain?'. The most common PVC plasticisers are selected from phthalate esters, phosphate esters, sebacate and adipate esters, polymeric plasticisers and citrates. Dibutyl phthalate was once widely used, but due to its high volatility it was readily lost and is partly to blame for the belief that all plasticisers migrate. Materials of a low migratory level can now be selected from the relatively large list of plasticisers. Plasticiser extenders which are used in some non-critical applications consist of chlorinated paraffin waxes and oil refinery by-products. The plasticiser content can vary according to the properties required. As a generalisation, plasticised PVC usually contains at least 20% of plasticiser. With some plasticisers there is an upper content limit of compatibility or loading capacity. Plasticisers reduce hardness, increase elongation, tensile strength and modulus, improve low temperature resistance but usually reduce resistance to chemicals and increase permeation. For a highly plasticised PVC the moisture permeability can be four to ten times that of an unplasticised PVC. Plasticisers can also migrate via interface contact with other plastics, e.g. into unplasticised PVC, nitrocellulose, etc. Exchange between product and pack can occur in both directions, e.g. certain labelling materials such as heat sensitive and self-adhesive labels when in contact with plastic materials. Both the plastic and the adhesives may contain plasticisers or migratory constituents. Most cellulosics use phthalate, sebacate, phosphate-type plasticisers (e.g. methyl phthalate (DMP) may be used in cellulose acetate). Plasticisers may also be found in polyvinyl chloride/acetate copolymers, polyvinyl acetate and polyvinyl alcohol formulations, polymethyl methacrylate, nylon and certain thermosetting resins.

Typical plasticisers include dimethyl phthalate (DMP), diethyl phthalate (DEP), dibutylphthalate (DBP), di 2 ethylhexyl phthalate (often known as DOP). Other plasticisers include epoxy-based materials, e.g. octyl epoxy stearate, and, more recently, polyurethane-based materials.

Fillers

A filler by definition is an inert solid substance. Examples include carbon black (up to 5%), chalk or calcium carbonate, talc, china clays, silica and magnesium carbonate. Fillers may reduce degradation of the plastic (carbon black may significantly reduce sensitivity to light) or be used simply to reduce cost. The maximum limit of fillers is around a 1:1 ratio, after which binding power with the plastic is lost. The more fibrous fillers such as fabric, carbon fibre, and glass fibres are usually found under the title of reinforcing fillers. Carbon black also provides some reinforcement properties. Fillers for thermosetting materials include wood flour, paper, glass fibre and natural fibres, i.e. cotton, fabric, etc. Moisture absorption, shrinkage and contraction vary considerably according to the fillers used. This is an important feature with closures, particularly if subjected to steam autoclaving, e.g. phenol formaldehyde caps are more stable than urea formaldehyde caps. The addition of fillers (excluding reinforcement fillers) to thermosetting plastics generally reduces physical properties and, depending on the actual filler(s) used, is likely to reduce chemical resistance and increase permeability. Occasionally coloured fillers may be used to achieve a dual role. Titanium dioxide is frequently used up to a 3% level but is frequently classified as an opacifier rather than a filler.

Filler reinforcements

Filler reinforcements are generally applied to products other than pharmaceuticals and are not covered in this chapter.

Toughening agents/impact modifiers

A few plastics which tend to be naturally brittle require an improvement in both their drop (impact) strength and their top loading (compression) strength. In the case of polystyrene, rubber is widely used as an impact modifier. Rigid PVC, particularly when used as a container, may suffer weakness when subjected to, say, a 3–4 foot drop test. Up to 15% of methyl methacrylate butadiene styrene (MBS) copolymer is usually added to improve impact strength. Chlorinated polyethylene has more recently been introduced as a PVC impact modifier. Vinyl acetate is frequently used as a modifier for PVC film. Polythene, LDPE–HDPE can have resistance to stress (environmental stress cracking), improved by the use either of rubber or polyisobutylene. These modifications have not as yet had any pharmaceutical applications.

Lubricants (may also be used as internal release agents)

Lubricants may be added either as an additive or at the fabrication stage as a processing aid. In general lubricants prevent adhesion with metal parts. Lubricants may be solids, such as waxes, stearates, i.e. fatty acid esters, fatty acid amides, or liquids such as liquid paraffins. Lubricants may also improve the flow and thereby lower the temperature of the moulding operation. For example, a silicone additive polydimethyl siloxane may be used in LDPE and HDPE films to improve flow. Stearamides are also used.

Lubricants may therefore act as either as an external or an internal agent. Depending on their chemical nature, a few may have secondary actions such as dispersing agents, plasticisation, or slip agents. These are usually included up to a 1% level.

Stabilisers

Stabilisers increase the stability of plastic either during processing or during the moulded life of the material. Heat stabilisers are essential to PVC, taking up any released hydrochloric acid from product decomposition. The broad categories of stabiliser used are found under 'Polyvinyl chloride' above. Stabilisers are frequently used to combat the combined effects of heat and light.

Ultraviolet absorbers

UV absorbers may be used for two reasons: to protect the plastic from UV degradation, and to prevent product degradation due to UV rays passing through the plastic. Chemically UV absorbers may be based on substituted phenols or benzophenones. Examples include 2-hydroxy-4-n-octoxybenzophenone, other hydroxy-benzophenones and compounds of oxalic anilide. These are usually added at a 0.1–0.2% level. Prevention of light penetration and protection of the plastic from light degradation can also be achieved by the addition of iron oxides and carbon.

Flame-retarding agents

To date flame-retarding agents have not consciously been used for pharmaceutical products, and are not covered here, except to note that electrical or electronic equipment involved in drug administration normally has to use flame-resistant materials for safety purposes.

Slip additives

Slip additives are widely used for films either made or used on relatively high-speed equipment where any non-slip or drag properties might be detrimental to output. The most-used slip additives are oleamide and stearamide; since these operate at the film surface they can be physically removed by abrasion. Although oleamide and stearamide are currently rated non-toxic, any solution contaminated by them may show a slight haze or milkiness. Thus a product with a clarity of solution test may have this feature jeopardised by storage in contact with a material containing these slip additives (e.g. LDPE liners or bags).

Anti-slip additives

These were primarily developed to provide good bonding for palletised loads of plastic sacks and bags. Without the additives plastic sacks would tend to destack and slide off when the pallet is moved or jerked. However, palletised loads can be stabilised by alternative methods, e.g. shrink and stretch wrapping.

Anti-blocking agents

Both reel-wound and sheet stacked materials may be difficult to separate due to blocking. This may be caused by the smoothness of two surfaces giving rise to surface adhesion. It can be prevented by the incorporation of finely divided silica or diatomacous earths at a level of up to 0.2%, e.g. mica.

Antioxidants

Antioxidants are fairly widely used at a 0.01–0.4% level to prevent or retard oxidative degradation of certain plastics. Polymers may be subject to various forms of oxidative attack during all stages of their life cycle, i.e. from polymerisation through processing to final end usage. The more used antioxidants include:

- hindered phenols and cresols (known as primary antioxidants and radical scavengers)
- secondary amines (known as primary antioxidants and radical scavengers)
- phosphites and thioesters (secondary antioxidants which operate as peroxide decomposers)
- butylated hydroxytoluene (BHT) and butylated hydroxyanisole (BHA) (typical primary antioxidants).

Variants of the above are found under many trade names.

Colourants

Colourants can be listed either under pigments, which are insoluble dispersible powders, or dyes which are liquid- or solid-based soluble materials. As well as simple colouring, new appearances are being achieved: pearlescent, tortoiseshell, marbleised, metallised effects, etc. Colouring a plastic may be achieved in several ways, i.e. masterbatch (solid or liquid masterbatching), dry colouring and precompounding, etc. Details of these are given below.

Masterbatching

SOLID MASTERBATCHING

Solid masterbatching consists of a high concentration of pigment in a carrier. The carrier can be the plastic with which it is to be compounded, a similar plastic or low molecular weight carriers. The ideal is a masterbatch which is miscible and dispersible with all types of plastic. The pigment level has conventionally been 10–20%. Recently more concentrated masterbatches with 40–60% pigment, usually in a carrier, have been made for use at an approximately 1% addition level.

LIQUID OR WET MASTERBATCHING

These are usually used as part of an automatic system whereby a supply of a liquid colourant is metered into the plastic. As a let down material, substances such as liquid paraffin may be employed. It is essential to ask what the diluent is.

DRY COLOURING

This term applies to two processes:

1 automatically adding a dry colourant by a metering system
2 the use of prematched blends with other ingredients so that a small quantity can be added with thorough premixing prior to moulding.

PRECOMPOUNDING

This involves the preblending and extrusion of pigments, fillers, additives with the moulding polymer. It is then a ready to use, prematched material. Pigments can include metallic materials (aluminium powder) and materials which provide opalescence.

While masterbatching systems have received little attention to date, there is now awareness of the importance of various constituents such as carriers of a similar plastic but of a different MFI, different types of plastic, paraffins, oils, etc., and certain added lubricants, etc. Even though they are present at low levels after dilution, knowledge is becoming more relevant. As an important step in knowing the constituents of a plastic, details on the master batch should therefore be included. Using a reputable masterbatcher (i.e. one aware of pharmaceutical concerns) overcomes the above risks.

Antistatic agents

Antistatic additives or agents operate by being present at the surface of the plastic where they attract a layer of moisture which acts as a conductor for electrostatic charges. They are normally incorporated at a level of 0.01–0.2% and are usually surfactants, i.e. cationic, anionic and non-ionic compounds.

Opacifiers

The most widely used opacifier is titanium dioxide at a level of 1–3%. Two types occur, Anastase and Rutile, with the latter being more widely used.

Whiteners – optical brighteners

Whiteners involve similar ingredients to those so well accepted in washing powders to give a 'whiter than white' appearance. Since this may relate to a degree of colourising, i.e. a very pale blue or violet, its presence can frequently be seen by viewing the inside of an apparently white opaque container. 'Whiteness' may be achieved by the addition of a material such as ultramarine.

Extenders

These are somewhat similar to fillers. They are used as a lower cost substitute for the plastic.

Internal release agents

These agents are somewhat similar to lubricants in that they provide release, particularly from metals, i.e. moulds. The substances include metal stearates, i.e. zinc, calcium, magnesium stearates, stearic acid and silicone fluids (0.25–1%), e.g. poly (dimethyl) siloxane.

Inhibitors

Not a widely used additive but may be used for specific purposes, e.g. as a copper deactivator or as a microbiological inhibitor.

Blowing agents

Cellular products may be formed by incorporating blowing agents. These are usually hydrazine derivatives which evolve nitrogen. A typical material example is expanded polyethylene which has been used as a closure wadding material. However, such materials may contain ammonia residues and lead to changes in product pH, hence alternative agents are used for expanded PE wadding.

Regrind

Regrind consists of reworked material, i.e. either natural plastic or plastic plus other constituents as per material being moulded. Regrind is usually used to specific levels, e.g. 10%, 15%, 20%, 25% maximum. However, continuous use of regrind may lead to some degradation of either the basic polymer or the other constituents. If regrind is not permitted a specific instruction has to be included in the specification. Some countries do not permit the use of regrind for certain types of product (e.g. for IV, injectibles.)

Degradable (biodegradable) additives

Some 20 to 25 years ago there was a popular belief that plastics should be made degradable and a series of additives were developed to achieve this end. These substances included photodegradable chemicals, chemicals slowly attacked by light and heat, starches which are subjected to microbial attack, e.g. edible substances, and water hydrolysable substances. More recently it has become preferable to reuse, recycle or incinerate plastic so that energy can be either conserved or recovered.

Residues in plastics

Residues in plastics, other than monomers, are not easy to define since each is dependent on the process of polymerisation. However, a list of residue headings can be identified as follows:

- catalysts, initiators or hardeners
- solvents
- suspending agents
- emulsifiers
- accelerators
- monomers
- dispersing agents, etc.

Catalysts vary according to the process of polymerisation, e.g. in the polymerisation of PE by the Ziegler process, triethyl aluminium and titanium tetrachloride are used. Certain polymers may contain peroxide residues from the use of benzoyl peroxide.

As an example of monomer residues and the possibility of toxicity risks, the case history of the vinyl chloride monomer (VCM) in polyvinylchloride (PVC) bears some study. Up to late 1973 PVC had been in use for over 40 years before the possibility of VCM being a carcinogen was established. Trials which followed earlier findings in 1971 showed the presence of both tumours and angiosarcoma of the liver, which is a relatively rare liver cancer. Further investigation established that deaths of workers or ex-workers employed on PVC polymerisation plants could be associated with long-term exposure to VCM. In the period 1976–1980 work to reduce VCM residues established the likely loss of VCM from a rigid pack (approximately 30% is lost to the atmosphere after 1 year) and the VCM equilibrium between pack and contents, and calculated the likely partitioning between product and pack. Latter extensive studies on food have shown VCM levels of the order of 0.005 ppm and less. It therefore now seems reasonable to meet the EU limit of 1 ppm (1 mg/kg) or less in rigid PVCs and a limit of 50 ppb (0.050 mg/kg) in food-based products. It can therefore be concluded that virtually all PVCs, whether plasticised or unplasticised, are now 'safe' (author's opinion) provided these limits are achieved. For those involved in the 'VCM' era there has always been difficulty in dealing with the emotive issue. That people have died on PVC polymerisation plants due to VCM monomers is not in doubt, whether the lower limits now imposed are necessary will probably never be established, but undoubtedly all have benefited from the early discoveries with animals when VCM was established as a carcinogenic substance.

Processing aids

Processing aids cover chemicals used for specific purposes to assist processing. Some are identical to those included under additives, e.g. lubricants, antioxidants, mould release agents. The last of these may be regularly sprayed onto moulds and may occasionally lead to poor label adhesion or oil-like contaminants.

Moisture content

It should be noted that certain plastics absorb moisture more readily than others. This moisture absorption may be related to the plastic itself or the constituents. Plastics with higher levels of moisture absorption invariably require 'predrying' as excessive moisture can boil off during moulding and give rise to imperfections. Moisture content may also influence permeability, particularly to moisture but also to oxygen and carbon dioxide (EVOH is a good example).

General properties

Any plastic constituent in addition to the function it serves must have heat stability, UV light stability, weather resistance, low solubility in terms of extraction, compatibility with other constituents and good dispensability. Where plastics have to be sterilised by irradiation, certain constituents may be degraded, or even continue to degrade after irradiation. Certain antioxidants are degraded by gamma irradiation.

Detection of constituents in plastics

Identification of constituents in plastics depends on a number of factors, i.e. the solubility or insolubility of the constituent in the plastic matrix, the fact that many are incorporated at relatively low concentrations, their reactivity and stability. The chemical identity and analysis for constituents may use both chemical and physico-chemical analytical procedures. These range from estimations on density, melt flow index (MFI), ash, melting point, observation of burning, visual characterisation to more sophisticated analytical techniques such as:

- infrared (IR)
- thin layer chromatography (TLC)
- high-performance liquid chromatography (HPLC)
- ultraviolet absorption (UV)
- mass spectrometry (MS)
- nuclear magnetic resonance (NMR)
- atomic absorption (AA)
- gas chromatography (GC)

- differential scanning calorimetry (DSC) and other thermal analysis techniques (TGA, DMA, DTA, TMA, etc.)
- multiple internal reflectance (MIR)
- attenuated total reflectance (ATR)
- Fourier transform infrared spectrometry
- gel permeation chromatography
- X-ray diffraction studies
- time of flight secondary ion mass spectrometry (Tof SIMS)
- X-ray photospectroscopy (XPS).

Chemical or physical tests can be broadly divided into those applied directly to the plastic and those involving some form of extractive procedure. When some constituents are segregated by the latter process they may be relatively unstable and rapidly degrade. To minimise such degradation it may be necessary to store extractives in the dark, in neutral glass, in light-resistant containers and/or under nitrogen. The possible degradation of constituents while they are still in the plastic cannot be ignored, i.e. when the plastic is gamma irradiated. It is therefore important to identify whether degradation has occurred either in the plastic or following an extractives procedure. Newer techniques include various methods of surface analysis, e.g. XPS, SIMS, AES, ESCA.

Fabrication processes for plastic films and containers

According to the end use of the plastic, different fabrication or conversion processes may be employed. Each may influence the type and the grade of plastic selected, the constituents therein and the processing aids to be used. It is essential for the packaging technologist to have knowledge of all conversion processes as this is critical to the design and constituents. The next chapter emphasises this latter point in that the final properties of a plastic may be influenced by the residues, additives and processing aids. The fabrication of plastic invariably involves a moulding or shaping process and although this was originally considered to involve heat and probably pressure, cold moulding or shaping processes are now finding commercial applications. With isolated plastics and processes, complex mouldings may need 'jigging' or annealing. (Jigging is where dimensional changes are restricted during cooling by placing in a 'jig'.)

Orientation

When materials are stretched just below or above their softening point the molecular structure undergoes orientation. If the stretch is the same in the machine and the cross direction then a biaxially oriented plastic is obtained. Depending on the degree of orientation, significant changes can occur in both the physical and chemical properties. For example, stretched or oriented films will return to their unstretched state when heated to a temperature at or above that used for the original orientation process. If such films are to be heat sealed then either a special heat sealing process has to be used (e.g. hot wire sealing in shrink wrapping which localises the heat applied) or a heat seal coating has to be applied to the material which will seal at a temperature below the shrink or deorientation temperature. If the oriented film is held under restraint while given an additional heat treatment then a heat set oriented film can be produced. The general properties which arise from orientation include improved clarity, reduced haze, greater rigidity and impact strength, better barrier properties and chemical resistance.

Orientation can be applied to films, sheets and containers. Recent examples in containers have used polyester, polyvinyl chloride and polypropylene. In these orientation processes, called stretch and blow in the case of containers, polyester and polyvinyl chloride achieve excellent clarity, and polypropylene considerably improved clarity. It should be noted that orientation of plastics with relatively low to medium melting points frequently will not allow autoclaving by steam or hot filling, since distortion or deorientation will occur.

The fabrication or conversion processes for plastics vary according to what is being produced, i.e. films, sheets, laminates, components or containers. Films or sheets are produced by similar processes. Laminates may be produced by adhering films to other materials or by coextrusion. The use of the latter, a process more ideal when high quantities are required of certain constructions, is increasing. Coextrusion can therefore combine the properties of several materials in thinner gauges, and frequently more economically than other alternative processes. However, normal lamination techniques have to be used if plies of paper or foil are involved (see Chapter 9).

Film and sheet forms

Films have a wide variety of uses, as bags, sachets, plies in laminates, etc., and can be produced by a number of processes, as follows.

1 Extrusion: either via a longitudinal slit (slot die) to give a flat film or via a circular die as a tube (lay flat tubing).
2 Solvent casting: for example, cellulose acetate dissolved in acetone. The liquid is metered onto a continuously moving belt which then passes through a drying tunnel where the solvent is driven off.
3 Calendering process: a process whereby molten plastic is passed through a series of highly polished (heated) rollers followed by a cooling roller nip.
4 Coextrusion: an extension of the extrusion process where two or more plies can be extruded in combination, i.e. as a multi-ply layer.

Although films and continuous sheet materials can be produced by the same processes, films normally have a gauge of below 0.010 inch or 0.25 mm.

Moulding processes

Moulding processes for solid, hollow components and containers include the following conventional processes:

- injection moulding (and coinjection moulding)/injection blow moulding
- extrusion moulding (tubing)/extrusion blow moulding
- compression moulding/compression transfer moulding
- thermoforming by pressure, vacuum, mechanical forming or combinations
- scrapless forming process (SFP)
- solid phase pressure forming (SPPF)

- dip moulding
- rotational moulding
- injection stretch blow moulding/extrusion stretch blow moulding
- reaction injection moulding (RIM)
- soft moulding

and variants of these.

Moulds and some moulding factors

Each of the above processes requires a form of mould or moulds, i.e. single cavity or multicavity, which involves capital expenditure. Depending on the design, the initiation costs will vary considerably. As the mould number increases, capital investment and machine complexity become more critical to a point where unit costs may pass beyond the minimum costs due to downtime, mould refurbishing, setting-up time, maintenance, production duration, etc. So although a two impression mould will give a lower priced article than a single impression, four than two, etc., the final choice has to be balanced against factors less obvious than simply output against downtime, labour, depreciation, etc.

For a more complex moulding (e.g. by injection moulding), 3–6 months might be necessary to produce satisfactory components from initial drawings, involving a detailed drawing, mould drawings, mould production, setting-up and approving the new moulds, evaluating out-turns to final approval for production purposes. In addition, extra time must usually be allowed for adjustment to moulds and retesting. Even when one mould from a single cavity tool has been approved it is equally important to check mouldings from all cavities from a multi-impression tool since heating and cooling cycles may have to be significantly changed from the former.

This not only may give rise to subtle changes, but mouldings may also change slightly (sometimes critically) when a new item is run over an extended production period. It should therefore be noted that the first-off item for a short run may not represent that achieved from normal running during continuous production. Technical discussions between the supplier/moulder and the user are therefore advised from initial choice of supplier through to satisfactory production. The options of adjusting items to drawings or alternatively drawings to match samples needs careful evaluation.

Where new company mouldings are involved, it may be advisable to proceed via a soft (or hard) prototype, single impression tooling stage, before being involved with the higher cost of 'hard' multicavity production tools. These prototype mouldings will usually take a similar time scale to produce, i.e. 3–5 months from a concept sketch stage. Soft tooling is only suitable for a limited number of items but is particularly useful for the testing of new device type concepts.

Although most moulding processes involve heating and cooling phases with or without the use of pressure, some newer processes have eliminated or reduced the application of heat (i.e. those involving mechanical forming under pressure or compression). The 'cycle-time' involving the heating and the subsequent cooling stages is usually critical to the cost in that it may influence not only output speed but quality and finish, etc. Some of the more important moulding methods are given below.

305

Injection moulding

Injection moulding is based on a reciprocating piston or screw process whereby a shot of molten plastic is delivered under pressure into a cooled mould, then held until hardened sufficiently to be ejected from the mould. The time taken by the total process to deliver a moulded article is known as the cycle time and the amount of plastic used per cycle as the 'shot', which must not exceed the weight capacity of the machine. In conventional machines the shot includes the articles moulded and supporting sprue and runners. In moulding smaller items, the sprue and runners may actually weigh more than the moulded articles, so it is therefore not possible to cost the material used without reference to the cost of this wastage which in certain processes may be used as 'regrind'. If this is not permitted, the scrap may be sold off at a substantially lower price. Newer hot runner techniques offer a means of reducing scrap which may then be limited to fairly short sprues. However, hot runners are more expensive to install and are not always economical or successful. The ultimate success of any injection moulding depends on:

1 the use of the correct grade of material
2 a well designed item
3 a satisfactory mould design
4 correct moulding conditions, temperature, (heating), cooling and cycle time.

If these are not correct, problems may arise from distortion (e.g. differential shrinkage between the flow and transverse direction), sink marks and voids (i.e. different rates of cooling between thicker and thinner sections), moulded-in strains (detectable in clear or semi-transparent mouldings by polarised light; cf. strains in glass), holding dimensional tolerances, gate brittleness, etc. Factors to consider in mould design include the following.

1 Adequate taper (where relevant) to allow extraction from the mould.
2 Minimum of changes in section thickness.
3 Avoidance of substantial undercuts.
4 Use of adequate radii to aid flow into and around corners etc.
5 Proper temperature control channels to maintain correct balance between heated plastic and cooling via metal mould.
6 Effective cavity layout, including sprues, runners, gate sizes and location of injection points, etc.
7 Proper venting of mould to allow escape of any possibly entrapped air.
8 Correct location of ejector points.
9 Control of shrinkage. Shrinkage is normally calculated as thou per inch. HDPE, for example, has a high shrinkage of 2.5 to 5.0%.
10 Mould finish. For a high-gloss finish a highly polished steel mould or a chromium plated mould is required and the mould temperature and material temperature are critical. Finishes or textured surfaces offering stippled, matt, satin, etc. are also widely available.
11 Mould layout becomes more critical in the case of multicavity mouldings where it is essential that each mould operates under similar conditions. Although it may

occasionally be necessary to 'blank off' a mould or moulds (e.g. damaged mould inserts), there is always a possibility that this may upset the delicate balance between mouldings.

Poor design and/or poor mould design may lead to other problems such as flashing, i.e. feather-like protrusions at mould joints, or between moving parts of mould, inserts, butting surfaces, etc., which in turn will lead to excessive manual trimming operations, or rejects. However, it must be stressed that good mould design practices will not overcome a poor component design. In understanding the manufacture and design of moulds it is essential to appreciate whether a mould can be adjusted to make a dimension smaller or larger. While it is not technically impossible to add metal to a mould, it is relatively simple, particularly prior to having a mould hardened or polished, to take metal off by grinding, spark erosion, etc. However, it must be noted that any moulding with a sunken or hollow area will require a similar protrusion (frequently called an insert) in the mould. Thus if the insert has metal taken off the internal size will reduce and if metal is taken off the main (body) of the moulding the size will increase.

As the more critical dimensions of a moulding may require proving by several adjustments to a mould, moulds will therefore be made to a maximum or minimum size at these critical areas and then be adjusted by taking metal off. Tolerances therefore cover such aspects as variable shrinkage, initial dimensional accuracy against a drawing and wear on the moulds during use. In the last case, wear will normally cause a metal-off situation whereby components will either slightly increase in size (body moulds) or reduce in size (inserts).

The option to use a hard metal for prototype tooling (i.e. in place of 'soft') may be worth considering, particularly as the quantity obtainable from a softer type metal may be relatively small and quantities cannot be guaranteed when the tool is refurbished or in some instances until a further new tool is made. With a hard mould, adjustments may be less easy or occasionally impossible but greater quantities for testing purposes (possibly for small tests markets or clinical evaluation trials) can be achieved. When new designs are involved it should be recognised that first drawings may be a best intention rather than a definitive recommendation. When first mouldings are received the option of adjusting the drawing (which is not then a specification) or the moulding must receive careful evaluation. Let it be stressed that the chances of either producing exactly correct drawings or mouldings at any initial stage (prototype or production tooling) are fairly rare, hence it is virtually essential to allow an adjustment phase in the programme. Computer technology can improve these initial design stages (CAD/CAM). The points considered above may also apply to other moulding processes.

Injection moulding is ideally suited to most types of component, e.g. various closure systems (screw, press-in, push-over), valves, metered dose pumps, plugs, and full aperture (wide mouthed) containers such as vials, tubes, tubs, jars. More complex mouldings can be used for more intricate designs which may employ split moulds, retracting core pins, travelling inserts, etc., all of which add to the initial mould costs. A simple single impression mould could cost £950 or $1,600, four impressions £3,250 or $5,300, and sixteen impressions £10,000 or $16,800, but an extremely intricate moulding could cost £29,500 or $49,000 for a four impression tool. Cost therefore reflects the complexities of the design and the moulding operation.

Coinjection moulding involves two or more materials into one mould.

Injection blow moulding

In this process a container is moulded in two stages. The first stage involves a hollow injection moulded parison during which the neck is formed, with an initial body shape around a pin or spigot. This is then transferred to a cooled finishing mould where the original parison shape is blown to the final shape. As with blow moulding of glass, the parison design is critical to quality and final container wall distribution. Since the neck section is injection moulded at the parison stage, better control can be achieved on this part of the moulding than with extrusion blow moulding. It is also possible to produce undercuts within the neck bore (for plug retention), and provide better control (e.g. eliminate sinkage) of the neck bore wall. The process is generally more expensive (e.g. mould costs) than extrusion blow moulding, hence it tends to be restricted to smaller sizes of containers. Many dropper and spray bottles (usually 40 ml and less) are produced by this process using multicavity tooling, i.e. six to twelve cavities.

Reaction injection moulding (RIM)

RIM is a relatively new process where the plastic is obtained by a reaction prior to the final injection process. A typical reaction is that which occurs between polyol and isocyanate.

Thermoset injection moulding (TIM)

TIM is another special process, which can enable thermosets to be produced more economically.

Extrusion blow moulding

Extrusion blow moulding is an extension of the extrusion process whereby an extruded tube is clamped in a cooled mould and then blown into a container. The tubular section may be of uniform wall section or variable wall thickness (usually achieved by cam parison controls). The latter permits the thicker sections to be positioned in the zones where the tube is to be blown out to the greatest diameter. In this way an irregularly shaped container can be blown with a more even wall section. The conventional extrusion blow moulding operations involve a nip or pinch off at both the base and the neck of the container. Since both of these involve a weld between opposing parts of the tube, the ultimate strength of any container depends on both these weld areas and the blowing operation. A container may be formed either neck-up or neck-down. Processing factors which may affect the final container are as follows:

1 process by which parison is cut off, i.e. knife, hot wire
2 the die design for tube
3 the blow-up ratio (the ratio of the parison tube diameter to the maximum diameter of the formed container)
4 material distribution – related to weight extruded, the temperature of the extrudate and the rate of extrusion
5 pinch off design – for both base and neck areas
6 surface finish, temperature (cooling) and venting of mould

7   blowing operation including blowing pressure and rate of blow
8   the design of the mould, particularly the avoidance of sharp corners with attention
     to adequate radii
9   finishing operations – any subsequent trimming or stripping operations, e.g. top-
     ping and tailing, may be done automatically or manually.

Among the latest techniques is the Japanese Culus blow moulding process which produces a preclosed tube from an extrusion process. It is argued that the absence of a base
pinch off eliminates the weakest part of a conventionally moulded bottle. The process
is suitable for single layer and multi-layer bottles with a wide variety of shapes.

Extrusion stretch blow moulding

Stretch, or more correctly bi-orientation, of a plastic offers considerable advantages in
terms of reduced weight, better rigidity, clarity and barrier properties. Stretch moulded
containers can be achieved by both extrusion and injection moulding techniques.
Extrusion stretch blow moulding normally takes place in three stages. A mould based
on a preform shape closes around the parison (tube) taking it to a second point where
following the insertion of a blowing pin the parison is lightly blown into the preform
shape. At this stage the neck is formed and any pinch off removed. The preformed
mould is held at a constant temperature (to suit the material) and then transferred into
the stretch blow station. Here a stretch blow pin passes into the neck, stretching the
container down to a predetermined point giving longitudinal orientation. Final blowing then occurs from the top of the blow pin, to give 'hoop' stretch followed by a cooling period. Materials such as PVC, PET and PP can be used in stretch blow moulding.
Sizes, although the process was originally associated with containers of over 1 l with
either a separate base or a petalloid base, are now getting smaller, with more conventional shapes, and the process is finding use in the pharmaceutical and cosmetic industries. In the case of PVC, bi-orientation provides sufficient resistance to impact as to
eliminate the need for an impact modifier (thereby reducing cost).

Injection stretch moulding

Whereas extrusion stretch moulding was originally suited to PVC, injection stretch
moulding became more widely used for polyester (PET). The process is somewhat similar to that described for extrusion stretch moulding except that the initial stage is an
injection moulded parison. This parison is then passed through a tempering phase
where it is cooled to the optimum stretching temperature. The preform is then mechanically stretched, followed by a stage where it is blown to the final shape. The stretch
blow moulding process just described is known as the 'single stage' process in that a
series of operations is carried out on a continuous basis. There is also a two stage/step
process which involves preform which is then cooled, stored and can be transported to
another operational area (e.g. in plant operation as part of filling line). The preform is
subsequently reheated, stretched and then blown into the final shape. Smaller injection
stretch blow containers are now used for a range of liquid products with PETP being
the currently preferred material. Greater use of injection stretch moulded polypropylene is also predicted.

Compression moulding

One of the earlier means of moulding, it is used for thermoset resins and certain rubber formulations, both of which undergo a 'curing' operation during the process. The powdered resin or rubber mix is placed into the lower half of a metal mould and the top half (female/male moulding) is brought together. The mould is heated and the molten materials are held under pressure (compression) until the hardening (chemical interaction) is completed. A catalyst is frequently used to accelerate the pressure, temperature, time cycle. During this cycle, gases and moisture vapour are released hence the mould has to be vented. Excess powder is usually added to ensure that the mould is completely filled, causing (with venting) flash at the mould joints, which is usually removed by tumbling or freeze tumbling. Since this gives rise to dust, mouldings frequently require an additional cleaning/washing process.

Compression transfer moulding (Thermoset)

This process is frequently used for more intricate mouldings. The thermoset powder is placed in a heated chamber, where it is liquefied and then transferred by a piston through a channel into a second mould, where the material is kept heated under pressure while the curing cycle is completed.

Although the above are the major moulding processes for thermosets, injection moulding can now be used for the selected thermoset moulding operations. The major use of thermosets still remains with screw closures. These are made on either a multi-cavity platen tool (up to 96 cavities) or a rotary type press which resembles a rotary tableting machine.

Thermoforming and blister (bubble) packs

Rigid blister packs may serve as a primary pack for a range of oral solid products (tablets, capsules, etc.), as a secondary display pack, to provide additional protection (physical and climatic) to a primary pack or as a security tamper-evident system for a product or pack. Soft blisters made from a flexible base can also be produced to contain liquids or semiliquids which can be dispensed by exposing a dispensing orifice.

Blisters can therefore extend beyond the simple solid dose form which is discussed in depth in Chapter 13.

Rotational moulding

Although rotational moulding is used for both plastics and rubber, pharmaceutical applications, other than for rubber mouldings, are unlikely.

Dip moulding

This moulding process is normally applied to a rubber latex or plasticised PVC (plastisol) whereby a solid shape is dipped into a mobile liquid. When the material has set the formed shape is stripped from the mould.

Ancillary processes involved in plastic conversion

These ancillary processes include deflashing, removal of prominent injection points, welding, heat sealing, general sealing, and the addition of coatings and/or the incorporation of special barrier additives. Decoration and printing are covered separately and may be part of a coating stage.

Welding methods

Welding methods are listed in Table 7.1. Ultrasonic welding is one of the most efficient methods of joining plastic parts, and different materials can be welded so long as they have a common monomer. While particularly useful for hard rigid materials, it may generate particles.

High frequency (HF) or radio frequency can be used on some flexible materials, e.g. PVC, PVdC, EVA and certain newer types of nylons and polyurethane coated materials. PVC blood bags and IV packs are made by HF welding methods in clean rooms.

Spin/friction welding primarily finds usage with engineering plastics such as acetal. It is occasionally used with plastic components found in packaging.

Adhesive and solvent bonding

Newer adhesives based on modified cyanoacrylates or chlorinated polymers, e.g. super glues, have increased the capabilities of adhesive bondings. These may occasionally be used on devices.

Improving the barrier properties of plastic

In the case of plastics, weaknesses in barrier properties can be substantially reduced by the use of glass-like or metal coatings based on silicon oxide, metal and metal oxides. These coatings use a range of techniques, e.g. dip coating, solvent, aqueous and aqueous dispersion coating, plasma enhancement, vacuum deposition. Carbon (diamond-like) coatings have recently become available (internal coating).

In addition to internal or external coatings, barrier enhancers can be incorporated into the plastic as additives. These can include various metal oxides, glass fibre, mica, etc. Incorporating a foil ply between layers of plastic is a further way of obtaining excellent barrier properties, e.g. multilayer laminated tubes, cold formed blisters, and additional overwraps should not be ignored.

Sterilisation of plastics

One of the early restrictions with plastic and pharmaceutical usage was associated with difficulties related to suitable sterilisation processes. The processes which can now be used include all conventionally available, i.e.

- autoclaving by steam sterilisation (moist heat)
- dry heat
- gamma irradiation

Table 7.1 Welding methods

Material	Ultrasonics	High frequency	Spin/friction	Hot plate	Hot gas	Adhesive/solvents
Acrylic/acrylic	E	F	E	E	E	F
Acrylic/styrene	F	NA	E	F	F	F
Acrylic/polyolefins	P	NA	P	P	P	P
Acrylic/PVC	P	NA	F	F	F	E
Styrene plastics/styrene plastics	E	E	E	E	E	E
Styrene plastics/polyolefins	P	NA	F	F	F	P
Styrene plastics/PVC	P	NA	P	P	P	F
Polyolefins/polyolefins	F	F	E	E	E	F
Polyolefins/PVC	P	NA	P	P	P	F
PVC/PVC	F	E	E	E	E	E

Approximate comparative welding times: ultrasonics 100; spin 150; friction 200; hot plate 600. Key to compatibility: E = excellent, F = fair, P = poor or unsuited.
NA = not applicable.
Taken from British Plastics and Rubber.

- accelerated electrons or beta irradiation
- gaseous treatment, i.e. ethylene oxide
- UV treatment
- heating with a bactericide (BP 1980)
- chemical treatment
- high-pressure sterilisation, i.e. 10 bar and more.

Steam autoclaving – moist heat sterilisation

Autoclaving with steam involves time/temperature relationships, i.e. 134°C for 3 min or 121°C for 15 min or 115°C for 30 min or such combinations of temperature and time which ensure sterilisation. It is advisable to carry out autoclave tests on any plastic as part of the development programme. Now that autoclaves have balanced or overpressure facilities, experiments have to be carried out in order that the correct conditions can be selected. It should be noted that distortion or extension (initially due to internal pressure in the pack) is likely to occur during the cooling cycle and it is during this period that additional pressure is required to overcome the internal pressure.

Steam autoclaving may be used for both filled (water-based) and empty packs and components which are subsequently assembled by aseptic processing. The plastics which can be steam sterilised include HDPE, PP, PC, PA and, under selected conditions, plasticised PVC.

Dry heat sterilisation

Dry heat sterilisation is rarely used for plastics, mainly because materials that can be subjected to temperatures of 160–180°C for 1–3 h are few and relatively expensive.

Gaseous sterilisation – ethylene oxide

Basically two processes are used: 100% ethylene oxide under negative pressure to ensure that any leakage is inwards, thereby reducing the risks of explosion; the alternative process uses ethylene oxide at a concentration of 10–15% with an inert gas diluent. Suitable diluents include nitrogen and carbon dioxide. Both methods need degassing processes to remove excess residual ethylene oxide levels which are absorbed by the materials. This may be done by a series of vacuum cycles, possibly with a raised temperature or natural degassing for, say, 7–14 days in a well-vented area either at ambient or a raised temperature. Testing for ethylene oxide retention is therefore advised for each different grade of plastic with extended periods of extraction until total extraction of ethylene oxide is proven. Extraction from LD polythene and plasticised PVC is relatively fast; it is relatively slow from polystyrene. Although ethylene oxide has low chemical activity and interaction with plastic or the ingredients of plastic are relatively rare, interactions with formulated products are occasionally found.

FDA recommendations have advised limits for ophthalmic and sterile injectable products. These limits include ethylene glycol from the hydrolysis of ethylene oxide and epichlorhydrin which results from the interaction of chloride ions with ethylene oxide. However, significantly lower levels are currently being advised, i.e. down to 2 ppm in Europe.

Gamma irradiation

25 kGy (2.5 Mrad) is the standard condition for the sterilisation of filled and packed products, packaging materials and components, and medical accessories. It is again advised that each material (type and grade) be thoroughly checked, by both an extractives procedure and chemical analysis of the plastic, before and after irradiation. Physical assessment is also advised, as most plastics when irradiated show an increase in the cross-linkage of the molecules which in the more flexible materials can be detected as a reduction in flexibility coupled with a reduction in impact strength and elongation. However, it should be remembered that irradiation may affect both the basic plastic polymer and any constituents included in the material. The fact that changes may not be apparent from visual examination does not preclude some form of chemical degradation. Smelling of components before and after treatment may occasionally indicate that a change has happened. Certain grades of LDPE have produced small quantities of formic acid/formaldehyde. Gamma irradiation has been used as a terminal sterilisation process where both product and pack are not affected.

Accelerated electrons (beta irradiation)

The accelerated electrons method is similar to gamma irradiation but milder in its effects on plastics. For this reason its usage is slowly increasing, with a number of plants now in use. Accelerated electrons or beta rays have lower penetration powers (compared with gamma irradiation) and sterilisation is normally achieved in seconds rather than hours. Effective checks are essential to establish whether any physical or chemical changes have any significance.

UV light radiation

This is not recognised by the BP or USP as a formal sterilization process. UV light is basically a surface sterilising process and is used in some sterile (class 1) areas to reduce any airborne contamination.

Hydrogen peroxide

Although not normally used for pharmaceuticals, hydrogen peroxide has been recognised by the FDA for the sterilisation of plastics (usually films) for the packaging of foods. A solution of 30–35% by volume hydrogen peroxide is normally used, with a residual limit of 0.1%. Filtered hot air is frequently used to remove and degrade hydrogen peroxide residues, sometimes in conjunction with exposure to UV light.

Heating with a bactericide (tyndallisation)

The British Pharmacopoeia 1980 included this as a sterilising process for aqueous products where the drug entity exhibits thermal instability but will withstand up to 100°C for 30 min. The process was subsequently excluded from the BP 1988.

Problems associated with preservative 'loss' with plastic materials are expounded under aseptic processes and preservative systems.

Aseptic processing and preservation

Sterile pharmaceutical products may be achieved by either a terminal sterilising process or an aseptic process. The former, although normally involving steam, may occasionally be done by gamma irradiation. This latter process needs more rigorous monitoring, since changes may occur not only to the pack but also to ingredients in the formulation. In aseptic packaging, sterilisation of the packaging components may be achieved by any of the processes previously described. Since the product formulation may vary according to whether the pack is unit dose or multidose and the latter has to contain a preservative system, loss of preservative into (absorption), or onto (adsorption) the plastic is a factor to consider. In order to ascertain whether such a loss may be critical, it is necessary to identify the general properties which may be required from a preservative system, i.e.:

1   to offer a high level of antimicrobial activity against all micro-organisms
2   to be effective over a wide range of pH and temperature and remain stable
3   to be free from toxic, irritant and sensitising effects
4   to be compatible with the product constituents and acceptable in odour, taste and appearance
5   to be readily soluble at the concentrations used.

Examples of widely used pharmaceutical preservatives include benzoic acid, benzyl alcohol, para hydroxybenzoates, 2 phenylethanol, phenyl mercuric nitrate. Whereas some have been known to suffer from absorption in certain plastics, others have been known to suffer from variable adsorption, which is far less predictable than absorption since it depends on the surface area involved.

It can therefore be concluded that all plastics are capable of sterilisation but need the selection of the most suitable process. Plastics will not support the growth of microbial contaminants unless the surface is wet or a high storage RH is involved. The bioburden may be increased by certain particulates, particularly if these consist of materials which will support growth. Material cleanliness and low particulate levels are therefore a prerequisite for a fully effective sterilisation process.

Clean manufacturing facilities plus adequate GMP back-up are now essential for producing many plastic containers and components for pharmaceutical applications.

Conclusions

Plastics undoubtedly have an increasingly useful role to play in both the packaging and administration of pharmaceutical products. To summarise, emphasis is placed on their advantages and disadvantages together with advice on the information required to prove their general suitability.

Possible advantages

1   Light weight.
2   Reduced volume. (these two result in significant savings in warehousing and distribution costs plus advantages to the consumer).

3 No corrosion problems.
4 Good resistance to mould and bacteria.
5 Generally inert chemically, but be wary of 'solvents'.
6 Usually have good impact strength; difficult to break, if breakage occurs fragments tend to be less hazardous than glass.
7 Wide design and decorative possibilities.
8 Offer a wide range of moulding processes, enabling designs to be produced with fewer assembly operations, resulting in less labour-intensive activities; can be produced by form, fill, seal processes thereby giving low particulate levels with low microbial levels, e.g. blow, fill seal.

Possible disadvantages

1 No plastic is totally impermeable to moisture, gases, etc.
2 Most plastics permit some passage of light. Even highly pigmented plastics and those with UV absorbers are likely to let certain wavelengths through.
3 Many are difficult to clean or are liable to attract dirt and dust under unfavourable conditions (electrostatic). This can be reduced by minimal or controlled handling.
4 May be permeable to, or subject to attack by, organic substances, particularly solvents.
5 Subject to adsorption and absorption according to formulation ingredients (see section on preservatives).
6 Light weight and thin wall sections may require specific production line handling.
7 Fully effective closing systems are sometimes difficult to achieve.
8 Certain designs may show panelling or cavitation.

No plastic will have all these advantages or disadvantages. A compromise between these factors will usually achieve an acceptable pack (for example shelf life could be reduced from 3 years to 2 years where a product shows some susceptibility to moisture). If in this example plastic offers certain plus factors, e.g. easier to handle and dispense, less risk in terms of safety, then the shorter shelf life compromise may well be worth while.

Setting the specification

To make certain that the plastic pack chosen has a high chance of success, it is perhaps worth concluding this chapter on plastics by repeating the list of points which need considering, i.e. a check list from which tests relevant to a particular pack should be selected.

1 Knowledge of formulation.
2 Information on plastic: type, grade, residues, additives, processing aids, details of masterbatching, if used; DMFs.
3 Toxicity/irritancy and the clearance of plastic and its constituents (reference to permitted lists including food grade approval).
4 Design and moulding process(es).

5 Physical and chemical analysis of plastic components against specification.
6 Handling onto, along and from production line.
7 Decoration, printing and identification.
8 Stress challenges – drop, impact, sterilisation, etc.
9 Cleanliness – microbiological and particulate.
10 Investigation tests with product accelerated tests.
11 Formal stability testing with product.
12 In-use tests, etc. (i.e. checking possible misuse, abuse by patient or user).
13 Storage, distribution and display (testing procedures).
14 Monitoring of complaints and customer reaction, interactions, comments.

As with all packaging materials, the ultimate specification is critical. Material purchase under warranty, provided the converting company operates a functional QC system and maintains good manufacturing practices, usually gives a good assurance that the material specified is supplied. In the long term this means that only specialist moulders with, for example, 'clean' production facilities will have the capability of reaching the standards required by the pharmaceutical, cosmetic and possibly the food industries. This may be coupled with minimum handling and possibly not supplying 'open' containers.

With the fast developments in the plastic industry, some of the lesser known plastics will either find future usage or already be used for devices, general medical instruments and apparatus or as implant aids. Certain plastics now involve alloys, i.e. mixtures of thermoplastics, and thermoplastic and thermoset resins. Improvements in what were the economic five plastics, i.e. polyethylenes, polypropylenes, polyvinylchlorides, polystyrenes and polyesters, are constantly occurring. Use of metallocene catalysts is likely to produce plastics of a controlled chain length.

Whether a moulding uses a virgin polymer or allows the use of regrind (plastic scrap from the moulding process) is a matter of an ongoing debate. However, as the continued use of regrind (i.e. regrind as regrind) can lead to some degradation, its use may have to be carefully controlled or a clause such as 'use of regrind not permitted' included as part of the specification.

Computer-aided design and computer-aided manufacture (CAD/CAM) may enable the lead times quoted earlier to be reduced.

Plastic technology is now reaching a stage where over 99% of pharmaceutical products could be packed in plastics within the next 5–10 years. How far this happens largely depends on the environmental debate. Thus when new products appear or old products are to be repacked, plastics rather than glass have now become the material of choice.

However, this choice initially starts with polyethylenes, the polypropylenes, the polystyrenes, the polyvinyls and more recently the polyesters. These relatively economical materials undergo continuing development and modification. For example, whereas LDPE was a hazy milky material where visual inspection might be considered suspect, higher clarity materials are becoming increasingly available. Antioxidant free grades of LDPE are also now offered (an EP requirement). The author therefore argues that most pharmaceutical products can be packed in these economical grades without resorting to the more expensive alternatives. If these economic grades lack certain barrier properties these can usually be overcome today by either suitable coating or overwrapping options.

Any new super-plastic, unless it matches the economics of the above, will take at least 10–20 years before it becomes a commercially successful material with wide pharmaceutical applications.

The emotive issues related to plastic and the environment have yet to be logically and scientifically resolved. However, predictable future trends which will increase the use of plastics in pharmaceutical applications are likely to include:

1   use of coextrusions for reel-fed blister packs
2   use of coextrusions for containers
3   increased use of unit dose packaging
4   extension of original pack (OP) dispensing which will increase the usage of smaller packs
5   greater use of combined packs and devices
6   increased usage of separate devices which will in the main be made from plastic.

Finally, recent guides offered by the FDA have identified the need for the following information when a plastic is used for parenterals (now similarly covered by EN 9090/III).

1   Name of manufacturer.
2   Type of plastic.
3   Composition, method of manufacture of the resin and the finished container, plus a full description of the analytical controls.
4   Physical characteristics (size, dimensions, whether flame treated, etc.).
5   Defect classifications (weight, seams, seals, wall thickness, pin holes, etc.).
6   Light transmission test, USP (particularly if product is photosensitive).
7   Tests (USP):

   • biological
   • physico-chemical
   • permeation.

8   Vapour transmission test (if appropriate).
9   Toxicity studies not included in USP:

   • sub-acute on extracts
   • cell culture.

10 Tests for leaching and migration.
11 Compatibility.
12 Sampling plan.
13 Acceptance specifications.

Although the list is substantial and useful, it ultimately should be possible to reduce it by increased knowledge and attention to QA and QC procedures.

It can therefore be concluded that a steady increase in the use of plastic for packaging materials, components and devices can be envisaged. Any trend to identify plastics suitable for pharmaceuticals (as already exists for foods) could possibly assist the industry, at least in the initial selection of materials. The fact that the quantities used by the pharmaceutical industry will never be large compared with, say, the food industry should make the industry aware that any increase in more stringent standards can only be achieved by an on-cost. Sharing standards with the food industry, whether it is related to materials or converted items, may produce an acceptable compromise.

However, it is inevitable that no textbook on plastics will ever be up to date, as technology and enterprise are constantly advancing. If this chapter creates an 'awareness' of the subject, the reader should be in a better position to keep abreast with new developments. There are, however, plastics which have not been mentioned together with variants of the moulding processes. Each plastic family also exists in many grades which, although initially quantified by melt flow index and density, may be far more complex as both homopolymers and copolymers may exist. Knowing the basics on polymers is essential to all activities involving polymers from creating designs, testing and approving them, right through to a successful product launch.

Although data sheets from polymer suppliers are a starting point for information on the properties of polymers, there is always a chance that materials may modify at least slightly during any conversion or treatment process. Such potential changes have to be checked by more and more sophisticated analytical methodology. This has to be supported by more in-depth knowledge of the polymers themselves.

Appendix 7.1: Processes used in the conversion of plastics

Extrusion and the extruder

Plastic granules fed via a hopper ((a) in Figure 7.1) are moved forward by a rotating screw (c) in a cylinder which has heating bands (b). The rotating screw compacts the material which undergoes plastication due to the heat and pressure. Although the process is usually continuous it can be made intermittent. In the continuous process the softened mass can be 'extruded' via a solid or hollow die to give a solid moulding, a sheet, a tube, etc., which is then cooled in water or air. The extruder is the work-horse of the plastic converting industry.

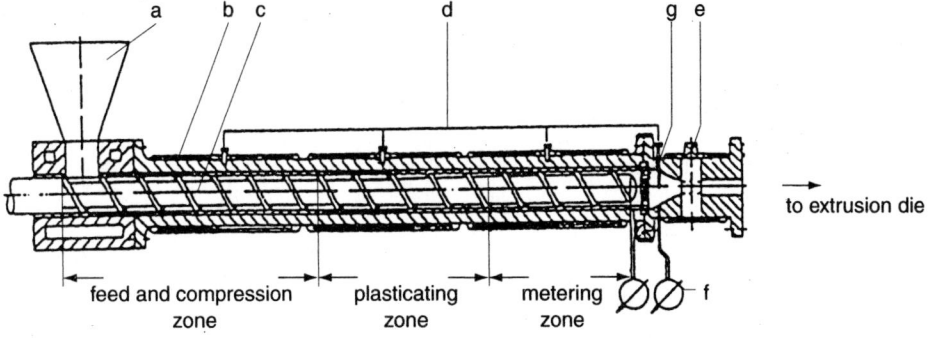

Figure 7.1 Design of an extruder plasticating barrel: (a) feed hopper; (b) heaters; (c) screw; (d) thermocouples; (e) back pressure regulating valve; (f) pressure gauges; (g) breaker plate and screen pack

Extrusion blow moulding

This is based on the unit in Figure 7.1. An extruded tube flowing downwards is enclosed by a cooled finishing mould with a nip-off/weld at the top and bottom of the bottle (trim/waste) where it is then compressed air blown and cooled to the final shape. The mould(s) may be neck up or down in a straight line or as rotating carousel (see Figure 7.2).

Extrusion blow moulding

See Figures 7.2 and 7.3.

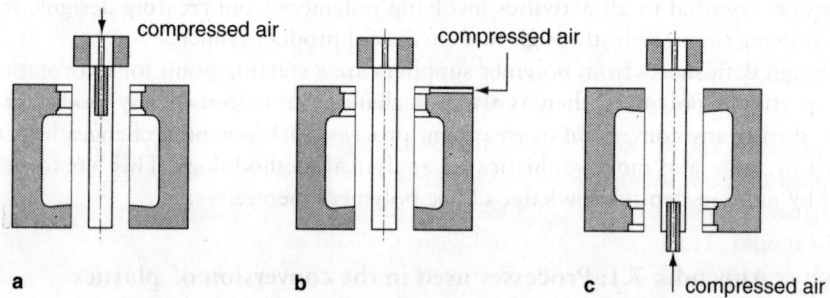

a   b   c

Figure 7.2 Blow moulding methods: (a) Plax method; (b) Mills/Pirelli method; (c) Kautex method

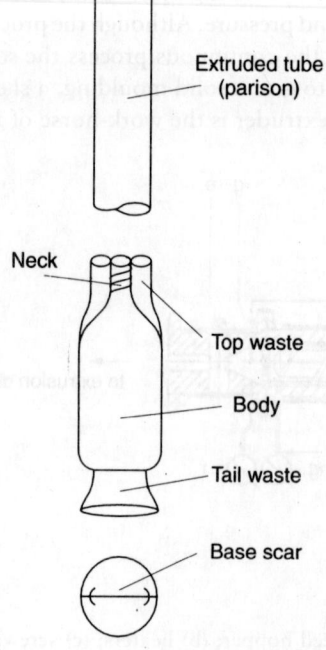

Figure 7.3 Extrusion blow moulding

Lay flat tubing or tubular film

This is a further extension of the extrusion process. A tubular film emerging from a circular die is internally pressurized with air. This extends the film which, together with the temperature and draw off rate, decides the material gauge and degree of orientation. The film may be blown upwards, downwards, or horizontally (Fig. 7.4).

Injection moulding

The basis of an injection moulding is a modified extruder where there is an additional reciprocating action which enables a 'shot' to be forced into single or multicavity moulds. The design of the extruding screw is critical to the operation (Figures 7.5 and 7.6).

Injection blow moulding

In this process a tubular-like shape is injected around a spigot or core pin (Figure 7.7). When released from the mould it is transferred to a second finishing mould where it is then further blown by compressed air to its final shape and cooled prior to removal from the mould. The operation is usually carried out on the rotating table principle. As in the process the neck of the container is moulded in the first stage, a higher quality is achieved compared with extrusion blow moulding. However, moulds are considerably higher in cost. As a result it tends to be restricted to smaller sizes, with particular application to pharmaceutical containers.

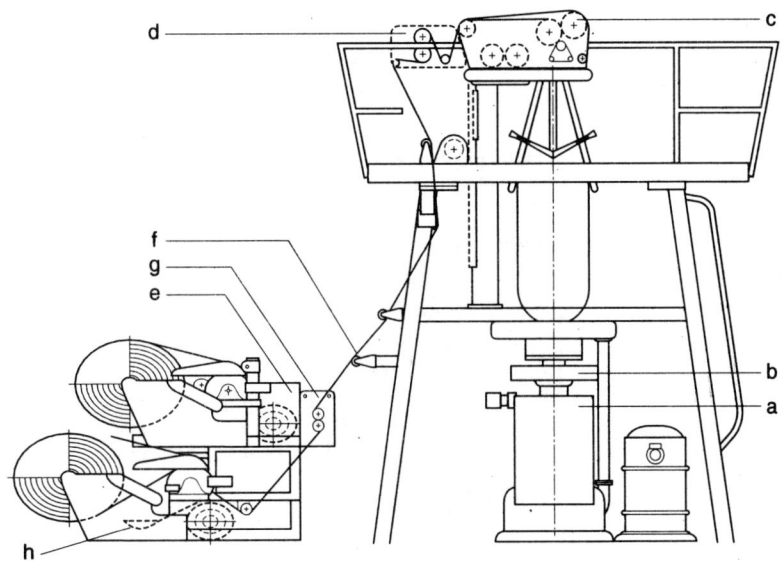

Figure 7.4 Tubular film apparatus: (a) extruder; (b) rotating blown film die; (c) haul-off unit; (d) pretreatment unit; (e) wind-up unit; (f) edge trimmer; (g) longitudinal cutter; (h) transverse cutter

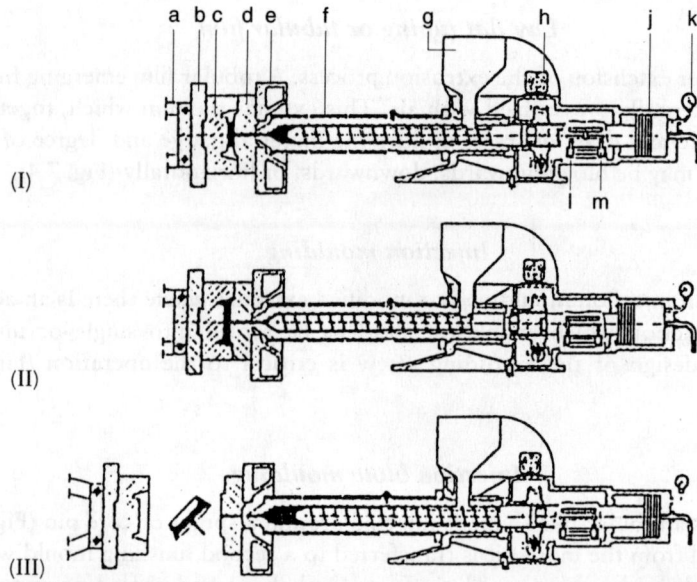

Figure 7.5 Injection moulding: design and operating sequence of a screw plunger injection moulding unit. (I) injection; (II) cooling (curing in the case of thermosets) under follow-up pressure; (III) ejection of the injection moulded part. (a) Clamping mechanism; (b) mould clamping; (c, d) injection mould; (e) mould clamping plate; (f) plasticating cylinder with screw plunger; (g) feed hopper; (h) screw drive; (j) hydraulic cylinder; (k) pressure gauge; (l) follow-up pressure limit switch; (m) screw stroke adjustment

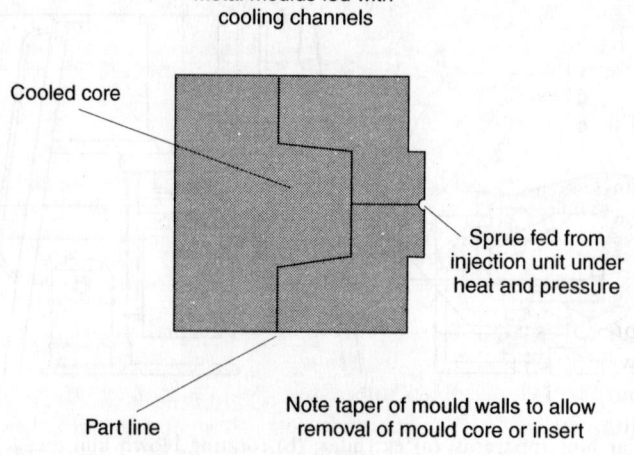

Figure 7.6 Typical two-piece mould for injection moulding

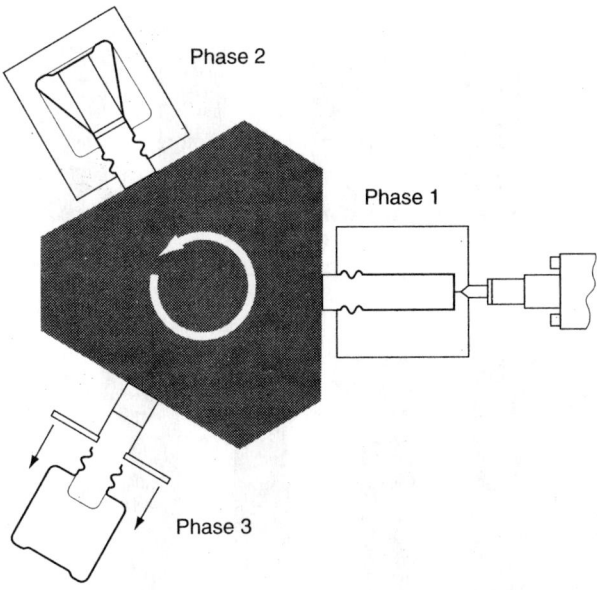

Figure 7.7 Injection blow moulding

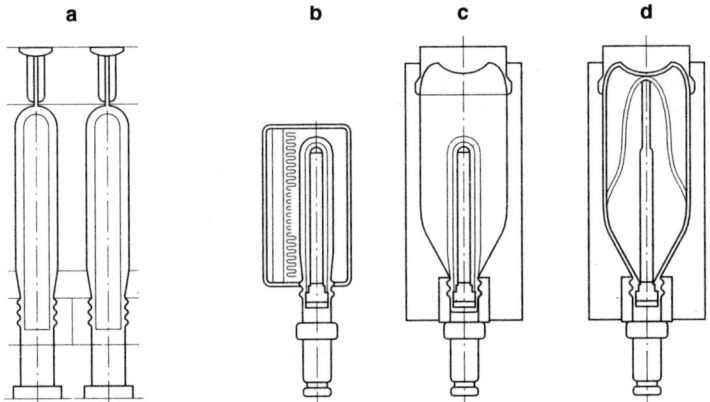

Figure 7.8 Injection stretch blow moulding

Extrusion and injection stretch blow moulding

Although both processes can produce reasonably good quality large containers, injection stretch blow moulding is more widely used for pharmaceutical containers. The first stage of moulding is basically as injection blow moulding. In the second stage the preform is conditioned to the specifically required temperature and then stretched in the finishing mould longitudinally and axially in that order. The first stretching operation is carried out by a descending rod and the second by compressed air (Figure 7.8).

In extrusion stretch blow moulding the first stage is similar to the first stage of

323

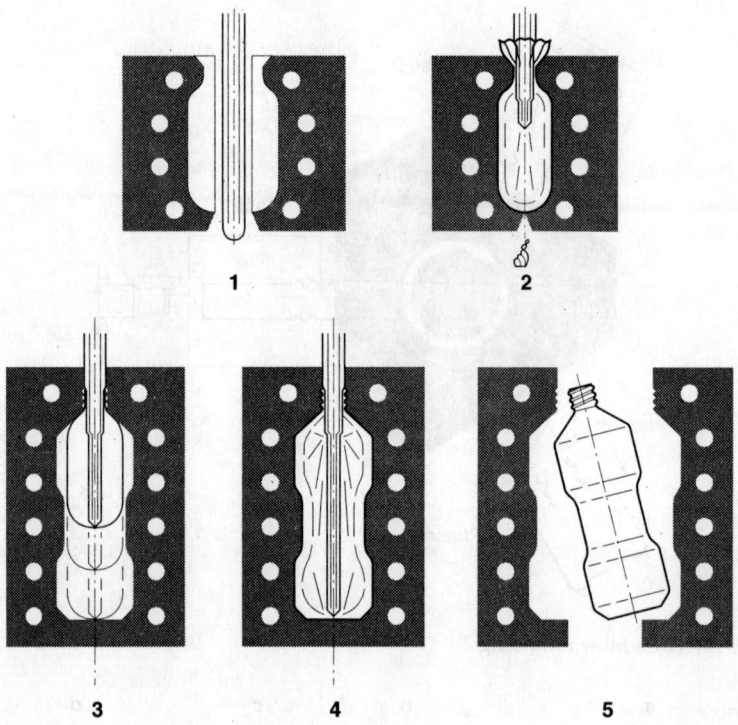

Figure 7.9 Extrusion stretch blow moulding: (1) extrusion; (2) blowing and conditioning; (3) stretching; (4) blowing; (5) ejection

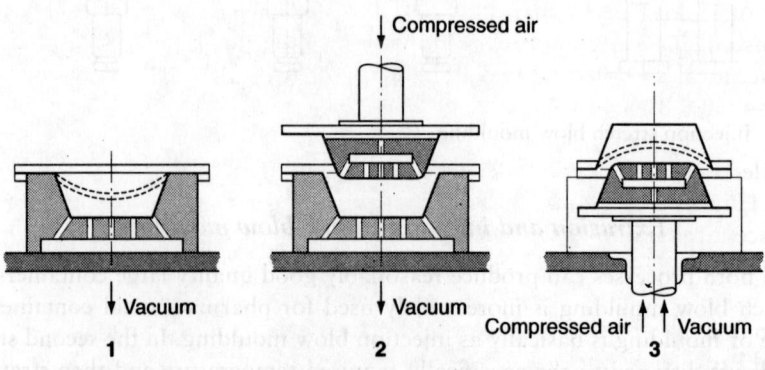

Figure 7.10 Thermoforming: (1) female mould, vacuum, no prestretching; (2) female mould, pressure forming with male or plug, prestretching; (3) male mould, vacuum, with pressurised air prestretch

extrusion blown, but the parison formed is conditioned to a specific temperature prior to stretching initially by a descending rod and then by compressed air (Figure 7.9).

Thermoforming

Thermoforming consists of softening a material and then shaping it in a mould by vacuum, positive air pressure, or mechanically or a combination of these. Forming can be into or over (drape) a mould. The material following softening by heat can be directly moulded or extended by vacuum or pressure prior to being finally formed (Figure 7.10).

References

Metallacene – catalysed Cyclo Olefin Copolymers
Vincent Sullivan – Medical Device Technology Oct 1998

Developments in Technology of Polymer
Mike Gaffrey, Development Engineer
Hoechst UK Ltd

Polymer Thin film Biosensors and their possible application in Medical Packaging Technology,
Lars Lindvold, Riso National Laboratory, Roskilde, Denmark
Pharmaceutical and Medical Packaging Technology 1998 Vol 8,
21-1-21-2 ISBN 87-89753-24-0

Security Applications by Injection Moulding of Micro Structures and Medical (Devices) Packaging
Henrich Gunstrip, Krukson Plast A/S Fredinchsvaerk, Denmark
Pharmaceutical and Medical Packaging 1998 Vol 8,
21-1-21-2 ISBN 87-98753-24-0

The use of Holograms in Pharmaceutical and Medical Packaging
Jan Stensborg, Centre of Advanced Technology, Roskilde, Denmark
Pharmaceutical and Medical Packaging 1998 Vol 8,
20-1-20-4 ISBN 87-89753-24-0

Static Electricity Fire Hazard, Restricted or Cleanroom Areas.
Martin Hughes. Stat attack, Buckinghamshire, UK
Pharmaceutical and Medical Packaging 1998 Vol 8,
19-1-19-2 ISBN 87-89753-24-0

Vitamin E, as an antioxidant choice for Polyethylene
Medical Packaging, Anthony O'Driskoll, Ciba speciality
Chemical Inc. Basel, Switzerland.

8

DEVELOPMENT AND APPROVAL OF A PLASTIC PACK

D. A. Dean

Background

As many pharmaceutical products are likely to generate some secondary effects or side-effects, it is important that the balance is clearly in favour of the effectiveness of the drug and that such secondary effects are kept to a minimum in terms of both the product and its immediate pack. The industry therefore devotes considerable resources to ensure that the pack more than adequately meets its primary function of economically providing presentation and confidence, information/identification, protection against ingress and egress, plus compatibility between product and pack, compliance and convenience, until such time as the product is used or administered. As a pharmaceutical pack is normally required to maintain a shelf life of 3–5 years, in-depth testing is essential. The pharmaceutical industry therefore requires in most instances a level of safety superior to that of a foodstuff. This is of particular relevance when one considers that drugs are normally taken only when a person is exhibiting symptoms of illness, hence any untoward additional side-effects are not only undesirable but against the general interest of public health.

Although glass and metal have traditionally been used for pharmaceutical products, it should not be assumed that they are inert or that they are the ideal packaging materials. Glass, for instance, is particularly hazardous when it breaks and alkaline glass can alter the pH of non-buffered aqueous solutions. The considerable increase in the use of plastic has been associated with user convenience features (e.g. squeezability), the more modern hence psychologically acceptable image, the greater ability to produce packs and devices in functional and complicated shapes involving less weight and frequently lower volume, at competitive and economically acceptable prices. New concepts, which would not be practical in glass and metal, have also assisted the progress of plastics and the pharmaceutical industry. Thus when it comes to new pharmaceutical products, plastics now stand a high chance of being used in spite öf the fact that all are to some degree permeable to moisture, oxygen, carbon dioxide, etc., and are often not as inert as competitive materials such as glass and metal.

Plastic packs have undoubtedly received greater scrutiny than many other types of pack such as metal and glass. Although in many instances this might be considered unfair, plastic can at least be used as an example of how a material can be thoroughly 'cleared' and approved in the widest pharmaceutical context.

Aspects which may need consideration in the development of pharmaceutical products can be identified from the following preliminary information.

Product characteristics (drug substance and product dosage)

Good knowledge is required of the physical and chemical properties of the 'product', the processes by which it is produced, and how it is used or administered.

Packaging aspects

1 Functional and aesthetic design.
2 Processes of manufacture and any assembly operations.
3 Selection of plastic type – general physical and chemical properties. Ideally food grade approved.
4 Selection of plastic grade – detailed physical and chemical properties, plus knowledge of constituents including any toxicity and irritancy aspects.
5 Compatibility requirements – with product, involving testing stages, i.e. feasibility stages (investigational) and formal stability stages.
6 Any specific performance requirements i.e. during use, including closure efficiency, warehousing, distribution and display, durability of identification/ decoration/print, etc.
7 Final studies of development versus production pack to identify any differences to the pack to be sold.
8 Identify additional tests necessary to check differences in (7).

Although certain of the above factors have been listed separately, in practice quite a few have to be considered in combination. For example, the practicability of any design has to be related to the process of manufacture and this may equally apply to the grade of plastic employed and the constituents found in the plastic. It is therefore intended to discuss some of the above factors on a broad basis and then consider the 'safety' and functional clearance of a particular plastic pack in greater depth.

Design can be considered as a relationship between size, shape, texture, colour, including opacity or transparency, the type of closure and the functional and aesthetic requirements of the pack.

Functional aspects which must be considered in the broadest context include the following.

1 Efficiency and ease of production for the supplying company, for instance, will production involve wastage due to deficiencies in the design i.e. quality of design?
2 How can container be effectively unscrambled and cleaned if necessary? (Note that trend is to produce clean containers and maintain clean.)
3 Minimum of production line problems during filling, closuring, labelling, cartoning, etc. (production efficiency).
4 Satisfactory stacking, transportation and handling.
5 Suitable for all aspects of patient usage, and general convenience.
6 Effective in terms of opening and reclosing. (Note possible conflicts between

child-resistance, tamper-resistance and difficulties for an ever increasing elderly population.)
7 Acceptable to packaging codes of practice, i.e. disposal, conservation of energy, recycling and reuse, minimum pollution risks, etc.
8 Meeting other legal or moral requirements, e.g. child resistance, tamper-evidence, etc., including product liability issues.
9 Compatible and suitable for the product.

The functional aspects of a pharmaceutical pack may range from simple containment, where this is a combined function of a container and its closure, to a pack which acts as a device to aid product administration. Rigidity or flexibility in the design of a container will relate to the type of material and distribution of the wall thickness, which require good radii and the avoidance of square or angular designs. Poor wall distribution, particularly where thin sections are involved, may reduce the product shelf life by increasing the effects of permeation and migration. Since some product constituents will diffuse through a plastic by solution in the plastic, followed by vaporisation from the external surface, rate of loss will largely relate to the solubility/diffusion coefficients and the wall thickness.

Design wall distribution will also be related to the physical strength of the container and its ability to withstand drops (e.g. breakage), long-term stacking (e.g. distortion or spilling), handling during filling, capping, etc. In the last of these the top pressure applied during capping may cause considerable container distortion. This may have to be overcome by alternative closuring methods or supporting the container neck.

The overall effectiveness of most containers relates to the design of the bottle neck and closure and the material from which the closure and container are made. Where a flexible material is used, a buttress thread (BS 5789, 1979) is recommended. However, if the material is substantially harder, e.g. HDPE, PP, or PVC, a conventional type 60° thread (BS 1918, R3/2 and R4 finishes for glass) can be employed.

The aesthetics of a container are of equal importance to ethical and OTC packaging. Ethicals must generally be elegant, simple with clear and concise wording which tones in well with the presentation. Although this may equally apply to some proprietary products, these tend to require greater eye appeal to attract a purchaser's attention.

Process of manufacture

Pharmaceutical containers can be produced by a number of moulding processes, and this may be carried out by a supplier or set up in-house to produce either a preformed container or one which can be formed, filled and sealed as a continuous operation. Often different moulding processes involve different grades of polymer.

Preformed containers can be manufactured by:

- injection moulding
- injection blow moulding/injection stretch blow moulding
- extrusion blow moulding/extrusion stretch blow moulding
- thermoforming by vacuum, pressure, with and without mechanical assistance
- cold forming by pressure or by plug (mechanical means).

All the above processes can also be used in a form fill seal process with, for example, thermoforming and cold forming blister packs. 'Rommelag' type bottle pack systems use an extrusion process where the container is formed by either blowing or vacuum (smaller sizes). Immediately after this, containers are filled, and the pack is sealed (welded) by using the residual heat in an extension to the main body of the container.

Decoration and printing

Decoration and printing are usually a separate process, although in mould transfers/labels or embossing/debossing may be added within the moulding cycle. The extra handling associated with pretreatment (flaming or corona discharge) and the relatively dirty nature of the decoration and printing processes is likely to lead to increased contamination unless very special precautions are undertaken. One option is to seal the containers at the manufacturing stage prior to printing and then later open them prior to filling. Printing or labelling after filling and closing is another way. Printing inks, particularly if plastic- or solvent-based, may also migrate into the product, or product excipients may permeate outwards, weakening the print key or causing changes to ink colours. (Printing inks need to have food grade approval.)

The main processes used on plastic containers, components, films, etc. are as follows:

- paper, plastic or laminated labels
- shrinkable or stretchable sleeves
- dry offset letterpress, gravure, flexography, (silk) screen
- hot die stamping and thermal printing
- transfer processes – therimage, letraset, dinacal, etc.
- cliché print, i.e. tampoprint, tampon transfer, pad printing
- non-contact processes such as inkjet and laser printing.

Materials and their properties

A basic knowledge of the chemistry of plastics, the polymerisation processes by which they are made, and their physical and chemical characteristics or properties is essential. Plastics can initially be divided into two groups, thermosets and thermoplastics. Most believe that thermosets tend to be restricted to wadded closures where there is no contact between the product and the closure, and the fact that certain internal coatings (lacquers) are thermoset-based is frequently forgotten. Thermosets such as urea formaldehyde, phenol formaldehyde (UF, PF), and occasionally melamine formaldehyde, which are used for closures with wood, paper, flour-based fillings, are all produced by condensation polymerisation where during the reaction a state of 'cure' is involved. Inadequate cure or overcure therefore reflects in substandard material and residues will inevitably remain which may occasionally migrate into a product. These residues may be phenol, formaldehyde and ammonia, in the case of phenol formaldehyde caps, if a phenol hexamine reation is used. Thus during the 'cure' both water and ammonia are released, some of which may be retained by the moulding.

Thermoset lacquers are also found in use as adhesive systems (including laminations) and as coatings for metal tins and tubes (i.e. epoxy resin, polyester and polyurethane-based polymers).

As indicated earlier, thermoplastics are far more widely used for containers, films and packaging components. Although a large number of different polymers can be identified, five basic types stand out as more economically viable than the others. These are:

- (PE) polyethylene LD, MD, HD and LLDPE
- (PS) polystyrene GP and various impact grades
- (PP) polypropylene and its copolymers
- (PVC) polyvinylchloride, plasticized and unplasticized
- (PET) polyester (even though the current price is significantly higher, i.e. around £1,100 per tonne, as it is usually moulded in thinner sections).

The cost of these starts in the region of £650 per tonne (for 10 tonne lots) and rises to around £850 depending on the type and grade. Each has grades approved for use in contact with food.

Price increases occur according to whether a material is natural, white opaque or coloured, or has other additives present. Additives are generally more expensive than the basic plastic.

In the past, equivalency between grades has usually been identified by comparing certain basic properties such as density and melt flow index (the amount of plastic which flows under given conditions of temperature, pressure and time). Although these are quite acceptable for many non-critical usages, further parameters must be considered particularly when the plastic is used for sterile products. This is because each plastic may contain different constituents and may be polymerised by a different process.

Of the economical plastics mentioned above, GP polystyrene is becoming less popular, as it is one of the most brittle plastics unless it is impact modified. GP or (GPPS) polystyrene has good clarity, is highly permeable (compared with most other plastics) to moisture and gases, has poor heat and solvent resistance. It crazes then disintegrates in contact with isopropyl myristate (which is used in some pharmaceutical formulations). It is, however, an excellent material to mould (low shrinkage)

Impact modified or toughened polystyrene is generally less transparent, more flexible, but poorer in water vapour and gas transmission.

Whereas low-density polythene tends to be used where a flexible pack is desirable, high-density polyethylene and polypropylene are finding a substantial usage where a rigid container with reasonable resistance to water vapour is required. These materials have generally good resistance to chemicals, including those preservatives, which are readily soluble in low density polyethylene. Both HDPE and PP can be steam autoclaved, with PP having around 20°C more latitude. Rigidity, crystallinity (a property related to moisture and gas transmission), chemical and particularly oil resistance, all increase from LD to HD. Low-density polyethylene may be prone to environmental stress cracking, unless a material of low melt flow index, i.e. less than 1.0, is used. Detergents, wetting agents and volatile oils all tend to be stress cracking agents.

Polypropylene can have its clarity and transparency improved by orientation, or by use of clarifying/nucleating agents.

Polyvinylchloride is rigid, transparent and, although it lacks the sparkle of polystyrene, is less brittle. Drop strength can be improved by the use of an impact modifier such as vinyl acetate or methyl methacrylate butadiene styrene (MBS). PVC is moderately permeable to moisture but has excellent resistance to oil and oxygen permeation. Plasticised PVC has high flexibility and is particularly useful when a collapsible pack is required. It is a poor barrier to moisture and a moderate barrier to gases, hence is usually 'overwrapped'.

Of the five economical plastics, PVC (both plasticised and unplasticised) tends to contain the most constituents and has recently been a prime target for environmentalists who associate its burning with the release of acid gases. LDPE is generally likely to contain the least constituents with PS, HDPE, PP being slightly worse. Identifying, quantifying and clearing these are discussed later. Permissible antioxidants are identified in the EP.

PET is usually the most obvious replacement for glass where oral liquids are involved. It is strong, has high clarity, moderate permeation to moisture, good gas barriers and good retention to certain volatiles such as camphor, menthol and alcohol. Use as a stretch moulding minimises thickness and generally further improves strength and barrier properties.

Other thermoplastics

The use of other plastics tends to be related to specialised needs and whether their advantages justify the additional cost, e.g. Aclar (trade name) may cost twenty times more than PET but is the nearest approach to an inert 'plastic' and is approximately ten times less permeable than Saran (PVdC – polyvinylidene chloride) which is widely used as a film coating. However foil, even when thin (0.006 mm and above) remains the best barrier material, with newer techniques of film metallisation, especially where two contact layers are used, coming a close second best.

Plastic grades

Once a plastic type has been broadly selected, the final grade can be decided. Food approved grades are the starting point for most pharmaceutical products. Grades are generally based on density, melt flow index, the fabrication process for which they have been made, final usage, and the additional constituents which they may contain.

These constituents may include additives: antistatic additives, UV absorbers, anti-slip additives, slip additives, colourants, opacifiers, plasticisers, stabilisers, antioxidants, etc., which may be added at the compounding stage to provide specific or modified properties. However, other 'constituents' may be present from the polymerisation and/or the converting processes. The polymerisation process may involve residues and processing aids. Residues (constituents which may remain from the polymerisation process) may include monomer(s), solvents, accelerators, catalysts, initiators, etc. Processing aids are additional substances to aid processing or restrain undesirable effects, e.g. antioxidants.

The converting or moulding process may also include the use of processing aids, e.g. lubricants and mould release agents. Masterbatching may contain lubricants, mould release and a carrier or base diluent which assist the manufacture of a concentrated masterbatch containing colourants.

From the above it is clear that asking the question 'what additives are included?' is unlikely to provide the full information related to the polymerisation or converting process. Checking the 'constituents' under specific headings provides more detail.

Toxicity and irritancy – safety aspects and organoleptic properties

Ideally no extractive from or loss into a plastic should be permitted, but in most practical circumstances some compromise must be reached. One is thus required to identify not only the level of migration, but whether any risks have been incurred in terms of the product's effectiveness or toxicity/irritancy. In respect of the latter, data is generally more readily available on toxicity aspects than irritancy. Packaging also must not bring about any 'deterioration in the organoleptic characteristics' (critical to many foods but of equal importance to certain pharmaceuticals). Attempts have been made to estimate the TRTC (taste recognition threshold concentration) of certain monomers, e.g. styrene monomer, and other constituents common to plastics. The level of transfer depends on the nature of the product, with oils and fats generally being more susceptible to detectable taint.

Stage 1 in the selection of a packaging material

There is still a certain reluctance for manufacturers, compounders and converters to declare constituents to the pharmaceutical industry, although there may be a reasonable willingness to provide this information to official regulatory organisations, i.e. by reference to a 'drug master file'. This situation is improving but obviously where constituents are not identified, greater clearance difficulties are experienced. Whether such information is freely given or not, it does seem relevant to pose three sets of questions, i.e. to the polymer manufacturer, compounder and converter.

Polymer manufacturer (for each identified grade)

1   What constituents (catalysts, accelerators, antioxidants, etc.) are used in the polymerisation process and what level of residues (particularly monomers) can be expected in the granules? (Note that granules are frequently produced via a multiple rod extrusion process through a 'town' water cooling bath, from which inorganic salts in 'hard' water may evaporate on the surface of the granules leading to contamination in the final moulding.)
2   What toxicity/irritancy data is available on these?
3   What levels of extractive for these residues can be expected using various solvents or simulants?
4   Details of analytical methods and accuracy/reproducibility of the methods, etc.

Compounder

1   What constituents are added, at what level and for what reason, i.e. colourants, dyes, opacifiers, UV absorbers, stabilisers, modifiers, etc.?
2   What toxicity/irritancy data is available on these and from whom (e.g. supplying companies)?

3   What levels of extractives can be expected?
4   Analytical methods and accuracy/reproducibility of the methods, etc.

It must be noted that not all plastics pass through a compounding stage or contain any additional constituents, e.g. possible virgin natural materials. However, constituents may be added by the polymer manufacturer, resin supplier (smaller quantities), via a masterbatching process or at the final conversion stage. Asking where constituents may be added is critical to obtaining information. A masterbatch containing 50% titanium dioxide prompts the question 'what is the other 50%?'.

Converter, i.e. laminate, film, bottle manufacturer

1   What processing aids are used by either direct addition to the granules or onto moulds (e.g. lubricants and antistatic agents)?
2   As 'compounder' above if 'compounding' occurs, e.g. colourants added immediately prior to the moulding operation.
3   What toxicity/irritancy data is available?
4   What levels of extractives can be expected?
5   Analytical method and accuracy/reproducibility of the methods, etc.

In an ideal situation these issues should be resolved between representatives of the pharmaceutical industry and the suppliers identified above, as part of the technical/economic validation.

Finally it should be noted that certain restrictions may have to be incorporated into the packaging material specification, e.g. 'No lubricants to be used', (magnesium and zinc stearate or similar lubricants may be incompatible with either the drug substance or certain excipients).

If the above information cannot be fully obtained then a formal guarantee must be sought that the polymer and the included constituents meet some level of food clearance (FDA, EU, etc.). This is normally accepted as the minimum information required before a plastic is considered further in the development stage of a pharmaceutical product. See Appendix 8.6 for details on EU listings related to plastic contact with foodstuffs.

Stage 2 – extractive tests, chemical and biological

This stage is only mandatory for certain types of product. The next testing phase is normally an extractive procedure, using a company in-house standard and/or an externally recognised standard covering chemical extractives and biological tests (toxicity/irritancy), using pharmaceutical simulants under selected conditions of time and temperature. These tests can generally be classified under three categories:

1   national regulations and compendial standards and guidelines (USP/NF extractive tests USA, JP, EP, etc.)
2   standards issued by standards institutions (e.g. BS 5736)
3   international guidelines proposed by the World Health Organisation (WHO).

The main proposals relate to injections and ophthalmic products (see Appendix 8.1), and the interpretation will depend on the product and the product usage.

Differences in approach between the BP 1988 and USP XXIII should be noted. The BP 1988 excludes details of extractive procedures although such tests were included in the BP 80 and are included in the USP XXIII. The BP argues that it only includes test procedures related to ongoing control of materials and products, whereas extractive procedures are intended for use in a developmental phase where a plastic is undergoing selection, i.e. 'extractives' are not intended for routine ongoing tests. It is presumed that once a plastic has been thumbprinted it can be routinely checked by some form of chemical analysis, i.e. IR, DSC.

Because an extraction test may be part of a compendial standard or a mandatory regulatory requirement, it is frequently believed that such a test procedure has total approval for the polymer involved. Although it may be one of the tests available, mainly because there are few alternatives, the usefulness of the procedure is not entirely proven. Therefore a material which passes both chemical and toxicity irritancy type tests is probably safe, bearing in mind that final clearance comes from the following compatibility tests (stage 3). Failing the test may not necessarily establish that a material is unsafe, but rather stimulates additional questions on the polymer, operators, test conditions, etc. Overall one must be reminded that a simulant, even if it appears to be relatively inert (water, saline, sodium bicarbonate solution, etc.) may produce different results to the actual product. Although implantation tests (see USP XXIII) may also provide useful information, this may again create data which are difficult to quantify. One must equally bear in mind the risk to the patient and the company – hence the philosophy that stages 1 and 2, which may be critical in the case of an IV product would involve fewer questions and less investigation for the clearance of a solid oral dosage form. Although extractive tests are not mandatory for all products, they can be a useful part of a databank if a particular grade of plastic is part of a company's inventory. Plastics classified under the USP 6 category, in theory, have the best safety clearance.

Stage 3 – product/pack compatibility and investigational testing

The third stage normally covers feasibility or investigational tests, i.e. the initial testing stages which are aimed at establishing the general suitability of a product–pack combination and involve some degree of accelerated conditions. Such tests normally include some cycling conditions, e.g. 15°C 50% RH, 37°C 90% RH with 12 or 24 hourly cycles and temperatures up to 50°C, but be wary of tests using temperatures above 45°C as certain pack properties can change and influence product changes.

One suggested accelerated test is to place an excess of cut-up pieces of the proposed plastic, immersed in the product, in a neutral glass stoppered container which is held at, say, 4°C, 25°C, 40°C for a period of 3 months. The product (and plastic) should be analysed at intervals for change and extraction. However, even a test of this nature is not all-embracing since total immersion eliminates possible change from air to air–liquid interfaces which occur in a pratical situation.

If there is no change in product or plastic, interaction is unlikely. However, if a change does occur it should act as a warning that something may occur under normal conditions in the long term. It is important that investigational tests cover any specially selected challenge conditions (light, cycling conditions, etc.) which it is essential to check but may not be covered by the formal stability tests. Such additional information has usually to be made available as a standard document and presented as part of any registration documentation (Expert Report under EU).

It is essential that the above tests acknowledge information built from challenges on the drug entity, and the preformulation and formulation stages. This background information should at least indicate the type of protection which has to be achieved by the pack. Compatibility between product and pack is therefore defined at this stage prior to the product–pack entering a formal stability stage. Data generated by feasibility tests may be used to predict an initial shelf life and provide support data for clinical trial supplies. Clinical trials and clinical trial data can also contribute towards the 'total data' which supports the product–pack ultimate shelf life.

Controls

The use of certain control experimentation is of particular importance during initial investigational research into a suitable pack. However, one should be wary of the word 'control' as its interpretation may have to change according to circumstances. If a product shows some deterioration in a plastic pack there must be immediate questions on whether this is pack- or product-related. Having a glass pack with an effective closure as a control will provide useful information, but raises the next question as to whether the glass bottle should be a bottle plus closure or a neutral glass sealed ampoule (e.g. the effectiveness of the closure in the former and an ampoule can become a pressurised system at higher temperatures). Higher temperatures normally accelerate change (all have heard of Arrhenius), and lower ones are less conducive to change. This immediately suggests that a refrigerator is a useful control condition for both the product and the pack. This is generally true, but there are circumstances where 4°C is an accelerated condition, i.e. plastics become more rigid and hence are under greater stress.

Holding adequate retention samples can also be part of control. An example is where a plastic bottle is put under test with a product. On removal of the polypropylene cap a yellow discolouration is found on the bottle neck. The questions asked can be: is it product-related? Is it a reaction between cap and bottle? Could it happen on an uncapped bottle (probably unlikely)? This situation could be resolved by testing bottles capped without product, together with separately stored retention samples of caps and bottles. How retention samples are stored and what they are stored in, etc., are additional questions which have to be asked.

Using effective controls, controlled conditions and well-controlled tests constitutes an important part of all investigational experimentation. It is an often neglected subject. Equally such experimentation should be supported by adequate statistical control. Take a situation where a wadded and a wadless (no liner) closure are to be placed on an HDPE bottle and then stored over a 6 month period in a cycling cabinet which cycles between 15°C 50% RH and 37°C 90% RH each 24 h. Question – devise a statisically controlled experiment to check any torque changes, indicating the number of samples required. Personally I would suggest the use of an induction sealed closure as the experimentation could be complex and costly for the information achieved.

Stage 4 – formal product–pack stability tests

These formal tests are normally scheduled over a period of 5 years, using a range of storage conditions, where the formulation and the pack are analysed at selected periods for changes, degradation, migration, etc., involving statistical evaluation such as regression analysis. The tests may include further biological and microbial challenge procedures, etc., to check that no significant changes have occurred in the product or pack.

Submission of data to regulatory authorities for product registration may commence once 6 or 12 months (ICH guidelines indicate 12 months) of good data has been obtained, on the understanding that this will be supplemented as additional data becomes available. Some authorities will allow a 2 year shelf life to be predicted from 12 months of 'accelerated' data. Guidelines drawn up by the CPMP within the EU, published as III/66/87/EN (now updated by ICH guidelines), identified certain climatic zones. (Table 8.1).

The work described above may be done entirely by the pharmaceutical company concerned or may be partially or fully contracted out. Whichever course is followed, it is important that all test procedures are properly documented and follow the guidelines established by GMP (good manufacturing practice) and GLP (good laboratory practice). This means, for example, that both product and pack components should be clearly defined, specified and identified (QC + type clearance) together with adequate testing procedures and the holding of retention samples, before they are entered into any investigational or formal test programme. Again attention to controls must be advised.

As a result, the data built up from all the stages, and supplementary clinical data, must be sufficient to satisfy:

1 the pharmaceutical company itself
2 worldwide or local regulatory authorities that the product and pack are compatible, that they do not incur any safety hazards, and that they maintain the shelf life declared on the pack and supporting documents at an agreed level of quality.

As pointed out, the above stages to 'clear' a plastic are supported by:

1 information on the pack or device constituents
2 extractive tests/product contact tests etc.

Table 8.1 CPMP climatic zone guidelines

Zone	Conditions	Area
I	21°C 45% RH	Temperate Europe
II	26°C 60% RH	Sub-tropical
III	31°C 40% RH	Hot dry
IV	31°C 70% RH	Hot humid

Expressed as kinetic mean temperature with recommendations that these conditions should be used in future stability programmes (see Appendix 8.14). Temperatures were subsequently rounded to 20°C, 25°C and 30°C.

3 short- and long-term stability tests between product and packaging/device components.

There are however additional activities (e.g. warehousing, distribution) whereby information is built up in order to establish the total stability/safety of the product, the clinical efficacy of the product/device and the functional acceptance of the product/pack/device in the hands of the ultimate user. (This is particularly relevant where the pack assists product administration: see Appendix 8.9 for further details.)

This total data philosophy covers information accrued from the time a new drug entity is discovered, through preformulation studies to final formulation in terms of physical, chemical, climatic and microbiological challenge so that the product characteristics, deterioration, degradation, etc. are established before it is placed into contact with a pack/device.

Comparison between foodstuffs and pharmaceuticals based on simulated extractive tests is inevitably difficult, because the site and mode of absorption may vary, because of the difference in the pre-storage period and the frequency of use, and the volume/weight of the product taken. With foodstuffs, the contact period between product and pack is usually shorter, but the quantity taken and frequency of use are greater, e.g. daily intake of margarine. Thus any EU extractive procedure may provide useful additional information for the pharmaceutical industry as part of stage 1 involving the screening of the material, but the simulants used may bear little relationship to the final pharmaceutical form. These tests are also more relevant to toxicity aspects rather than to irritancy. For food extractive tests see Appendix 8.6.

An additional fact to consider is that the pharmaceutical usage of any plastic tends to be relatively small when compared with other industries: food, motor, etc. This situation poses considerable problems to both the pharmaceutical industry and the polymer manufacturer or the converter when any information is requested, as invariably the in-depth data required is out of proportion to the profit made. Attempts to overcome this problem have been suggested (the industry pays for the information, or information within the industry is pooled), but so far little progress has been made towards a satisfactory solution.

This general lack of information creates problems between the product and the pack, where on one side considerable analytical resources are put into product identity, purity and impurity (the last of these now being of the greatest relevance) whereas on the other hand the constituents of the plastic cannot be fully identified. This situation inevitably creates an ongoing argument as to whether such in-depth information on the plastic is relevant or irrelevant, particularly if the total pharmaceutical clearance programme does not highlight any cause for concern. Personally I believe that in-depth knowledge can only improve the long-term relationship of suppliers and users. This must also be a two-way process where the pharmaceutical industry must provide more information to the supplier. The fact that many suppliers will provide such detailed information to a regulatory authority (this information is essential in Sweden and the USA) may seem a reasonable compromise, but let us again not forget that the information in total must satisfy both the regulatory authorities and the pharmaceutical company itself (the latter is the more important, since if it has not convinced itself, how can it convince others?!).

Additional discussion

In terms of the differences in attitude towards glass and plastic, glass is generally considered inert and safe as it has been used for thousands of years and proved by time, whereas plastics, being modern, are under constant surveillance. Therefore one could suggest that if glass had been discovered today, it would have had a more difficult task to establish itself when faced with the more stringent types of tests now applied to plastics.

Another current example of 'attitudes' involves thermoplastic and thermosetting resins. The stringent tests referred to previously are invariably carried out on any thermoplastic which forms part of a primary pack. However, thermosets and in particular thermosetting lacquers, enamels and adhesives are rarely exposed to an extractive-type procedure, since they are not always recognised as plastics.

We must also recognise that there is a danger for test procedures to grow to a point where they are either meaningless or unnecessary. This does not imply that every enthusiastic investigator is unscientific, but tries to recognise that the introduction of any new procedure is only based on the facts available at that time and relies much on any subsequent publicity which it receives in order to become established. Procedures once established frequently become far too difficult to replace.

Having made such a comment, it is equally important not to be complacent. Thus any system generally adopted by the pharmaceutical industry must be subjected to constant review, in order that adequate standards of safety can be achieved at a reasonable cost. Although this is likely to mean a need for more in-depth knowledge on the plastic and modifications to the currently recognised extractive procedures, it seems extremely unlikely that the last approval stage (formal stability or shelf life tests) can ever be replaced. However, new computerised data retrieval systems will enable greater confidence to be maintained provided the input of data at all stages is optimised.

It must be reiterated that each use of a plastic, as either a pack or a device, must be carefully evaluated against a background of the product and its use, paying particular attention to the following.

1   Type of product:

   • contact phase – volume
   • contact area – during storage, transit and in use.

2   Storage conditions at all stages of its shelf life. Note that refrigerator conditions are likely to be far less encouraging to extraction, hence may offer a degree of control.
3   Shelf life and length of time product is in contact with pack. Pack upright, inverted, etc.
4   Mode of administration and the risks of absorption of any extracted constituents via that route.
5   Dosage level, frequency of use and application, i.e. treatment period – continuous, intermittent or temporary. (Is product seasonal, stored partly used until next year?)
6   Misuse/abuse by patient or children, etc.

Finally, the possibility of product migration into the pack (e.g. loss of preservatives) coupled with permeation of oxygen, carbon dioxide and moisture must also be considered as a factor which could cause changes in the migratory nature of constituents in the plastic.

Oxygen may cause slow oxidation of a plastic resulting in a slight change in the constituents extracted after storage. CO_2 permeation, being roughly five times faster than oxygen, will frequently cause a pH shift with unbuffered products with an equilibrium value pH of 4.3–4.6. Hence a shift in pH leading to further changes in levels of extraction must not be overlooked. Irradiation can also cause plastic constituent changes (see sterilisation and Appendix 8.11).

General performance requirements

Since the functional aspects may vary according to how a pack or device is used, some general headings will be considered first.

Closure efficiency

Closure design needs consideration for effectiveness during use, i.e. opening and reclosing, problems associated with stacking (top pressure), torque control range if a screw closure, the effects of time and temperature, dimensional tolerances and compliance, etc. Tests to differentiate loss via the closure, or through the main body of the container, are frequently necessary. Even with moderately permeable materials, moisture loss or gain can be greater through the closure system if it is not effectively designed or closed. Plugged bottles systems may be particularly prone to seepage due to climbing film-type effects, and sinkage behind the threads in the bottleneck bore encourages capillary-type seepage. This especially applies to certain extrusion blown bottles. Injection blow moulding may be necessary to overcome this problem, as it provides a better controlled neck finish and can eliminate thread sinkage in the bottle bore.

Decoration permanency

Print and colour may suffer from discoloration (fading or darkening), surface rub or abrasion, print or label lifting due to poor adhesion or key, and lack of product resistance. Various types of test are available to check these. Discoloration may be checked by direct exposure to sunlight or artificially accelerated conditions, e.g. xenon test. With the latter, 'fade' may be compared with changes based on the British Wool Scale. It is advisable to check the temperature as occasionally discoloration is increased by the combined effect of temperature and light. Light may also cause changes to the plastic material itself. ICH Guidelines define tests using specific light sources.

Print key may be checked by the Scotch tape test, where a strip is applied to the surface to be tested and is then removed in a standard way with observation for print lift.

Product resistance consists of applying the product to the print or decoration (controlled temperature), at the end of which the product is cleaned off in a rubbing motion to see whether any decoration is removed.

Solvents in inks may also permeate into the products and occasionally product ingredients may change the permanency of the ink if they pass through the plastic. Similarly, labels adhesives may also contain migratory constituents. (Special checks are essential on pressure and heat sensitive adhesives.)

Environmental stress cracking

Environmental stress cracking is less prevalent today (except in Third World countries) and more readily understood. Stress cracking is a phenomenon related to internal stress arising from the moulding operation or externally applied stress, which in conjunction with a stress cracking agent may lead to a plastic (e.g. low-density polythene) cracking. Most detergents or wetting agents act as stress cracking agents. In the Hedley test the container is filled with the product, the closure applied as normal then stored at 60°C for 48 h. If no cracking occurs, the test is passed. If the storage is then extended to 7 days the point of cracking (if it occurs) indicates the weakest point(s) in the moulding. Plastics may also be given a stress crack value based on the Bell telephone test (hours taken for a crack to appear). Those with the higher figures are less stress crack prone.

Typical stress conditions may be created by capping (tension between bottle and cap threads), plugging (expansion of the neck bore), top pressure occurring during stacking, etc.

Warehousing and distribution

Warehousing and distribution hazards include impacts, compression and vibration. One or a combination of these may distort the container, loosen or tighten the closure, and cause deterioration to the decoration. Thus any of these aspects may have to be tested by simulated laboratory tests or actual warehousing/travel tests.

Outer or transit packaging can occasionally contribute to changes in the primary pack or the product. External wrapping materials may contain various migratory constituents, e.g. when a shrink or stretch film is in intimate contact with a primary pack or plastic components of a device. Odorous board, adhesives, printing inks on external packaging have also been known to cause flavour and/or odour changes.

Conversely, a laboratory test on single (exposed) primary packs may show a moisture loss or gain which is significantly reduced when the same pack is stored in bulk, i.e. the outer packaging reduces the exchange by adding barrier materials and slowing down the atmosphere circulating around the pack(s), thereby changing the effective gradient between the inside and outside of the pack.

Use and misuse by the patient

Tests necessary to indicate how a consumer uses or misuses a pack or device are critical to total assessment. A point to consider is that air can enter the pack by an increasing amount as a product is used. Occasionally this ingress may give rise to excessive product deterioration, thus proving that either the pack size must be limited or air ingress restricted, e.g. the individual protection offered by a unit dose pack may be the preferred answer. A closure system may occasionally deteriorate or become less effective during use. Returned clinical trials may help in this evaluation, particularly where microbiological contamination may be involved.

Consideration of misuse may challenge the way a product should be stored, i.e. upright, upside down or on its side, and may require testing.

Sterilisation

Sterilisation may give rise to adverse actions depending on the process and the particular grade of plastic, pack, etc. This means that if a pack is to be sterilised, either as a terminal operation or as part of an aseptic process, careful checking for possible changes is essential. Textbooks which make general statements should be treated with caution, as individual grades of plastic may react differently.

The three most likely processes are:

1   steam sterilisation – autoclaving at 121°C for 15 min or 115°C for 30 min
2   gamma irradiation and accelerated electrons (normally associated with aseptic processing)
3   ethylene oxide (normally associated with aseptic processing).

All of these may give rise to changes with the product or pack or both. For example, terminal autoclaving by moist heat may cause physical or chemical changes to the product or the pack. Whether the pack is distorted frequently depends on the product volume to vacuity ratio (i.e. ullage or airspace), since this may give rise to either extension or dimpling of the package. A pack which becomes extended (by excessive internal pressure) puts stress on the closure or seal, or container. A dimpled pack normally results from a negative pressure situation and is particularly likely to occur in packs which have thinner sections. The use of overpressure or balanced pressure autoclaves is essential to control dimpling, when moist heat sterilisation is employed. The overpressure employed will have to be adjusted according to a wide range of variables, i.e. plastic, temperature, pack size, shape, wall distribution, content versus vacuity, etc.

Gamma irradiation of 25 kGy or above and accelerated electrons tend to cause similar changes to the product/pack. These processes are normally used as part of an aseptic process to sterilise the pack components before use, since many products tend to degrade if terminally sterilised. Some contact lens solutions and normal saline products can be satisfactorily gamma irradiated in a suitable plastic or metal pack (aerosols).

Although 'irradiation stable' lists of types of plastic and specific grades are sometimes available from suppliers, this in no way clears a plastic for gamma irradiation until a company has satisfied itself that either no change occurs or changes are acceptable. Occasionally chemical changes may be related to either the polymer or the constituents within the polymer. Further details on this are given in Chapter 7 and Appendix 8.11. Note that irradiated samples should be analysed immediately or the samples kept in well-sealed impermeable packs (e.g. glass containers), i.e. avoid containing them in polythene bags to await analysis, as volatile products of degradation can be lost to the atmosphere. Irradiation under nitrogen significantly reduces degradation.

Various attempts have been made to phase out ethylene oxide treatment as a sterilisation process, but it is still used. Ethylene oxide largely relies on the material being permeable to the gas under certain conditions of time, temperature, moisture and pressure. Plastics which do not have a solubility coefficient for ethylene oxide may prove difficult to sterilise or proof of sterilisation may be difficult. The residual levels of ethylene oxide remaining also depend on the affinity or solubility of ethylene oxide for that particular type and grade of plastic. Aeration after sterilisation may be under vacuum or by simple storage with good air circulation for periods of up to 1 month (7–14 days is more normal). Since ethylene oxide degrades to ethylene glycol and epichlorhydrin (when chloride ions are present) and both of these exhibit degrees of toxicity, it is advisable to check for all three products. Any remaining ethylene oxide in the plastic will ultimately partition between the product, pack and external atmosphere. Again, treated containers should be stored in well-sealed impermeable packs when awaiting analysis. As analytical methods become more sensitive to the likely residues, lower limits are likely to be imposed. Since ethylene oxide is not inert, product interactions cannot be ruled out.

It can be concluded that a pack may be affected by most of the sterilisation processes hence thorough testing is essential in terms of possible changes in physical and chemical properties and appearance. Loss of preservatives may also be critical at a sterilisation stage.

Panelling or cavitation

Occasionally plastic packs may show partial collapse or indentation, a phenomenon known as panelling or cavitation. This may be caused by the following.

1   Hot fill plus effective closuring creating a partial vacuum on cooling.
2   Adsorption of a gas (usually oxygen) from the pack headspace.
3   Absorption of a product constituent which causes the inner section of the wall to swell, thus causing distortion.
4   Loss of volatile constituents through the plastic; may be an extension of (3).
5   Pack extension due to incorrect pressure balance during the autoclaving cycle – may be called dimpling if mild. Often associated with uneven wall thickness. The above cannot be predicted and are only discovered after storage.
6   Pack partially collapses during cap application.

The reverse of cavitation can also occur, e.g. on a nitrogen flushed product – gases (oxygen/carbon dioxide) enter the pack causing the bases to be bowed outwards.

Impact resistance

Plastic packs which are likely to crack on impact may be checked by a drop test procedure, e.g. a percentage must not break when dropped from a selected height onto a standard surface. The pack is dropped in a defined way (usually down a tube) onto its base or closure.

Clarity or transparency (light transmission)

May be quantified by the amount of light which passes through the container. Some pharmacopoeia tests require a certain level of light transmission to be achieved in order that particulate contamination can be checked. USP XXIII provides a useful test procedure for light transmission.

Light exclusion

This is the opposite to light transmission in that the greater part of the light must be filtered out. This test may define the wall thickness (i.e. 2 mm in the case of glass). Exclusion of light may be achieved by inclusion of colours, fillers, UV absorbers, or in combination with a carton or overwrap. Only carbon black pigmentation gives 100% light exclusion.

Electrostatic

Most plastics are prone to electrostatic unless special precautions are taken to reduce it. Static is increased by dry product filling, hot filling and operating in a dry atmosphere (more likely to happen when conditions external to the factory are dry, i.e. during freezing weather). Cleaning 'plastics' and then drying by heat can create conditions of high electrostatic attraction, and if the air surrounding the materials is not adequately filtered the component can be even dirtier after the alleged cleaning process. Static can be reduced by:

1   moisturing, i.e. using higher conditions of RH
2   earthing, or ionising the surrounding atmosphere
3   washing with the correct detergent, anionic or cationic (i.e. surface antistatic)
4   adding an antistatic agent to the plastic.

(3) and (4) generally work by attracting a layer of moisture to the surface, thereby allowing the charge to be conducted away.
  Electrostatic can be measured either directly by sensitive equipment or by checking the dust patterning with a fine carbon cloud under standard conditions.

Pretreatments for printing (and labelling)

Components can be pretreated by:

1   gas flaming
2   high-voltage corona discharge
3   chemical treatment (this may be similar to surface sterilisation as used for some food packaging processes).

Containers are normally pretreated by flaming and films by corona treatment. Pretreatment can be checked by wetting the surface and observing the affinity of the surface to water (untreated surfaces retain the water as droplets) or actually measuring the angle of contact, which is reduced when the surface is oxidised. Pretreated surfaces effectively last for 3–6 months. Surface treatment may also enhance the effectiveness of some of the constituents which operate at the surface of the container, e.g. antistatic slip and anti-slip.

Development versus production pack

Before any pack reaches production, differences between the pack tested and the pack to be marketed must be identified and cleared. It is virtually inevitable that there will be some differences. One of the most likely lies in the labelling, decoration or printing of the pack. If it is subsequently decided to label a pack by, for example, a thermoplastic or a heat seal label, these must be thoroughly checked since all contain constituents (in the adhesive system) which may possibly migrate into or through the plastic. Migration from self-adhesive labels has been reported whereby formulation excipients, including the preservative BKC, can be degraded. Effects from other external influences, even the lacquer used for a collapsible carton, should not be ignored. In another instance, the addition of an overwrap has been known to nullify stability on an exposed bottle in that an ingredient which 'escaped' from the latter was retained when overwrapped and the carton suffered discoloration. Differences often occur between a single impression prototype tool and a multi-impression production tool. It is important to identify any differences and then to ascertain requirements for additional testing.

Conclusion

The ultimate task of the pack is to produce confidence in the product in terms of convenience, preservation and protection from the environment, while ensuring that the product remains satisfactory in the fullest sense, i.e. integrity, identity, uniformity, safety, effectiveness, etc., all at an economically acceptable cost. Undoubtedly pharmaceutical packaging does receive greater attention to detail than any other form of product.

Although the types of test procedure will broadly continue to follow the stages identified in this chapter, the ultimate intensity of the procedure must be related to the type of product and the route by which it is administered, etc. (see Appendix 8.8 for a suggested intensity of testing table). The use of a declared 'food grade' plastic is therefore the minimum standard for a pharmaceutical product. Reference to Toy Regulations may also provide useful information especially where coloured materials are employed.

As the cost of clearing any product–pack combination is inevitably high, it is extremely important to define adequately the product, the pack, and the processes involved in these clearance schedules, and to finish with:

1 a product specification including process of manufacture
2 a pack specification covering the pack and its component parts
3 a specified means of bringing the product and pack together, i.e. the packaging process as defined by standard operating procedures.

The future control of the product and pack (and changes) then revolves around these specifications. In the case of a plastic pack or plastic components it may be necessary not only to define tightly certain critical factors in the specification, but to purchase under a certificate of warranty. Regular QC checks are likely to include melt flow index, density and IR identity and the use of DSC (differential scanning calorimetry). The last of these is a particularly useful means of providing plastic identification and an indication that the thumbprint is as per the original clearance tested material. Surface analysis testing is likely to become increasingly necessary with some products. As an additional insurance, a selected number of production batches are placed on an 'ongoing' product stability test annually. This monitoring system ensures that the stability profile (and shelf life) of the product does not change with the passage of time.

Changes in product, pack or process inevitably involve some form of retesting schedule, the intensity of which varies according to the nature of the change. ICH and EU guidelines provide suggestions.

Note that adequately defining the product, the pack, etc. means that provisional specifications should be written prior to any testing being carried out. Each item should also be thoroughly checked by in-depth QC procedures so that all materials used in investigational and formal tests can be fully identified.

It can therefore be concluded that 'plastic' packs and devices supplied by the pharmaceutical industry normally pass through a thorough and rigorous test procedure, but even so, such procedures will continually improve. If possible, loopholes in the present systems must be identified by more attention to the internal storage containers, piping, filters, etc. which are usually found in factory production areas and the bulk containers used to supply the industry with drugs and other excipients, as these receive far less attention than the pack destined for the 'patient'. If these are plastic contact materials, they will require some form of ongoing review.

In addition, work related to the clearance of the pack, the establishment of total integrity and GMP cannot be isolated into apparently watertight compartments such as product development, pack development, production, marketing, QC, as all must operate as an effective team with a high degree of communication and co-ordination. A packaging co-ordinator or a suitable 'generalist' with an ability to give an overview is therefore essential to success, but to date this has been recognised by only a few companies.

Finally let it be stressed that this chapter has been written to give a degree of both alertness and understanding. It in no way sets out to say that any approach is the ultimate, since test procedures must be constantly reviewed and updated. If a company technologist says 'we have done it this way for the past 20, 10 or 5 years', or 'we have always used this test', it is quite likely that they are not up to date and are not being fully effective. Virtually all stages identified in this chapter must be treated as long-term information gathering. Extractive tests fall into this category by providing the best information available at that moment. To date there are no records of people dying from using 'plastics', but rather from the processes by which they are synthesised (e.g. VCM). However, the industry must remain responsible particularly in terms of product/pack liability and at the same time remain commercially viable. Efforts to push testing to a point where it is carried out for testing's sake, or because someone has devised a test, must be resisted. Finally, tests to clear a pack initially must not be confused with tests to clear component deliveries, i.e. an in-house QA/QC situation. Tests must therefore be reviewed against their applications in a development and/or a QA/QC function.

The appendices

Some appendices are included so that the background on which procedures have been developed can be understood. Developing the future by ignoring the past can rarely be advised. 'Fresh' ways of evaluating pack (device) plastic suitability are essential to the future success of the industry. Five years ago this success as related to plastic and pharmaceuticals was easy to predict. Today, with growing environmental concerns, such predictions are less clear. The sophisticated world continues to be innovative, with emphasis on combination or composite materials (as offered by coextrusion etc.). Reuse and recycling of these mixed materials is certainly far from clear, so how will this apparent conflict be resolved? Who will predict?! Five years ago the author awaited a balance (on plastic testing/investigations) to be achieved between the practical side of industry and the more theoretical side of academia. Today the environmental issues add further complexity to future progress, and may influence a swing back to simple, single materials, or lightly coated materials.

It should be noted that many of the factors which need consideration when a pharmaceutical product is to be launched in a plastic pack share common ground with pharmaceutical and medical devices. Appendices (8.1, 8.3, 8.4 and 8.5) indicate the various proposals on the testing of plastics for pharmaceutical products. Appendix 8.2 provides a typical type of clearance programme for a multi-dose sterile product in a plastic pack.

EU activities on plastics for pharmaceuticals and foodstuffs are covered in Appendix 8.6. The need to extend the principles of GMP to the suppliers of plastic materials, containers and components is highlighted in Appendix 8.7. Appendix 8.8 introduces how the risk related to the product form can be expected to be reflected in the intensity of the tests necessary to approve a product–pack system. Additional factors which may change the level of testing are also discussed.

Appendix 8.9, in identifying how packs are becoming increasingly complex and sophisticated (e.g. to assist in product administration or as special devices), indicates the various types of additional testing which are now essential to approval. Appendix 8.10 lists support papers written by the author with reference to plastics.

Appendices 8.11, 8.12 and 8.13 open up a relatively new topic where a possible technical gap between the information given in polymer supplier data sheets and the properties of the plastic used in the final pack can be identified.

Finally, it is inevitable that some new guidelines will have appeared since this chapter was written. One area of constant advance is the ongoing publication of ICH guidelines, e.g. testing for the effect of light. However, even these guidelines will need review once some experience of their use has been obtained, and this point has been made previously about all test procedures. Testing at the ICH condition 40°C 75% RH provides a severe challenge to many packs, and there are various ways by which this challenge can be addressed (see Appendix 8.14).

Appendix 8.1: WHO guidelines

The World Health Organisation has proposed international requirements for plastic containers for pharmaceutical preparations. These include guidelines on selection of plastics/code of practice, covering the following.

Infusions and injections

- Physico-chemical on aqueous extracts.
- Non-volatile residue, heavy metals, buffering capacity, reducing substances.
- Biological *in vivo*.
- Acute systemic toxicity in mice (aqueous/alcoholic, oily extractants).
- Intracutaneous test (rabbits). Cardiovascular (cat) toxicity – infusions.
- Biological *in vitro*.
- Haemolytic effect of aqueous extract.

Aqueous ophthalmic preparations

- Physico-chemical on aqueous extracts.
- Non-volatile residue, buffering capacity, reducing substances.
- Biological test on aqueous extract.
- Eye irritation in rabbits on repeated instillation (Draize test).

The above is based on the 26th WHO Report and subsequent updates.

Appendix 8.2: Programme evaluation example

The following is a suggested programme for the evaluation of a plastic container for a liquid multidose injection product (not lyophilised).

1 Establish suitable grade of plastic. Determine that the plastic and constituents meet food grade standards. Discuss residues, additives and processing aids, etc. which may be present with relevant parties. Check available safety data. Note – additive content should be low and certain heavy metals absent (Cd, Pb, etc.).

2 Apply physico-chemical tests (on plastic or extract) and biological tests (on extract).

(a) Metallic additives – BP 1980 Appendix XIX A200–202 USP XXIII Containers.
(b) Non-volatile residues, residue on ignition and buffering on purified water injection extract – USP XXIII.
(c) Reducing substances on autoclaved water extract.
(d) Turbidity test (autoclaved) and freedom from froth.
(e) Acute systemic toxicity on sodium chloride injection extract using mice – see USP XXIII Containers.
(f) Intracutaneous test on rabbit. Sodium chloride injection extract – see USP XXIII.
(g) Eye irritation in rabbits – repeated instillation (Draize test) reference possible irritancy effects – USP XXIII.

3 Establish critical product characteristics by preformulation studies followed by challenge test on proposed formulation.

4 Actual injection stored in final plastic pack.

(a) Initial feasibility tests can use a similar plastic container and the product manufactured on a development scale – some accelerated testing may provide relevant data, i.e. temperatures up to 45°C. (May be used to provide stability data for clinical trials – IND stage in USA.)
(b) Formal long-term stability tests.

   (i) Usually carried out on up to three batches of product made on a production scale and packed in the container in which the product will be sold.
   (ii) Programme to cover 5 years.
   (iii) Test periods 0, 3, 6, 9, 12, 18, 24, 36, 48 and 60 months.
   (iv) Storage conditions 4°C, 25°C, 25°C 60% RH, 40°C, 40°C 75% RH for full period and possibly 45°C for 3–6 months. Conditions to be humidity controlled (and continuously recorded).
   (v) To check product and pack at related intervals for chemical change, i.e. purity/degradation/loss of active ingredients and primary constituents (e.g.

preservatives). Preferably by analytically specific methods. Degradation products not to exceed 1% with clear identification of major degradation substances. Recheck microbiological effectiveness (i.e. USP XXIII challenge test EP or BP 88 challenge test) at 0, 12 months, 24 months, 36 months, and sterility. Check plastic for chemical change, absorption, adsorption of ingredients, etc. (by extraction if necessary).

(vi) Physical change (do not overlook the importance of appearance, flavour, odour, colour, etc.).

(vii) At selected intervals and conditions (e.g. 25°C and 40°C after 12 months and 24 months etc.) check for possible changes in toxicity (BP 1980 toxicity test B on A201). Rechecks would also be advised on possible irritancy (Draize test).

(viii) In cases of pack change, i.e. glass to plastic, it may be possible to use the previous pack as a control. However, a control (i.e. sealed neutral glass ampoule) should always be considered for all stability or feasibility programmes. Storage of the pack without product may be necessary for comparison purposes in some circumstances. Pack change comparison could use 3–6 months at 40°C 75% RH with four periods of analysis, using previous pack as control, but this would need to be supported by a full stability programme.

5. Write up specifications for plastic, pack and pack components. Agree with suppliers.

6. Carry out ongoing stability on production batches using 25°C plus controlled RH. As per ICH recommendations.

Pack components, products, etc. need to be checked and cleared by QC, using written specifications, prior to use in any test programme. All procedures and activities need to be identified and recorded and fully validated.

These QC/GMP type activities are equally important during any stability programme in that when product samples are removed for analysis, the pack should be checked:

(i) at time of removal from test environment
(ii) when it is opened
(iii) after the product samples have been taken.

This should be a comprehensive examination by a trained packaging technologist. Simply opening a pack without observations may destroy evidence associated with possible pack deficiencies. (Analytical out-riders may be associated with pack deficiencies.)

Appendix 8.3: Examples of national standards for plastic containers for pharmaceuticals, USA and UK

USA

- FDA: General guidelines; Guideline for the Packaging of Human Drugs and Biologics – February 1987.
- USP XXIII, Containers (currently under review – new draft 1998).
- Biological Tests for Parenterals and Ophthalmics: reference should be made to CFR (Acceptance of Plastics and Constituents for Foodstuffs).

UK

- BP 1988, General Guidelines – Specific Tests for Large Volume Parenterals.
- DHSS (1973) Ref. 008 and 020. Specifications for Blood Bags and IV solutions – with Specific Reference to PVC (updates scheduled).
- BS 1679 (pt IV) Plastic Containers for Tablets and Ointments (currently under revision).
- BS 5736 (1979–1989) Parts 1–9, Evaluation of Medical Devices for Biological Hazards.
- EC/EP 1989 – then 1999.
- EP: Polyolefines.
- LDPE: See monographs.
- PVC/PP/HDPE etc., EP 1989.
- 9090/111: see summary in Appendix 8.8.

Appendix 8.4: Examples of national standards for plastic containers for pharmaceuticals, Europe and Japan

France (Pharmacopoeia Francaise Xth edn 1982)

- General Statement of Interaction.
- Parenterals – Biological and Physico-chemical tests.
- Ophthalmic preparations – Transparency and Neutrality.

Japan (Pharmacopoiea 10th edn 1982)

- 500 ml (or larger) aqueous infusion containers only apply.
- Physico-chemical and water permeability tests.
- Biological tests.
- Note – Japan Pharmaceutical Affairs Bureau Notification covers ophthalmics.

Nordic Pharmacopoeia

- Transfusion tubing
- Containers for blood, aqueous solutions, infusions, injections, irrigation solutions.
- Biological (pyrogenicity, acute toxicity, haemolytic) and physico-chemical tests.

National Swedish Pharmaceutical Laboratory

- Submission on standard form.
- Composition and properties of plastic and constituents.

Switzerland (Pharmacopoeia Helvetica)

- Must meet food requirements.
- Parenterals and ophthalmics – colourless, translucent, chemical tests, permeability to water and micro-organisms.

Note: The European Pharmacopoeia has now replaced many of the national ones.

EU – *General rules covering medicinal products*

- Directives 65/65/EEC, 75/318/EEC, 75/319/EEC, 89/341/EEC, 89/342/EEC, 89/343/EEC, 89/381/EEC.
- There are further CPMP guidelines issued as 'The Rules Governing Medicinal Product in the European Community', found as volumes I, II, III and IV.

See Chapter 3 for updated information.

Appendix 8.5: Bibliography

1   J. Cooper, *Plastic Containers for Pharmaceuticals. Testing and Control*. WHO, Geneva, 1974.
2   WHO Expert Committee on Specifications for Pharmaceutical Preparations (26th Report). Technical Report Series 614, Geneva, 1977.
3   *British Pharmacopoeia*, 1980/1988/1993.
4   *United States Pharmacopoeia* XXIII, incorporating the NF.
5   *Pharmacopoeia Helvetica* VI.
6   *Pharmacopoeia Francaise* Xth edn, 1982
7   *Japanese Pharmacopoeia*, 10th edn, 1982, p. 762–770.
8   *Nordic Pharmacopoeia* 1970.
9   National Swedish Pharmaceutical Laboratory.
10 Deutscher Normenauschuss (German Norm), DIN 13098, 13099, 58368.
11 *The International Pharmacopoeia*, Vols 1 and 2, 3rd edn, WHO, 1981.
12 CFR (USA) Code of Federal Regulations.
13 Japan Pharmaceutical Affairs Bureau Notification 958. Testing Methods for Plastic Containers.
14 European Pharmacopoeia 1980, subsequent edns 1982, 1989, etc.
15 *Pharmacea Fennica* (Finland) 1984.
16 Biological Reactivity Tests, *in vitro* and *in vivo*, USP XXIII.
17 Pharmacopoeial Forum, p. 4804, 11 Jan., Feb. 1989.
18 ASTM E813–83 (USA).
19 ISO/TC 194/WG I, Feb. 1990. Medical and dental materials and devices – Biological Evaluation pt. I, Selection of Tests.
20 Guidelines for Submitting Documentation for the Stability of Human Drugs and Biologics, Feb. 1987 (FDA). Currently being updated and expanded.
21 *Contemporary Biomaterials* by Boretos and Eden, published by Noyes. References: Acute safety tests, Acute toxicity tests, Implants and histopathology.
22 Some biological clearance references (packaging and product): BP 1980/1988/1993; EP 1989, various sections on plastics (constantly being updated); BS 5736 pts 1–9, Evaluation of Medical Devices for Biological Hazards.

Appendix 8.6: The pharmaceutical industry, plastics and the EU

A European committee (under the EU) has introduced monographs on plastic for certain pharmaceutical packaging applications as part of the European Pharmacopoeia. These identified certain plastics, and their ingredients which could be 'permitted'. It is now becoming increasingly evident that a 'permitted' list is possibly restrictive to free trade and biased towards the grades of plastics and their associated ingredients which have been 'approved'. A view that the information is advisory rather than mandatory is being seen by some countries as a means of either accepting the broad principle or circumnavigating the original intentions. The UK BP commission maintained that some form of performance standard would be preferable, i.e. an approach which is generally adopted by most UK-based companies.

Although it is generally accepted that only plastic materials and their associated constituents declared as 'food grade' should be used for pharmaceutical products, the 'global migration' approach currently being adopted in Europe has also come in for criticism. The aqueous extractive procedure causes little concern, but the rectified olive oil extractive procedure is not only difficult to carry out but relatively poor in terms of reproducibility. In addition, olive oil, being a naturally occurring product, is difficult to control.

In defence of this approach it must be noted that dependence on FDA approved materials is not foolproof, since many substances included are based on a committee consensus of opinion rather than detailed toxicological evidence. However, records of deaths from using plastics (excluding the polymerisation or compounding process) are virtually non-existent and reports of adverse affects relatively rare. The latter tend to be related to toxicological and pharmacological work on ingredients where mutagenicity, carcinogenicity, etc. have been shown, and such ingredients were excluded from use even though the risk of these being extracted may be nil. In general quite a few of the recorded adverse affects tend to be related to the plastics used internal to the body (implants, catheters, tubing, etc.).

It therefore can be concluded that there is considerable confusion in Europe associated with the use of plastics for pharmaceutical applications generally. The following 'food' legislation has been introduced:

- 90/128/EEC: Details of limits (10 mg/dm^2).
- 82/711/EEC: Details of tests.
- 85/572/EEC: Details of simulants.

These, together with various amendments in each case, cover the extractive test procedures, based on an upper limit of 10 mg/dm^2. Plastics and the constituents which they may contain are partly covered by a list system as mentioned earlier.

Appendix 8.7: The plastics industry and GMP including traceability

The extensive testing carried out by the pharmaceutical industry to clear a plastic and identify the constituents is of no avail if the polymerisation, compounding and fabrication processes are not controlled by some code of practice. The *Orange Guide on Good Manufacturing Practice (GMP)* and the recent EU guidelines could equally be applied to the plastics industry. Some of the more basic aspects would relate to the following.

1 Clear batch identification of all materials (polymers and constituents).

351

2 Documented control on materials received/issued incoming and outgoing materials (i.e. traceability).

3 Identification of what batch is used in what process to allow trace-back to an original 'supply' batch.

4 Clear flow paths from raw to finished materials with 'hold' and quarantine areas.

5 Materials and finished goods to be identified by name, batch number, date, etc., and to pass through a 'hold' or quarantine area (while under inspection) to a clearly defined storage area when status is confirmed.

6 The QC operation identified above in (5) would also include status labelling which indicates the various stages, e.g. green (pass), red (failed).

7 All materials to require a specification by which they can be identified, ordered and controlled.

8 Materials used in any process must also undergo checking operations to ensure that (a) materials are correctly labelled, (b) correct materials are issued, (c) the correct quantity is issued.

9 Retention samples should be kept for specific items and any change (process or materials) should be carefully monitored, and referred to customer.

10 Material segregation to be organised and controlled to prevent admixtures. (Particularly important for regrind.)

11 Item segregation to be organised and controlled to prevent admixtures from adjacent machines.

12 Machines to operate under acceptably clean conditions to minimise airborne contamination.

13 Items emerging from machine to be exposed for a minimum of time, i.e. direct feed into suitable (clean) PE bags etc.

It should therefore be concluded that the pharmaceutical industry will ultimately require a reasonable guarantee that the material tested, approved and specified remains identical in terms of formulation, purity and general quality. Buying under warranty may be an acceptable way of achieving this, coupled with a good GMP approach by the plastics company.

Note: In the UK the Pharmaceutical Quality Group (Institute of Quality Assurance) have devised Supplier Codes of Practice which link GMP to ISO 9002 Quality System certification.

Appendix 8.8: Risk versus intensity of testing

It is logical that the risk (to patient/user and company) should bear some relationship to the intensity of the tests involved in the clearance of the materials from which the pack is made.

Intravenous (IV) solutions head Table 8.2, as with the large volumes involved even a small level of 'extractive' will be rapidly in contact with the most sensitive body organs, i.e. heart and brain, e.g.

1000 ml extractive 0.1% = 1 g (IV solution)
20 ml extractive 0.1% = 20 mg (nasal spray)

Table 8.2 Intensity of testing required (in reducing order)

Group A
- Sterile products
- Large volume parenterals (LVPs)
- IV solutions
- Irrigation solutions
- Dialysis solutions, etc.

Group B
- Small volume parenterals (SVPs)
- IV additives
- Intravenous
- Intramuscular injections
- Subcutaneous injections, etc.

Group C
- Implants
- Ophthalmic products (multidose and unit dose)
- Nebulisation solutions
- Wound care products
- Non-sterile products, i.e. transdermal patches, vaginal-rectal products, local and topical products, liquid oral products, solid oral products

This example confirms a need for different intensities of testing according to the product category/route of administration. This will also be influenced by:

- the product-to-pack contact area
- the nature of the product (chemical–physical characteristics)
- the contact time and temperature (etc.).

Table 8.2 suggests a product 'intensity of testing' order, which is headed by sterile products. However, the position in this order may change according to any special product characteristics, contact area, contact time, temperature, etc. The table is therefore given to create a greater awareness of how 'risks' to 'benefits' might be considered. Some 'other factors' are given as a separate list below.

Intensity of testing: other factors

1. Patient type, i.e. elderly, adult, child, neonate.
2. Treatment – position in general may vary according to nature of treatment, i.e.

   - pre-operation
   - post-operation
   - intensive care.

3. Size of product-to-pack contact area.
4. Nature of product, e.g. oils tend to be more extractive than water-based materials (e.g. rubber/plastics). See also EN 9090/III (Appendix 8.13).
5. Storage conditions/period (temperature, RH, time, etc.).
6. Processing factors (terminal versus aseptic processing etc.).

Appendix 8.9: Pharmaceutical packaging with emphasis on administration aids and separate medication aids/devices

Introduction

An increasing trend towards 'drug delivery systems' has meant that packs which assist product administration, separate devices which aid medication, and the use of implantations have been steadily growing. Examples cover squeeze packs, pump systems, aerosols, dermal patches, lung inhalation systems involving powders and solutions, etc. These sophisticated and complex designs to aid drug administration have brought a need for a new level of knowledge associated with their production, efficiency in use, cleaning techniques and procedures, etc., coupled to the overall product stability. For example, although a product may be chemically stable, it will possibly only remain effective if its physical form and the performance of the device do not change throughout storage and use. Analytical test procedures therefore have to be supplemented by either 'user' assessments or simulated laboratory tests, in order to establish that the dose delivered remains in the right form (e.g. particle size distribution in the case of inhalations), the right concentration and quantity, etc.

In certain instances, this work becomes part of the stability programme so that 'drug delivery' parameters can be checked at the various time/storage intervals and conditions. This is also likely to involve the hygiene side of medication, i.e. whether there are any microbiological risks to users, how are these minimised (usually by cleaning) and, if a disinfecting agent is advised, whether it is safe, particularly if residues cannot be avoided, etc.

Although less complex, products which are reconstituted may also fall into a similar category, particularly as the pack may have to play two roles, e.g.

1   Retaining a dry powder or crystalline product in a stable form for the main shelf life.
2   Providing limited shelf life – usually as a liquid product, from reconstitution to completion of the medication period.

Subtle changes to plastic packaging components (e.g. swelling or shrinkage due to temperature or solvent absorption) may also influence the 'dose' dispensed (e.g. top pressure on a dropper plug has been known to reduce the orifice size, thereby changing the size of the 'drop'). See also Chapter 2.

The elderly patient

In this area there is already a conflict between tamper-evidence/resistance; child resistance; and packs which require easy access and reclosure by those who are infirm, elderly, arthritic, poor of sight, etc. This conflict also extends to OPD (original pack dispensing) and the increasing use of controlled dosage packs (i.e. special packs for the elderly population). Since many of these packs place several products in a common area, identifying those products to be taken at, say, 8.00 a.m., 12 noon, 5.00 p.m., 9.00 p.m., etc., any possible interaction between the various products must be considered. The fact that these packs have to be made up by a dispensing activity conflicts with the concept of OPD (where the original pack reaches the patient) as either original packs have to be broken down or bulk packs of products become a necessity.

The fact that monitored dosage packs are useful to elderly compliance does not appear to be in dispute. However, there are certain question marks against the direct admixture of several products, e.g. whether checking this is a development, clinical, medical, stability/analytical function has to be decided. Most of the packs used are based on plastics.

This also raises questions on the suitability of dispensed packs and their shelf life. The fact that a pharmaceutical company spends significant costs, time and effort in establishing a product–pack shelf life and that this can be put at risk by transfer to a different pack (the pharmacist thereby accepting responsibility) appears questionable in terms of modern 'product liability'.

Patient usage

As packs, administration aids, and separate medical application devices become more complex, the possibilities of misuse or abuse obviously increase. This in turn brings increasing demands for good clear instructions and assessment, either as part of a clinical trial or by special user/laboratory programmes capable of identifying misuse and/or abuse.

Under such programmes even packs or systems which do not assist administration may need some form of assessment (e.g. blister packs and the elderly). However, with reclosable packs, the user may never replace the closure properly, hence a different question may have to be addressed, i.e. whether the product will be adequately protected during its use period! Opening and reclosing a pack under an adverse atmosphere is a further possible 'risk'. Syrup-based products often cause closure sticking problems, hence may need special tests.

Some initial conclusions

One initial conclusion is that storing a packed product under a static climatic condition and chemically analysing any change is no longer an adequate test for 'fitness for purpose'. This is particularly true where the pack may 'change' under the conditions of storage or use, or where the pack assists in the administration of the product, or where the product is administered via a separate device. In the last case, subtle product changes may alter the dose delivered to the patient, or the device may also change with use and time (e.g. wear) and cause dosage problems. Product and device therefore have to be assessed together and independently, and hence may require shelf-life limitations.

Support documentation for company and regulatory clearance (of products, packs and devices)

It should be increasingly evident that the total data required to clear a product, pack and device is becoming more and more complex from both a company and a regulatory point of view. Boundary areas, as associated with previously apparently well-defined disciplines, are also becoming less easy to define. What is becoming more important is that there is an overviewer who can see the total picture and can make certain that all pertinent tests and procedures are identified and adequately carried out, with the results recorded and signed by an authorative person. This type of background is particularly important where the 'risk to user or patient' is high, e.g. large and small volume parenterals, implants, eye products, sterile unit doses, wound care products.

Although less information and testing may be necessary where the risk to patients is lower (topical application, oral products), it has already been indicated that the need for further 'tests' in this area may also increase.

Finally, it should be stressed that 'packs' used in all stability trials should be 'examined professionally' both before and after they have been opened and sampled for analysis. Again this may need to be formally written up as an authoritative document.

Documentary support to product registration will therefore increase rather than reduce in the future. Where possible, such documents should follow some common form of layout, for example:

1   what each sets out to achieve (objective)
2   a clearly expressed conclusion
3   adequate support detail free from ambiguity, recording results of tests carried out
4   full details of what product–pack was used
5   comprehensive records of test procedures, conditions, etc.
6   cross-references to book records and person(s) carrying out tests and when
7   authoritative signature(s) of approval with title(s) etc.

A well-presented report will make registration easier and more effective, and improve confidence between company and regulatory authorities.

Some examples of products requiring supplementary testing procedures are given in Table 8.3. The list is not comprehensive, as further examples can readily be added, but it should indicate some of the supplementary types of investigations which may be needed for certain products, both before and after storage and use.

Appendix 8.10: Other articles by author

1   Unit packaging of pharmaceutical preparations, *Institute of Packaging Symposium*, 27 September 1973.
2   *The Pharmaceutical Industry – Plastics and Packaging*, BPF, 1975.
3   *Blister and Strip Packaging*, Institute of Packaging, 1977.
4   Foil in pharmaceutical packaging, *BAFRA 77 Symposium*, published in *Manufacturing Chemist and Aerosol News*, February 1978.
5   The unit dose packaging of liquids and semi liquids, *Interphex Conference*, 1978.
6   The Pharmaceutical Clearance of a Plastic Pack/Device. GMP *Conference – Powder Technology*, October 1980.
7   Quality control and pharmaceutical packaging, *British Journal of Pharmaceutical Practice*, Vol. 2, No. 10, March 1981.
8   Plastics and the pharmaceutical industry, *Frost and Sullivan Symposium*, 1981.
9   Polyethylene – pharmaceutical and medical applications, *PRI Polymer Conference*, June 1983.
10 Plastics for toiletry and cosmetic products, *Toiletry and Cosmetic Journal*, 1983.

Table 8.3 Products requiring supplementary testing procedures

Product	Test
Multidose injections (vials)	• Multiple piercing of rubber bung, e.g. fragmentation, coring, resealing. • Volume extracted (how).
IV solutions	• Check against 'giving sets' for fit, flow, removal of particulates, leakage, collapse (if collapsible), air ingress, etc.
Inhalations (generally)	• Particle distribution, blockage, losses by impaction, changes in dosage throughout pack. • Influence of different inhaler systems, if relevant, etc.
Metered dose pump systems, e.g. nasal spray	• Actuations to prime. • Retention of prime. • Dose variation (device). • Number of doses per pack. • Particle size range. • Blockage. • Drying-out of solution. • Non-available residue • Microbial risks – contamination.
Eye drops, i.e. multidose/unit dose	• Variations in drop size. • Drops per pack. • Efficiency of closure in use. • Drying-out of product. • Drop size change in use/after storage. • Loss of preservative during use. • Non-available residue. • Microbiological 'grow back'.

11 Packaging and product stability, *CPA Conference*, Holland, November 1983.

12 Design of powder inhalers (Newman, Dean and Young), *The Practitioner*, November 1983.

13 A new era in unit dose packaging, *Unit Dose Conference*, IOP, 8 October 1986.

14 Stability aspects of packaging, *Drug Development and Industrial Pharmacy*, Vol. 10, Nos 8 and 9, 1984.

15 Sources of particulate contamination in sterile packaging, *Pharm. Technology*, August 1985.

16 Assessment of performance, testing and quality of conventional screw (plastic) closures, *PRI Conference*, 28 April 1986.

17 Handling and performance characteristics of plastic screw closures (production lines), *PRI Conference*, 28 April 1986.

18 Tamper evident and tamper resistant packaging, *TEPCON Conference*, April 1987.

19 The manufacture of clean materials, containers and components for the packaging of pharmaceuticals, *IOP One-day Conference*, 2 December 1987.

20 Historical survey on the use and growth of plastics in the pharmaceutical industry, *PRI Conference on Update on Plastics*, 7 December 1988.

21 *Combination materials, flexibles, laminations, etc.*, March 1989.

22 *Closures and closure systems for rigid plastic packs*, IOP, July 1990.
23 *Overcoming permeation and diffusion problems by the use of overwraps*, 1990.
24 The sterilisation of plastics. An introduction and overview, *IOP Conference on Sterilisation of Plastics*, 4 December 1990.
25 *Pharmaceutical packaging with emphasis on administration aids and separate medication devices*, ECEC, 1991.
26 *Assessment of closure efficiency*, PRI/IOP, January 1991; IOP, January 1991.
27 *Making an effective seal, heat sealing*, IOP, January 1991.
28 *Pack–material selection for the packaging of toiletry and cosmetic products*, CPA, USA, August 1991.
29 *Package printing and decoration*, Version VI, February 1991.
30 The expanding role of the pack (and the test procedures associated with registration), *BIRA Conference*, September 1991.
31 An introduction to the filling of liquid pharmaceutical products, *IOP Conference*, December 1991.

Appendix 8.11: Possible processing effects on plastic materials, containers and components

Plastics subjected to processing procedures, either as part of a conversion operation or at a subsequent stage associated with product manufacture and packaging, may incur temporary or permanent changes. Whether these changes are critical to the product will depend on the product and the risks incurred. In the case of pharmaceuticals, toiletries, cosmetics, etc., some in-depth investigations may be required to quantify the significance of any deviations from the chemical, physical or physico-chemical properties of the preprocessed material. Examples of possible changes are indicated below.

Plasticised PVC 'bags' undergoing steam autoclaving

When autoclaved under pressure in a steam autoclave, plasticised PVC interacts with moisture/heat and becomes quite hazy and milky. After cooling down, the PVC reverts to its normal clarity. There is, therefore, a temporary period during which the PVC has different physical and possibly physico-chemical properties.

It should therefore be noted that a number of plastics may change during a steam autoclaving process where temperatures of 100–135°C (achieved by pressure) can be reached. This applies to both single and multilayer material, and includes adhesive layers. Overpressure autoclaves are usually essential to prevent physical distortion during cooling.

Gamma irradiation

Irradiation (usually at 25 kGy) can have various effects on plastic including physical and chemical changes which may be permanent, temporary, or ongoing. Physical changes are most frequently associated with cross-linkage, which usually reduces flexibility and increases rigidity (slightly).

Chemical and physico-chemical changes can be related to both the polymer and the constituents in the polymer (residues, additives, processing aids, etc.). Chemical degradation to any of these may be identified as colour changes, surface changes, odours, taints, as well as by chemical analysis. For example, certain grades of LDPE have been known to generate both formaldehyde and formic acid (as end breakdown products) when subjected to 25 kGy gamma irradiation. Antioxidants can also be degraded.

Since gamma irradiation may modify the surface of a plastic, initial stress lines (due to molecular chain fracture or cross-linkage) may become a propagation point for long-term cracking, particularly when stored under 'hotter' conditions. This surface modification or change usually depends on the presence of air or oxygen. Carrying out irradiation in a nitrogen atmosphere, or having an oxygen impermeable layer on the plastic surface, reduces the above problems.

Surface treatments

A major application of surface treatments is for print key or adhesion related to printing, labelling, etc., by oxidative-type surface treatments. These include corona (films), flame treatments (containers), each of which can give a marginally different effect.

Surface treatment can also affect the amount of 'bloom' or surface migration of various active surface agents (lubricants, slip and antislip additives, etc.) and either subsequent 'migration' into a product by surface abrasion or chemical removal, solubility, etc.

Electron beam or beta irradiation

As a generalisation, electron beam treatment creates similar effects to gamma irradiation, but usually on slightly reduced scale, since depth of penetration is less.

Changes – crystalline versus amorphous

Processing involving heating and cooling may influence the ratio of crystalline to amorphous material, thereby modifying the characteristics of the polymer involved.

Conclusions

The above examples are only the tip of the iceberg. There are many process procedures that can modify the properties of plastic. The more obvious ways in which plastic performance can be influenced include:

1 changes in the solubility of the absorbing materials in the polymer
2 changes in the solubility of the absorbing materials in the surface layer
3 changes in the surface conditions
4 opening-up of molecular structure by swelling (increases permeation)
5 movement of internal constituents to the surface (or vice versa)
6 changes in mass or density
7 molecular changes due to degradation, including chain fission.

If any of the above (or combinations) occur, changes may arise to physical, physicochemical properties, e.g. in terms of diffusion, permeation and migration/leaching.

Thorough retesting is therefore sometimes essential to detect changes between the 'processed' and 'unprocessed' (as supplied initially) plastic.

Appendix 8.12: Pharmaceutical supplement

Summary – plastics and pharmaceutical packaging

Since the worldwide need for pharmaceuticals is still steadily expanding, there is a continuous growth of pharmaceutical packaging with a particular emphasis on plastics. This growth is especially vigorous where packs also act as administration aids or devices, in special blow/form fill seal operations and in general areas where innovation is involved. Coupled to these activities are gradual changes in the intensity of testing, together with a greater interest in traceability, effective validation, safety, efficacy, quality, etc. As the knowledge requirements also have to increase in order to meet the above demands, it may be useful to have a check list on what problems can arise between pharmaceuticals and plastics as seen 'today'. The following list is not in any order of importance, as problems will change according to the product and circumstances involved.

1   Permeability to moisture.
2   Permeability to normal gases, oxygen, carbon dioxide, nitrogen.
3   Absorption of moisture/solvents.
4   Physical and chemical changes due to processing activities (conversion, pretreatment, sterilisation, etc.).
5   Changes due to ageing/exposure against time and the environment (light, oxygen, temperature, etc.).
6   Potential for environmental stress cracking.
7   Absorption and adsorption of product constituents, e.g. certain preservatives.
8   Constituents' migration from the plastic to the product.
9   Exclusion of light.
10 Removal of constituents present at the surface of the plastic, by physical abrasion.
11 Shrinkage/sinkage – related to plastic, thicknesses, design, etc.
12 Dimensional and visual assessment.
13 Level of electrostatic charges.
14 Evaluation of closure efficiency.
15 Total compatibility with the product.
16 Material cleanliness, i.e. material bioburden/particulates.
17 Aroma/flavour.
18 Identification, i.e. checking supply of correct materials, by chemical or physico-chemical analysis of the bulk material, or the surface of containers.
19 Constituents identified in terms of residues (from polymerisation process), processing aids, additives, masterbatch constituents.
20 Identification of process(es) of manufacture/conversion, as these may influence properties.
21 Food grade approval via any relevant food regulations.
22 Colour measurement to obtain a reference standard (usually light and dark limits) for pigmented (opaque) and dyed (translucent/transparent) materials.

23 Resistance to pH changes – may arise from pH shift or changes.
24 Resistance to impact forces (drops, forces, puncture resistance, etc.).
25 Resistance to vertical forces – top compression as experienced during capping, stacking, shrink wrapping.
26 Heat softening and heat deflection/distortion temperatures – reference hot processing etc.
27 Flame/fire-resistant – relevant to electrical instruments and devices.
28 Resistance to creep or cold flow – materials may change in shape, dimensions, etc., related to a pressure force (stress) and temperature/time.
29 Resistance to sterilisation process (dry heat, moist heat, irradiation, UV, etc.).
30 Degree of orientation (may influence percentage of shrinkage on heating).
31 Extractives. Tests may be derived from directives, compendial standards, World Health Organisation, etc., with limits/standards based on chemical or biological test procedures. Such tests can provide useful comparisons but final approval can only be based on tests where contact between product and pack is involved.

The above list indicates a range of factors to be considered when developing a plastic pack for a pharmaceutical product. The level of in-depth testing required will inevitably vary according to the risks to both the user/patient and the company, e.g. product liability.

Each factor identified can be expanded as a topic in its own right. A few examples are given below.

Absorption and adsorption of preservatives

Certain preservative systems can be lost from certain plastic packs by 'sorption' and solubility in the plastic and, if they are also volatile, by evaporation from the external surface which is in contact with the atmosphere. Reports, particularly as references in textbooks, often suggested that phenol could not be used as a preservative in low-density packs. Subsequent work, many years later, established that the solubility of phenol in polyethylene was relatively low and that sufficient phenol for adequate preservative efficacy could be retained by a number of methods, i.e. coating LDPE internally or externally, or enclosing the pack in an additional barrier overwrap (e.g. paper/foil/PE or similar foil-bearing barriers).

Other preservatives which suffer from sorption in LDPE include benzyl alcohol, chlorbutol, chloroform, chlorocresol, 2 phenyl ethanol. Sorption also occurs with HDPE and PP but usually to a lesser extent. PVC is less prone to preservative absorption and has been employed to retain certain volatile preservatives (2 phenyl ethanol).

Adsorption, where the preservative attaches itself to the surface of a plastic, tends to vary according to the type of plastic, constituents in the plastic, surface treatment, surface area of the plastic. Adsorption has been found with most mercurials, including Thiomersal, benzalkonium chloride and bromide, etc. Small amounts of chlorhexidine, benzoic acid and hydroxybenzoates have also had losses reported for certain plastics.

It should be noted that although preservative loss can be quantified by chemical analysis, the microbial effectiveness of the preservative remaining can usually only be evaluated by a preservative efficacy challenge test.

Absorption of moisture

Since all plastics are to some degree permeable to moisture it is inevitable, particularly at higher humidity levels, that plastics may contain traces of moisture. Certain plastics, especially those based on OH groups, e.g. polyvinyl alcohol, ethylene vinyl alcohol and others (some nylons), can absorb sufficient moisture to cause problems during moulding. Such polymers need to undergo a predrying operation prior to moulding. In general, the higher is the moisture content the higher the permeability to moisture, gases, and odorous vapours. EVOH, for example, is an excellent barrier to gases and moisture when very dry, but these barriers significantly reduce as the moisture content in the polymer increases. As a result of this EVOH is usually sandwiched between two moisture barrier polymers such as LDPE or PP. Plastics which absorb moisture are less prone to electrostatic problems.

Sinkage and shrinkage

Plastics show a much higher coefficient of expansion (and contraction) than metals. This means that the material contracts during the cooling cycle of a moulding operation, hence most moulds have to be made larger than the component drawing dimensions if the defined size is to be produced. The level of shrinkage typically varies from around 0.5% to 5%, e.g. the polystyrenes (PS, HIPS, SAN, ABS) are in the lower level while HDPE/PP tend to be towards the upper level with the other plastics somewhere in between. Calculating shrinkage becomes increasingly complex with difficult three-dimensional objects which exhibit many changes in thickness. For simplicity of design an item of uniform section is far easier to produce than a complex three-dimensional design. Thicker sections may typically show areas of sinkage as found within the bottle neck bore of many extrusion blow moulded bottles, i.e. behind the thicker sections of the external thread. In complex designs this sinkage, coupled to changes in section thickness, can lead not only to sinkage, but to distortion and possible twisting of the component. Although this might be overcome by putting the component in a jig which restrains movement during final cooling, this can be an expensive, labour-intensive process. Although the 'pressures' employed in injection moulding can reduce sinkage and distortion, good effective mould design is essential to quality mouldings. However, the final quality will also depend on the machine cycle (pressure, time, temperature, etc.), hence this must ultimately be equated with cost.

The level of sinkage/shrinkage is also influenced by other factors such as fillers, pigments, melt flow index, density and cooling rate. It should be noted that materials which are oriented, either purposely or accidentally (e.g. in a moulding, operation), will shrink significantly if they are heated above the temperature used for the orientation process. Amorphous materials show less shrinkage than crystalline polymers.

Extractives and general compendial tests

Extractive tests based on various simulants are offered in such compendial standards (past and/or present) as USP, EP, JP, WHO, and BP. These tests, in which extracted solution(s) are subject to chemical analysis and biological assessment, give information on the materials extracted and the general safety of the extracted solution. Although attempts are being made to standardise methodology worldwide, there are currently differences between the requirements in the USA, Europe, Japan, etc. Some of these are summarised in Table 8.4; in the EP 1989 they are covered under V1.1.2. etc.

Table 8.4 Requirements for plastic materials

V1.1.2.1. pages 1–8	Materials based on poly(vinyl chloride) i.e. materials based on plasticised poly(vinyl chloride) for containers for human blood and blood components and for containers for aqueous solutions for intravenous infusion. (1989) Covered by V1.1.2. (1–7)
V1.1.2.1.2 pages 1–5	Materials based on plasticised poly(vinyl chloride) for tubing used in sets for transfusion. (1991)
V1.1.2.2.	Polyolefins
V1.1.2.2.1. pages 1–3	Polyethylene – low density, for containers for preparations for parenteral use and for ophthalmic preparations. (1992) Note – no additives.
V1.1.2.2.2. pages 1–5	Polyethylene – high density, for containers for preparations for parenteral use. (1990)
V1.1.2.2.3. pages 1–5	Polypropylene for containers for preparations for parenteral use. (1990) Covers homopolymer and copolymer. Limit of not more than three stabilisers (antioxidants) from a list of nine.
V1.1.2.3. pages 1–6	Ethylene–vinyl acetate copolymer for containers and tubing for total parenteral nutrition preparations. (1993) Limits level of vinyl acetate – 25% maximum containers, 30% tubing. Limit of not more than three stabilisers (antioxidants) from a list of five. Identifies limits for oleamide and erucamide, calcium and zinc stearate, calcium carbonate, potassium hydroxide, silicone dioxide. SILICONES
V1.1.3.1.	Silicone oil as a lubricant. (1985)
V1.1.3.2.	Silicone elastomer for closures and tubing. (1985)
V1.2.3.	RUBBER CLOSURES
V1.2.3.1.	Rubber closures for containers for aqueous preparations for parenteral use. (1989) There are two basic types – Type I: meet strictest requirements Type II: offer certain requirements but cannot meet all the requirements of Type I.
V1.2.2.	PLASTIC CONTAINERS
V1.2.2.1.	Plastic containers and closures
V1.2.2.2.	CONTAINERS FOR BLOOD and BLOOD COMPONENTS
V1.2.2.2.1.	Sterile plastic containers for human blood and blood components.
V1.2.2.2.2.	Empty sterile containers of plasticised poly(vinyl chloride) for human blood and blood components.
V1.2.2.3. pages 1–2	Plastic containers for aqueous solutions for intravenous infusion. (1990)
VI.2.2.4 pages 1–5	Sterile single use plastic syringes. (1991)

Appendix 8.13 (based on EN/9090/III): Typical pack/packaging information normally required

Primary or immediate packaging

1   The nature of the packaging material, indicating the qualitative composition.
2   Description of the closure (nature and method of sealing).
3   Description of the method of opening and, if necessary, safety devices.
4   Information on the container (single or multidose) and dosing devices.
5   A description of any tamper-evident closure and child-resistant closure.

The above has to be supported by supplementary data, i.e. development pharmaceutics which justify the choice of pack and include:

1   tightness of closure
2   protection of contents against external factors
3   container/contents interaction
4   influence of the manufacturing process on the container (e.g. sterilisation conditions).

Packaging material (primary or immediate packaging)

Specifications and routine tests, covering:

1   construction, listing components
2   type of materials identifying nature of each
3   specifications, which may vary in detail according to product nature and route of administration.

Routine tests are likely to include:

* identification, appearance, dimensions, performance, bioburden, etc.
* scientific data listed under general and technical information
* plastic (general information)

    1   name and grade as used by manufacturer
    2   name of plastic manufacturer (parenterals, ophthalmics)
    3   chemical name of material
    4   qualitative composition
    5   chemical name(s) of monomer(s) used.

Material should have food grade approval, otherwise additional toxicological data will be required.

Plastic (technical information)

1   Characteristics: general description, solubility in various solvents.
2   Identification usually by infrared for the material, the main additives, any dyes.

364

3 Tests including general tests, mechanical tests, chemical/biological (extractive procedures using suitable solvent).
4 Name of manufacturer/convertor.

Appendix 8.14: Summary of ICH guidelines on stability and possible influences on the 'pack'

Although the ICH guidelines make reference to 'stress conditions', involving low and high temperatures, low and high humidities, freeze–thaw, varying light intensities, including cycling conditions, storage at a fixed temperature and humidity may not fully challenge the pack (and the product). A pack may therefore withstand continuous storage at 25°C/60% RH, 30°C/60% RH, 40°C/75% RH, etc., but fail under cycling or higher temperature stress conditions. However, packs are more likely to change if exposed to a multiplicity of challenges, e.g. temperature and RH changes, vibration and compression (on a production line, in storage or distribution), the influence of oxygen, light. Changes arising from these challenges may subsequently be reflected in the stability of the drug substance or the product dosage form.

It is therefore important to bear in mind some of the differences between fixed static climatic conditions and the real world where fluctuations in temperature, humidity, light, etc. may be further influenced by such physical challenges as varying degrees of vibration and top compression, as identified earlier. The author therefore believes that the ICH guidelines put additional emphasis on the role of the packaging technologist who must more thoroughly investigate any deficiencies which may arise in the pack and possibly jeopardise the shelf life of the product. Information detailing such challenges will likely need to be presented as a formal document as part of the regulatory submission, rather than being included in any formal stability programme.

Packs which are to some degree permeable to moisture (as are most plastics) will lose or gain moisture according to whether they are exposed to a high or low relative humidity respectively. 40°C/75% RH may be particularly severe on a fully exposed blister pack and give an artificially low shelf-life prediction. The same condition may offer little challenge to moisture loss as the vapour pressure inside the pack may virtually be at equilibrium with the external atmosphere (plastic containers).

Packs removed from a simulated climatic condition also need to be checked for any signs of change/deterioration

1 prior to opening
2 during opening (peel strength, closure, torque/force, etc.)
3 after product removal.

This is particularly relevant where extremes of temperature and cycling conditions are involved since closure efficiencies may vary according to the storage temperature. This can be critical where a product in its pack is allowed to equilibriate with bench conditions before it is subjected to analysis, so a trained packaging technologist is essential to these examinations.

Finally, it is likely that the severest ICH conditions will imply that more effective barrier packs will be essential for certain products (some blisters). As the guidelines only test the primary pack, the fact that the secondary (transit) packaging can contribute to the total shelf life has not been considered. Although a packaging technologist might argue with this, it seems unlikely that the guidelines will be changed in the near future. As a result trends may be towards better barrier materials, coated materials or the addition of various overwrap options. This is yet another challenge to tomorrow's technologist.

It is therefore important to be aware of guidelines but at the same time to be 'wary' of any deficiencies that may be associated with them.

Appendix 8.15: Future polymers for pharmaceuticals

Needs for improved properties may involve the use of coatings for the well-established economic polymers, the additional use of protective overwraps, or the use of new potential polymers. The last of these are likely to include:

- PBT (polybutylene terephthalate)
- COC (cyclic olefin copolymer which includes Resin CZ from Daikyo Seiko and Topas from Ticona Mitsui); use for the former has already been found for vials for expensive lyophilised biotechnology products
- LCP (liquid crystal polymers) used either on their own or as blends with other materials (PE and PET)
- PEN (polyethylene napthalate) currently being used with PET to achieve hotter fills.

Another alternative is the use of Metallocene catalysts to produce polymers with improved control of MFI and chain length distribution.

9

FILMS, FOILS AND LAMINATIONS (COMBINATION MATERIALS)

D. A. Dean

This chapter covers single layer, multi-layer and combination materials found as films, foils, laminations, coextrusions, coatings, etc.

Single ply materials

Although a proportion of 'flexibles' are multi-layer materials, a number of flexible packaging materials are found as single plies. Single ply materials are found in the form of paper, and those plastics which either do not require an additional coating to achieve a heat seal or can be employed as a direct wrap. Examples of these include various grades of polyethylene and plasticised PVC, which have to be high-frequency welded. A few foils may be used uncoated. (Note that most foils are varnished, lacquered or wash coated to improve scuff resistance or to assist print key.) Other single (monolayer) plastics may also be found as wraps which are restrained by a secondary feature (such as a tie or tape) or rely on special properties, e.g. cling films, for their retention around a product. Cling films, skin wraps, etc. involve such materials as thin gauges of plasticised PVC, Surlyn ionomer, modified grades of low-density polyethylene and Saran (PVdC) copolymers. Thus the use of single ply materials should not be ignored, particularly as these are frequently seen as being more environmentally friendly (i.e. multi-layer materials are always more difficult to recover or recycle). Of the single ply materials listed above, paper needs special mention since it was one of the earliest wrapping materials and still has significant use worldwide.

Polyethylene, as LDPE, LLDPE or a mixture or blend involving combinations of LDPE, MDPE, HDPE, EVA, etc., finds a wide usage in bags, sacks, sachets, overwraps, shrink wraps, stretch wraps, etc. Most deep freeze packs, for example, use LDPE or an LDPE mixture which is produced from a reel on a form fill seal type machine. However, as many of these packs are up to 100% printed, even ink of 2–5 µm could be considered as a separate layer which modifies some of the physical and chemical properties. As all polyolefins need a surface (oxidative) treatment to ensure a good print key, this or any other surface treatment process may further modify the film properties.

Another use of single ply plastics is found in window cartons (cellulose acetate, polyester, regenerated cellulose, OPP, PS, etc.) and in plastic cartons (PVC). The use of thermoformings as bubble and blister packs for toiletries, pharmaceuticals, etc. and trays, soaps, etc. frequently falls in a grey area as to whether they are forms of flexible or rigid packaging. Frequently the final category is decided by the lidding material.

As mentioned earlier, foil can be found as a single layer material and applied as an overwrap using the dead fold characteristics of soft foil. Thin foil can be partly strengthened by embossing, but due to its extensibility it tends to demand an additional support ply.

Since it is sometimes difficult to identify whether a material is a single ply or a multiple ply, most students should examine a range of thinner materials to try to establish any constructional differences. However, many apparent single ply materials, e.g. biscuit, confectionery and chocolate (bar) wraps are actually multi-ply materials: these frequently use a type of OPP (oriented polypropylene – especially the pearlised variety) where a special (coextruded) outer and inner heat seal ply has been added. MAP and CAP food materials are likely to have an 'anti-mist' coating.

Finally, the use of recycled paper/board requires mention since continuous recycling leads to shortening of the fibres and a steady reduction in physical properties.

Although only a few single layer materials may appear to be used for pharmaceuticals, the largest use is likely to be found in shrink and stretch wrapping. As these may confer some barrier properties as well as acting as a means of collation and tamper-evidence, they are expanded on below.

Shrink wrapping

If molecular orientation is introduced into a plastic, by extension under certain conditions, it will undergo deorientation or shrinkage, back to roughly its original dimensions, if subsequently reheated to the temperature above that at which it was earlier oriented. This property is normally achieved in a film by either the stenter process or the extrusion lay flat tubular process. The stenter process, which usually involves extrusion-casting, has one advantage in that the oriented film can be heat set (somewhat similar to annealing), thereby giving an improved degree of dimensional stability (reduces deorientation when heated). It is, therefore, more widely used for heat sealable, wrapping films which are not used via a shrinking process. In both cases the orientation operation occurs at a temperature just below or above the softening point of the material in question. The most common shrink materials are low density polythene, polypropylene, polyvinyl chloride or ethylene vinyl acetate copolymers.

As the name implies, shrink wrapping utilises an oriented plastic which, when placed around an object, can be heated to a temperature where it returns, or tries to return, to its original dimensions – thereby forming a tight shrink wrap. Shrink wraps may be employed to wrap individual products, cartons, groups of cartons, packs in trays, etc. They can thereby be used to add to individual protection, act as a tamper-evident feature, improve certain barrier properties, act as a waterproof covering, or as a means of collating and protecting a number of items.

The shrink wrap material may be applied in two basic ways.

1   As a *full overwrap* – to provide a total wrap – where all of the item or items are enclosed by a film, i.e. an all-round wrap.
2   As a *sleeve overwrap* – a sleeve wrap where the ends of the longer direction are open and therefore exposed.

The shrink wrapping process involves several functions:

1   placing the film around the item(s) to be shrink wrapped
2   sealing the film
3   passing the unit through a heated (shrink) tunnel, arranged to give uniform heating, and avoiding hot and cold contact areas.

To create a total wrap, an L sealer or a fold-heat seal is usually required, while in the case of a sleeve wrap, a single longitudinal seal is used. The method of sealing is usually via a heated wire which may be used in conjunction with an impulse and pressure system or an impulse and radiant heat system.

While orientation gives a broad improvement in physical and chemical properties of plastics, i.e. improvements in clarity, tensile strength, inertness and reduced permeation to gases (oxygen, carbon dioxide), moisture, etc., these properties are lost once deorientation occurs.

Shrink films

Low-density polyethylene

Oriented LDPE is the most widely used of the shrink wrap materials. It has good strength, toughness and tear resistance. It also has good low-temperature resistance, hence is suitable for parts of the world with well below zero conditions. LDPE is a reasonable moisture barrier but is a relatively poor oxygen and carbon dioxide barrier.

Special grades of plastic need to be selected for satisfactory shrink films which need to cover a wide range of shrink ratios (machine versus cross direction). In the case of lay flat tubing, the ratio is achieved by bubble blow-up, rate of draw-off and other factors. Grade factors which are of special significance include density and melt flow index. Higher density materials have poorer puncture, impact and seal strength but have a higher shrink strength and lower percentage shrink. The melt flow index also relates to shrink strength, i.e. a lower MFI gives a higher shrink strength.

The incorporation of vinyl acetate into LDPE provides a softer material which shrinks at a lower temperature. Shrink temperature is around 108–115°C for LDPE.

Oriented polypropylene

This material offers high clarity, very good tensile strength and has high shrink energy. This means it should not be used on flimsy materials (e.g. light weight cartons) as this can give rise to distortion. OPP requires a higher temperature for orientation, hence needs more heat to give controlled shrinkage. However, PP has a much narrower deorientation range than LDPE and can prove more difficult to heat seal effectively. The shrink temperature is high, around 130–140°C.

Polyvinyl chloride

Both unplasticised and plasticised PVC shrink films are available. Plasticised material feels softer to touch, is less brittle, has a lower softening point and shrinkage.

Unplasticised PVC has good surface gloss and clarity, but tends to be brittle, of poor impact strength and rather easy to tear once initiated. Shrink temperature is around 90–100°C.

Multi-layer materials

Multi-layer materials are used for special reasons, e.g. where an already shrink wrapped material has to undergo a further (secondary) shrink wrapping operation. This means that a different material is essential to prevent sticking, e.g. coextruded LDPE/EVA/PP where the PP inner layer will not stick to LDPE. Usage of multi-layer materials is limited.

Shrink wrap applications

Pallet shrink wrapping

This can be achieved using a preformed shroud (or hood), two single webs or a pre-cut tubular form from a lay flat reel. In each case the perimeter should only exceed pallet size by around 7–12%. LDPE is the most widely used material, of 75 to 200 μm gauge.

Transit wrapping

This may involve the collation of packages of similar or variable shapes. The most popular form uses either a direct shrink wrap (e.g. multi-packs) or a shallow tray which is usually made from corrugated board or solid board. Thermoformed plastic trays with a formed base (and/or a lid/cover) are also widely employed (e.g. bottles and aerosols). These systems offer restriction to pilferage and due to the see-through nature of the film may avoid the need for external labels. (Internal labels may be necessary if stock is controlled via a bar code.) Although LDPE has the major use, PVC may occasionally be used for its higher clarity. Gauges of 25 to 100 μm are usually employed.

Display wrapping

Shrink wraps may be used on a number of materials (products) and packed items (e.g. cartons) to maintain cleanliness, to prevent or restrict pilferage or access to the product, to provide good surface gloss, etc. PP and PVC are used for their excellent clarity and sparkle. PP, however, has a narrower deorientation range and higher temperature than LDPE and PVC, hence may be more difficult to control. LDPE is available in high-clarity grades and has a 'soft feel' (similar to plasticised PVC). Gauges of 25–40 μm are widely used.

In the above applications, either a sleeve wrap or a total wrap may be employed. The total overwrap has the advantage of excluding dirt and dust; it can also be a significant barrier to moisture. In the case of the total wrap, holes are initially required to allow any air to escape.

Reel materials

Reels may be unwound and used in different ways. L sealers usually use a single reel of a centre folded film.

In other systems two reels are used and these are welded together by a transverse sealing jaw. This is presented as a curtain to a moving product, so it is then enveloped by the curtain.

Shrink terminology

- Percentage free shrink – ratio measured in both the transverse (cross) and machine directions of the shrunk film versus its original dimensions.
- Shrink ratio – ratio of machine direction to cross direction shrinkage.
- Shrink energy – energy built into the film by orientation which is subsequently released during shrinkage.
- Retained shrink – shrink retained when film is tightly wrapped around an article (after shrinkage has occurred).
- Shrink strength – various oriented materials have different shrink energies, hence forces applied to the enveloped item vary.
- Film slip – this is the reciprocal of the coefficient of friction.

$$\text{Film yield} = \frac{\text{area of film } (m^2)}{\text{weight of film (g or kg)}}$$

Stretch wrapping

Stretch wrap films are elastic in nature, hence possess a memory. The film must have high elasticity, and once in position must not relax and lose tension (i.e. become loose).

Film materials

Linear low density polyethylene (LLDPE) is the predominant stretch wrap material, but films based on LDPE combinations, EVA and plasticised PVC are also found. Stretch materials can be produced by various processes, i.e. from lay flat tubing, casting, etc. The latter process gives orientation in the machine direction which assists stretch in the wrap around direction. Cling properties required for grip may be achieved by incorporating a cling additive or coextrusion to the outer surface(s) of a more tacky material, e.g. EVA.

Use of stretch films

Stretch-materials are usually applied in one of two ways. In the first of these, the material is extended by tightly wrapping it around an item or group of items in such a way that stretching occurs between the item and the unwound reel, i.e. it is extended at the point of application.

This process usually relies on the item or load rotating (e.g. a pallet) while the film reel is held vertically so that it can operate with a spiral motion. With simple hand wrapping, the operator walks around the item, applying layers which overlap in a spiral motion. Since these processes can only be applied to the sides of a pallet, a top sheet inserter may be employed to cover the top. This is then held in position by a stretch layer. The level of stretch achieved depends on the material employed, the uniformity of the load and the process employed. If a material is over-stretched i.e. the natural yield point is exceeded, the film becomes less puncture resistant and may break. Limits of stretch by these processes are around 50–60%.

Cling films usually can be categorised under stretch films.

In the second method, material is mechanically pre-stretched before application, using materials that can be stretched over 100%. This is partly because a pre-stretching process has a better control over the stretching operation, which occurs between two rollers placed near the reel of film. Since these two rollers are fitted with variable gears, the degree of stretch can be both controlled and altered. The width of the reel is maintained during this stretching process, which alters the properties of the film and increases the yield (lowers material used, hence reduces material cost). Improved methods of stretching are now available and can stretch the material three fold, i.e. up to 300%, by using motorised units.

Applications of stretch wrapping

Pallet stretch wrapping

This is the most popular use of stretch wrapping, hence it is frequently compared with shrink wrapping in terms of advantages and disadvantages. All the methods previously outlined are employed with LLDPE being the predominantly used material, in conjunction with a pre-stretching operation. Gauges of 15 to 50 µm are usually employed.

Stretch bundling

Stretch bundling can apply to single products or packs, or groups of somewhat irregular loads. The film is normally stretched around the 'product' to give a tight wrap with up to 25% stretch. The material finishes with an adhesive or heat seal. Modified LDPE, VLDPE or EVA are normally used.

Other applications for shrink and stretch materials

Skin packaging

Skin packaging employs material properties which are similar to stretch wrapping in that the film employed may stretch in the process. However, heat and vacuum are usually employed, hence stretch may also approach an orientation operation. In terms of material, Surlyn ionomer and Saran may be used as well as the more conventional materials.

Shrink sleeving

Shrink sleeving made from lay flat tubing or welded tubing is widely used as a tamper-evident overwrap to enclose either a whole container or neck and closure. Materials include PVC, polypropylene and polyester. Shrink sleeving can improve container barrier properties or light exclusion.

Cling film

Cling films are usually elastic-type materials which will undergo stretch. The originally used cling films were based on plasticised PVC and PVdC (Saran) films. More recently, LLDPE and LDPE, particularly as mixtures with other plastics, are being widely employed.

Shrink versus stretch wrapping

Each of these has advantages and disadvantages which are given in Table 9.1. Further comparisons could be made against fibreboard outers which offer advantages in stacking strength and cushioning properties. This is often more important during transportation as in many warehouses stock is racked and not stacked two or more high. Both shrink and stretch wrapping offer significant cost savings over fibreboard if circumstances permit their use.

Table 9.1 Shrink versus stretch wrapping

Shrink	Stretch
Equipment more expensive, involves sealing, wrapping plus heat shrink tunnel.	Lower cost, frequently smaller.
More energy: orientation plus heat energy to shrink.	Less total energy stretching, no heat.
May not be suitable for heat sensitive items.	Can even be used under cold (refrigeration) conditions.
May distort under transit conditions.	Retains load more tightly.
Shrink in shrink wrap (two or more) may stick together.	Virtually no film-to-film sticking.
Shrink film will take up uneven contours more readily.	Will create areas of higher tension due to irregular products.
Needs different film widths for a range of sizes.	Needs fewer reel widths for a range of sizes.
Can be printed using distortion printing where shrinkage is uniform and well controlled.	Easier to print as stretch is mainly in one direction.
Can provide better weather protection etc., particularly if a total wrap.	Less protective, may not be totally waterproof.
Adds to general protection (climatic).	Lower climatic protection.
Uses (generally) more film (heavier gauges).	Uses less film.

Combination materials covering flexible and rigid applications (or multilayer materials)

The above heading has been selected to include all variants which may be now used for both flexible and rigid applications. Whereas previously these may have been introduced under 'flexibles', 'film, foils and laminates', etc., the use of new technology such as coextrusions, metallisation and different coating techniques has produced some confusion as to what terminology should be employed, so the word 'multi-layer' may be more appropriate.

General properties

Basically these combinations employ a range of materials to achieve certain specific functions, i.e. to offer:

1 support to other plies
2 barrier properties
3 heat sealing or sealability, including cold sealing
4 ease of decoration or printing
5 reflectivity when desirable
6 a means of bonding two or more materials together
7 ease of opening
8 security in the form of child-resistance, tamper-resistance or tamper-evidence
9 improved machine ability or improved machine performance
10 cushioning
11 acceptable cost
12 minimal use of resources (renewable or non-renewable)
13 suitability for disposal.

Certain materials, depending on caliper, grammage, grade, etc., may serve several functions. It is therefore only possible to indicate the primary function of some materials.

Base web materials

Base web materials may consist of or include:

1 paper
2 regenerated cellulose
3 plastic film
4 aluminium foil
5 coatings

- protective
- heat seal or cold seal
- surface appearance or texture (may also be protective)
- metallisation
- adhesive or tie
- waxes – surface or wax impregnation

6 plastic coextrusion and extrusion.

General construction – specifying

It should be noted that combination materials are specified (from the outside inwards) by weight (g/m^2), gauge or caliper. Most are made as a 'reel'-fed operation and into 'sheets' if required.

Printing processes

Printing may occur before, during or after 'combination' and then the material is covered by a clear coating or a clear film. Although virtually any printing process could be employed, flexography and gravure are the main contenders for reel fed materials. More recently offset lithography has increased in use.

The base web materials and the role they may play are now covered in greater detail.

Paper

Paper may be made from mechanical or chemical pulp. The latter is preferred due to its purity, white colour (if bleached), strength, slow ageing, etc. Paper is usually below 300 μm in thickness; above this caliper the material falls into a 'board' or 'carton' category.

The advantages of a paper ply are as follows.

1   Basically of a non-toxic origin (be aware of 'dioxin') – starting with relatively pure cellulose fibres and water.
2   Relative low cost with ready availability. (Wood is preferred origin, but other sources are used.)
3   Available in a wide range of types, substances, finishes, etc., depending on fibre length and the method of finishing. Typical papers include:

- opaque glassine
- vegetable parchment
- MG sulphate
- tissue
- MG bleached Kraft
- super-calendered (SC) bleached Kraft
- coated papers
- glazed imitation parchment (GIP).

4   Various additives can be incorporated at the beating, refining or finishing stage, i.e. the paper can be modified to suit specific uses (improve opacity, printability, etc.).
5   Can be printed by a wide range of processes, especially prior to lamination.
6   Can readily be coated by emulsion, lacquer, solvent, or extrusion-based processes, etc.
7   Can be laminated to other materials with a low-cost aqueous adhesive due to its absorbent (porous) nature.
8   Has good rigidity and strength – hence makes a good supportive material.
9   Porosity can be adjusted to allow diffusion of gases, steam, etc. for sterilisation while maintaining a barrier to bacteria and moulds.

10 Opacity can be varied according to the fillers used. It can also be coloured or tinted.
11 Paper shows a degree of compression, hence acts as a slight 'cushion'.
12 Paper can readily be torn or cut open.

The main disadvantages of paper are as follows.

1 Paper is moisture sensitive and contains on average 7% moisture under 'normal' storage conditions. Changes in moisture may induce temporary 'curl' or distortion, or 'boil-off' when heated.
2 Paper has no moisture-resistant properties (unless specially treated), hence no barrier properties against moisture, gases, etc.
3 Has no heat seal or cold seal properties, hence special coatings or films are required for effective sealing.
4 Has poor transparency and gloss when compared with certain coatings and plastic films.
5 The porous nature of paper with air entrapped between the fibres acts as an insulator. This makes heat transfer more difficult, particularly on high-speed heat sealing equipment.
6 Paper is usually thicker than plastic films, hence gives less coverage for the same weight.
7 'Grain' in machine or cross direction confers various property changes.

Summary

Paper is widely used in laminations to give support and add strength; it is readily printed, easily opened, biodegradable, etc., all at a relatively economic cost. It is usually used within the range of 10 to 90 g/m^2. For further detail see Chapter 5.

Regenerated cellulose film (RCF) (Cellophane, Rayophane, Diophane, etc.)

The process of manufacture is detailed in Chapter 7. Natural RCF, apart from natural clarity, is similar to paper in its general properties, although it is a continuous film and not fibrous in nature, e.g. it is moisture sensitive and not heat sealable. Moisture permeability can be improved by coatings which can also confer heat sealability. These coatings, which may be applied to one or both sides, are usually based on nitrocellulose or Saran (PVdC).

These materials are covered by various earlier used codings:

- DMS – one side coated with nitrocellulose lacquer
- MSAT – two sides coated with nitrocellulose
- MXXT/S – solvent coating of PVdC, both sides
- MXXT/A – aqueous dispersion coating of PVdC, both sides
- MXDT – single side coated PVdC

The coding definitions include:

- M, moisture vapour coating
- S, heat sealing
- D, one side coated
- X, PVdC coated
- F, extra flexible
- Q or P, high moisture permeability but heat sealable
- H, tropical
- QF, quick freeze
- PT or P, plain, transparent, colourless, non-moisture-proof
- C, coloured.

However coated, the base film remains moisture sensitive and gains or loses moisture via the raw (cut) edges. This means that the material shows a degree of dimensional instability and reels of material if stored under incorrect conditions will expand (dumb-bell reels) or contract at the edges. Most regenerated cellulose materials contain humectants and plasticisers aimed at resisting changes in moisture levels. Reels should, however, be stored flat and under controlled climatic conditions to avoid reel distortion affecting machine performance.

Summary

Although regenerated cellulose plants still exist, worldwide usage has significantly reduced due to the better dimensional stability properties of various polypropylene-based films. However, regenerated cellulose still finds usage for certain special applications, e.g. overwraps.
   Cellulose derivatives are also found in other forms, as detailed below.

Cellulose acetate (e.g. Clarifoil)

Like regenerated cellulose this is a clear sparkling film with a high gas and moisture permeability (i.e. the film breathes), but has poor chemical resistance and is difficult to heat seal. Like RCF it has poor dimensional stability and has been used for window cartons and an external glossy film for laminations.

Films and coatings based on plastics

Films are continuous, thin, clear, coloured or opaque materials derived from organic polymers. Most polymers are synthesised whereas the 'cellulose'-based films mentioned previously are mainly of natural origin.
   Films are usually less than 250 μm thick with most lying between 12 and 50 μm. Films can be produced from a number of processes:

- extrusion – from a slit die (flat die extrusion) or lay flat tubing (cylindrical die)
- extrusion plus calendering
- regeneration casting – as regenerated cellulose
- solvent casting
- calendering
- coextrusion – involving two or more materials.

377

Most of these processes are described in Chapter 7 and only exceptions are covered here, e.g. solvent casting involves a polymer dissolved in a solvent. The solvent is subsequently evaporated from the cast film by heat, thereby leaving a film. Cellulose acetate film is made by such a process.

Calendering is basically a rolling or roller process (like an old-fashioned mangle) where a plastic is heated and then rolled with heated and then chilled rollers. The caliper is controlled by the gap between the cylinders.

All manufacturing processes may be combined with other operations such as slitting, surface treatment (usually corona discharge), printing. Differing properties may be created in the plastic according to the conversion process.

Orientation

One special additional process is called orientation, where a plastic film is stretched at a temperature below its crystalline melting point in the machine or cross direction or both. The latter is called biaxial orientation. These orientation processes increase molecular alignment thereby improving strength in the direction of stretch, improving clarity, reducing permeation to moisture and gases and usually improving chemical resistance. When subsequently heated above the temperature of orientation, most oriented films will revert to their original dimension.

Oriented films are usually coated with a heat sealant which seals at a temperature below the orientation temperature, otherwise the film will shrink in the heat seal zone, crystallise and possibly become distorted (cockle) and brittle. Oriented films can be 'heat set' by special treatments.

General properties of films

Appearance

Films vary in transparency (haze); most are transparent with a glossy surface. Reverse side printing usually improves appearance and eliminates rub – but beware of process solvents affecting product. Films may also be tinted or pigmented (opaque).

Strength and flexibility

Most films are flexible and fairly strong. Some resist tear but usually tear easily once a tear point is initiated (slit, V-shaped notch, etc.). Most plastic films remain reasonably consistent for several years under reasonable storage conditions. Films generally age more rapidly when exposed and not in reels.

Heat seal

Most films can be sealed by some means – direct heat, hot air, ultrasonic, HF or RF, etc. Some need special heat seal coatings.

Protective properties

Generally all plastic films are water-repellent (water-resistant). Various degrees of barrier are offered against water vapour permeation, gases (organic and inorganic), oils, solvents, aromatics, preservatives, etc. All films, if free of pinholes, provide a barrier to moulds, bacteria, etc., i.e. are a hygiene barrier.

Permeation is usually measured as:

- gas: $cm^3/m^2/24$ h, at $25°C$
- moisture – $g/m^2/24$ h, 90% RH 38°C (tropical) per 0.025 mm thickness
  – $g/m^2/24$ h, 75% RH 25°C (temperate).

The USA tests use 100 in^2 instead of m^2. The 'total' barrier depends on a number of factors such as caliper, area, gradient on either side of barrier, temperature and any damage due to creasing, printing, etc., including diffusion/solubility factors associated with permeant and film.

Films show different resistance to oil, solvents, perfumes, preservatives, acids, alkalis and other organic and inorganic substances.

Other special features

Other special features include shrink films, stretch films and cling films. These features are, however, unlikely to be used in combination materials although oriented plastics are used in cold formed blister packs.

Special individual films and their uses

All plastics are to some degree permeable to moisture, vapour and gases, but are considerably superior to untreated or uncoated paper. The following material factors may require consideration in the selection of a plastic film, but it should be noted that only some of the factors listed below are subsequently considered under the general review on each plastic:

- weight per unit area (g/m^2) and/or caliper
- yield and cost (depends on caliper/density)
- transparency – light transmission; haze
- tensile strength and tear resistance
- ageing characteristics – under light, oxygen, temperature, light and low-temperature performance, softening point/melting point
- water vapour permeability
- gas permeability – note that permeation of N_2, O_2, CO_2 is usually of a 1:4:20 ratio
- odour permeability (organic and inorganic)
- resistance to water, solvents, oils and fats, etc.
- ease of printing (choice of process/ink/need for pretreatment)
- ease of heat sealing (temperature range, dwell time, pressure)
- freedom from static or level of static
- odour and taste characteristics (food grade acceptance)

- adsorption/absorption of preservatives
- non-inflammable
- presence of additives, processing, aids, etc.
- slip characteristics/coefficient of friction (critical for form fill seal machines)
- toxicity (risks for food grade acceptance
- irritancy
- blocking – tendency for two layers of laminate to stick together
- dimensional stability – important with print registration
- stress crack resistance
- extractives
- melt flow index (MFI)
- converting characteristics – each process may modify the basic polymer in a small way e.g. sealability, by heat, high frequency, ultrasonic or impulse sealing; so they also need consideration.

The polyolefins

These include the

- polyethylenes (PE), density 0.90–0.96
- polypropylenes (PP), density 0.90–0.91.

Polyethylenes (polythenes) include materials designated as low, medium, high, and linear low: PE (LD, MD, HD, LL, VL, UL).

Low density (0.915–0.925) offers a reasonable barrier to moisture but is a poor gas barrier and odour barrier, is permeable to oil, perfumes, etc. and tends to absorb or adsorb certain preservatives. Some grades, particularly with a high MFI, are prone to environmental stress cracking (ESC) when under a stress (in-built or applied) and in contact with a stress cracking agent (e.g. detergents, wetting agents). LDPE may be modified by the addition of EVA which increases its flexibility (it is already a very flexible material), widens and lowers its heat sealing range and optimises heat sealing speed. (LLDPE is steadily increasing in use and can generally be used where LDPE is referred to.)

As density increases (MD 0.925–0.935, HD 0.935–0.965), the material increases in rigidity, improves in barrier and chemical properties, becomes more difficult to heat seal (higher temperature), reduces in transparency and increases in haze. HDPE is approximately a threefold better moisture barrier than LDPE of equivalent thickness. Polythene surfaces need pretreatment prior to printing or adhesive lamination.

Uses for the films include:

- heat seal inner ply in laminations, sacks, shrink and stretch wrapping, etc.
- LDPE is frequently used as a lamination ply to bond two materials together
- HDPE is employed in boil-in-the-bag applications.
- All have applications as bags.

LLDPE is actually a copolymer of ethylene, with butene, octene or hexene. It is finding increasing use due to economies of polymerisation and film strength. It provides the strongest heat seal of the PEs, has more extensibility and a capability of being down-gauged. Other ethylene polymers include the following.

Ionomer (Surlyn) is a methacrylic acid and ethylene modified molecule with a metal ion (sodium, zinc, magnesium). Easy sealing, soft, strong, grease-resistant clear film, and seals well in contact with contaminants. Puncture-resistant, with a high hot tack. Approximately double the price of LDPE, but can be used in thinner gauges. Can be used in the inner ply of laminates, at approx. $\frac{2}{3}$ gauge of LDPE and as a skin pack over sharp or pointed objects.

Other ethylene copolymers

EMA, ethyl methyl acrylate, is a random copolymer consisting of a polyethylene main chain with methyl acrylate side branches. One main application is the film used for surgical gloves. It is more flexible than LDPE, less crystalline and much softer with a rubbery elasticity. It also has low softening and heat seal temperatures, good strength but poor optical properties. It can accept high pigment and additive loadings and is therefore widely used as a carrier for masterbatches.

Cast polypropylene (PP) is extensible, moisture-resistant, clear and seals at temperatures above those used in steam sterilisation. Oriented PP is strong and can be used in thin gauges. Unless coated or coextruded the film cannot be heat sealed without distortion. OPP is very clear, but can also make an opalescent film. Has a similar degree of inertness to HDPE.

Unless PVdC coated or metallised, OPP is a poor gas barrier and needs pretreatment prior to printing.

Oriented PP is used for overwrapping cartons, generally as a replacement for regenerated cellulose. Cast PP is used as the seal layer for packs designed to withstand autoclaving. Special grades of PP are now available for blister packing. Woven PP with across and diagonal plies are used for sacks and bags. Trade names: Propophane, Propofilm.

Polyvinyl chloride (PVC, density 1.35–1.40)

Clear, good gas barrier, does not heat seal. Found in the following forms.

- Plasticised PVC – rarely used except as bags (IV solutions, blood) or as pillow packs. Sealed with special adhesives, or by HF/RF welding. Plasticised film is highly moisture permeable.
- UPVC (unplasticized PVC) – may contain a low level of modifier (vinyl acetate). Has a low permeability to oxygen but is moderately permeable to moisture. The material is fairly rigid and is not heat sealable.

PVC is used in overwrap film, shrink film, shrink sleeving, thermoforming for all types of blister and bubble packs. Plasticised PVC IV bags are usually PP/Nylon overwrapped to reduce moisture loss.

Polyvinylidene chloride (Saran, PVdC, density 1.65–1.70)

PVdC is a soft cling type film but very strong. Difficult to handle. An excellent barrier to moisture, gases, grease and odours generally. Has a fairly narrow heat sealing range unless modified. May discolour slightly and embrittle slightly with age.

PVdC has limited use as a film but may be used as a central core in some co-extrusions. Often used as a coating material, e.g. on other films as a good barrier and heat seal.

Polystyrene (PS, density 1.05)

Relatively highly permeable to moisture, and fairly permeable to gases. Used for thermoforming (non-barrier usage) and as a shrinkable film on a limited basis. Relatively brittle material unless impact-modified when clarity reduces.

Used mainly in blister-type packs (and as bubbles on cards for display) and OPS for some labels.

Fluorochloroethylenes

Chlorinated and particularly fluorinated derivatives of ethylene usually offer high inertness and good barrier properties. One film, Aclar (trade name) based on poly-monochlorotrifluoroethylene (PCTFE), is the most moisture-impermeable commercial film currently known. For a similar thickness it is approximately ten times less permeable than PVdC. Derivatives generally have high melting and softening points. Found both as homopolymers and copolymers. For detail see Chapter 13.

Polytetrafluorethylene (PTFE, trade name Teflon)

PTFE is a very hard, chemically inert, low-friction material. It is mainly used to coat machine parts (to reduce friction) and heat sealing jaws to aid clean release. It is not used as a lamination film but has been used as a coating on closures (densities up to 2.2).

Polyvinylidene fluoride (PVdF)

More inert than PVdC; may find some application, but is more expensive.

Polyvinyl fluoride (PVF)

Has high weather resistance, but again, high costs restrict packaging applications.

Polyester (polyethylene terephthalate, PET; density around 1.38)

Usually found as a cast film. It can readily be oriented and heat set. It can be produced in thin gauges (down to 12 μm) as it is an extremely strong and tough material. Polyester is also clear and glossy.

It is heat seal resistant unless produced as a coextrusion or coated. A good barrier to most gases and volatiles, but only fair to moisture. It is easily metallised. Found as PETP and PETG (Kodak), Pet G contains an additional glycol molecule.

Often used as an outer ply to laminates and makes a good abuse-resistant layer. Use of metallised polyester is increasing as single and double metallised layers. Difficult to tear – needs a tear propagation point.

Thicker grades can be thermoformed (medical and pharmaceutical applications) and subsequently sterilised by steam autoclaving, gamma irradiation, etc. Non-oriented PET has a high melting point, around 250°C.

Polyamide (Nylons, density around 1.1)

Although various grades are available, Nylon 6 is mainly used for films (also 6:6 and 11). Generally flexible and tough at low and high temperatures. Only fair in resistance to grease and oils, with low gas permeability and a poor moisture barrier (due to absorption of water). Can be heat sealed in spite of high temperature and steam autoclaved. It can also be thermoformed. Usually slightly hazy although oriented nylon is clear. Usual gauges 25, 50 μm with orientation producing films down to 12 μm.

Combined with polythene to give various thermoformed packs for cheese, bacon, etc. Also used as an outer ply for boil-in-bag applications and as an outer ply in some cold formed blisters.

Polyvinyl alcohol (density 1.25)

PVOH is a water soluble film, with good gas, odour and grease barrier. Used as a water soluble sachet, but usually needs protection from moisture.

Polycarbonate (PC)

Another tough, clear film. Withstands steam sterilisation. Rather expensive. Only fair moisture resistance but good scuff resistance. Used in some laminations.

Polyacrylonitrile (PAN, trade name – Barex)

Good gas barrier. Only fair moisture barrier. Clear but not as clear as some other films, i.e. polystyrene, polycarbonate, polyester.

Polyurethane (PU)

Strong and rubbery. Frequently used as an adhesive or tie layer. Widely used as foams.

Ethylene vinyl alcohol (EVOH, trade name – Eval)

Good gas and odour barrier. Good moisture value when dry, but as moisture is absorbed, moisture barrier properties reduce. Relatively expensive. Usually used as a central ply in coextrusion processes. Replacing foil layer in some laminated tubes. Good barrier to certain flavours: peppermint, spearmint, etc.

Spun bonded materials (Tyvek)

Very tough with paper-like appearance. Used in medical packaging as a steam sterilisable porous material, (excludes bioburden). Based on HDPE. Has high strength.

Pliofilm – rubber hydrochloride

Was an excellent sealing medium but had few other properties to recommend it. Still available on a limited basis. Deteriorates rather rapidly with age.

Coatings

Coatings are an alternative means of adding properties which are not present in the base material: improved barrier, heat or cold sealing, improved appearance, adhesion, etc.

Types of coating processes

- Water-based – usually as a dispersion or emulsion coating, e.g. PVdC, cold seals.
- Solvent-based – followed by evaporation, e.g. heat seal lacquers, high-gloss lacquers, primers and key-coats.
- Vapour – e.g. vacuum metallisation.
- Molten materials – are applied hot then allowed to set, e.g. waxes, hot melts, plus extrusions or coextrusions and such new coating processes as plasma enhancement, sputtering, vacuum deposition, etc. (see below).

The application of coatings

Other than the newer coating methods mentioned above, many coating methods apply a liquid-based material to a solid web. These coatings may be applied either as a continuous (overall coating) or by a pattern system which may involve a 'printing plate' principle. Coating processes may apply excess, followed by controlled removal of the excess (e.g. by a 'doctor' blade system) or by a controlled (premetered) amount being applied directly (Figure 9.1)

Deposition can also be obtained by electrostatic spray or electrodeposition.

Typical examples of coatings are as follows:

1   Nitrocellulose, which was one of the earliest coatings used, as per MS regenerated cellulose film.
2   Saran or PVdC (usually a copolymer of vinyl chloride and vinylidene chloride). Applied by either solvent or aqueous dispersion coatings, with high coating weights (up to 180 g/m^2) requiring a number of coatings. Dispersion coating generally tends to have better moisture barriers.

PVdC may be used as an internal barrier-sealing ply or an external layer for protection and gloss.

Lacquers and waxes

1   Widely used as an external coating to provide a protective coating to the print, and to provide a product-resistant finish. UV cured lacquers, varnishes and inks can offer a very high gloss.
2   Microcrystalline waxes may be used for barrier properties or as a heat seal. They

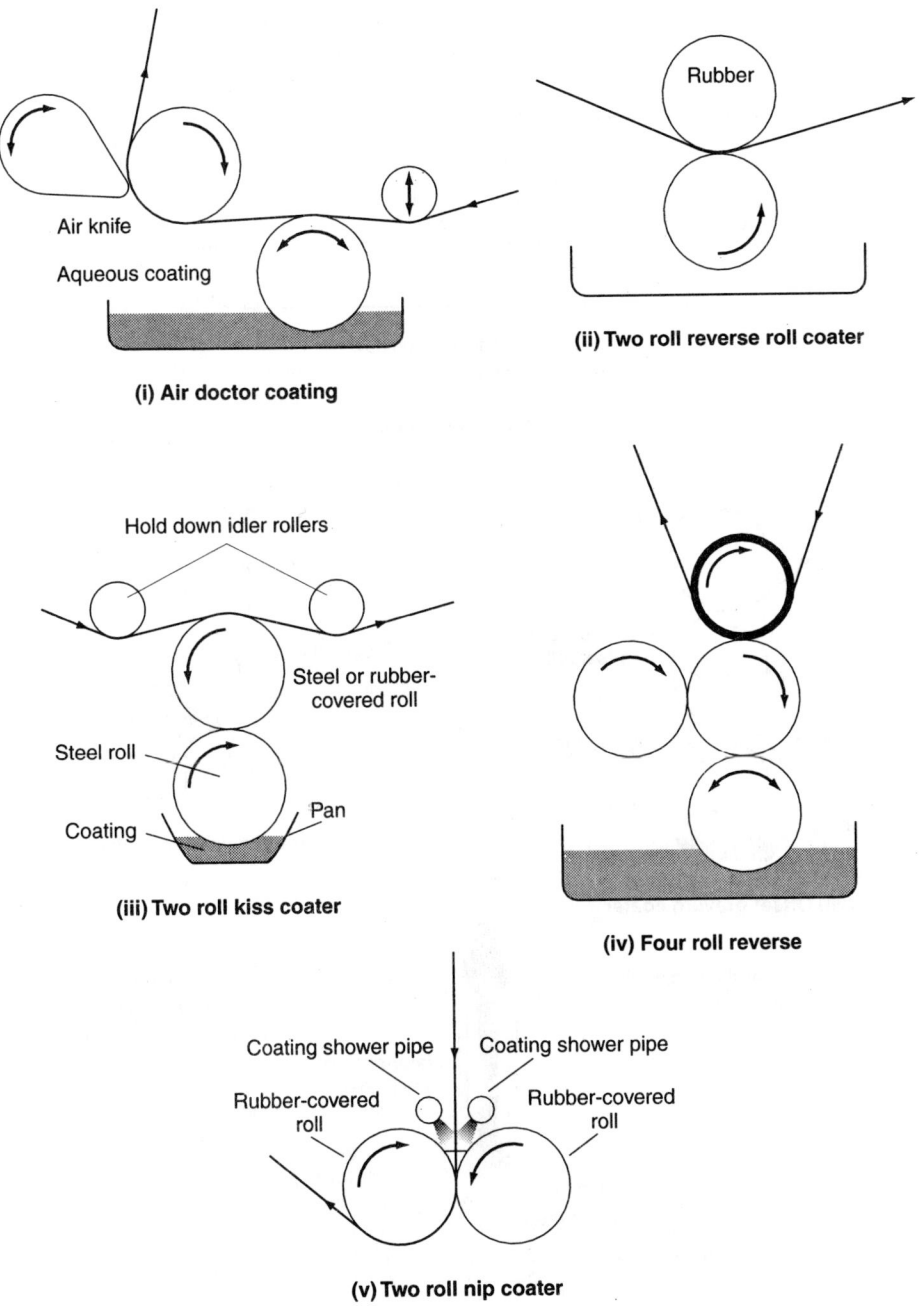

Figure 9.1 Liquid coating processes: (i) excess application technique; (ii–viii) predetermined (measured) systems; (ix) for higher viscosity materials

Coating reservoir
Carton blank
Conveyor
Overflow catch pan
Overflow coating

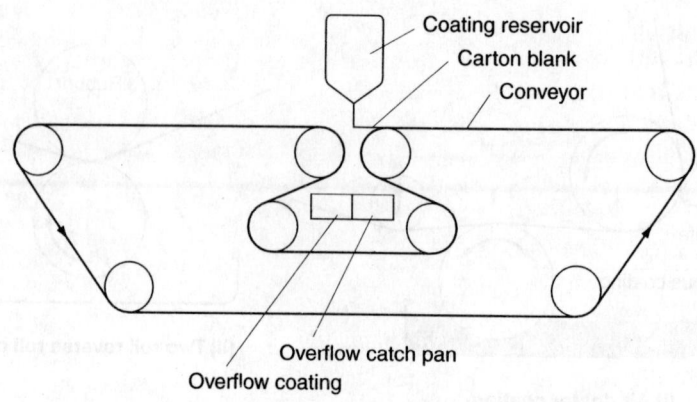

(vi) Curtain coater

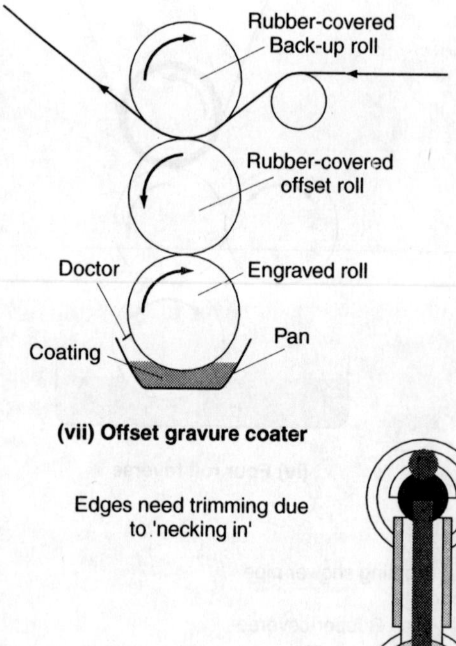

Rubber-covered
Back-up roll
Rubber-covered
offset roll
Doctor
Engraved roll
Coating
Pan

(vii) Offset gravure coater

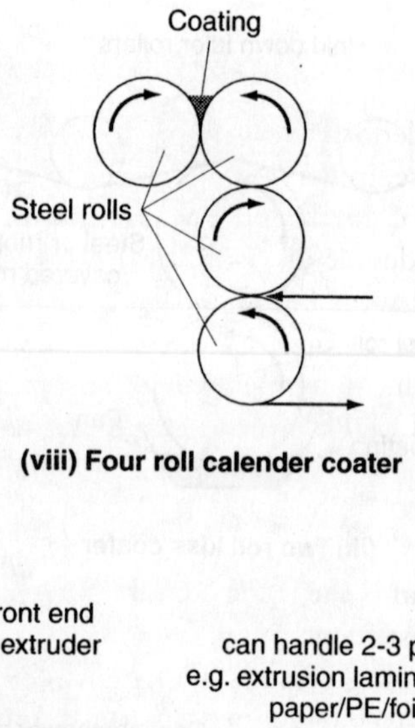

Coating
Steel rolls

(viii) Four roll calender coater

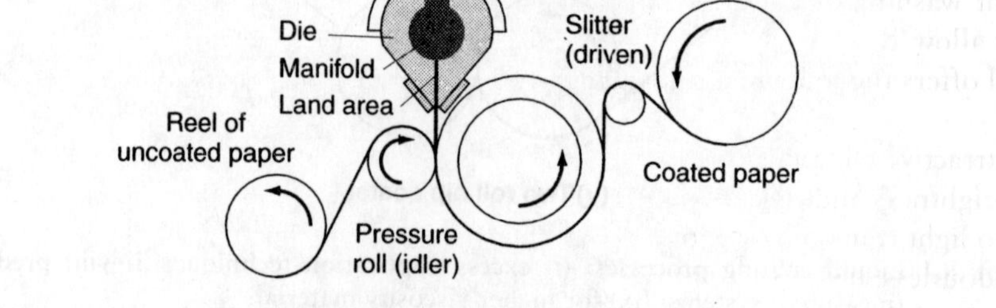

Edges need trimming due
to 'necking in'
Front end
of extruder
can handle 2-3 picas
e.g. extrusion lamination of
paper/PE/foil
Water-cooled
chill roller
(driven)
Wind-up
Die
Manifold
Land area
Slitter
(driven)
Reel of
uncoated paper
Coated paper
Pressure
roll (idler)

(ix) Extrusion coating paper

may be used as either a surface layer or as a total impregnation (paper). Known as wet and dry waxing respectively.

3   Hot melts and adhesives. May be used in a lamination process, but are usually considered as coatings. Hot melts may confer some protective properties, even when used for adhesion purposes, as they are based on plastics, i.e. are 100% solids.

Extrusion coatings

Extrusion is a process where plastic film is delivered hot onto a substrate ply. A more economical way of attaching a ply of plastic and widely used for LDPE. Is less practical with certain other plastics due to risk of degradation (PVC) or the high temperatures employed. Direct extrusion and coextrusion enables use of thinner gauges of materials typically down to 12 μm.

Coextrusion coatings usually employ materials of similar viscosity, softening or melting points, whereby two or more layers can be joined together internally or externally by extrusion dies.

Vacuumised treatment, e.g. metallisation

Used to deposit a coating of aluminium onto the surface of films. Gives foil type appearance, reflecting light and heat and reducing moisture and gas permeation. Covering of particles is not continuous and can be demonstrated by holding up to light when the degree of visibility enables items to be identified through the film. Using two metallised webs laminated with metallised area to metallised area contact gives much superior protection. Lamination to a flexible substrate reduces cracking of the metal layer which can happen when the material is creased or flexed, i.e. by the addition of an LDPE or LLDPE layer to give PET/metallised/LDPE.

Foil – aluminium

Aluminium is the most abundant metal on the earth's surface, but it is one of the most costly constituents in a laminate.

Foil is obtained from metal of 99% purity and above. The gauges range from 0.006 mm to 0.040 mm. The foil is annealed to give a soft foil with a 'dead fold' property. Hard tempered (non-annealed) foil occasionally finds special applications, i.e. push-through lidding for blister packs. Lubricants are removed from hard foil by either solvent washing or controlled heating. For any nominal gauge +8% variation is normally allowed.

Foil offers the following properties:

* attractive metallic appearance
* brightness and reflectivity (light and heat)
* no light transmission; total barrier
* odourless, tasteless, non-toxic
* hygienic (process of manufacture eliminates any microbiological contamination; it will not support growth of bacteria or mould)

- excellent barrier to moisture and gases – even pinholed varieties offer better protection than plastics and papers (particularly when laminated to a plastic ply).
- can be printed and embossed.

The disadvantages of foil are that:

- it is not heat sealable
- in thin gauges it is extensible, hence needs a support layer
- under unfavourable conditions foil may corrode, either in contact with 'chemicals' or due to bimetallic corrosion (e.g. in contact with a ferrous metal)
- surface oxidation causes loss of lustre
- perforates or pinholes relatively easily with thin grades, when creased, folded or excessively flexed.

Where thin foils are used in laminations the bright or dull side needs to be nominated. Matt usually gives the best adhesion. This may also be improved by the use of a key or primer coating, also called wash coatings, weight 0.5 to 2.0 g/m^2.

Pinholes and moisture permeation

Foil of 0.038 mm is guaranteed pinhole-free; 0.017 mm can be considered commercially free for most purposes. Lower gauges gradually increase in the likely number of pinholes, e.g. 0.009 mm foil may contain 100–700 pinholes per m^2 and 0.012 mm foil 30–150 per m^2. If these are laminated to plastics then the permeability relates to the area of pinholes and type of plastic when equated against the total area of foil. Hence the permeation figures remain low unless the perforations are increased or enlarged during the lamination and subsequent machining operations on the packaging equipment. For this reason pick-up on finished packs is more relevant than direct permeation figures on the basic packaging material. Gas permeation is usually greater than moisture, hence could be more critical.

Foil strength

Soft aluminium foil has a fairly low tensile and tear strength, so it is essential that very thin gauges are supported by paper or film. In general, foil of 0.025 mm and below has to be supported. For example, 0.025 mm foil laminated to 30 g/m^2 LDPE is a widely used strip packaging laminate. In theory, 0.015 mm foil laminated to 30 g/m^2 LDPE would be a more economical proposition. However, at this caliper any undue stretch would be likely to perforate and tear the foil. Hence it is possible to reduce the foil caliper only if support is increased, i.e. by the addition of a paper ply. Thus if cost savings are to be made the final laminate would probably be either

- 37 g/m^2 GIP/0.012 mm foil/30 g/m^2 PE, or
- 44 g/m^2 GIP/0.008 mm foil/23 g/m^2 PE.

Foils used on the external ply are invariably given a light coat of lacquer to reduce scuff and improve slip. However, if paper is a middle ply any excess moisture may literally 'boil off' during the heat sealing operation. Paper as an external ply is therefore generally preferred.

Foils of 0.006 mm and 0.007 mm are now offered and may be incorporated into a variety of laminations. Special thicker foils of 0.040 mm (40 μm) and above (up to 60 μm) are used for some cold forming operations.

Summary

Flexible packaging foil is usually coated with heat sealing material or laminated to other plies that include a heat sealable layer. Lacquered, sometimes embossed, foil is used to lid containers, e.g. blister packs. Foil is used in a wide variety of laminates. However, it cannot be used in any coextrusions, hence alternative barrier materials have to be used.

Laminations and lamination processes

Laminates are combinations of various plies created to obtain the properties which are not provided by one material alone. They use the minimum of materials (thin gauges and low grammage), and are cost-effective. However, they conflict with certain environmental issues, as recycling and/or reuse is either impossible or difficult.

Two widely used laminations are paper/foil/polythene and paper/foil/Surlyn. In these constructions the paper provides strength, brilliance and printability, the foil provides an excellent barrier to moisture, oxygen, light, odour and flavour (loss or gain), and the polythene or Surlyn gives heat sealability. These are widely used for strip and sachet packaging.

Lamination processes

Lamination may be achieved by adhesives, extrusion and coextrusion (Figures 9.2 and 9.3).

The more traditional method to make laminates uses separate plies combined with adhesives, which can be divided into groups – molten, water-based and solvent-based. Wax and polythene extrusion are the main molten laminants. Water-based glues are often used to combine paper and foil. Solvent-based adhesives include the polyurethanes, but recent developments use water dispersions and molten curing systems to replace the solvent systems. Cross-linking reactions develop high heat and product resistance in all these adhesives.

Extrusion consists of extruding a film from a slit die where the hot film may be nipped in contact with a second material and then cooled to give a bond between the two (or three) materials. Extruded LDPE is widely used both as a film in its own right and as a ply which combines plies on either side of it. Circular die extrusion can also be employed without the 'nip' stage in slit die laminating, i.e. it involves true coextrusion.

Coextrusion produces a multi-ply material directly from the individual resins. The method is limited to thermoplastic materials such as polythene, polypropylene and nylons. Thin layers of extruded bonding resins are necessary to combine many of the resins. Coextrudates have to be surface printed and the outer film cannot be reverse printed as it is often used with more conventional laminates with a film outer ply.

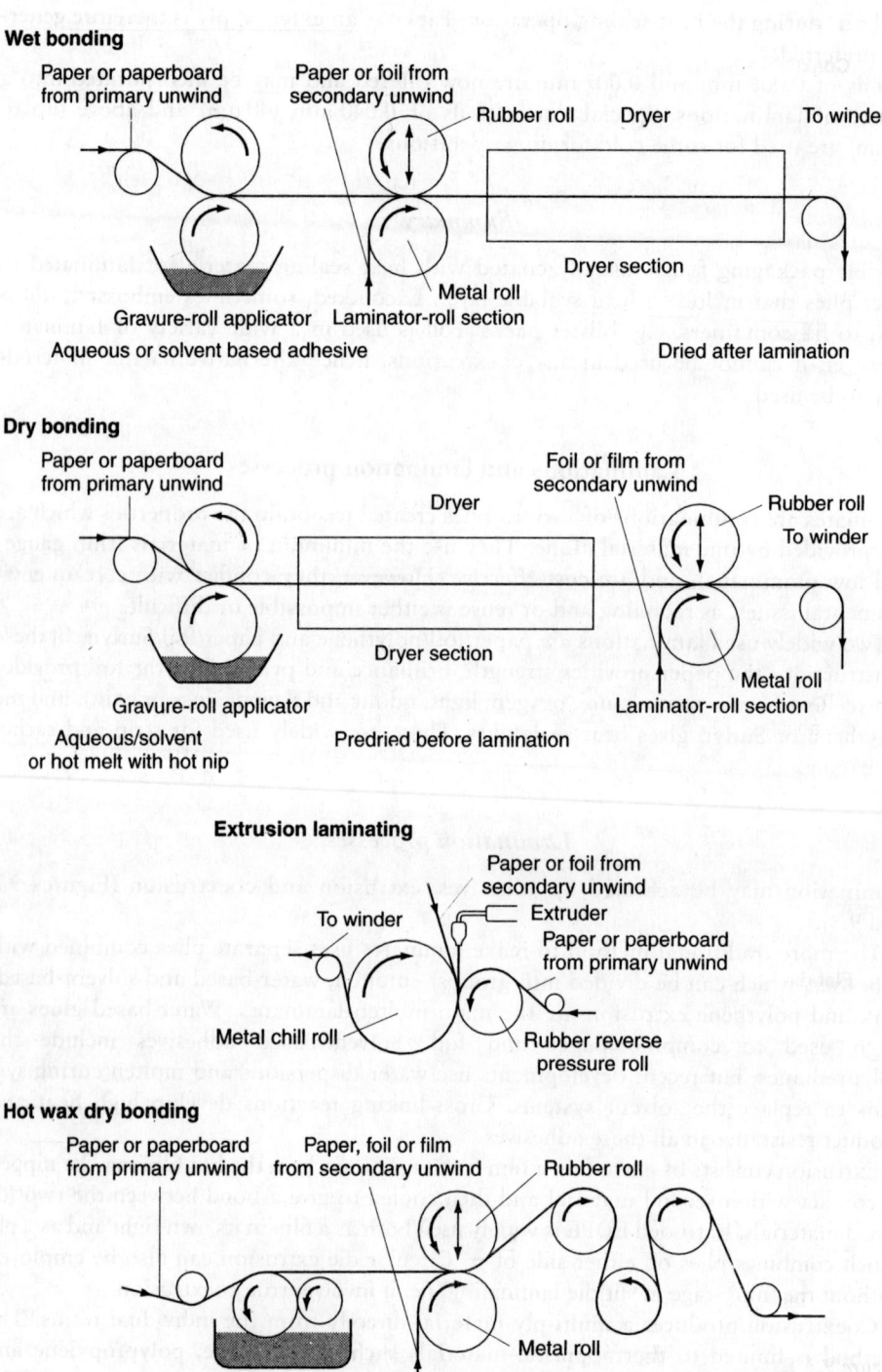

Figure 9.2 Lamination: wet and dry bonding

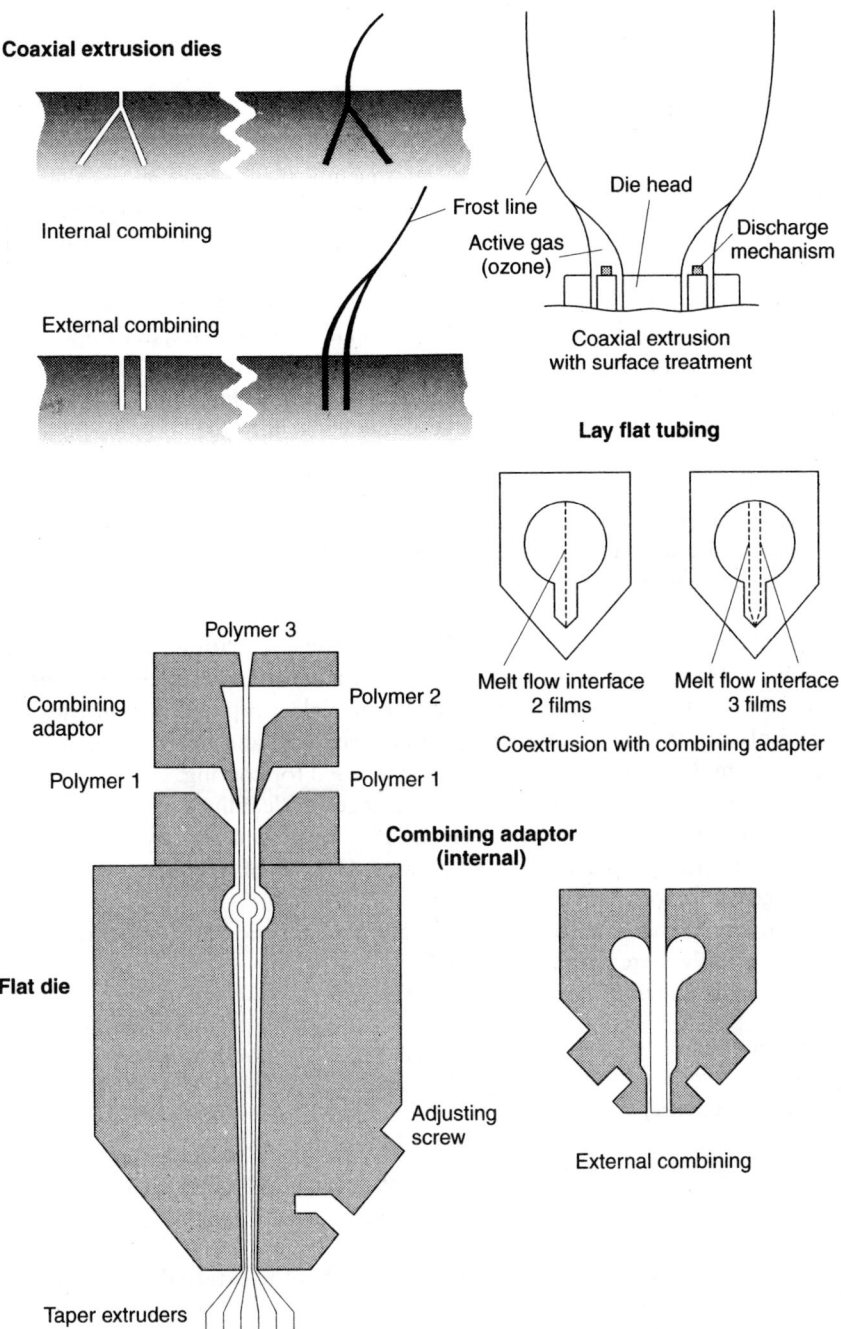

Coaxial extrusion dies

Internal combining

External combining

Frost line

Active gas
(ozone)

Die head

Discharge
mechanism

Coaxial extrusion
with surface treatment

Lay flat tubing

Melt flow interface
2 films

Melt flow interface
3 films

Coextrusion with combining adapter

Polymer 3

Combining
adaptor

Polymer 2

Polymer 1

Polymer 1

**Combining adaptor
(internal)**

Flat die

Adjusting
screw

External combining

Taper extruders

Figure 9.3 Extrusion and coextrusion processes

Adhesives – traditional

Various types of adhesive may be employed, i.e.

1   aqueous – with paper-based materials or where moisture can be lost from or through one web
2   solvent – loss of a volatile carrier by heating and special ducting
3   hot melts – advantage of virtually instantaneous set once heat is removed
4   hot wax – similar to hot melt except that wax remains pliable for a longer period.

(1) and (2) are termed 'wet' bonding while (3) and (4) are known as dry bonding processes. However, the second type (solvent) can also be used as a dry bond, where the solvent adhesive is applied to the substrate, excess solvent is evaporated off and then the second ply is bonded to the tacky adhesive via a nip roller.

Adhesive coatings may be applied by several means, i.e.

- excess of coating is added to the web and the surplus is removed by means of a rigid knife, flexible blade, or air jet knife, i.e. 'doctor' systems
- a controlled amount is applied to the web by means of rollers (roller coating), brushes, a calender, or by curtain coating.

A coating may be achieved by passing the ply between a coating roller and a back-up roll (usually rubber) or by kiss coating whereby the tensioned web makes contact with a coating roller. With certain more difficult materials a nip roll system (hot or cold) may be employed. In this instance the area between web and roller is flooded with the coating medium. Gravure cylinders may also be used for coating.

In general, hot melts offer production advantages in cleanliness of operation and the elimination of solvent extraction problems. Hot melts can also be modified to contribute to the barrier properties of the laminate. Control of heat and cost are the main disadvantageous factors.

More modern systems include polyurethane and acrylic-based adhesives and two-part curing adhesives are gaining popularity.

Examples of the various laminations used include:

1 OUTER PLY	CENTRE PLY	INNER PLY
PAPER	FOIL (barrier)	POLYTHENE OR SURLYN
(strength, appearance)		(heat seal)
2 OUTER LAYER	CORE	INNER LAYER
COPOLYMER (heat seal)	POLYPROPYLENE	COPOLYMER (heat seal)
	(strength/barrier)	

Laminate 2 has the advantage that it will seal to either the external or internal layer to itself, i.e. an overlap seal can be achieved.

Coextrusion is the latest process by which a series of plies can be joined together in the hot state. This may involve direct adhesion between plies or the use of extruded 'tie' or 'adhesive' layers. These bonding layers are frequently only a few micrometres thick and involve relatively low grammage levels. However, coextrusion is only cost-effective as a long-run process since set-up times can be lengthy.

Table 9.2 Provides a comparison between laminates and coextrudates

Laminates	Coextrudates
Versatile, include thermoplastic, paper and foil.	Limited to thermoplastic materials of similar viscosity. Exclude paper, foil, metallisation.
Sandwich print and coating can be used for good appearance and protection.	Surface print and coating only can be used.
Various adhesives can be employed. Cross-linking adhesives are often used, giving good heat and product resistance. Older adhesive systems are more prone to delamination.	Thermoplastic adhesives have to be used with limited product resistance. Some layer combinations do not require adhesives or tie layers.
More rigid.	Less rigid (especially cast).
Extra cost is necessary to pre-make individual layers before laminating. These layers also have a certain minimum thickness (limitations related to producing and handling this material).	Most cost-effective, especially for long runs. Thinner layers of more expensive materials can often be used. Setting-up operation needs greater expertise and may be lengthy, with various levels of wastage.

Decoration and printing

Materials may be surface printed, reverse side printed (if transparent) or sandwich printed (between two plies – either surface or reverse side). Two basic printing processes are usually employed:
   Flexography and gravure (offset lithography may eventually come on stream).

Flexographic and gravure or photogravure printing

Flexography was a relief process on a rubber or composition type stereo mounted on a printing cylinder. Originally suffered from squash-out but better control on registration means that good half tone printing can now be achieved.

Gravure printing employs an intaglio process whereby the print area lies below the surface of the plate in small cells. The tone or colour depth may rely on the depth of etch (i.e. amount of ink which lies in the cells) and/or the number of cells per linear inch. All gravure is basically half tone (solid line gravure plates are used in some tampon or cliché processes).

Gravure printing plates are expensive, £750–1,000 per cylinder (per colour), so four colour printing will involve an outlay an of £3,000–4,000. Make ready is also fairly lengthy, hence long runs are necessary to offset the high cost of the setting-up. Gravure gives very high-quality reproduction. Lower cost plate making processes have recently become available via the use of laser technology.

Both flexographic and gravure are reel-fed (web-fed) printing processes. Both can use solvent type inking systems which are suitable for non-absorbent materials such as films and foils. Drying processes usually employ heated drying tunnels where the solvent is removed (and reclaimed). Special UV inks and UV curing systems, IR drying systems, etc. are also available.

With the flexographic process, water-based inks can be used on paper (original aniline dye process) where adsorption forms part of the drying process.

The choice of printing process depends on the design, the number of colours, the quality, the printing surface, the length of run, etc.

Heat sealing – peelable, semi-permanent, permanent

Basically any heat sealing operation depends on the correct combination of temperature, dwell time, pressure and removal of heat, with pressure being the least critical (note that if pressure is excessive, sealant can be squeezed out of the seal zone).

However, for an effective seal consideration must also be given to the following.

- Sealing jaw pattern (line, cross-hatch, etc.) may involve two matching patterns or one side smooth.
- Area or width of seal zone (if too narrow, the seal may not be totally effective).
- Condition of machine, evenness of seal pattern, alignment of jaws.
- Type of temperature control and operational range (thermostat control is better than simmerstats, ±7.5°C possibly drifting to ±15°C with time). Electronic control is most accurate, say ±2.5°C.
- Product contamination – can interfere with sealing.
- Material to specification, e.g. no excessive caliper variation.
- How seal is achieved – platen or tangential contact (i.e. roller process where only a point of contact is made as distinct from a platen process where an area is sealed by a flat contact).
- If made from a reel process (which is usual), how resulting pack is removed from web by guillotining or punching. Hence accuracy and tolerance of cut are important so that an adequate heat seal margin is maintained.
- Number of joins in reel (should be flagged).

As a general rule 5 mm margins are recommended, but with push-through blister packs 3–4 mm is fairly normal.

Failures in heat seal can occur because of creases in the seal area giving rise to capillary leakage. Such capillaries are more likely to cause microbiological contamination than product losses. Under fluctuating temperatures the pack may breathe.

Seal defects may be detected by vacuum, pressure, pack deflection or gas sniffing.

In the case of multi-ply packs some plies (particularly the foil) can be perforated but, as other plies may be continuous, leakage will not be detected by a vacuum test. However, this perforation may be sufficient to affect product life. This type of leakage may have to be detected by visual means (microscope) or by careful separation of the plies by suitable solvents. The other alternative is to subject the pack to a cycling climatic test, i.e. 15°C 50% RH and 37°C 90% RH with 12 h cycles.

In some instances the heat seal ply of a lamination has to be peelable. These should be checked for peel strength over the shelf life of the product as in some instances the peel strength may reduce and so jeopardise the seal or increase it to a point where a permanent non peelable seal is obtained. The use of pattern lacquers also assists peelability.

Sealing can also be achieved by impulse, ultrasonic and RF/HF (radio or high frequency) methods and by cold sealing (pressure sensitive) type materials. See Chapter 11 for fuller details.

Lamination selection

Any laminate may consist of a number of plies selected from paper, cellulose, films, foil, coatings, tie layers, metallisation, etc. From previous pages the permutation possibilities are enormous. However this choice is restricted by:

- quantity/commercial availability
- technical requirements
- cost of base materials
- cost of lamination processes
- cost of printing cylinder and process (origination)
- the amount of laminate required (quantity)
- the yield (and from which choice the cost per area of laminate is derived).

One of the more complex laminates used consisted of clear LDPE/LDPE white/paper/LDPE/LDPE copolymer/30–50 μm, EVOH or Al foil/LDPE copolymer/LDPE clear. As another example, many laminated tubes now consist of five layers e.g. two plies LDPE/40 μm foil/two plies LDPE.

By listing some of the more widely used flexible (lamination) materials it will be seen that certain materials are rarely used in laminations except for very specific and very specialised cases. For the purpose of this list, 'paper' will cover any variety.

- paper/PVdC and PVdC/paper/PVdC
- paper/LDPE and paper/Surlyn
- regenerated cellulose/LDPE
- foil/LDPE and foil/Surlyn
- foil/heat seal lacquer
- paper/foil/LDPE and paper/foil/Surlyn
- polyester/foil/polyethylene or Surlyn
- Nylon/polypropylene.

Note: Reference to specific gauges has been deliberately avoided, as final choice may depend on the many factors mentioned earlier. Surlyn is slightly more expensive than LDPE but gives a better seal if seal area is likely to be contaminated with the product. It also seals at a lower temperature, allowing increased output speeds.

Examples of pharmaceutical applications

Strip packaging

1. 82 g/m^2 (25 μm) Al foil/30 g/m^2 LDPE or 25 g/m^2 LDPE. Gives excellent moisture, gas and light protection. External foil image.
2. 30 g/m^2 glassine/ink/poly/67 g/m^2 Al foil (20 μm) 25 g/m^2 LDPE. Good protection – more subdued metallic image.

Sachet packaging

1   59 g/m^2 paper/14 g/m^2 PVdC – here PVdC provides protection and heat seal.
2   37 g/m^2 paper/glue*/24 g/m^2 Al foil (8 μm)/25 g/m^2 LDPE. Provides a good barrier and LDPE as heat seal medium.
3   24 g/m^2 foil/glue*/44 g/m^2 paper/37 g/m^2 LDPE. Similar to (2) but with foil external. See Appendix 9.1 for a typical QC specification for a Laminate material.

Blister packaging

Tray:

1   UPVC, 100–300 μm
2   PVdC coated (30–100 g/m^2), PVC or PET or PP (150–300 micron).

Lidding:

1   hard foil (18–20 μm), heat seal lacquer (3–15 g/m^2)
2   soft foil (25 μm), heat seal lacquer (6–12 g/m^2).

Food and confectionery packaging

The latest feature in food packaging is the retortable pouch as a replacement for an open topped can. At the moment economics are improving as the cost of steel and tin-plate rises. However, filling speeds for pouches are considerably lower and additional strength outers (for stacking) add to the cost.

Retortable pouches can be made from combinations of foil, polyester, nylon, polypropylene, HD polythene, provided the laminant (or the process of lamination) employed will withstand the autoclaving conditions of temperature and moisture. Due to the flat shape of the pouch and high surface area, sterilisation times can usually be reduced compared with cans.

An important factor in both pharmaceutical and food packaging is that materials employed have FDA clearance with reference to any hazards. This may be checked by reference to the supplier and by obtaining full details of the formulation of each film employed.

The above are included as the pharmaceutical industry often follows the food industry when new materials are involved. This is sometimes economically sound where quantities are not sufficiently high to support the development of a specific material for the pharmaceutical industry, e.g. a retortable material in the food industry could be applied to a non-retortable use.

Other points

Laminates can be fabricated in a vast number of combinations and therefore the choice of the correct technical material may appear to be extremely complex. However, if the

---

* 12 g/m^2 LDPE is an alternative, extrusion laminated.

choice is restricted to what is adequate rather than perfect for a given purpose, it is possible to introduce a reasonable degree of standardisation and therefore obtain further economic advantages from larger demands.

An additional factor must also be considered. How do laminates compare with other competitive materials (such as glass, metal and plastic containers) in terms of disposal, pollution, reuse and conservation of the earth's natural resources? There is no doubt that combinations of plastic, cellulose, foil, etc. do present a disposal problem and although two of these can be incinerated, the economics of recovering the foil is relatively poor. The overall economics of using laminates can be compared with other materials by quantifying the packaging costs and disposal/reuse costs. This approach does not include any 'convenience' value associated with each type of pack.

However, since most are reel-fed materials involving form fill seal activities, the space required for the storage of incoming materials is significantly less than for preformed containers which store air. There is also a significant saving in weight and space in many circumstances.

Life cycle analysis is expected to help in the long term the environmental aspects associated with the future of packaging. Life cycle assessment can also be applied. However, each involves factors which are difficult to accurately quantify.

Virtually all forms of flexible packaging find some use in either pharmaceutical or medical products. Pack forms include:

- conventional strip and blister packs
- cold formed foil blisters
- specially selected strip and blister packs with additional child resistance
- sachets and pouches (single and compartmental)
- sterilisable sachet and pouch systems
- a wide variety of overwraps.

Although the majority of the above will use conventional types and combinations of material, some will use specific or specialised forms which are solely related to pharmaceutical or medical products. Strip and blisters tend to fall into this latter category and are covered in Chapter 13.

Products and instruments requiring sterility need special mention, as both the materials and the processes offer a number of combinations. In total these can cover all the previously mentioned methods for obtaining a sterile pack, i.e. terminal sterilisation by steam autoclaving, or gamma irradiation, or the aseptic approach using dry heat, moist heat, gamma irradiation, accelerated electron or gaseous treatment, plus newer on-line aseptic processes. The last of these, which are currently being developed as a total in-line system for the food industry, are normally reel-fed. The material is sterilised by UV or chemically by hydrogen peroxide or any similar sterilising chemical process, provided it is non-toxic with a low level 'residue'. In the USA hydrogen peroxide has been approved for the sterilisation of food materials with a residue limit of 1 ppm. This or a similar system is likely to find pharmaceutical applications.

Although certain products can be terminally sterilised by moist heat, gamma irradiation or accelerated electrons, these tend to apply to relatively few pharmaceutical applications where flexibles are involved (the last two are more widely used for medical instruments in pouches or sachets).

Moist heat is only a practical process where the product contains sufficient moisture and the seals are robust enough to withstand the temperature and pressure of the process. Stresses on the pack can be reduced by autoclaving under water and/or by using a balanced/overpressure autoclave. The latter is normally programmed to provide an external pressure during the cooling cycle in order to balance the internal pressure within the pack and thereby prevent the seals of the pack from rupturing. Paper plies (unless treated to repel water/steam) are usually excluded from pharmaceutical packs which are sterilised by steam. However, special paper plies with low porosity to prevent penetration by bacteria are available which are steam sterilisable, provided some degree of 'wrinkling' is acceptable.

Plastic 'papers' such as Tyvek, a porous spun bonded HDPE, are particularly suitable as an alternative to a sterilisable paper. Where non-porous plastics are involved sterilisation can be achieved by gamma irradiation, accelerated electrons, or gaseous treatment. Gamma irradiation can cause critical changes to some plastics, e.g. a less flexible material, discoloration or the release of gaseous substances. The last of these may give rise to organoleptic changes or increased risks with toxicity or irritancy, with a possibly greater emphasis on irritancy or allergenic type substances. Gamma irradiation can also change the structure of adhesives and alter the bond strength. It has been used to improve the peelability of some semi-permanent bonds.

Although ethylene oxide readily penetrates most plastics, attention has subsequently to be paid to any degassing phase and the level of residues associated with ethylene oxide, ethylene glycol and epichlorhydrin.

To conclude, it is likely these pharmaceutical applications for new combinations of flexible materials will follow those of the food industry, although occasionally there will be concepts which are specifically developed for pharmaceutical products. The purchasing power of the industry (compared with foods) will frequently restrict progress.

Increased growth in the materials currently used (listed below) is therefore more likely than a surge in the use of raw materials.

1   Foil:

- soft aluminium foil, 0.006–0.038 mm (as a ply in combination with other material)
- hard aluminium foil, 0.015–0.025 mm (as a ply in combination with other material)
- special foils for cold forming, 0.040–0.060 mm.

2   Paper: tissues, Kraft, bleached Kraft, glassine, glazed imitation parchment (GIP).
3   Plastic plies:

- LDPE, MDPE, HDPE, LLDPE (and combinations of these)
- Surlyn ionomer
- nylon and oriented nylon
- polypropylene (PP and OPP)
- Aclar
- Saran (PVdC)
- ethylene vinyl acetate
- polyester

- cellulose acetate
- regenerated cellulose
- polycarbonate
- ethylene vinyl alcohol
- polyvinyl chloride.

4   Coatings:

- metallisation
- polyvinylidene chloride
- nitrocellulose
- various heat seal coatings, washes, lacquers and varnishes
- solvent coatings
- silicon oxide and carbon coatings.

Conclusions

It is clear from the preceding text that polymers and coatings can provide a wide range of properties. Since most heat sealed (or cold sealed) flexibles are tamper-evident, this is obviously a positive feature which can encourage further unit dose type packaging. UK investigations have also established that, provided the materials are opaque or dark tinted and reasonably substantial (i.e. not flimsy), most strip and blister type packs offer reasonable child-resistance. This is generally as good as reclosable child-resistant packs where there is always a risk that the closure is not properly reapplied and any removal usually exposes a child to a greater quantity of a product.

It can therefore be concluded that there are many good reasons why the use of flexibles for pharmaceutical products should enjoy continuing success.

Other alternative coating processes

These alternative processes include metallising with metals other than aluminium, e.g. Camvac offers a coating of aluminium oxide on a material called Camclear. More recent additions include silicon oxide, (SiO_x) coatings, carbon like coatings, etc. Such coatings and volatile polymer coatings can be applied by a range of relatively new techniques found under the following headings: vapour, vacuum or electron beam deposition, sputtering and plasma enhancement, etc. (Figure 9.4). Coatings may involve gases, fine particles or a liquid which is usually deposited on the exposed material to be coated when it is passed over a chilled cylinder in a vacuum chamber. The thickness or weight of material deposited varies from very thin (measured in Angstrom) to that measured in microns.

Metallisation

This consists of fine particles of aluminium or other metals. Gain in barrier properties is often 20× or 40× but this reduces to 4×/5× if the material subsequently becomes severely creased and the surface is broken. Virtually any material can be metallised, e.g. PET, LDPE, PP, paper. They have a highly reflective surface but can be seen through against a bright light. Metallised materials can be laminated by wet or dry laminating systems, directly coated, etc.

a Evaporation

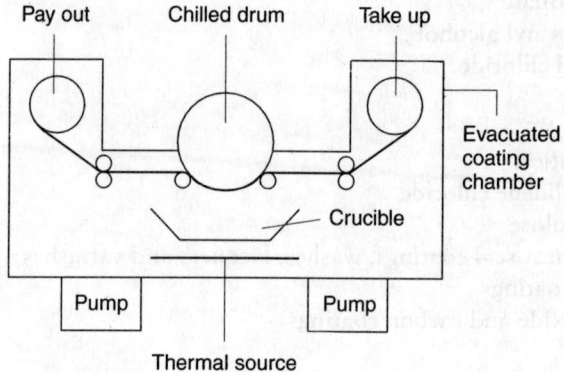

b Sputtering

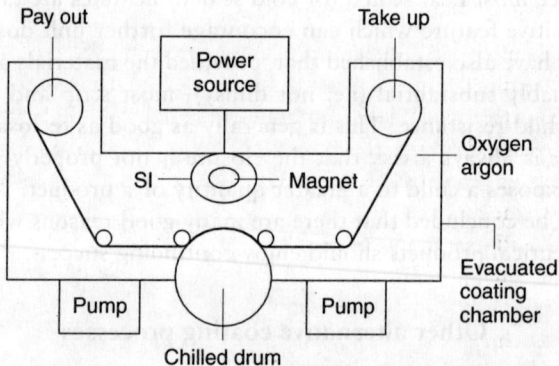

c Chemical plasma deposition (CPD)

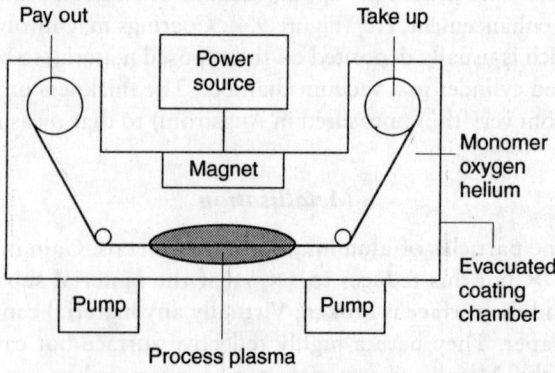

Figure 9.4 Alternative coating processes. In (A), the crucible contains material to be evaporated (aluminium, SiO/SiO$_2$, etc). Evaporation is by resistive heater or electron beam gun

Silicon oxide (SiO$_x$) coated materials (thickness 1500–3000 Å)

These are produced by several conversion processes (evaporation, sputtering, chemical plasma deposition). Evaporation is the same method as that used to create metallisation using aluminium. A material is heated in a crucible by either a resistive heat or an electron beam gun (hence the name electron beam deposition), whereby the material evaporates and subsequently condenses on a chilled film in a vacuum chamber. In the case of SiO$_x$ coatings, the aluminium used in metallisation is replaced by SiO/SiO$_2$.

Sputtering (coating thickness 400–500 Å)

This process relies on an electromagnetic powered source which, together with an ionised gas mixture of argon and oxygen, causes the argon to bombard a silicon source whereby silicon atoms are created and subsequently attach themselves to a chilled substrate. The level of SiO$_x$ created is controlled by adjusting the oxygen content. This process is the least economical (high energy required).

Chemical plasma deposition (CPD) (coating thickness 300 Å)

Although this can use a chilled drum, it is not essential, as the process involves a relatively low heat loading. The process again uses a vacuum chamber provided with a helium–oxygen mixture and a silicon-based monomer such as tetramethyldisiloxane or hexamethyldisiloxane. An applied power creates a plasma which activates the oxidation of the silicon gas, creating reactive chemical molecules which form the SiO$_x$ coating on the film surface.

In general the CPD method, as used by Airco Coating Technology, gives the lowest deposit, a clearer film (others may have a yellow tinge), a better bond (chemical rather than mechanical), a more extensible material (stretches further before the surface ruptures), and this is achieved at a relatively low power input and a reasonable output speed.

SiO$_x$ can be applied to films such as PET, PP, nylon and PE. O$_x$ usually lies between 1 and 2 (but excludes 2, i.e. SiO$_2$). Improvements in barrier properties are up to 120× for oxygen and 45× for moisture, but severe creasing can cause a reduction. It has been shown that CPD coated SiO$_x$ films will withstand autoclaving (moist heat) of 121°C, or perhaps above.

Diamond-like carbon (DLC) (coating thickness in micrometres)

This is the newest coating process to emerge and has been applied to PET and PP films. The coating shows high hardness, transparency and impermeability, reducing moisture permeation by 40–60× and oxygen by up to 100×. In the process of manufacture acetylene is ionised in a vacuum chamber, releasing carbon onto a film.

Fluorination

Fluoride treatment of HDPE conveys improved resistance to solvent-type organics. Use for certain pharmaceutical products is under test, with manufacture of single and multilayer material including coatings.

Appendix 9.1: Packing material specification

STANDARD NAME: LAMINATE PRINTED ABC		DATE:	CODE REF:

SUPERSEDES SPECIFICATION:	CODE:	DATED:	NEW DESIGN:

REASON FOR REVISION:

GENERAL DESCRIPTION:	Paper/Foil/Polyethylene laminate, sachet front, printed ABC
MATERIAL DESCRIPTION:	$37g/m^2$ paper/12.5g. m^2 LDPE/0.012mm soft aluminium foil/$25g/m^2$ LLDPE. Paper to be spirit varnished.
CONSTRUCTION:	Four ply laminate, foil extrusion coated with LLDPE. Paper to foil extrusion laminated with LDPE on bright side of foil. Reel to meet no 3 on standard unwind chart of National Flexible Packaging Association.
SIZE/CAPACITY:	Reel width 100mm to be within $\pm$ 1mm of nominal width, core diameter 76mm. Maximum reel diameter 400mm
DRAWING NUMBER:	Reference/date
DECORATION/ PRINTING:	Printed as per artwork... .. Varnished except for batch no area, incorporating APE registration mark, to be within $\pm$ 0.5mm of nominal distance. Text correct to proof previously approved ref... ... ... Colour to be within agreed colour tolerances and matching Pantone colour references.
SPECIAL TESTS:	See cross references to master manual for printed laminates, i.e. heat sealing, adhesion strength, varnish test, rub resistance, fade resistance of print.
ACCEPTABLE QUALITY LEVELS:	Critical 0% Major 0.65% ALSO SEE NOTES ON REVERSE Minor 4.0%

MODE OF PACKED FOR DELIVERY AND IDENTIFICATION

Rolls to be individually wrapped, fitted with core plugs to prevent core damage and palletised. Alternatively, they may be packed in strong boxes fitted with core rods. The rolls to be sufficiently well packed to prevent movement and impact damage. Rolls to be wound sufficiently tight to prevent telescoping. All packs to be correctly identified externally and within core.

AUTHORISATION:	
SUPPLIER:	DATE:
RECEIVING COMPANY:	DATE:

SUPPLIER

Notes

1. Where PHARMACEUTICAL COMPANY X HAS APPROVED BUYING SAMPLES FOR GOODS, any orders for goods of the same description subsequently placed by the Company shall unless otherwise indicated, be deemed to be placed on the basis of such buying samples as well as on the description and/or specification, and in all such cases the goods shall conform both to such buying samples and the description and/or specification.

2. The supplier shall effect no physical or chemical change to the product or its method of manufacture without the prior agreements in writing of the Company.

3. The Company reserves the right to revise or amend the specification after formal notification to the supplier.

4. The right is reserved to reject individual reels at the time of their use, should a fault appear within the confines of the reel.

5. Sampling, inspection and classification of defectives is conducted strictly in accordance to . . . . (The AQL's for this are shown overleaf).

6. Visual defect classifications

CRITICAL

a) Admixtures
b) Print defects which result in non compliance with Statutory Regulations

MAJOR

a) Print defects which result in the illegibility of the text
b) Defects which are likely to materially affect the usability of the laminate when used on automatic packaging machinery
c) Defects which are likely to result in the product not meeting the required standard

MINOR

a) Print defects which do not affect legibility of the text but are a departure from normal commercial standards
b) Colour variation outside of the established tolerances
c) Defects which are not likely to materially affect the usability but are a departure from normal commercial standards

AUTHORISATION:	
SUPPLIER:	DATE:
RECEIVING COMPANY:	DATE:
SUPPLIER	

10

METAL CONTAINERS

P. L. Corby and D. A. Dean

Introduction

Although the use of metal in packaging appears to be on a slow decline, the trend towards continuing reduction in weight has meant that more containers are being made from the same overall weight of metal. It therefore remains generally competitive with other materials, particularly as it can be manufactured and filled at high speeds. However, metal is being increasingly challenged by plastics, glass and composite materials which involve a wide range of coating processes such as metallisation, silica oxide and carbon.

With pharmaceuticals, metal, particularly tinplate, was at one time widely used for pastille tins, ointment tins and various built-up containers for powders, tablets, capsules, etc. As the early use of tinplate declined, aluminium containers had a period of success, but other than aerosols, are now reducing in usage mainly because of their high cost compared with plastics and glass. However as raw materials vary significantly across the world and processing equipment, once installed, has to justify its initial expenditure, metal usage can vary from country to country.

The main metals currently in use are the following.

1   Tinplate, with various types of base steel and coating weights. Since tin is now a high-cost material, lower coating weights are frequently supplemented by lacquers, enamels, print coverage to add to protection from potential corrosion.
2   Tin-free steel where additional protective coatings are essential, i.e. enamels and lacquers.
3   Aluminium and various alloys of aluminium.
4   Aluminium as a foil, often laminated to other materials.
5   Metallisation involving the deposition of aluminium or oxides of aluminium onto other materials such as paper or plastic.
6   Stainless steel.

The main uses of the above in the pharmaceutical industry today include the following.

1   Tinplate

   • Built-up containers made from a number of components with a range of possible closure features, e.g. ring pull, diaphragm seal, aerosol.
   • Lidded shallow drawn containers with a rolled edge.

2   Aluminium and various alloys

- Impact extruded rigid containers – especially aerosols. Also used for rigid tubes.
- Impact extruded collapsible tubes.
- Shallow drawn containers.

3   Aluminium foil, usually as laminations for blister, strip, and sachet packaging.
4   Metallisation, often used as a more economical substitute to foil but has lower protective properties.
5   Stainless steel, i.e. a chromium (12–14%) and nickel (up to 0.7%) steel widely used for mixing vessels and manufacturing equipment.
6   Other metals – tin is occasionally used for collapsible tubes.

Metal closures are still in wide use, being manufactured from tinplate, aluminium and alloys of aluminium, and these cover screw closures, various forms of lidding, aerosol valves, overseals (e.g. for vials), etc.

Metal containers

Metals were first used as containers as early as 4000 BC, and probably before that. The first metals used were those found in their native state requiring only gathering and hammering into shape. These included gold, silver, copper, and white gold (electrum). Some very early examples of pottery vessels were obvious copies of metal prototypes, as they show simulation of seam lines and rivets.

Since the modern era of packaging dates from about the time of the industrial revolution of the eighteenth and nineteenth centuries AD, the metals we need concern ourselves with today are almost exclusively steel, tinplate and aluminium. Tinplated sheet iron was developed in Bohemia in 1200 AD and kept a jealously guarded secret for several hundred years.

Aluminium was not isolated until 1825 and remained a rare curiosity until the late 1880s, when a practical method of extraction from bauxite was developed. From that time on its price steadily dropped. Its widespread adoption in packaging came in the mid-1940s, when techniques for rolling and decorating thin aluminium foils were perfected.

Metal containers are strong, relatively unbreakable, opaque, and impervious to moisture vapour, gases, odours and bacteria, providing they are pinhole-free. They are also resistant to both high and low temperatures. However, metals require the application of coatings and lacquers to prevent chemical reaction and corrosion from the inside or outside. Special coatings and coating techniques have therefore been developed for this purpose, e.g. tinplate is in fact a coated material.

Metal containers are available in a variety of shapes, sizes and styles ranging from small elongated collapsible tubes and shallow drawn containers to large built-up containers including steel drums of up to 110 gallon capacity. Many of these containers are in direct competition with equivalent containers produced in glass or plastic, e.g. collapsible metal tubes compete with laminated and plastic tubes and rigid metal tubes compete with glass or plastic vials.

Although metal containers exist in many different styles, most are parallel sided and of relatively simple cross-section, e.g. square, rectangular, oval or circular, the majority being circular. This is due to limitations in manufacturing techniques which do not apply to glass or plastic. However, the technique of building-up metal containers from sheet by means of seaming confers one advantage over glass and plastic in that right angles can be easily achieved. Blown glass or plastic containers require radii, particularly at the base of the container, in order to avoid excessive thinning (Figure 10.1).

The use of sheet material also allows decorating before container fabrication instead of after, with fewer limitations than for processes applicable to finished containers. Furthermore this enables the decoration to be carried right up to junctions and around curvatures which would otherwise be difficult, if not impossible, to decorate.

It is in the field of aerosols that metal containers have predominantly established themselves. Although glass, plastic and plastic-coated glass aerosols are finding their own specialised applications, metal aerosols are likely to retain the bulk of the market as long as cost advantages are offered.

In common with glass and plastic containers, the performance of a metal container is partly governed by the nature of the closure involved. Some of these closures are similar to those used on glass and plastic containers, e.g. plastic and metal screw closures and frictional closures such as plug or slip lids. Others, which are mainly used on metal (or metal composite) containers, are lever lids and permanent mechanically seamed-on closures.

THREE-PIECE CANS

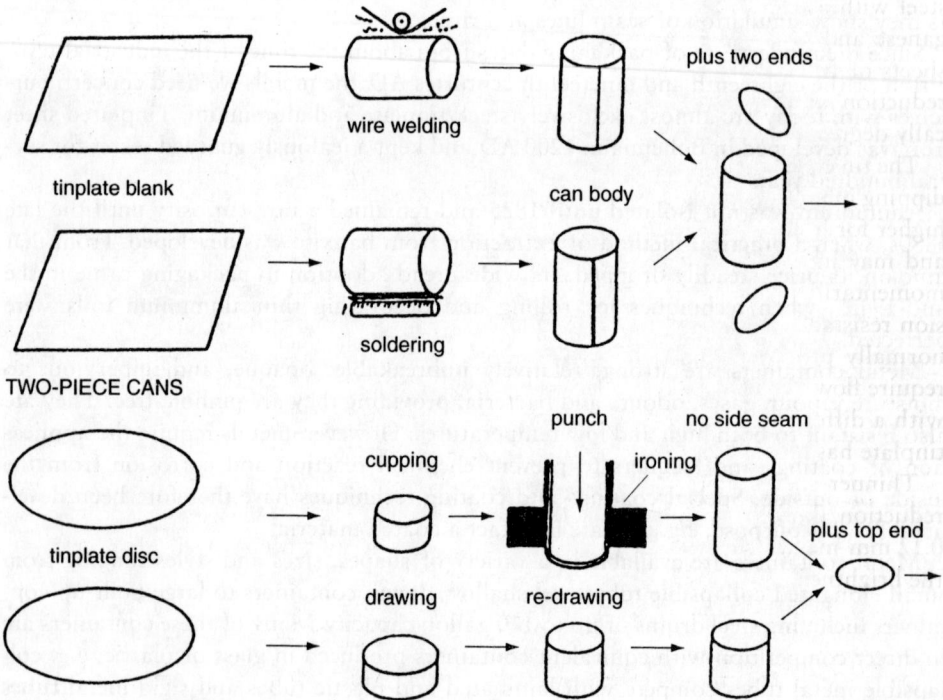

Figure 10.1 Some methods of can manufacture

Modern packaging metals

Tinplate and associated materials

Tinplate is mild or low-carbon steel sheet or strip which is coated on both sides with commercially pure tin. Other steel-based materials which are occasionally used in packaging are steel itself, blackplate, galvanised and stainless steel. Blackplate is uncoated steel which is highly susceptible to corrosion and is of limited application. Galvanised steel is produced by coating the steel with zinc by hot-dipping or electro-plating. The materials in this group are mainly restricted to making larger containers, e.g. drums for bulk chemicals. Stainless steel finds wide usage in the pharmaceutical industry, mainly as types 316 and 304.

Within the past three decades tin-free steel (TFS) has been developed. This material consists of a mild steel base – exactly as used for tinplate – but with a coating of chromium–chromium oxide only about 1/30 as thick as an average tinplate coating. The function of this coating is merely to protect the steel base from corrosion prior to fabrication. TFS containers need to be coated on the inside and outside with one of many organic coatings in order to make them at least as corrosion-resistant as uncoated tinplate containers. To date the main usage of TFS has been for can ends.

Manufacture of tinplate

The steel base, which contains small amounts of carbon (also known as a low carbon steel with a carbon content of less than 0.25%), sulphur, phosphorus, copper, manganese and silicon is rolled from ingots into slabs and then into continuous strip or sheets of from 0.20 to 0.25 mm thickness. The process is known as 'continuous cold reduction' and involves pickling in hot dilute sulphuric acid, oiling, rolling, electrolytically degreasing, annealing and tempering to the required hardness.

The tin coating is then applied either by electroplating or by the older process of hot-dipping in molten tin, to a coating thickness less than 0.002 mm for electro-tinplate but higher for hot-dipped tinplate. Electro-tinplate is produced in a continuous strip form and may include a flow-brightening operation whereby the newly applied coating is momentarily melted and then allowed to cool, giving a bright surface and better corrosion resistance by improving the continuity of the tin coating. Hot-dipped tinplate is normally produced in sheet form although occasionally strip is used, and does not require flow-brightening. Unlike hot-dipped tinplate, electro-tinplate may be produced with a different coating weight on each side, known as differential tinplate. Electro-tinplate has almost entirely superseded hot-dipped tinplate for can manufacture.

Thinner sheets down to about 0.15 mm may be achieved by an additional cold-reduction (known as double reduced tinplate) before tinning. Thicknesses down to 0.12 mm may be achieved by cold-reduction after tinning (i.e. re-rolled tinplate), but the brightness and protectiveness are reduced.

Specification of steel and tinplate

Steel contains a small percentage of other elements, the quantity and proportion of which can be varied to produce four chemical sets of steel: MC, MR, L and D. The degree and type of cold-reduction and annealing or tempering affect the formability of the steel sheet. In the USA, as many as nine different hardness of temper classifications are available. There are five recognised commercial finishes of tinplate, namely bright, matt, silver, stove, and shot blast, all of which are achieved by the use of textured work rolls during the final stages of temper rolling. With the exception of matt finish, each requires flow brightening after electro tinning.

Several different systems are used to express the thickness of steel and these vary according to whether it is being used with or without a tin coating. The thicker sheets of steel which are used for drum manufacture are specified in terms of gauge rather than thickness, the gauge being defined in terms of the area covered per unit weight. A comparison of the US and UK systems is given in Table 10.1.

Thinner gauges of tinplate are specified in terms of their nominal thickness, which ranges from 0.31 mm down to 0.12 mm in 0.01 mm steps. In practice the thickness is calculated from the weight per unit area divided by the density rather than by direct measurement. Although tinplate is a combination of steel and tin, the actual difference in density is relatively small (0.5 g/cm^3) and the proportion of tin present is very low (~1%). Therefore for practical purposes the density of tinplate can be taken as identical to that of steel (7.85 g/cm^3).

The tin coating on tinplate is more conveniently expressed as the coating weight per unit area (as g/m^2) for each surface separately. These figures are prefixed by the letter E for electrolytic (equally coated) tinplate, D for differential tinplate and H for hot-dipped tinplate. There are standard coating weights for electrolytic tinplate in the UK (1.1 to 14.0 g/m^2) and on hot-dipped tinplate (11 to 22 g/m^2).

Prior to metrication the coating weight was expressed in terms of the total weight applied in lb per base box (as in the USA). The base box being defined as the total coated surface area of 112 sheets of size 14×20 inches, i.e. $31,360 \text{ in}^2$ (20.2325 m^2) of tinplate or $62,720 \text{ in}^2$ (40.465 m^2) of tinned surface.

Thin nickel coatings are being developed as a cheaper alternative to tin and may be plated electrolytically down to one-tenth the thickness of a conventional E 2.8/2.8 tin coating.

The type of solder used with tinplate is normally tin/lead but antimony has replaced lead where there is a possible extractive hazard, e.g. for aerosols containing aqueous formulations. Efforts are being made to reduce the lead content of solder for health

Table 10.1 Comparison of commonly used steel gauges: USA and UK

Gauge no.	UK Birmingham gauge		US manufacturer's standard gauge	
	Imperial (in)	Metric (mm)	Imperial (in)	Metric (mm)
14	0.079	1.99	0.075	1.90
16	0.063	1.59	0.060	1.52
18	0.050	1.26	0.048	1.21
20	0.039	1.00	0.036	0.91
22	0.031	0.79	0.030	0.76
24	0.025	0.63	0.024	0.61
26	0.020	0.50	0.018	0.46
28	0.016	0.40	0.015	0.38
30	0.012	0.31	0.012	0.31

reasons. The tin coating is essential for soldering, since tin-free steel cannot be soldered. Leadfree solders are now available but these are largely being replaced by welding.

The protective value of the tin coating increases with coating weight. The more corrosive chemicals and certain pharmaceuticals require use of coatings at the top end of the range.

Differential tinplate may be used, e.g. where higher corrosion resistance is required inside the ultimate container, or conversely used with the heavier coating on the outside, e.g. for shipment of inert materials to tropical regions. The drawing and wall ironing process also requires the heavier tin coating on the outside for lubrication.

The heaviest tin coating is extremely thin and rarely completely continuous, so the risk of external corrosion can be reduced by application of an enamel, and possible chemical reaction with the product can be eliminated by internal lacquering.

Can enamels and lacquers

A wide range of internal lacquers developed for the heat processed food industry also find uses in the pharmaceutical and cosmetic field. The lacquers, which include acrylic, phenolics, polyesters, epoxy and vinyl resins, are normally applied via an organic solvent which is subsequently evaporated during curing. The use of aqueous carriers and powder coatings has also been developed. Ferrolite is a plastic coated metal using polypropylene, polyester, etc.

The choice of resin is based mainly on satisfying product compatibility requirements such as resistance to acid or alkali, and freedom from flavour or taint. The resin must adhere well and have sufficient flexibility to withstand the container fabrication process. It must also be resistant to damage if the container is soldered. On shallow drawn or formed foil containers, protective coatings are applied to the foil or sheet prior to container fabrication. On deep drawn or extruded containers, coatings are applied after fabrication. With soldered or welded cans the opposite internal area can be protected by a 'side-stripe', after fabrication.

Aluminium

Aluminium sheet is used for drawn or formed one-piece container bodies and also in the fabrication of multi-piece built-up containers.

The first stage in the extraction of aluminium from bauxite is to extract the aluminium oxide (alumina) which comprises 40% to 60% of bauxite, by a chemical process. The alumina is then dissolved in molten cryolite (a double fluoride of sodium and aluminium) at 1100°C and separated into oxygen and metallic aluminium by the passage of a direct current. The reduction operation requires almost 8 kW h to produce 1 lb of aluminium, having started with about four pounds of bauxite.

The molten aluminium which accumulates at the bottom of the reduction cell is regularly syphoned off and cast into rectangular moulds to cool and solidify. The resultant ingots are then scalped to remove 4–5 mm of the rough exterior which may contain aluminium oxide inclusions. In order to relieve internal stresses resulting from casting and to distribute any alloying constituents more thoroughly, the scalped ingots are homogenised by reheating to about 600°C for 24 h.

Aluminium can be produced up to 99.99% purity, but this is not only expensive but mechanically weaker than aluminium of a lower purity. Therefore a small percentage of other elements is included, e.g. 0.4% iron, 0.2% silicon, plus traces of copper and manganese. Where maximum rigidity is required, e.g. for formed containers, an alloy containing 1.25% manganese is used such as NS 3 in the UK or 3003 in the US. The latter also contains up to 0.2% copper.

Sheet rolling

The first stage is hot rolling whereby ingots are heated to 550°C and passed back and forth through vertical roll mills, resulting in a considerable increase in length as well as reduction in thickness. When the thickness has been reduced to about 20 mm the material is passed in line through a series of mills known as 'tandem' mills to differentiate them from the original reversing mills. Each succeeding mill stand rotates at a higher speed to accommodate the elongating metal. Water-soluble lubricants are continually sprayed onto the surface of the aluminium to avoid excessive temperature rises and build-up of aluminium powder or oxide.

The material emerging after continuous hot rolling is coiled up and then cold rolled to complete the reduction. The thickness of material is approximately halved with each pass. Heat generated during cold rolling is removed by spraying on a mineral oil blended with organic load-bearing additives such as oleic acid, palm oil or higher alcohols. This also serves to prevent sticking of the metal to the rolls. If intended for foil the coils are annealed to relieve built-in stresses and submitted to additional cold rolling. Unless hard temper foil is required, the material is annealed again to make it flexible and at the same time to remove the remaining film of rolling oil.

Sheet to be used in container manufacture is rolled to the desired initial gauge. In the case of formed semi-rigid foil containers the final gauge of the finished container is in the region of 0.1 to 0.2 mm, depending on size. In such containers there is very little change in gauge in the forming operation. In rigid formed containers, such as drawn cans, body stock sheet gauges are about 0.25 mm and stocks about 0.32 mm. In the drawing process gauge is substantially changed.

Properties of aluminium

Aluminium is very malleable and ductile and easily formed into containers. During the process it is subject to work hardening which can be used to advantage in producing rigid containers. Alternatively the formed containers can be annealed to restore the softness and flexibility, e.g. in producing collapsible aluminium tubes.

Aluminium is light in weight with a density of 2.7 compared with steel (and tinplate) at 7.8. Although the density of aluminium is slightly greater than that of glass, the ability to utilise very thin wall sections enables lightweight containers to be fabricated which are easy to handle and reduce shipping costs. The metal surface is highly reflective and bright in appearance, enabling striking decorative effects to be achieved.

Chemically aluminium is odourless, tasteless, non-toxic and sterilisable. It is relatively resistant to corrosion but forms a layer of the denser oxide which, being relatively impervious, inhibits further attack. The formation of this oxide is exploited in anodising to form a more permanent barrier, often with the inclusion of colours to give copper or brassy effects.

Since aluminium is subject to attack by strong acids and alkalis it is frequently coated or lacquered. The aluminium surface is receptive to lacquers, inks and enamels, enabling components to be protected internally and decorated externally.

Decorating metal containers

Although it is possible to modify the planar surface of a metal container by indentation inwards (debossing) or outwards (embossing), the term 'decoration' usually refers to one or other of the printing processes. This may be preceded or followed by a coating process: roller coating, spraying, anodising, etc. However, it is the print process itself which is mainly responsible for identifying the container and enhancing its presentation.

The vast majority of metal containers built-up from sheet materials are decorated in the flat prior to fabrication. The process most used (offset lithography) was used for printing on metal long before it was adapted for printing paperboard. A process which is basically dry offset lithography is also being increasingly used.

Metal containers produced by impact extrusion must be decorated as the last stage rather than the first stage. The process normally used is rotary dry offset letterpress. Drawn containers may be decorated either before fabrication (by offset lithography) or after fabrication (by dry offset letterpress). The choice depends on the depth of draw and the amount of distortion which can be tolerated. Deep drawn components are invariably decorated after forming.

Any of the metal containers discussed can be labelled instead of printed. Labelling is often used for small quantity and short runs, and is also advantageous when a packer requires several print variations on otherwise identical containers. In this instance the packer is usually able to operate on a smaller stock holding of empty containers and has greater flexibility to meet changing market requirements. 'Labels', include paper- or plastic-based materials, and stretch–shrink sleeving.

Screen printing

The screen printing process – or silk screening as it is still sometimes called – is a sten-cilling technique which employs a screen mesh instead of a solid stencil. The screens nowadays are more normally made of nylon, polyester or steel. The resultant thick ink film has a good body and high gloss. The main pharmaceutical application of screen printing is for steel drums where small quantities of a given design are often required. Where the design is very simple, stencilling itself can be used. Both screen printing and stencilling can be carried out either in the flat or on the finished drum.

Offset lithography

Offset lithography is a planographic process and depends on the chemical modification of the surface of the printing plate so that only the image areas accept ink and the non-image areas accept water.

For litho printing metal it is usual to apply an opaque coloured (often white) base coat in order to provide a suitable background for printing. This base coat or enamel is normally applied by roller coating but can also be printed, e.g. to leave uncoated areas for a metallic effect, or for printing with transparent inks. The surface of tinplate is superior to tin-free steel or aluminium for this purpose. If the tinplate is ultimately to be soldered a strip is left free of enamel and print to avoid unsightly scorching. (This can still be achieved with roller coating.) Metal sheet for drum manufacture is more often roller coated overall and then 'touched up' by spray painting after the soldering operation.

Nowadays the most commonly used enamels are synthetic resins, e.g. vinyls, acrylics, epoxy resins, which are usually stoved after application. Sometimes a priming coat is applied before the base coat to facilitate subsequent forming operations.

After the base coat application, the metal plate is printed either half-tone or solid depending on the design. Either one or two colours can be applied in a single pass using either transparent or opaque inks, followed by baking for about 10 min at about 240°C. The heat drying mechanism is a combination of polymerisation and oxidation plus some evaporation. The printed sheets are then over-varnished by a roller coater and baked once again. The over-varnish is usually a synthetic resin similar to the base coat but without the pigment. Some machines can apply the varnish in line over the wet inks, the process being known as trailing varnish. UV curing of inks and external coatings is now being widely used, with a considerable saving in energy and a reduction in emissions of volatile solvents into the atmosphere.

The varnish film must be tough enough to protect the print during fabrication as well as during container handling and usage. The base enamel, inks and varnish must be flexible enough to withstand the forming operation without cracking, and physically stable and colour-stable to withstand repeated baking, e.g. the base enamel of a six colour job could be stoved up to a total of eight times.

The process described above is sometimes referred to as wet offset lithgraphy and uses bimetallic plates, e.g. copper on steel, prepared by photochemically etching away the non-image areas so that the steel base is exposed, leaving the copper image areas slightly raised. On application of water by the damping rollers the hydrophilic steel attracts a film of water and at the following inking station the hydrophobic copper attracts the oily ink. The alternative dry offset process utilises a plate of a single metal, e.g. steel covered with a photosensitive compound. This is again etched away so that the non-image steel areas are slightly recessed, but damping rollers are not used although the equipment is similar.

Offset lithography is used to decorate metal sheet for shallow drawn containers and lids since the resultant distortion is inherently small. When deeper one-piece containers, e.g. drawn and wall ironed aerosol cans, are printed most of the decoration is normally on the sidewall. One technique used is known as distortion printing. The original design is printed in the flat in a condensed or distorted fashion which is calculated geometrically so that when the three-dimensional can is formed the print becomes elongated and assumes the correct dimensions. More usually the containers are printed after fabrication in the same way as extruded tubes.

Rotary dry offset letterpress

This is a relief printing process in which the image areas are raised above the level of the non-image areas and transferred from the inked printing plate to the metal surface by means of an intermediate resilient rubber surface.

This process is used to print cylindrical containers. Since the tubes must be supported on a mandrel during the printing process, it is essential that one end of the tube be of unrestricted aperture. This is one of the reasons that 'monobloc', DWI and DRD cans are necked-in after decoration and the bodies for two-piece cans are printed before seaming on the end. The other reason is to allow the decoration to go beyond the shoulder and right into the seam itself. A base coat of white enamel is first applied to the container by roller coating and set by partial baking, which aids keying of the inks at the printing stage. The base coat can also extend marginally around a corner radius, e.g. at the base of a rigid tube or over a bead or shoulder where present. However, the next operation of printing itself is restricted to the cylindrical surface as the actual (relief) printing plate is wrapped around a cylinder in a similar manner to a lithographic plate.

Each tube is supported separately on a mandrel which can rotate freely on its axis. The inking stations apply their separate images to the same rubber-faced blanket cylinder and the composite image is transferred to the tube in a single revolution of the latter. The printed tubes are then dried again. The tubes are held on pins for both the initial base coat baking cycle and the print baking cycle. A period of 4 min at 170–230°C is normally adequate, depending on the nature of the enamel and the inks. Where there is a possibility of the product reacting with the decoration, an over-varnish is applied by roller coating, and set by baking.

The decorative effects which can be achieved by offset letterpress printing are much more limited than those available by offset lithography on sheet materials. The design is limited to a maximum of six colours and a second pass is not possible.

It is not advisable to print wet on wet. If it is desired to achieve an effect of one colour superimposed on another, it is preferable to reverse the required image out of the first (background) colour and to 'fit' the second colour into this area. With very fine type matter where 'fitting' is impractical, a darker colour may be superimposed directly onto a lighter background, but if this dark colour appears elsewhere on the design there will always be a difference in shade.

Full colour half-tones cannot easily be produced by offset letterpress since they would inherently involve wet on wet printing. However, screened work in a single colour is possible, e.g. to achieve a black and white photographic effect. More recently half-tone work has successfully been completed, but there is a problem in achieving a gradual fade-out of any colour. Hence, designs tend to feature a relatively sharp edge around the half-tone section. Another point to be borne in mind is that a design which involves lining up a strip of colour running around the entire circumference of the container should be avoided, because lining up is difficult as the tube may not be truly cylindrical and in any case it is rotating freely on its mandrel; also, where the overlap occurs there is a double ink film which can mar the desired effect, particularly with light colours. It is therefore preferable to leave a gap rather than insist on an overlap. This is a typical example of the importance of producing a design capable of reproduction by the printing process which will ultimately be used.

Types of metal containers

Metal containers can be classified into several general categories based on methods of manufacture, as follows.

1. One piece seamless containers

    - formed foil or sheet
    - shallow drawn
    - drawn and redrawn/drawn and wall ironed
    - impact extruded.

2. Multiple piece built-up or fabricated containers

    - open top
    - closed top
    - aerosols.

Formed aluminium foil containers

By definition, a formed aluminium foil container is made by forcing the material to assume a shape with little or no metal 'draw'. Corner folds help provide some rigidity and prevent leakage. Folded back edges provide strength, avoid finger cutting, and better accept a matching lid. Folded containers cannot be made round or oval. Few if any of this type of container are used for pharmaceutical packaging.

A later type of formed container was made by using matched male and female dies with sufficient clearance between them to permit the metal to slip and form wrinkles rather than be stretched. A much greater versatility in shape is available in this container. Smooth drawn flanged containers which accept a peelable lidding have been used for unit dose packs of liquids and semi-liquids. These packs may be lacquered or unlacquered.

Shallow drawn containers

The term 'drawing' in container manufacture refers to the process whereby an article is formed by drawing or pressing it from a sheet of the material, using matching male and female dies. Both tinplate and aluminium are used. Decoration can be carried out in the flat prior to forming and thus has more in common with built-up containers than impact extruded seamless containers.

Obviously drawing puts a severe strain on the metal sheet, and the amount of distortion which can be tolerated depends on the thickness of the metal and the ability of the surface finish, e.g. tinplate coating or decoration, to adhere firmly to the base metal. The containers produced by drawing are relatively shallow with a maximum depth up to half the diameter if circular. Metal screw caps and aluminium roll-on cap shells are also produced by the same process.

Tolerances are so close that flanges and bottoms are smooth and walls are nearly wrinkle free. Vacuum or compressed air may be used to assist the forming operation. In one extreme example, aluminium containers are air formed using either a female die only or a female die and a plug assist. The open end is tailored to receive its closure by curling it inwards or outwards and beads may be added around the container to strengthen it and to assist in locating or removing the ultimate closure. The base of the container is often inset slightly for added strength and to protect any decoration.

Shallow drawn containers are produced in two basic shapes – round and rectangular. Round containers are used for packing viscous pharmaceutical ointments and creams which may be difficult to fill or dispense from collapsible tubes. Since the containers have full apertures and vertical side walls, filling may be accomplished with wide bore filling tubes.

Rectangular containers are more normally used for packing discrete items such as tablets, pastilles, surgical plasters and dressings. However, it should be noted that even so-called rectangular containers must have rounded corners. The depth of draw is in practice limited to twice the corner radius.

Both tinplate and aluminium sheet may be used to produce shallow drawn containers, the choice depending on cost versus product resistance. Dry products and non-aqueous creams are usually satisfactory in tinplate, whereas aqueous creams are better packed in aluminium. Alternatively, lacquered tinplate can be used for aqueous creams but there is always a chance of corrosion at any raw edges. Tinplate is stronger than aluminium for a given thickness.

Deep drawn containers

Deeper containers or more complex shapes can be produced either by drawing and redrawing or by a combined drawing and wall ironing process.

In the draw and redraw (DRD) process, sheet material – prelacquered if required – is fed to a cupping press where it is stamped out into a disc then formed into a shallow cup. The cup then passes to the second drawing stage where the depth is increased and the diameter reduced. The process is repeated as many times as may be necessary prior to trimming and flanging.

Since the DRD process is carried out on prelacquered sheet, TFS can be used. There is little or no reduction in gauge, the sidewall and base remaining essentially the same as the starting gauge. This feature makes the process ideal for food cans where the finished container must withstand both internal and external pressure created during retorting and cooling.

The alternative drawing and wall ironing (DWI) process also begins with a simple drawing stage, but is followed by ironing of the sidewall to increase the depth of the container while maintaining the diameter. This results in a substantial reduction in gauge, e.g. material starting at 0.25 mm or more may be reduced to 0.1 mm on the sidewall, and is ideal for certain aerosols where the internal pressures make the can stronger after it has been filled and sealed. The process is applicable to either tinplate or aluminium. When used on tinplate the tin coating serves as lubricant. Internal coating by spraying is carried out after forming.

Both DRD and DWI cans are seamless and hence more aesthetically pleasing than built-up cans. Technically they are more secure, as there is no side seam or base seam at risk. Beads or corrugations may be added to the sidewall of both types of can for strengthening purposes. This is essential for the DWI can to enable it to be used for foodstuffs. Frequently the base of the can is domed upwards to maximise the resistance to internal pressure, e.g. for aerosols.

Closures

The closures used for shallow drawn rigid containers are slip lids for round containers and either slip lids or hinge lids for rectangular containers. They are produced from the same materials and by the same technique of drawing as the containers on which they are used.

When used on round containers, slip lids normally rely on forming a closure between the side wall of the container and that of the lid. Hence the effectiveness of the closure is governed by the difference in diameter of the two components, their relative rigidity and the depth of engagement. The lid itself – which is often domed – may stand considerably proud of the upper rim and allows brimful filling.

An outward curled rim is frequently used on containers for ointments and creams, keeping the raw edge away from the product and away from the customer's finger. The lid itself may also feature a similar outward curled rim. The use of curled rims is more common with tinplate than with aluminium, since cut edges are sharper and there is a higher risk of corrosion.

When slip lid containers are used for aqueous creams or ointments with volatile constituents, a glassine or foil laminate membrane is often placed across the rim of the container resting on the product. This serves to reduce losses on storage and in use and the membrane can also carry additional instructions to the customer or patient. Sometimes this membrane is sized to overlap the rim so as to become entrapped on closuring. In this case allowances must be made when specifying tolerances of fit for the container and lid. The slip lid should support the weight of the filled pack when it is lifted by the lid.

Although slip lids are also used on rectangular drawn containers, the geometry of the two components does not allow as tight a fit as is possible with round lids. Hence moisture sensitive tablets or pastilles are better packed in round containers. Alternatively a slip lid of the type commonly used on both round and rectangular tobacco containers can be used. This is usually referred to as a vacuum sealed lid but more accurately described as a differential pressure lid. The lid itself incorporates a flowed-in PVC or EVA gasket to form a closure with the upper rim of the base.

In production the filled container – with the lid loosely applied – is fed into a vacuum chamber where a vacuum is first applied followed by a top loading to force the lid into intimate contact with the container rim. When the external pressure is restored to atmospheric, the 'vacuum' within the container maintains the seal. The effectiveness of the closure can be checked visually or automatically by observing a depression in the lid due to the pressure differential. The container is opened by releasing the vacuum with the aid of a coin slot built into the base. Both container and lid are constructed of tinplate rather than aluminium and in a fairly thick gauge in order to withstand the pressures applied.

Hinge lids are restricted to rectangular containers. Hinge lids are unsuitable for products which are at all moisture sensitive, but they can be used for dressings or adhesive plasters. The hinges may be formed from matching tabs and slots formed in the container and lid, or involve a separate wire hinge entrapped within a curled under extension to the lid and whose ends slot into two notches in the container sidewall.

Both slip lid and hinge lid rectangular containers often have retaining pips or ridges to give a more mechanically secure closure. A strip of pressure sensitive tape can be used as an extra safeguard, i.e. for tamper-evidence and accidental opening. For additional protection and lid security, a complete band of tape can be applied around the junction of the container and lid.

Impact extruded containers

The impact extrusion process is used to produce open-ended collapsible tubes from softer metals such as tin and lead. When aluminium is used, it work-hardens during the forming process and the resultant tubes must be annealed to regain flexibility. Alternatively aluminium tubes may be left in their work-hardened state as rigid containers. Impact extrusion is a particularly useful process to produce containers with a high length to diameter ratio, e.g. up to 7 : 1. A slug of the metal to be formed is held in a female die and is struck by a punch which has the same form as that of the inside of the ultimate container. Upon impact the metal flows up the outside of the punch. A stripper plate then removes the extruded container on its return stroke.

Although any parallel sided shape can be produced, the most common shape is cylindrical. The slug to produce a cylindrical tube is a metal disc approximately equal in diameter to the finished tube. The thickness of the disc governs the volume of metal available to form the tube base and wall. The clearance between punch and base of die governs base thickness. Hence a container could, if required, be produced with a thick base and thin wall section.

Rigid impact extruded aluminium containers

Full aperture rigid extruded aluminium containers are suitable for packing a wide range of dry pharmaceutical products, e.g. powders, tablets and capsules. Although not as inert as glass, they are lighter, more compact and unbreakable and the addition of an internal lacquer is normally adequate to prevent product–container reaction.

An advantage over glass is that relatively small quantities of containers can be printed economically, which obviates the need for labelling. However, in order to effect a true cost comparison, differences in production line speeds must be considered as well as basic container prices.

Containers with restricted apertures suitable for packing liquids can also be produced by first extruding a cylinder and then necking or spinning it in at the open end. Seamless containers in a range of sizes are used for the bulk shipment of expensive items such as perfumes, essential oils, antibiotics, vitamins and hormones. These containers can be designed with no sharp corners so that they can be easily cleaned and sterilised by autoclaving if required.

The use of 'Monobloc' cans produced by this method is usually restricted to smaller sizes for cost reasons, but in countries where aluminium is cheaper relatively large aerosols are produced. Impact extrusion is also used to produce open-ended cylinders onto which bases are seamed, e.g. general purpose liquid containers and two-piece aerosol cans. In this case a ring slug is used rather than a disc, and the lower end is formed in the shape of the shoulder during the extrusion process, e.g. as for collapsible tubes.

Aluminium for impact extruded rigid containers is usually of 99.5% or 99.7%+ purity. A slab of aluminium is rolled down to the required thickness and the slugs stamped out. These slugs are lubricated then fed from hoppers into horizontal or vertical automatic impact extrusion presses where the container is made. The wall thickness for rigid containers is usually in the range 0.2–0.4 mm. After forming, the container is trimmed to length and the appropriate finish applied. This can be a simple inward or outward curl, a screw thread or an outward flange for double seaming. 'Monobloc' aerosol cans are sometimes given an inward domed base for added strength and stability.

Organic fatty chemicals used as lubricants in the extrusion process are washed off in caustic soda and the containers rinsed and dried in ovens. The containers can then be spray lacquered internally with a vinyl or epoxy type lacquer and decorated externally.

Closures

The simplest form of closure for a full aperture container is a friction fitted wadless polyethylene closure, of the snap-on type or the plug fitting type. The rim of the container is usually curled outwards to avoid sharp edges and facilitate closuring, and is ideal since it does not impinge on the fullness of the aperture for filling or dispensing. Friction fitted caps can also be fitted with an integral bellows or spiral device to eliminate the need for separate foam pads or cotton wool packing. To improve protection against moisture ingress a variation of the bellows type of closure can be used in which a small quantity of silica gel is incorporated in a compartment in the cap.

An alternative method, which provides a greater degree of protection than a simple snap-on cap is to apply a screw finish to the container so that it will accept a prethreaded plastic or metal cap. The actual neck finishes applied to metal containers, and hence the caps used, are not identical to those applied to glass. Aluminium caps are usually preferred for compatibility and appearance reasons in that they can be made to match the container itself. Like the container they can be plain or lacquered internally and externally and decorated or embossed/debossed with a logotype. Due to their relatively shallow depth, caps are produced by drawing rather than impact extrusion.

Although such aluminium caps may be fitted with any of the commercially available cap liner materials, it is becoming increasingly common to use a flowed-in PVC or EVA liner. Smaller sizes may incorporate a complete disc whereas larger sizes only require a circular gasket to mate with the rim of the container.

To achieve an even distribution of the compound and ensure the optimum seal, it is preferable that the cap has a circular channel into which the gasket is flowed. Closure efficiency is further improved if the rim of the container is curled inwards to give a smooth edge and gives an effect similar to a body bead in strengthening the container where it most needs it, and facilitates the capping operation. Size for size the efficiency of the closure obtained by this method is similar to that for a glass bottle with a foil-faced cap liner. Such closures are preferable to desiccant closures for products such as gelatin capsules.

Where the ultimate in protection is required, aluminium containers can be flanged and fitted with seamed-on aluminium easy-open ends. These containers are tamper-evident, but once opened the product must be used within a short space of time, unless polyethylene overcaps can be used during the use of the product.

An alternative tamper-evident feature consists of a foil laminate diaphragm which is heat sealed across the aperture of the can before capping. Child-resistant closures are being developed for aluminium tablet containers similar to those used on glass and plastic bottles and vials. Carnaud Metal Box is marketing a version of the Pop-Lok closure developed by Safety Packaging Corporation, NJ, USA. This closure is of the friction fitted plug type and operates on the press and lift principle. If the container were required to be tamper-evident as well as child-resistant this could be achieved by combining with a foil diaphragm as described above.

Reduced aperture containers for liquids are usually fitted with screw caps similar to those described above for full aperture containers for dry products. The larger containers used for bulk chemicals are often fitted with additional safety devices such as tinplate or polyethylene wells or shives and crimped-on tamper-evident overcaps for extra security. At the other and of the scale is the miniature aluminium bottle of capacity 4 ml which is used in the UK for a breath deodoriser and has a polyethylene neck insert swaged into the open end of the container, enabling a conventional screw closure to be used.

Impact extruded collapsible metal tubes

Collapsible metal tubes are used extensively for packaging a wide range of pharmaceutical and cosmetic creams, pastes, ointments, jellies and semi-liquids.

Metal tubes are impermeable to moisture, gas, odour and light provided they are adequately closed. They are convenient for a customer or patient to use and as the contents are expelled by squeezing the tube, there is no tendency for the walls to recover their original shape when the pressure is released. Consequently the risk of air entering the pack and reacting with the product or causing it to dry out is minimised. Internal coating may be necessary to prevent chemical reaction. The joint properties of impermeability and collapsibility are advantages over most plastic tubes, which are not only permeable but also tend to snap back into their original shape after each application.

The properties of metal and plastic have been combined in the form of a laminated tube, which consists of a polyethylene/aluminium foil/polyethylene or similar laminated body fitted with a polyethylene nozzle and is less permeable than a conventional polyethylene tube with less tendency to draw air back. To date the main usage of laminated tubes has been for toothpastes, but wider pharmaceutical applications are now found.

The basic extrusion process used for metal collapsible tubes is identical with that used to produce rigid aluminium containers except that the slugs used are rings rather than discs and the female die which holds the slug is shaped so that the metal is forced downwards into the die to form the shoulder and nozzle as well as upwards around the plunger (Figure 10.2).

The formed tubes then pass to a trimming machine where they are cut to length, a thread cut or rolled on the nozzle, and the face of the nozzle orifice cleaned. The shoulder, which is relatively rigid, may be decorated, e.g. with concentric rings, if required. The tubes are then ready for the finishing operations of internal coating, enamelling, printing and capping.

Whereas rigid containers can only be produced from aluminium, collapsible tubes can be produced from any of the softer metals such as aluminium, tin, lead and tin/lead alloys. Aluminium tubes must be annealed after forming and finishing, otherwise they are too springy. This process also serves to remove all traces of lubricant.

Tin is the least reactive of the metals available, is very bright and is also non-toxic. However, it is inherently expensive and its usage is therefore restricted to pharmaceuticals such as antibiotic and some ophthalmic ointments where maximum protection is

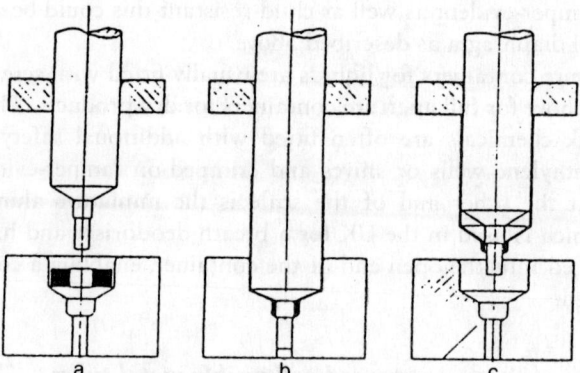

(a) Pierced slug in die of impact extrusion press
(b) Impact of punch
(c) Retraction of punch: tube removed by stripper plate

Figure 10.2 Collapsible metal tubes produced by impact extrusion

required. Lead-based tubes are now not recommended for pharmaceutical products, for toxicity reasons.

The majority of collapsible tubes are made from aluminium, which is relatively cheap but subject to attack by some acidic or alkaline products. The widespread use has been made possible by the development of internal coating systems which are sprayed into the tube immediately after forming it. A wide range of coatings are used including vinyl, epoxy and phenolic resins. The use of epoxy and phenolic resins is restricted to aluminium tubes due to the high curing temperatures required. Most internal lacquering systems involve two coatings, the first being partially dried before applying a second coat and drying completely. Needless to say, where lacquers are used it is essential that they be pinhole-free for the whole length of the inside of the tube, including the interior of the nozzle. After the internal coating has been applied the tubes are enamelled externally, baked, printed and the print dried by heating again. It is essential that the enamel and print – as well as the internal coating – be flexible or the tube may become unsightly when the product is dispensed.

The finished tubes are then capped automatically and packed into shipping outers for dispatch to the packers. Tubes are normally packed open end upwards, for ease of removal, in fully divisional slip lid fibreboard outers, sufficiently rigid to protect the tubes from denting in transit and impeding the filling and closing operation. It is also important to avoid contamination of the open tubes during transit and in storage.

An interesting development which is claimed to save over 75% in storage space was the conical tube developed by the Metal Closures Group in the UK. The tube is extruded as a parallel sided tube and then expanded mechanically at the open end to form a slightly tapered shape. Empty tubes can be nested for shipment to the packer where a special dispensing unit is necessary to feed them into the filling and closing machine. The tubes are also flared slightly at the open end to minimise mechanical damage of the decoration between tubes.

Closures and closuring

A collapsible tube has two closures, one formed at the open end by the packer after the product has been filled, the other at the nozzle through which the customer expels the contents of the tube. The majority of reclosable tubes are fitted with screw closures or flip-top variants on screw closures.

Thermoset caps are fitted with any of the commercially available cap liners used in caps for glass bottles and rigid metal tubes. The choice of liner facing depends on satisfying product compatibility requirements. Injection moulded polyethylene and polypropylene closures have gained ground, since a separate liner is unnecessary due to the inherent softness of these materials. Sometimes a pattern of concentric rings is embossed in the sealing surface to deter leakage. Alternatively an internal plug may be incorporated in the cap so as to form a seal with the nozzle bore (Figure 10.3).

Various shapes of cap are used, the most common being the straight taper or flowerpot style. Full skirted caps are occasionally used so that the tube may be displayed standing vertically on its cap without a carton. Most metal tubes are in fact individually cartoned after filling to facilitate handling, storage and inclusion of a leaflet, etc.

Although the tube filling and closing machine may incorporate a device for tightening any loose caps, the main concern of the packer is to ensure a leakproof permanent seal at the open end after the product has been filled. This is achieved by shaping the tube, folding it over on itself and crimping it. In general the effectiveness of the closure increases with the number of folds. However, it should be borne in mind that the more

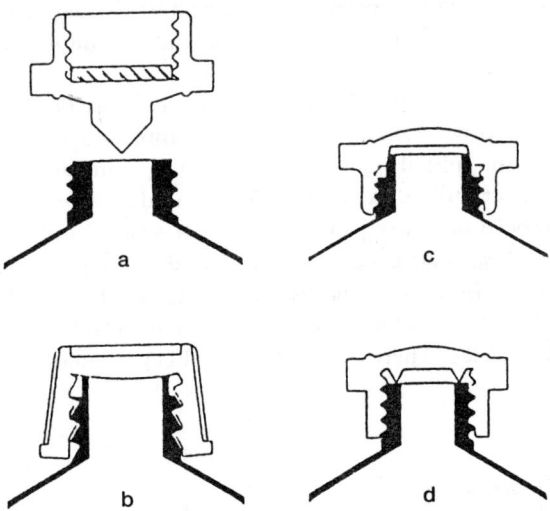

(a) Membrane sealed with 'v' thread and spiked piercing cap of urea, wadded
(b) Buttress thread and polythene wadless cap
(c) Urea wadless cap on 'v' thread
(d) Urea wadless cap on 'v' thread and with special sealing device

Figure 10.3 Caps for collapsible tubes

complex folds require a greater length of tube. A saddle fold requires 10 mm more than a double fold (Figure 10.4).

With printed tubes it is essential to leave an adequate unprinted section at the end of the tube so that the design is not obscured when the fold is made. The base enamel can be continued virtually to the end of the tube where a registration mark is usually incorporated, and picked up by a photoelectric cell on the filling machine to ensure that the tubes are closed and crimped in the appropriate position relative to the printed design. Provided the design is not too complicated, it is possible to arrange for it to be repeated three or more times around the circumference of the tube so that registration of the crimp is not necessary.

The crimp pattern which is applied on the final fold often incorporates a space for batch and expiry marking. Care is needed to ensure that the enamel or metal – particularly the harder metals such aluminium – is not pierced by the debossing action. As an additional insurance against leakage at the end fold, a band of anti-seeping compound is often applied by the tube manufacturer just inside the open end of the tube. Various compounds are used including wax, rubber, latex, pressure sensitive materials and vinyl lacquers. These must be checked for product compatibility in the same way that the tube material and internal coating is tested. Sometimes heated closing jaws are used to obtain the maximum benefit from vinyl-type lacquers.

Nozzles

Collapsible tubes are produced in a range of standard diameters, the length being selected to suit the required fill volume and method of closing. The nozzle and orifice size are governed by the viscosity of the product and the amount to be dispensed per application.

Many pharmaceutical products require special applicator nozzles which are permanently attached to the tube. Alternatively, separate applicators may be supplied for fitting onto the end of the tube (by screwing or pushing) immediately prior to use. With many products, contact with a metal applicator is undesirable. Elongated plastic nozzles have therefore been developed which are either swaged into the tube shoulder in place of the normal metal end or subsequently fitted as a separate component.

When used for ophthalmic tubes the plastic nozzle has the added advantage of eliminating the risk of metal spicules which occasionally result from machining screw threads onto metal nozzles. There is a mandatory FDA standard on particulate conta-

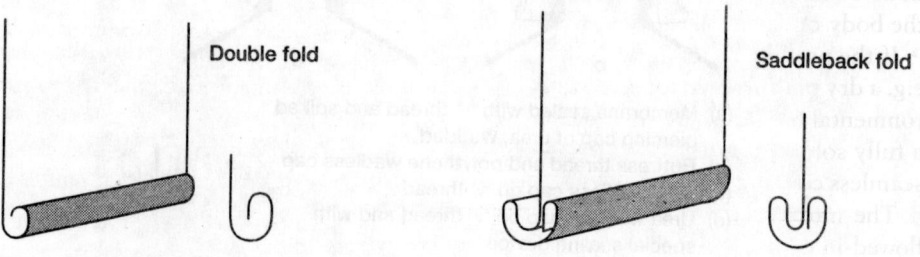

Double fold   Saddleback fold

Figure 10.4 Metal tube-end closures: typical folds

mination of eye ointment tubes including both metal particles and other foreign matter. Special precautions are therefore taken in the production, cleaning and packing of tubes for pharmaceutical applications. Ultrasonic cleaning is sometimes used. Having produced clean tubes, it is then essential to prevent recontamination by careful outer packaging, e.g. by using die-cut non-fibrous divisions and special masking tape to cover the open ends of the tube. Depending on construction, eye ointment tubes are usually sterilised by irradiation or exposure to ethylene oxide prior to filling.

If the ultimate in protection is required, a membrane of metal less than 0.1 mm thick is left across the nozzle face and provides visible tamper-evidence. Sometimes a special double-ended cap is used, incorporating an integral piercing device. The tube is pierced by removing the cap, reversing it and screwing it back onto the tube until the inverted cone pierces the membrane. If the product is of the unit dose type a membrane tube is used without a cap or threaded portion, e.g. taper or torpedo ended tubes. In this case piercing of the nozzle must be carried out with a pin or similar device. Alternatively a break-off style tip can be used.

Built-up containers

Built-up containers consist of at least two components, namely a base and a side wall, which are mechanically secured together by a seamed joint. With the exception of aluminium extruded bodies, the side wall itself also involves a seam. Frequently a third component is affixed permanently to the side wall and it is this extra component which accommodates the closure itself.

Before discussing built-up containers and their closures it is necessary to define the most common forms of seam.

Seams

The seam which joins the two edges of the rectangular blank together to form the container body may consist of a lap seam, a butt seam, a locked seam or a 'Mennen powder' seam. Both lap and butt seams require the addition of a joining compound to make them mechanically secure. The locked seam is strong in tension but weak in compression and is therefore used for containers which need to withstand internal pressures, e.g. aerosols, whereas the 'Mennen' seam is used when the container needs to withstand compression, e.g. talcum powder containers (Figure 10.5).

The seam of the base to the body may be a simple crimped seam, a single seam or a double seam. The double seam is the most secure mechanically. The seam of the end to the body or side wall is often referred to as a chime.

If the product is not difficult to contain, and there is no problem of moisture ingress, e.g. a dry product or viscous liquid, and does not require complete protection from environmental hazards, a dry jointed container seam may be adequate. At the other extreme a fully soldered or welded can will offer the ultimate in protection, i.e. equivalent to a seamless container. The process of soldering or welding also aids mechanical strength.

The most common other method of seam treatment is by lining the ends with a flowed-in compound such as rubber latex or synthetic rubber during manufacture. On subsequent double seaming these compound lined ends are capable of giving hermetic seals. The alternative is to treat the joint after forming with a solvent-based lacquer

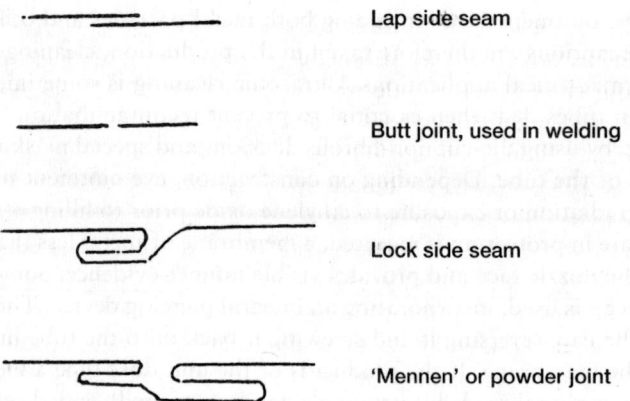

Figure 10.5 Typical metal joints used in tinplate containers

(known as doping or solutioning). If the joining compound is applied during the seam forming operation it is known as cementing. Solutioning and cementing are usually encountered with side seams.

Can dimensions are expressed in terms of nominal diameter (or base dimensions if rectangular) × height. By tradition the first digit is in inches and the second pair in six-teenths, for example, 202 × 408 represents a cylindrical can of diameter $2\frac{1}{8}$ and height $4\frac{1}{2}$ inches.

Container fabrication – the open-top can

The actual process of forming the container is probably best described by taking the open top food or beverage can as an example. Sheets of metal (0.12–0.30 mm thick), pre-printed and lacquered if required, are slit first in one direction and then at right angles to produce blanks of the correct size. A stack of these blanks is fed into the bodymaker where each blank is notched at one side and slits are cut in the other side after which the seam hooks are formed.

The body blank is formed into a cylinder over a mandrel and the hooks are engaged and rolled closed to form the side seam, which is then soldered or welded. A recent development consists of making a cylinder long enough for three bodies, which is parted across previously made score lines into three separate can bodies. Speeds of up to 900 bodies per minute can be achieved, compared with around 500 for the conventional method.

The exact shape of the blank is dictated by the necessity of forming a locked seam for the whole length of the cylinder except for the two extremes which are left as a lap seam. The open ends of the cylinder are then flanged outwards. There are thus two overlaid thicknesses where the seam is flanged rather than the four which would have resulted if the locked seam had been extended for the full length of the cylinder. This is extremely important for the next stage, which is double seaming the base into position. The base or end is previously punched out and a lining compound flowed into the rim. The base is supported by an internal chuck while the body flange is held in position and the double seam is made by a series of rollers. During this operation the body flange is doubled back on itself to form a hook which engages with a similar hook in the base to form the double seam. Although the seamer is able to cope with the change from two or four thicknesses of side wall, it would not be able to accommodate the increase from four to eight thicknesses if the flange consisted of a locked rather than a lapped seam (Figure 10.6).

If the metal is TFS rather than tinplate then a variation of the process is used, since TFS cannot be soldered. Instead the side seam can be made by welding, which gives much higher output speeds. The welding system employs a rectangular blank with no notching or hooking and a simple lap seam (1 mm overlap is adequate). The width of the visible side seam is only 4 mm compared with 20 mm for a soldered tinplate can, resulting in a smaller blank and a saving in tinplate. The finished seam is usually given a side-stripe of lacquer internally and externally for protection. Welding using butt edges is now preferred.

The cementing system also involves a simple lap seam, although the actual overlap is greater (6 mm). The joint is made mechanically secure by applying a strip of plastic (usually Nylon) at one edge of the body blank before forming it into a cylinder. The two overlapped edges are heated to about 300°C to melt the plastic, which then acts as a cement when it cools. Once the side seam has been made the body is flanged and double seamed exactly as for the soldered can (Figure 10.7).

Cans are tested by air pressure on rotating wheels, and faulty ones are automatically rejected. The tested cans are then packed in cases, cages, pallets or directly onto freight cars according to the customer's preference, with end closures shipped separately. Non-cylindrical containers, e.g. rectangular or oval cross-section, are more difficult and slower to make.

Open-top cans themselves are not widely used in the pharmaceutical industry, since by their nature these packs are not reclosable although polyethylene overcaps are sometimes provided for this purpose. An easy opening feature may be incorporated by means of a ring pull device in the lid.

Similar full aperture cylindrical cans are occasionally used for dry pharmaceutical products in conjunction with simple friction closures such as slip lids or plug lids. The open end of the container is usually rolled over to avoid a raw edge. Although these two-piece containers are easily opened and reclosed, the efficiency of the closure is reduced by the presence of the side seam. Consequently they are only used for relatively non-moisture sensitive products, the seams being left untreated. The same considerations apply to rectangular cross-section cans, but there is the additional possibility of applying a hinged lid closure. In general, if the best performance is required from any of these frictional closures it is preferable to use a container with a continuous rather than interrupted side wall. Alternatively, a third (seamless) component can be seamed onto the body, making a three-piece container. The simplest example of this technique is the lever lid or ring and cap container.

Ring and cap containers

In the pharmaceutical industry, ring and cap containers, lever lids or multiple friction containers are mostly used for powders – health salts, dietary supplement powders, etc. – which are only moderately susceptible to moisture pick-up but require an easy and effective reclosure.

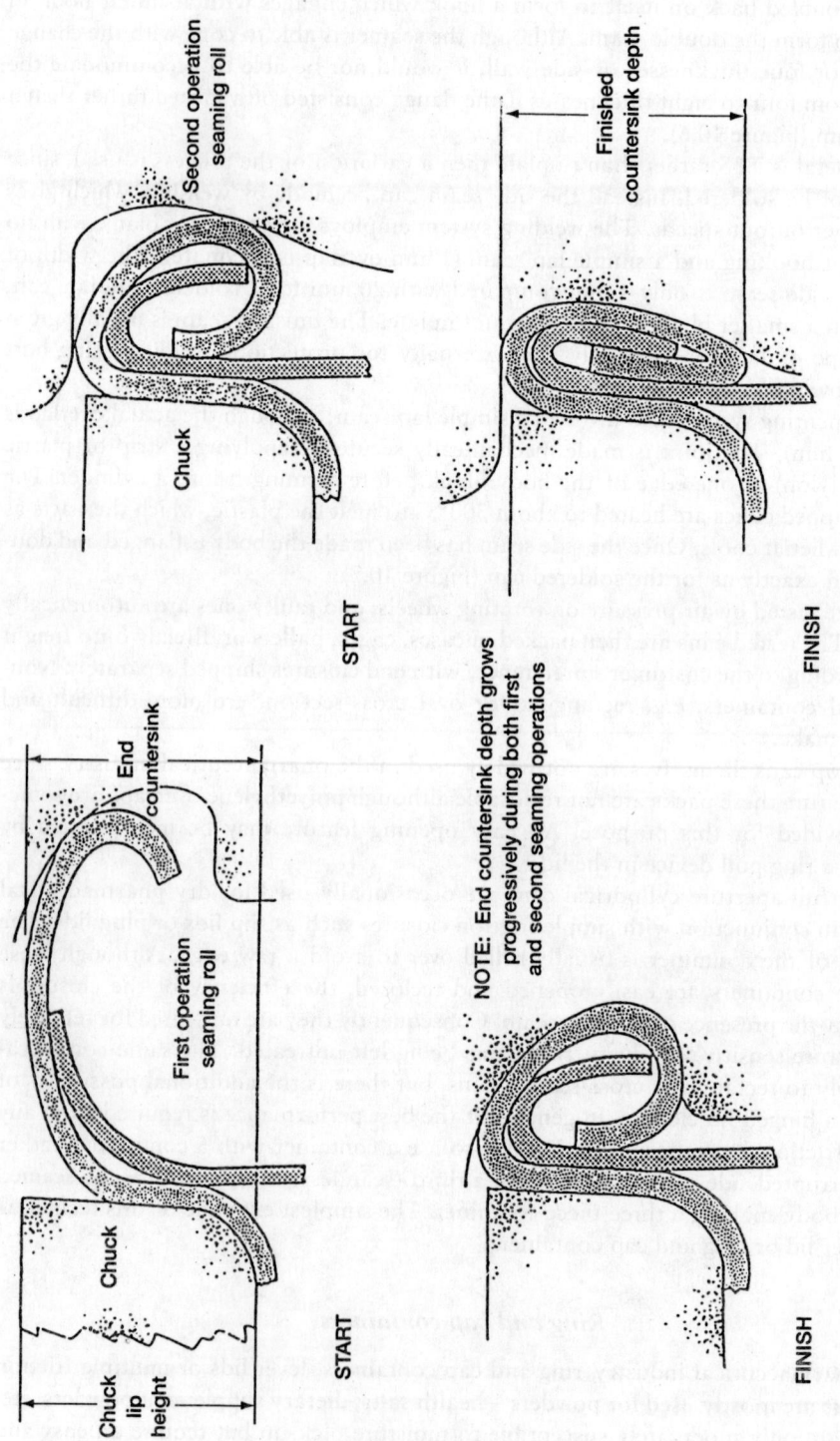

Figure 10.6 Two stages of double seaming

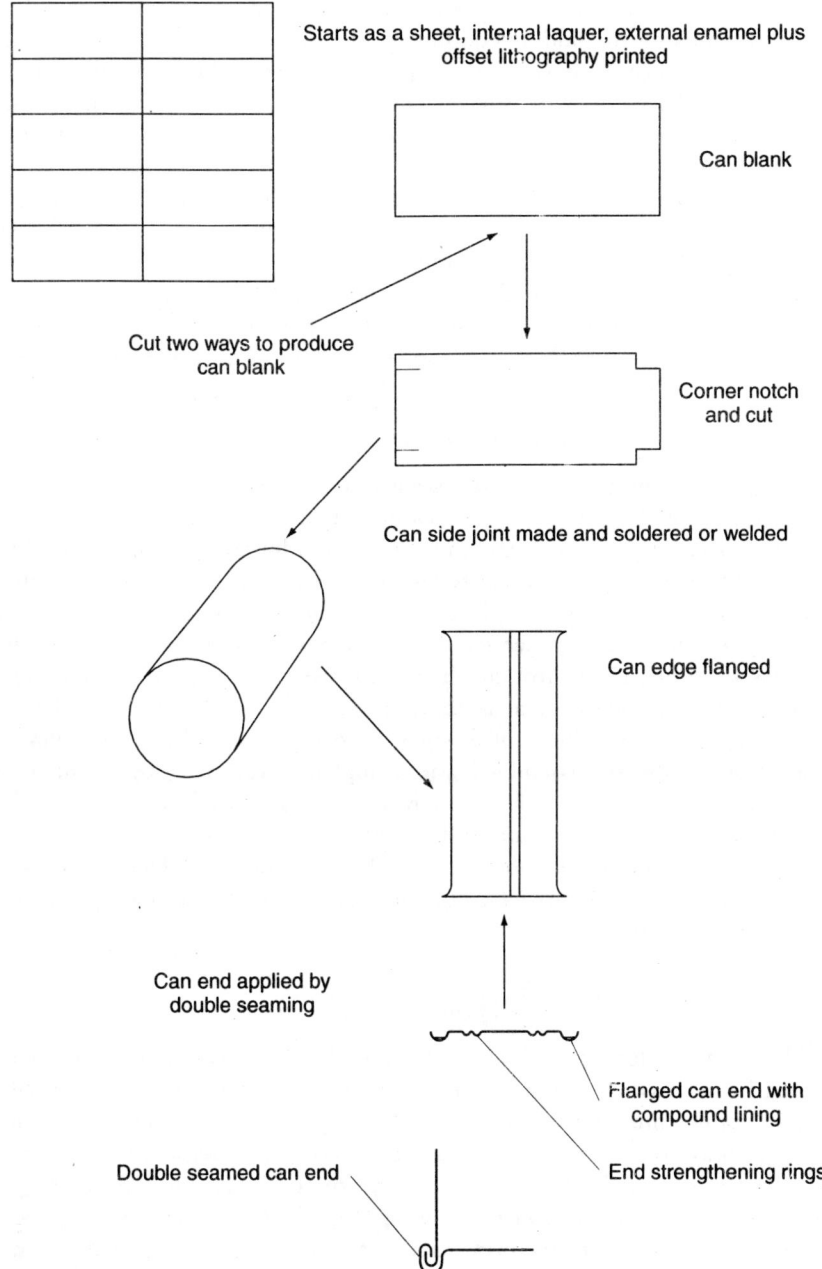

Starts as a sheet, internal laquer, external enamel plus offset lithography printed

Can blank

Cut two ways to produce can blank

Corner notch and cut

Can side joint made and soldered or welded

Can edge flanged

Can end applied by double seaming

Flanged can end with compound lining

Double seamed can end

End strengthening rings

Figure 10.7 Three-piece built-up can (tinplate)

The containers are usually constructed in tinplate with double seam base and 'Mennen powder' side seams since the container needs to be capable of withstanding considerable compression when the lid is applied. The seams themselves may be dry or treated, depending on end use. Since both the ring and the cap are seamless, a very effective frictional closure can be achieved. The amount of interference can be varied and depends on the lidding equipment, the quality of closure desired, and the relative ease with which the customer is required to open and reclose the pack. If necessary, lids can be secured with special clips or spot soldered, the latter adding a degree of tamper-resistance. Sometimes a double ring is used to ensure a more effective closure.

A more elegant method of achieving tamper-evidence is the addition of a diaphragm affixed to the lower side of the ring. In this case the can is supplied to the packer with the diaphragm and lid in place and the other end open for filling. The packer then double seams on the end which will become the base of the closed container. The diaphragm may be simply paper or, if an additional barrier is desired, foil can be used.

Note that the lever lids discussed are applied only to cylindrical containers.

Talcum powder containers

The principle of attaching an extra component so that the packer can add the final closure is also illustrated by the talcum powder container. Talcum powder containers have a simple cross-section, e.g. round, rectangular (with radiused corners) or oval. They are usually constructed of tinplate for cheapness with a single seam base and 'Mennen side seam', both seams being untreated since the container is only required to be relatively siftproof. A shoulder is then either seamed on or pushed on to give a friction fit, and incorporates a central orifice through which the packer fills the powder then plugs with a two piece rotary plastic or metal sprinkler closure. If the shoulder is of the pushed-on variety the packer has a choice of filling and closing as described or receiving shoulders and closures already assembled and completing the pack by pushing on the shoulder. The second alternative has the advantage of giving a larger filling orifice and is preferred where metal closures are to be used since these are not as easy to apply as the plastic type and are probably best left for the container manufacturer to assemble. On the other hand, open two-piece containers with no shoulder lack rigidity and can be very prone to transit damage.

Liquid containers

Reclosable containers for liquid products are usually three-piece containers, the closure itself being formed with the third component. A common example is the cylindrical cone top container fitted with a screw neck to which a conventional cap is applied. Similar necks may be fitted to rectangular section containers with flat rather than conical tops. Press caps can also be used on this type of container. The principle of a press cap is essentially the same as a screw cap except that the tension which is applied to the resilient cap liner is built into the press cap. Since the press cap is opened, as the name implies, by simply pressing on the top of the cap, it is necessary to provide overseal protection against accidental opening and spillage. This type of closure is more frequently encountered with bulk containers.

Nowadays the smaller sizes of round and rectangular section containers for liquids are often fitted with plastic dispensing closures. It is also possible to produce two-piece screw top containers in aluminium in a similar manner to that in which two-piece aluminium aerosol cans are produced. In this case the base, which may be either flat or domed, is invariably constructed in aluminium so that the resultant container may be used for corrosive chemicals without further internal treatment.

Three-piece aerosol cans are constructed by seaming a cone onto the body of a two-piece built-up tinplate can. The can itself is constructed in a similar way to an open top can but with a strengthened locked and lapped side seam so that it will withstand internal pressure. The base of the container is domed upwards for the same reason and is invariably compound-lined and double seamed onto the side wall.

Shipping containers

Built-up metal containers are used for the storage and transport of a wide range of bulk chemicals, e.g. dry powders and liquid. Although the heavier gauges of tinplate can be used for containers of up to about 5 gallons capacity, from this size upwards steel is invariably used.

In the USA steel drums are defined as single-walled shipping containers of capacity 13–110 US gallons, whereas containers of less than 13 gallons are called pails. (In the UK pails may be referred to as kegs.) Pails are constructed from steel of 29 gauge to around 24 gauge. Lightweight drums up to 55 gallons are constructed in steel ranging from 26 to 20 gauge. Heavy drums vary from 18 to 14 gauge. If the ends of drums are constructed of a different gauge from the sidewall, the gauge of the sidewall is quoted first and then the ends, e.g. a 20/18 drum has 20 gauge sidewall and 18 gauge ends. Specifications for pails and drums for packaging dangerous or hazardous products such as acids, flammables, explosives and poisons are governed by the US Department of Transportation regulations.

Steel containers are fabricated from sheet steel in much the same way as open-top cans are made from tinplate. Apart from the obvious difference in size and hence production rate, the main difference in their construction is the nature of the seams. The side seams may be merely folded over if the container is intended for dry products or welded to provide strength and liquid-proofness.

The welded cylinder is then flanged, ready to accept the base and top if applicable. At the same time circumferential corrugations or beads are added to increase the strength of the container. With large drums a pair of extra prominent beads are often applied to serve as rolling hoops. The base may be double- or treble-seamed into position using a seaming compound or solution as for open-top tinplate cans. However, in order to ensure liquid-proofness, a peripheral weld is often applied just inside the double seam itself. In addition the end seam is sometimes protected from mechanical damage by reinforcing it with a band of metal around the chime. With large drums the ends may be welded to the side wall and a reinforcing band either shrunk on or welded into position.

There are two basic types of container, namely open-headed (or full aperture) and tight-headed. The former are used for dry products, semi-solids and viscous liquids whereas the latter are used mainly for liquids. The term 'tight-headed' implies that the top of the container is permanently secured by the drum manufacturer, apertures for filling and emptying being provided in the lid itself. Pails and small drums for liquids usually have only one aperture in the lid but larger drums invariably have two apertures, the second (often smaller) aperture serving as a vent when dispensing the contents. A variety of closures is used including press-caps with overseals, lever type closures, and internal or external screw-threaded closures in metal or plastic. The most commonly used closure is probably the 'Tri-Sure'. This consists of an externally threaded bung fitted with a plastic or rubber gasket plus an overcap.

Closures for open-headed pails and drums are full-diameter lids. The seal is usually effected by a rubber or plastic gasket contained in a channel in the lid. The closure is then completed and made mechanically secure by means of a separate metal closing ring fitted with a bolt or lever type fastening. The lids of pails sometimes incorporate lugs which are mechanically clinched to the upper flange of the pail.

Since pails are small enough to be handled manually, steel handles are often attached for this purpose. It is also common to reduce the diameter of the bottom or top chime to facilitate stacking. These containers are widely used in the pharmaceutical industry for the in-house handling of tablets. Tight-headed pails with one closure only are often fitted with specially shaped tops which have a raised portion instead of a recess above the double seam. This is known as an interrupted chime, and its purpose is to allow the pails to be stored in the open without the risk of water accumulating in the head and penetrating the closure by capillary action.

Although all the containers discussed so far in this section are cylindrical or near cylindrical, small containers are sometimes made with rectangular cross-sections in order to save space in storage. A number of proprietary designs are available, but the best known is probably the 'Jerrican'.

The inner surfaces of drums and pails are usually treated, epoxy and polyurethane resins being the most common. Instead of applying the lacquer to the base sheet it can be sprayed inside the drum after fabrication to ensure that all seams are adequately protected. This is particularly important for welded drums where the welding process destroys the original coating on the sheet. The container is then stoved to cure the resin. The efficacy of the coating depends to a large extent on correct surface preparation, e.g. mechanical roughening or phosphating. A phosphate coating is frequently used externally prior to decoration. Galvanising is used for heavy duty multi-trip drums. In this instance the complete drum is immersed in a bath of molten zinc.

If the product demands complete protection from metal contact, a polyethylene liner can be used. The liner can be applied *in situ* by a sintering process or formed as a separate blow-moulded bottle. The resultant container is more accurately described as a composite container rather than a steel drum, as it combines the virtues of plastic and metal in one container.

Aerosols

Aerosol containers may be produced by any of the main methods for manufacturing metal containers, i.e. by impact extrusion in aluminium, by building-up from tinplate, or by drawing and wall ironing. Since the technology of all metal aerosols, as well as those constructed in other materials, is similar irrespective of the method of construction, it is convenient to group them together under one heading.

The number of aerosol fillings in the UK is approximately 1.25 billion pa, with slightly less in France and Germany giving a total of well over 3 billion for Western Europe and approaching the US figure of 4.0 billion. Total worldwide consumption is over 10.0 billion units. Of these about half are attributable to hairsprays, personal deodorants, antiperspirants, perfumes and other pharmaceutical or cosmetic products.

In this market the choice of container is often based on shape, appearance and possible decorative effects provided that the basic compatibility requirements can be satisfied. Internally applied epoxy–phenolic lacquers are commonly used to prevent interaction between the container and product. Built-up tinplate containers may have an epoxy phenolic side-stripe in addition to protect the seams. Tinplate aerosols account for nearly 90% of the aerosol market in the UK and the USA, the balance being mainly aluminium. The proportion of aluminium aerosols is much higher (~50%) in the rest of Western Europe.

The built-up tinplate container is the cheapest form of aerosol but was initially considered unacceptable for most pharmaceutical products due to the unsightly appearance of the soldered side seam. However, the development of reduced width side seams by jet soldering, cementing or welding e.g. soudronic weld, makes the built-up container a more attractive proposition. Most of the built-up aerosol containers produced in the UK nowadays have welded side seams. Alternatively the side seam can be concealed by applying a printed wrap-around label to the finished aerosol.

Aluminium aerosols are inherently more expensive than tinplate but can be made in one piece with neither side seam nor bottom chime. However, for practical or economic reasons these 'Monobloc' containers are usually restricted to the smaller sizes of aerosol. Larger sizes are produced in two pieces, i.e. with a continuous side wall and a seamed-on base. In the past few years the process of drawing and wall ironing has enabled continuous side wall containers to be produced from both aluminium and tinplate sheet. Unlike two-piece extruded body containers, these containers have no base chime but instead have a seamed-on cone. When two different metals are involved, e.g. aluminium body and tinplate base, additional product compatibility checks must be carried out due to the risk of electrolytic corrosion. Again special coatings are available to inhibit this effect.

Components and types of aerosols

The principle of all aerosols is that a liquefied gas in a pressurised container will provide a constant pressure while the container is being emptied. The essential components of an aerosol beside the container itself are the product, propellant, and valve assembly. The valve is designed to dispense the product in the required manner while maintaining both the product and propellant hermetically sealed until the product is expended. The fact that the product is sealed in the container and protected from air and other outside contaminants has obvious advantages in the field of pharmaceuticals. The intimate mixture of propellant and product in a true aerosol results in a rapid expansion of the propellant as it leaves the valve orifice. This breaks up the product into small particles giving a fine mist, coarse spray, foam, or dust according to the nature and relative quantity of the product and the propellant and the type of valve.

The cup is usually formed in tinplate and incorporates a grommet or flowed-in compound lining (usually nitrile rubber) to ensure a leak-proof seal with the cone. Except for the smallest 'Monobloc' containers, the cone is invariably fitted with a standard 1 inch aperture. The method of closing the valve cup into the cone – known as crimping, clinching or, more correctly, swaging – consists of mechanically expanding the valve cup just below the curl of the cone so that the joint is mechanically secure and when filled the pack is able to withstand pressures of up to 150 lb/in^2. The swaging process is naturally critical, and the swage depth and diameter must be closely controlled to avoid leakage (Figure 10.8).

In the centre of the valve cup is mounted the valve housing into which fits the valve stem itself. This is maintained in the 'off' position by a stainless steel spring. The valve is opened by depressing or tilting the actuator or button when the product is dispensed via a dip tube. A seal between the valve housing and cup is usually affected by a neoprene or nitrile rubber gasket. The spray is influenced by valve design, product/propellant system and also the dip tube bore.

A wide variety of propellants originally included the fluorinated chlorinated hydrocarbons, paraffin hydrocarbons such as propane and butane and inert gases. Originally the use of fluorochlorohydrocarbons was predominant but there has been a trend to the straight paraffin hydrocarbon or alternative HFAs. The main disadvantage with hydrocarbon propellants is their flammability and the need for special filling plant. Most of these gases in the liquefied state fulfil the function of a true two-phase aerosol, i.e. for a given temperature they provide a fixed pressure as the product/propellant mixture is expelled, providing there is always some liquid propellant left. The pressure is usually within the range 10–70 lb/in^2 at 21°C and mixtures of propellants are used to achieve the desired pressure. Compatibility with the product formulation is obviously the other main requirement. The liquid propellant may be either in solution with the product (the vast majority of aerosols) when it produces a true aerosol spray or in an emulsion with the product whereby a foam is produced. With powder aerosols the product is dispersed in the propellant itself with the assistance of a dispersing agent.

There is another class of aerosols, known as single phase aerosols, in which the propellant is a compressed inert gas, for example carbon dioxide, nitrogen and nitrous oxide. With this type of pack a high pressure is used initially (90–150 lb/in^2) since the internal pressure diminishes as the container is emptied. A single phase aerosol is more acceptable as a foam dispenser for toothpaste and hand cream than a spray pack, but if used inverted all the gas will be released quickly (unless it is specifically designed to be used inverted) and the product will remain with no means of dispensing it.

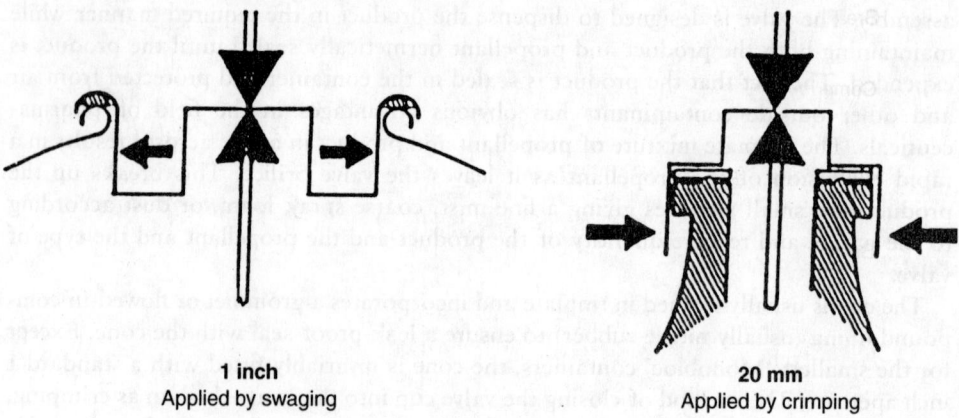

1 inch
Applied by swaging

20 mm
Applied by crimping

Figure 10.8 Aerosol cups

There is a third class of aerosols which use a three phase system consisting of separate layers of liquid propellant, product (usually aqueous) and propellant vapour. These often operate at low pressures.

Valves

The type of valve used is selected according to the formulation, the propellant system and the way in which the product is to be delivered. There are five main types of valve, namely spray, foam, stream, metering, and drop dispensing valves. Spray valves themselves can be classified according to the proportion of propellant in the formulation and the nature of the active ingredient. The metering valve type is used in pharmaceuticals in conjunction with a specially designed applicator cap for throat, lung inhalations and nasal sprays. A unique pharmaceutical application is the pain relieving spray which relies entirely on the cooling effect of 100% propellant vapour. Suspensions of antiseptic powders or talcum demand yet another type of valve, as do spray-on bandages. Compartmental aerosols have been developed for products which are basically incompatible with conventional propellant systems. The product is contained either in a plastic bag or on the upper side of a piston. Product filling is accomplished in the normal manner from the top but the propellant is filled through a small valve in the base of the can. One example of the former is the Press Pak produced by Cebal.

Currently metered dose inhalations are showing significant growth, particularly for the treatment of asthma (Figure 10.9).

Filling and packaging

The process of filling aerosol containers involves four main operations, namely product filling, purging, swaging, and propellant filling, the order of which may be varied. There are two filling methods, 'cold filling' and 'pressure filling'.

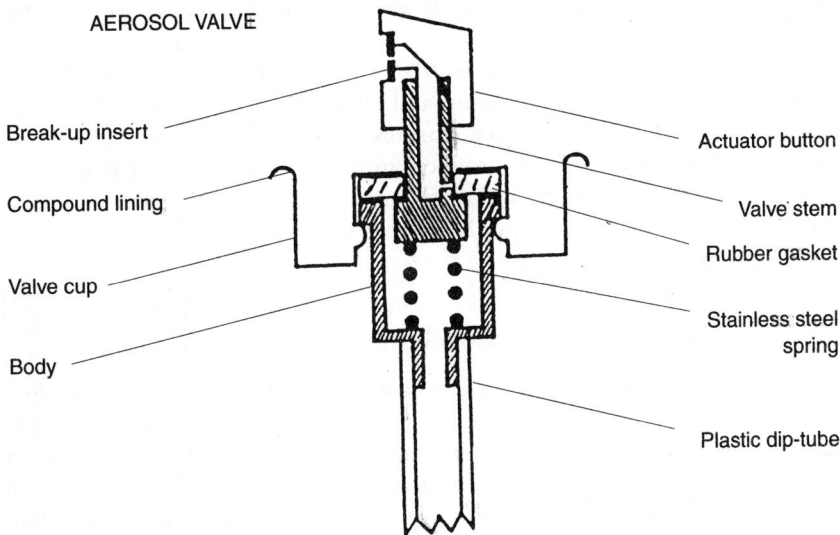

Figure 10.9 Aerosol valves

In cold filling both the product and propellant are refrigerated and filled volumetrically as liquids through the 1 inch aperture before the valve is swaged into position. (This process is self-purging.) The product formulation must be able to withstand cooling. Pressure filling also begins with product filling but the propellant is handled as a gas. After the product has been filled – allowing for headspace – it is purged with propellant vapour and the valve swaged or clinched in position. The bulk of propellant is then filled either through or around the valve system. Special valves are available to allow filling – through the button. A variation of pressure filling – known as under cup filling – is first to fill the product and then, with the valve loosely in position, to draw a vacuum on the container, inject the propellant under the cup and finally swage the valve cup onto the container. Pressure filling equipment is more expensive than cold filling equipment, but the running costs are lower.

With all these processes, removal of the headspace air by vacuum or purging with propellant vapour is essential, as otherwise the internal pressure would be lowered.

After filling and closuring, the containers are tested in a water bath at 55°C or above to check for leakage. The containers are then dried, and the buttons applied. All containers are spray tested in a special spray booth. Unprinted containers are then labelled and covers applied. At this stage some products are trayed off, then check weighed for losses following a storage period (allowing for swelling of gaskets).

Sometimes a two-part cover is used where the inner section serves as an actuator and the outer section is rigid and performs the usual function of a cover in preventing accidental spraying by top pressure. The capped and labelled aerosols are then either packed into outers with or without divisions, or shrink wrapped.

Cautionary wording such as 'Pressurised container, Protect from sunlight, Do not expose to temperatures exceeding 50°C, Do not puncture or burn, even after use, Do not spray on a naked flame or any incandescent material' is mandatory in many countries. If the spray emitted when the valve is operated is adjudged to be flammable according to the appropriate standard test method, then this must also be stated. Such warning statements are often required on the outer packaging as well as the unit container.

Another requirement which is likely to become of increasing importance with aerosols is the demand for child-resistant and tamper-evident closures. Although current FDA legislation only requires such closures to be applied to oven cleaners, it may well be extended to other aerosol products including some pharmaceuticals, and a number of approved child-resistant closures are already available. Most of these closures rely on the user either replacing the overcap or rotating the cap to a safe position for their effectiveness.

Conclusion

Metal containers still play a very important role in packaging, accounting for one-quarter of the total sales of all packaging materials. In the total UK production of metal containers, 10% is aluminium, the remainder being mainly tinplate. To put this figure into perspective it is worth noting that only 4% of total steel production is accounted for by packaging end uses. Although the proportion of aluminium used for packaging is considerably higher at 16%, it does not reach the dominant levels achieved for glass, paper or even plastics.

Notwithstanding the relatively small contribution of metals used for packaging compared with other uses, efforts are constantly being made to reduce the amount of material used for each application. For example, the use of thinner steel base materials and lighter weight tin coatings helps to conserve the world's resources as well as reducing costs. The development of replacements for tin coatings and the extended usage of tin-free steel will help in prolonging supplies of this scarce resource. Alternative manufacturing techniques such as DRD, DWI and the use of welding rather than soldering all give material savings.

Most packaging is non-returnable and is destined to end its life – or at least its primary life – in the refuse bin. Although nearly all packaging ends up as rubbish, by no means does all rubbish consist of packaging. A study in the UK by Incpen (Industry Committee for Packaging and the Environment) has shown that packaging materials account for only 28% by weight of domestic rubbish. The contribution of metals to this is about the same as that for glass at approximately 8%. It should be borne in mind that these estimates are based on weight and do not take into account density considerations, the presence of hollow-ware or compaction.

The fact that most packaging is one-trip is particularly true with pharmaceuticals, where the hazards of contamination and admixtures far outweigh other considerations. Hence the emphasis on recovery and recycling of the basic materials rather than reusing containers is to be welcomed.

Although tin comprises less than 0.5% by weight of tinplate, its recovery is now an economic proposition, but mostly from the waste which occurs at various stages of production. The recovery of metals from domestic mixed waste is naturally more difficult owing to the difficulties of sorting and general contamination.

Another factor governing the viability of recycling is the energy content of the material concerned. As energy becomes more expensive it will become increasingly more attractive to recover those materials such as aluminium which are not in themselves scarce but where the energy content is relatively high.

Supplementary notes on foil (aluminium) and its use in packaging applications

In the early 1930s foil could be found as tin foil, lead foil (widely found as a lining in tea chests), and aluminium foil. The fact that the general public picked up the word 'tin foil' and carried it forward from generation to generation has caused a certain amount of embarrassment, in that virtually all uses of the earlier 'tin foil' have now been replaced by aluminium foil. The USA, however, still uses tin foil as a cap lining material, with small similar usage in Europe.

Most aluminium is derived mainly from an ore called bauxite, which produces approximately 1 tonne of aluminium from 4 tonnes of ore and is a high energy intensive process. As a result of this, aluminium is widely produced and used in those countries which have the cheapest energy supplies, e.g. hydroelectric power. Aluminium is one of the lighter metals with a density of 2.7 (note that glass lies between 2.25 and 2.5, covering neutral and soda glasses).

The production of aluminium foil

Aluminium foil is produced from a billet or ingot of aluminium hot rolled to a strip with a thickness from around 5–6 mm down to 0.4–0.5 mm (foil strip). Since aluminium undergoes a phenomenon called work hardening, the coiled foil strip is subsequently annealed to reduce the hardness. This is then cold rolled to around 0.038 to 0.025 mm when, to produce even thinner gauges of foil, two plies are brought together for the final rolling processes. When these two layers are ultimately separated, gauges of 0.006 (6 µm) to 0.025 (25 µm) are achieved with one side (outside) bright and one side (inside) matt.

Foil rolling involves high speeds (1000 to 2000 ft per minute), high pressures (0.25 to 0.75 t/in^2), and long areas as the material halves in thickness and doubles in length during each pass. Lubricants both ease the rolling action and help to remove the heat generated by the rolling processes.

If soft foil is required (note that further work hardening has occurred in these processes), the material is again annealed. Since the foil is constantly lubricated to aid the rolling process, the final annealing burns off the lubricant which would otherwise make coating, lamination, printing, etc. difficult. In the case of hard foil the lubricant is removed either by a lower heating treatment or by solvent (more expensive). The annealing temperature for aluminium lies between 400 and 500°C. The lubricant used in the rolling process includes various oils such as cocoa butter.

The thinner gauge foils are considered commercially free from pinholes at 17 µm and above. Pinholes occur from small particles of dust and grit which contaminate the foil during the rolling process. A typical figure today for 0.009 mm (9 µm) soft foil would be 200 per m^2. Typical foil yields at these thinner gauges (see Table 10.2) are:

- 9 µm – 29,000 in^2/lb
- 12 µm – 22,000 in^2/lb
- 25 µm – 10,400 in^2/lb.

The properties of aluminium foil

These properties generally apply to both hard and soft foil.

1 Foil normally carries an extremely low bioburden and, provided it is dry, does not support microbial growth.

Table 10.2 Aluminium foil caliper/gauge/area

Europe		USA		
Thickness (µm)	Yield (g/m^2)	Thickness (Mil)	Yield	
			(lb/in^2)	(lb/m^2)
6	16.3	0.24	0.105	0.036
9	24.4	0.35	0.155	0.054
25	68	1	0.96	0.15

All data are approximate. Foil yield might vary if either side carries a wash coating. 1 Mil = 0.001 in.

2 Foil provides a good printing surface (usually by flexography or gravure printing). However, ink adhesion may deteriorate with storage time, hence the surface is often coated with a primer or wash coating of $1-2 \text{ g/m}^2$, e.g. nitrocellulose and vinyls.
3 Light in weight.
4 Exhibits dead-fold characteristics – stays relatively flat when folded.
5 Impermeable to moisture, gases, etc. if pinhole-free.
6 Excludes light (i.e. totally opaque).
7 Reflective to both light and heat.
8 Relatively resistant to corrosion, oils and greases.
9 High yield in thin gauges.
10 Taint and odour resistance.
11 Readily attached to other materials (laminations, heat sealants, etc.).
12 Alternative surface finishes, e.g. embossed, mechanically grained, extra bright, matt both sides, anodised, etched.
13 Non-toxic – broad inertness.
14 Non-magnetic, good electrical conductor.
15 Good heat conductor (cold and heat).
16 Does not burn/heat-resistant (cf. plastic).

There are also a few negative features.

- May be extensible in thin gauge – hence may stretch and perforate.
- Not heat sealable unless coated or laminated.
- Creases fairly easily – may increase level of pinholes and perforations.
- Scuff and rub resistance – foil will abrade fairly easily (foil to foil, foil to product, etc.), producing dark particles.
- Foil can be attacked by stronger acids and alkalis.
- Foil may corrode in contact with other metals as an electrolytic cell is set up when the product (or condensed moisture) acts as an electrolyte. To minimise corrosion risks, storage in a warm dry place is recommended.

Uses of aluminium foil

Aluminium foil has found a wide range of packaging applications. These include foods, drinks, pharmaceutical, toiletry, cosmetic, etc. Foil, although primarily used for its barrier properties, is widely used for its quality image and decorative appeal coupled to effective machinery handling. Gauges normally range from around 40 μm down to 6 μm, with soft foil being predominant. A few applications for hard foil are found, with a major use being as a lidding for pharmaceutical push-through blister packs. The tensile strength of hard to soft foil is usually of the ratio 8 : 3.

Unsupported foil

Early use of aluminium foil (well before the introduction of plastic and plastic coatings) involved unsupported foil, but this has limited use in the pharmaceutical industry.

Supported foil

The extensibility of foil has already been quoted as one possible disadvantage whereby the material would show stretch and possible perforation. This results in most foils being supported by the use of cellulosics including paper and board, plastic films or coatings, etc.

The fact that foil has no heat seal properties initially limited expansion of foil usage (until plastic heat sealants became more readily available). Early heat sealants included waxes and microcrystalline waxes, either on their own or as coated or impregnated paper. Subsequent to the use of wax, other heat seal (HS) coatings and then the seal plies (polyethylene and pliofilm) were developed. Heat seal coatings (as distinct from materials which also act as a barrier ply) are usually less than 25 g/m^2 whereas film plies used as a heat sealant usually start around 20 g/m^2. Weights for a coating start around 4 g/m^2 and are offered in 2–3 g/m^2 ranges up to 25 g/m^2 as previously quoted. For further details on how foil may be bonded to other materials (wet and dry bonding, extrusion coating, etc.), see Chapter 9.

Where foil is laminated to paper, attention must be paid to both the composition of the paper and moisture content if subsequent corrosion is to be avoided. Ideally the moisture should be 7% and less, and chloride and sulphate controlled so that the pH (acidity) is not below 5. If the foil is laminated by an adhesive, similar factors apply.

Example of foil usages are:

1   general overwrapping (as an additional moisture barrier)
2   sachets for a wide range of products, e.g. various powders, liquids, shampoos
3   diaphragm seals for various containers by adhesion, heat seal or induction sealing
4   linings for closure facings (waxed or unwaxed)
5   seals and labels
6   lined carton systems for solids and liquids (Hermatet, Cekatainer, Tetrapak, Combibloc, etc.)
7   linings (inner or outer) for composite container packs (spiral or convolute windings)
8   strip packs/blister packs
9   push-through lidding – hard or soft foil
10 cold formed foil blisters
11 tear tapes (as used on various film wraps)
12 hot foils stamping – special printing 'foils'
13 collapsible tubes – laminated materials.

In these applications foil is contributing to such aspects as tamper-evidence/resistance, child-resistance (sachets, strips, blisters, pouches, etc.) and high barrier packs, and many have special features related to the use of aluminium foil. Some of these special features are identified below.

Selecting a gauge or foil

Foil gauges down to 6 μm are now available. However, the amount of 'support' required tends to increase as the gauge reduces; e.g. 0.025 mm foil laminated to 30 or 25 g/m^2 LDPE is a widely used strip pack laminate. In theory an 0.018 mm foil laminated to 30 g/m^2 LDPE would be a more economical proposition. However, this combination would likely exhibit stretch, hence would possibly tear and perforate the foil. As a result it is necessary to increase the tensile strength of the support ply, e.g. by the addition of paper. Thus if cost savings are to be made the final laminate will probably be:

- 37 g/m^2 GIP (paper)/0.009 or 0.007 mm foil/25 g/m^2 LDPE or Surlyn
- 44 g/m^2 GIP (paper)/0.008 or 0.007 mm foil/25 g/m^2 LDPE or Surlyn.

Opinions vary on the gauge of foil to use as the outer paper (printed) may have an anti-scuff overlacquer which also adds to the overall strength of the material. Paper/foil/heat seal is generally preferred.

Since the above has moved from a double-ply construction to a multi-ply lamination (the paper to foil may be an adhesive or extrusion coating), the latter is more costly to produce. As a result of this, any change to the new combination is only likely to be economical (how increase in cost of manufacture is counterbalanced by the reduction in material costs – i.e. savings on foil) if the thinnest gauge of foil 'acceptable' is employed. What is 'acceptable' depends on the product properties (is it extremely moisture or oxygen sensitive?) and the handling characteristics of the processing equipment.

Pinholes and pinhole theory

The significance of pinholes in foil has a relatively small influence on the overall barrier properties, provided the pinholes are 'filled in' on either or both sides by a plastic film or coating. Pinholes normally occur randomly and are usually less than 25 μm (0.001 inches) in diameter. Due to the random nature, a proportion fall in the seal area and non-seal area of most packs. Where the pinhole falls into the latter, the permeability relates to the area of the pinholes and the permeability of the film(s) involved.

If the water vapour transmission rate for LDPE is 3 g/m^2 per 24 h at 38°C 90% RH for 25 μm, then permeability for a single 50 μm pinhole is likely to be as follows.

Area of pinhole (a circle) = πr^2

One pinhole = 3.1416 × (0.025)^2 mm
              = 0.00197 mm^2

Moisture permeation over 1 year (as mg)

$$\frac{0.00197 \ (mm^2)}{1000 \times 1000 \ (m^2)} \times 3000 \ mg \times 365 \ days = 0.00215 \ mg$$

i.e. permeation through a defined single pinhole is 0.00215 mg per year or a negligible amount, and for a sachet containing five pinholes per side (ten in total), permeation over 5 years is in theory only 0.11 mg. For example, with a layer of LDPE on both sides of the foil permeation should be even lower. Further details on pinholes can be obtained from the PIRA/BAFRA report published in 1974 and entitled *Barrier Properties of Aluminium Foil*.

In general, a foil-bearing laminate containing a few pinholes is an excellent barrier material and significantly superior to most economical plastic materials. This picture only changes if the foil lamination become perforated by handling operations which may include creases and creasing. If creases into a heat seal area lead to capillary-type leakage this may also reduce the overall barrier properties. Capillary channel leakage is more likely to be highlighted by temperature changes in cycling conditions (the pack expands and contracts, hence undergoes a breathing action) which are less likely to occur if stored under a controlled condition environment, e.g. 25°C 60% RH or 40°C 75% RH, i.e. ICH conditions.

Permeability to gases may be more critical than moisture. Gas permeabilities of plastics generally follow the ratio of 1:4:20 for nitrogen to oxygen to carbon dioxide and are usually significantly greater than moisture permeability.

Laminates for collapsible tubes

The use of laminates for collapsible tubes is an example of the success of a new approach. The fact that the word 'collapsible' has been maintained indicates that the pack may be subjected to rather severe handling. It is for this reason that the usually central foil ply is 40 μm thick. Most laminated tubes are five to seven plies with the decoration being a sandwich print.

Two conversion processes are available to produce laminate collapsible tubes which involve a cylinder of the laminate to which an injection or compression moulded shoulder and nozzle are attached. A rondelle (a specially shaped disc) is frequently added to the latter to reduce any permeation risks via the plastic shoulder and nozzle. Foil of 40 μm, widely used in these constructions, is currently being challenged and replaced by a layer of EVOH, SiO_x or diamond carbon type coatings.

Foil lined carton systems

The use of foil lined carton systems for both dry and liquid products is another success story. Since in most instances the cartons are sealed by heat (the inner ply is a heat seal), the 7–9 μm foil may be attached to either the outside or the inside of the carton board. Foil lined carton systems may be employed for certain oral powder or granule based pharmaceuticals.

Diaphragm or membrane seals on plastic, glass and metal containers

The advent of the Extra Strength Tylenol poisonings in 1982 in the USA put new demands on tamper-evident/resistant packs. As a result of this, diaphragm or membrane seals increased in popularity for two reasons.

1 Diaphragms can be applied by adhesive, heat seal or induction sealing after product filling.
2 As well as being an excellent tamper-evident feature this can also make a very good primary seal on glass, metal and plastic containers. This is a particularly useful closure adjunct for plastic closures on plastic packs. If a foil diaphragm is the effective primary seal then closure torque (long-term) becomes less critical.

Of the three methods mentioned for making a diaphragm seal, induction sealing is proving particularly successful. Although the ultimate seal between the diaphragm and the closure relies on plastic, it is the foil ply which acts as a receptor to the induction waves, causing the creation of heat which softens the plastic sealant. Foil is therefore an essential component of induction diaphragm sealing, normally carried out via the closure which has the diaphragm or membrane lightly adhered within the cap. Induction sealing only applies to plastic caps, which should be retorqued after the operation.

Cold forming

Another more recent technology is the cold forming of a foil sandwiched between two plastic plies. The process involves the forming of a relatively shallow, well radiused draw by a mechanical (cold) stretching action between male/female dies, or air pressure forming into a female mould. The outer plastic plies are usually oriented polypropylene or nylon and the inner ply is PVC, polyethylene or a heat seal lacquer. The middle foil ply needs aluminium of a special crystalline structure to permit the flow of the foil without perforation. For this, a foil within the gauges of 40–60 µm is employed. Cold formed packs of this gauge, if correctly formed, give 100% protection in terms of moisture, gases, odour/flavour pick-up (or loss), etc. The latest advanced forming technology (AFT) uses a double forming process which reduces the blister size.

The preforming of foil based materials also occurs in certain strip packaging operations and for the tropicalised blister packs (i.e. a conventional blister is covered on the plaster (blister) side with shaped foil tray), thus enclosing the whole pack in foil.

Blister packs

Pharmaceutical blister packs are mainly used with a foil lid which may be 'push-through' (as used in Europe) or peelable (as used in the USA). Push-through foil lidding is made from either hard foil (15–20 µm) or soft foil (25 µm). Laminations using these may also be used to increase child-resistance.

Overwrapping laminations – incorporating aluminium foil

Various combination materials are available to improve moisture and gas protection, which are either used as an internal liner or bag or as an external overwrap. Most incorporate heat seal plies and use support materials such as nylon, polypropylene or more likely polyester which are recognised for their tensile strength and resistance to tear. Overwraps may involve large sachets, large bags, pouches, flowraps, grocery wraps, etc., all of which act as moisture or gas barriers. In certain instances this may allow the use of more economical or standardised primary packs.

Metallisations and coated plastics

Although the continued use of aluminium foil appears assured, it is facing increased competition from special coating processes which are being used on a range of plastics. These processes include metallisation which involves the vacuum deposition of aluminium particles, coatings of silicon dioxide, etc., using such methods as sputtering, electron beam deposition and plasma coating, and the incorporation of certain 'solids' into the plastic (e.g. mica particles).

Although each of the above improves the general barrier properties of the plastic, handling and creasing may lead to significant barrier reduction in certain situations. However, these improvements are being consistently developed, hence may create a longer term threat to the relatively high cost of many foil-based materials. For example when two metallised layers are laminated together, e.g. PET/metallisation/metallisation/PET/LDPE, a barrier approaching that of foil can be achieved – but at a cost which is similar to that of a foil bearing laminate.

Conclusions

The usage of foil, in spite of down-gauging (use of thinner gauges), has steadily increased, mainly due to the constant discovery of new packaging concepts. Since foil is relatively expensive due to the initial high cost of aluminium ($1450, £900/t) it is under increasing challenge from other materials. However, foil (for its thickness) remains an excellent barrier material, which, supported by its other assets, keeps it as an effective packaging material. Foil (and aluminium-based materials) can be recycled with a recovery value of around £600 per tonne. At the present moment the future of foil as a packaging material appears assured.

11

CLOSURES AND CLOSURE SYSTEMS

D. A. Dean

Introduction

With the majority of pharmaceutical products, the closure is an integral part of the pack, hence the word 'pack' covers both the container and the closure system. The latter may involve a unit dose or multidose where an included feature (e.g. heat seal, weld, peelable seal) or a separate feature (e.g. screw cap, lever lid) defines how the system functions. Because in most circumstances the pack is only as effective as the closure employed, a successful marriage between container and closure is essential to the product shelf life and its acceptance during use. In some instances a closure may serve a relatively simple function, i.e. act as a dust cover; at the other extreme it has to be hermetic, i.e. it permits no exchange between the product and the external atmosphere. This differs from a sterile closure system which retains sterility, i.e. prevents contamination from micro-organisms but may permit exchange by permeation of gases, moisture, etc. Sixty years ago there were relatively few closure systems, whereas today there are literally thousands. Closures and closure systems have as a result become both more sophisticated and more complex. This is particularly true when the closure assists in the administration of the product and/or where it incorporates special features to improve safety and security (tamper-evidence, tamper-resistance, child-resistance, etc.). This broadening role for closures and closure systems must cover the full life of the product (storage, transportation, display and use).

A primary function for even the simplest of closure systems is to retain or contain the contents. Safety and security may be necessary to prevent hazards resulting from leakage, seepage, spillage, prevention of pilferage, exposure to the wrong persons (e.g. children) or loss of quality, purity, etc., by some source of contamination, impurity, etc. Closures may also form part of the overall design of the pack and enhance the decorative appeal (image/presentation), act in a functional role during use (e.g. reclosables) or actually assist in the administration of the product (e.g. aerosol valve). Closures also act in a protective/preventive role by restricting ingress (odours, taints, moisture, oxygen, carbon dioxide, mould, bacteria, etc.) and egress (loss by evaporation, loss of moisture, perfume, flavourings, volatiles, etc.).

To the above design and functional factors, must be added those associated with cost and production line efficiency, i.e.

1 application at a required speed
2 equipment availability at an acceptable cost

3 minimum downtime and wastage/losses
4 specific pack/closure or preferably a range of packs (of differing designs and materials, involving packs and closures)
5 meeting the required performance standards
6 acceptable cost, including cost of closure components
7 maintaining any additionally required functions associated with dispensing, tamper-resistance resistance, tamper-evidence, child-resistance, etc.

A closure is therefore an essential part of any basic pack and as such must assist in providing a product with protection, presentation, identification/information and convenience on an economical basis until such time as the product is totally removed from the pack. The latter may be a once-off operation (i.e. it is a one-use or unit dose system) or multiple use in that the product is used over a period, thereby creating the need for a reclosable pack. In all instances the time between the creation of the packed product and its ultimate removal/use while it is still in a satisfactory state represents the shelf life of the product.

In the case of reconstituted products the closure may have to serve two somewhat different roles, i.e. prior to reconstitution where a powdered or crystalline product is involved and after the constitution when the product is in a liquid form. Convenience in use has increased in importance with the growing elderly population who may have impairment of movement, poor co-ordination, poor sight, etc. There is therefore inevitably some conflict between the need for ease of opening/reclosure and child-resistance, tamper-resistance, etc. and the fact that many closure systems are becoming more sophisticated by their administration functions.

The closure itself must be clean and sufficiently inert so that it does not affect the product by absorption/adsorption (from the product), interaction or permitting migratory substances to pass from the closure into the product. A closure may also be called on to provide protection against any hazard which may face the product during its shelf life, e.g. climatic, chemical, biological and mechanical hazards. Although the above references to closures may appear to cover only the primary or immediate pack, they are also important to the secondary pack. For instance, a fully taped (H seal) and glued case is more robust than a partially taped case – the better closuring system making for a more rigid unit, which will more effectively withstand both transit and stacking.

Since the closure is an integral part of the total (primary) pack, it cannot be considered in isolation. Thus when the environmental issues are fully considered, more attention will be required on the closure component (e.g. the public is encouraged to remove metal caps from glass bottles before the latter are deposited in bottle banks). Using closures made in the same materials as the containers has been suggested as being environmentally friendly. These, however, can create technical problems.

The initial conclusion is that any pack is only as good as the 'closure' system employed. Not only are closures becoming more complex and sophisticated, but the total functions which they serve are more diverse than many people realise and frequently they do not receive the attention to detail that they deserve. This broad chapter on closures therefore highlights the diversity of the systems employed, and the importance to the pack design, presentation and treatment.

The basis of closure systems

Closures may be achieved by a number of basic means or a combination of two or more, as follows.

Pressure

1   Mechanical pressure, e.g. top, side, internal pressure on a container finish ideally involving a seal between a fairly rigid material and one which is more resilient. Includes screw closures, plug seals, lever lids, etc., which create an interference fit between two materials.
2   Atmospheric pressure (pressure and vacuum): although a similar mechanical seal occurs to (1), this is initially achieved by a pressure differential (e.g. vacuum sealed tin).

Temperature

1   Welding/heat sealing – involves the direct and indirect application of heat, usually under pressure, for a given time (dwell) followed by a cooling period, so that a bond is made between two materials.
2   Electrical, e.g. ultrasonic, high-frequency/radio frequency, impulse, induction sealing. Basically a modification of the heat seal process.

Adhesion

Achieved by aqueous, solvent, hot melt, etc., adhesives or self-adhesives, cold seal materials. Solder is a metallic adhesive system. Solvent bonding is a chemical adhesive system.

Closure evaluation and performance against egress and ingress for reclosables

Closures usually have two stages of evaluation. These involve:
1   initial developmental evaluation by which pack and closure are selected and approved (note that this involves factors in addition to egress and ingress)
2   ongoing evaluation whereby incoming closures, production produced finished packs, display, use (and any subsequent customer complaints) are monitored and assessed, i.e. the basis of normal QA and QC.

In order to define the 'seal or closure effectiveness' for any closure system, some clarification of terminology is essential. One basic means of assessing a closure is by loss or gain as measured by weight or volume, as follows.

Loss from product (egress)

Although loss can occur to solid-based, gaseous or liquid-based products, only liquid-based are dealt with here.

- Leakage: liquid (or contents) positively found on external surface of the pack or closure.
- Seepage: example is where there is no obvious sign of leakage but liquid (or dried contents) may be found on container finish (threads) or on inner surface of cap.
- Evaporation: loss is normally detectable only by weight change. Occurs between seal area and possibly the main body of the container.
- Permeation: difficult to distinguish from evaporation but weight loss occurs by permeation through the sealing media, the closure and possibly the body of the container, if these are permeable.

Note that since evaporation/permeation involves the loss of the 'solvent', this may also be detected, by analysis or other leak detection techniques ('sniffing').

Gain to product, i.e. ingress

Usually associated with moisture pick-up, but can be related to any movement inwards by solid, gaseous or liquid substances. Moisture gain is detectable by weight increase or product analysis.

Microbiological ingress

Critical to sterile products, i.e. ingress of bacteria, mould or yeasts, and requires special detection techniques.

Gaseous exchange

Ingress or egress of gases such as oxygen, carbon dioxide, nitrogen may be associated with product deterioration or organoleptic changes. As with the above, loss or gain may occur via leakage/seepage or permeation mechanisms. Gas permeability increases as the temperature rises where plastic materials are involved.

Terminology related to closure efficiency remains fairly loose in terms of both ingress and egress. The USP XXIII offers tests for tight and well-closed containers based on the rate of moisture ingress into closed containers containing a desiccant under selected conditions of temperature and RH. Correlation between such movement inwards and outwards and that associated with flexible materials also requires further quantification, especially when measured by modern leakage detection instrumentation. The latter involves detection of pressure changes based on positive and negative pressure systems and the detection of various gases by a range of 'sniffing' systems. The means of generally defining closure efficiency requires further quantification.

It should also be noted that closure evaluation can rarely be assessed by one simple test, as the seal or fit between components may change with time and the surrounding climatic conditions. Typical evaluation stages could involve:

1 immediately closure has been applied
2 after a period of storage, possibly followed by transportation (involving compression and vibration)

3   at point of use
4   during and after periods of use.

Closure assessment and control: some general factors

Closures and closure systems may depend on or be influenced by a number of factors:

1   documentation/information/specifications
2   people (processing and usage)
3   machinery/instruments
4   the materials, container and closure
5   the environment – storage and application
6   warehousing and transportation
7   the product.

For instance, the apparently simple operation of applying a screw cap to a screw finish on a container can be broken down to well over 100 possible influencing factors. Examples of these are as follows.

Torque

An application torque may be given as between x and y lb ft ins or N m. The removal torque will change according to how long after application a check is made, the environment in which it has been stored, the type of materials used, etc. Hence removal torques may differ considerably after 10 min, 2 h, 24 h, 7 days, etc. – therefore the time factor between application and removal may have to be assessed and documented. Such changes are usually greater when plastic caps are applied to plastic containers.

However, a closure and container which provide a satisfactory marriage may still not be fully satisfactory, if either the container partially collapses or compresses during application of the cap or top pressure during stacking, or vibration plus top pressure during transportation causes unacceptable loosening of the closure. This is related to thorough testing during the development stages.

Information

Incorrect use and interpretation of information, the keeping of inadequate or inaccurate records, poor investigational techniques, improper adjustment or validation/ checking of recording instruments and machines, are a few examples how people may influence a closure system.

Wear

Machinery wear, changes due to vibrational effects, excessive speed, etc. may give rise to machine-dependent problems. Although it may be frequently assumed that a fitter knows his or her machine, it does not necessarily mean that he or she understands every process, as this ultimate detail may only be established by high-speed photography. Such an investigation may show distortion of components, excessive or short

447

throw, vibration, etc. Another common feature is that fitters (or even engineers) with excellent machine training may lack adequate training on material aspects, closure specification, etc. Regular monitoring of instruments associated with the machine or those used for measuring is important. Operator training is essential to any effective operation, plus regular validation of all instruments.

Materials

The materials employed for the container and the closure have a significant influence on the design, the process by which they are made and the performance. The materials may include the following.

- Metals – tinplate, tin free steel, aluminium, aluminium alloy, etc., and even stainless steel (vessels for bulk storage must also have effective closure systems).
- Glass – neutral, treated and soda glass. Although it is mainly used for containers, glass stoppers can still be found.
- Plastics – based on both thermosetting and thermoplastic polymers. Note that these have higher coefficients of thermal expansion than metal.

Since most closures put large dependence on their surface properties, these may be modified by the use of coatings, lacquers, etc. With plastics the constituents may be either at the surface (slip additives, lubricants, etc.) or migrate to the surface with the passage of time. These surface agents may also be changed or modified by processing, flame treatment, etc. The trend towards improving the barrier properties of plastics by coatings, e.g. fluoride treatment, silica oxide coating, may also influence closure performance. The process by which a closure is manufactured may introduce design restrictions (e.g. shape and depth of thread in the case of metal). In the blow moulding of plastics, injection moulding invariably gives better control over the neck dimensions and quality compared with an extrusion blow moulding process. Quality of design is therefore a major factor to consider in closure performance.

Environment

The environment may be critical to both the closure and the product as both may suffer from expansion and contraction due to temperature or RH changes. Other factors should not be excluded as a source of problems. For instance, static problems can increase with thermoplastic caps if the RH is low. This is particularly likely to occur during cold weather. The answer may be humidification of the atmosphere, avoiding addition of an anti-static agent to the plastic, avoiding a hot fill or neutralising charges by earthing or electrical means (ionised air). Artificially created environmental conditions may also cause problems, e.g. applying a 'cold' closure to a hot filled product.

Warehousing and transportation

Certain closure systems may be changed by top pressure from stacking and/or the effects of vibration or the combination of vibration and compression during transportation. For example, cartoned cylindrical containers are likely to rotate during transportation, thereby possibly reducing the closure torque. Top pressure may also weaken the seal impression on a variety of closure systems.

User or usage tests

The overall performance of a closure must include the 'use' period. Thus although a closure may enable a product to reach its point of use satisfactorily, it still has to serve certain functions such as tamper-evidence/tamper-resistance, child-resistance, reclosure, etc., in use.

Interaction between closure and pack (e.g. the black slurry which may occur with aluminium collapsible tubes), and possible adhesion between closure and pack (e.g. as may occur with sugar- or syrup-based products), are typical of what could occur if usage tests were omitted. Simulated use tests are particularly important with aerosols, pump systems, etc., which combine the closure with a dispensing system.

The product

The product factors which may need consideration include viscocity, cleanliness of fill, whether product froths or is corrosive, coefficient of expansion, volume to vacuity or ullage ratio, etc. Note that alcoholic based products have a higher coefficient of expansion than water, hence need a higher level of vacuity. Vacuity levels normally lie between 2% and 10%. Certain more volatile materials and chemical based products will create internal pressure according to the vapour pressure exerted for a given temperature. In certain instances, e.g. with peroxides, hypochlorites and similar products, pressure may be controlled by the use of venting closure systems.

Initial approach to closure assessment and control

The above examples should establish that any closure or closure system requires an in-depth knowledge of a number of areas, which are usually identified from experience rather than being found in textbooks.

An example of this lack of basic information can be found in the standard 40 cm^3 oval nasal spray bottle which usually consists of an LDPE bottle, LDPE plug, dip tube, and a thermoset or thermoplastic cap. The cap may incorporate one of four types of primary seal, a spigot (which fits into the plug orifice), a half ball (which fits into a recess or socket in the plug), a raised ring, or a flat sealing surface.

The cap is also usually shaped to make a secondary seal on the plug shoulder, this being a means of centralising the cap and preventing excessive top pressure on the plug tip (thus avoiding distortion of the plug tip and closure of the orifice by cold flow). In practice even some of the existing packs tend to leak or seep, particularly if subjected to excessive changes in temperature or when transported in 'pressurised' holds in aircraft. Although this may be due to a combination of incorrect tolerances on the components and/or the use of insufficiently controlled capping torques, finite causes are difficult to establish without large-scale statistically controlled programmes (on a scale usually not acceptable to industry in terms of time and human resources). Factorial experimental design at the suppliers should reduce this risk. 'Quality' of the container neck will also vary according to whether it is moulded by an injection blow or an extrusion blow moulding process.

Evaluation therefore requires a logical and basic approach which in the case of 'reclosables' could follow the following stages, using egress as an example.

1   Evaluation of drawings, i.e. for containers, closures, closure fitments (plugs etc.) involving all relevant tolerances. Study of these drawings may establish that a closure can or may be either ineffective or suspect. What cannot be done by the study of drawings is an evaluation of the level of efficiency. This can only be done by the tests described later.
2   Checking samples with drawings. If they do not match, decide whether the drawings should be altered to actual dimensions or the samples readjusted to the drawing dimensions. (Note that decisions partly depend on whether tooling is new or established.)
3   Product egress. Depending on the material from which the pack is made, egress may occur via the closure and the pack. If this does arise, then it will be necessary to measure:

    (a) total loss from pack
    (b) loss from closure
    (c) loss from container component.
    Although (a) should equal (b) + (c), possible constituent absorption/adsorption cannot be ignored.

Rate of loss will be related to temperature, the vapour pressure of the product in the pack and the vapour pressure of the product constituents in the surrounding atmosphere. In the case of a water-based product, the product will have both a vapour pressure and a relative humidity above the liquid, each of which will change according to the temperature. Actual loss will be related to the 'gradient' between the product 'headspace' and the external atmosphere, i.e. the greater the difference between the two, the greater will be the 'loss' (in theory).

However, temperature increase will generally change the internal RH/vapour pressure differently and independently to the external atmosphere, hence the rate of loss will vary as conditions change. Constant storage at one condition (e.g. 25°C 75% RH, 30°C 30% RH, 37°C 90% RH) will therefore not be easy to equate with 'actual' conditions. Product vapour pressure and RH above the solvent will also depend on whether 'salts' are dissolved therein, since the presence of a solute in a solvent lowers the vapour pressure. Note the vapour pressure of a substance (liquid or solid) is the pressure exerted by its vapour when in equilibrium with the substance.

Relative humidity is defined as the vapour content as a percentage of the concentration necessary to give vapour saturation at a given temperature. It also can be expressed as the ratio of the vapour pressure of the water vapour contained therein to the saturated vapour pressure of water vapour at the same temperature. A rise in temperature therefore reduces the RH (provided there is no addition of water vapour) and a drop in temperature raises the RH until such time as 100% RH or dew point is reached. Excess water then condenses out – i.e. there can be an internal 'shower effect' within the product or pack. RH can be measured by a wet and dry hygrometer or other instruments.

Atmospheric pressure

One atmosphere is defined as a pressure exerted at a sea level temperature of 15°C (1013.25 mbar) or the pressure exerted by a mercury column (of defined density and under defined gravity) of 760 mm height. Examples of some typical vapour pressures over a range of temperatures are given in Table 11.1.

Actual 'loss' will only be optimised if the solvent emerging is immediately removed (i.e. is swept away by air or a moving atmosphere). Build-up of the solvent in the external atmosphere will therefore slowly retard rate of loss, as the external concentration rises.

From this it should be seen that if an aqueous product is stored in a permeable pack, moisture loss will relate to the external environment and whether it is 'static' or is subject to motion or movement. Storage at, say, 37°C 90% RH will be relatively restrictive to moisture loss, whereas 37°C 30% RH will have a significantly greater 'gradient' and losses could be relatively high (particularly if held in a venting cabinet with a fan).

Egress or loss may relate to any substance (liquid, solid or gas) which exerts a vapour pressure under normal storage conditions, which usually lie between (−20°C) deep freeze conditions and somewhere around +55 to 60°C. However, moisture loss (and gain) is critical to many products, hence requires special consideration. As mentioned previously, whether loss is solely via the closure and/or pack depends on the materials employed for each. In order to separate the loss from each it may be necessary to carry out controlled experiments where either the container or the closure is covered or coated with an impermeable material (wax dipped or foil covered and sealed) so that permeation from one can be quantified.

This is particularly relevant where plastic packs and plastic closures are employed. In the latter case it may additionally be necessary to seal off the closure as loss may occur both through or around the seal, and through the cap itself (particularly if a wadless system is employed). In such instances 'weight loss' is the normal way of assessment. This is usually more accurate than assessment by chemical or physical analysis unless the loss of moisture causes a readily measurable physical or chemical change.

One final point related to loss is that loss may occur as total product (leakage or seepage), or by permeation coupled to evaporation. Each of these loss sources needs some form of quantification (see above). It should be noted that if product degradation and solvent evaporation occur similarly, chemical analysis may falsely indicate that no change has occurred, i.e. proportional compensation will mislead the conclusion.

Table 11.1 Typical vapour pressures (mm mercury) at various temperatures

Material	Temperature (°C)							
	−30	−20	0	5	20	80	100	120
Water	–	0.8	4.6	–	17.5	–	760	–
Acetone	11.2	–	–	89	185	–	2790	–
Benzene	–	–	–	–	·77	760	–	–
Ethylene glycol (antifreeze)	–	–	–	–	–	–	–	39

Loss by evaporation – use of Lyssy dynamic water vapour tester or similar instruments (e.g. Mocan–Permatran W)

There are a range of instruments which can electrolytically detect the rate at which moisture is given off into a dry stream of nitrogen which either is passed over packs containing a water base or passes through a permeable membrane (having a humid atmosphere on the opposite side). This procedure has an advantage over actual weight loss tests, which need time for equilibrium to be established (particularly if the pack is paper labelled or contains a paper-based wad). Normally the Lyssy dynamic water vapour tester will provide rate of loss figures for a given temperature within 24 h of the experiment start.

Vacuum tests

Whether a pack will leak can also be checked by some form of vacuum test. The vacuum may be drawn on the pack containing the product, or a product of lower surface tension to encourage loss, or held in a dry vacuum chamber or by placing an empty pack under water (the water normally contains a dye and a wetting agent) and again applying a vacuum. In both types of test, product (or air) out or liquid in may detect a defective closure system. The level of vacuum drawn, the time it is held, and the way it is built up and released vary from company to company.

Vacuums employed normally range from 15 to 25 inches of mercury (380–633 mm) and are held for 30 s to 10 min. Rate of vacuum release may also vary (fast, slow). In each of these tests the packs are sealed as per normal production.

Pressure tests

This test can only be applied to flexible packs, as the pack is put under positive pressure by some form of weight/force. A full pack is employed and loss detected by actual leakage. Also, a filled container can be stored on its side for 24 h at 38°C (after filling at a lower controlled temperature) (see CAN/CSA – 276. 1-M 90 (Canada) using a three-quarters full container). A positive air pressure test (using a full pack in a reinforced chamber capable of being pressurised) can also be employed.

Combined pressure and vacuum tests

In actual practice a pack may suffer from positive and negative pressures due to changes in environmental air pressures. This may occur due to either transportation via air in pressurised and unpressurised aircraft or changes in air pressure by ground height.

If a product starts at sea level, each rise of 1000 ft will involve a negative pressure differential of $(-)0.475$ lb/in^2, i.e. 0 to 10,000 ft $= -4.75$ lb/in^2. It should be noted that pressurised aircraft are pressurised to 8,000 ft, i.e. a negative pressure of $(-)3.8$ lb/in^2. Since unpressurised aircraft can fly up to, say, 24,000 feet (16,000 ft may be more normal), negative pressure of $(-)11.4$ lb/in^2 (16,000 ft $= -7.6$ lb/in^2 may be found (the figures given are pressure changes).

Typical heights and pressure differential conditions are:

- London – sea level, 0 lb/in^2
- Johannesburg – 6,500 ft, –3.1 lb/in^2
- Mexico City – 7500 ft, –3.6 lb/in^2

Note that normal atmospheric pressure is approx. 14.7 lb/in^2, and the above are again quoted as pressure changes.

Products being moved by air or between sea level and higher areas can be exposed to both negative and positive pressure differentials. These may cause pack distortion with flexible materials and generally increase the risk of product leakage or seepage. Marginally suspect closure systems may therefore have problems under the situations indicated above. Pressure differentials may be further influenced by temperature changes, particularly those which arise from the conditions associated with moist heat sterilisation, i.e. 108–135°C in the presence of 'steam'. In the case of flexible materials, an overpressure or balanced pressure autoclave is essential to prevent pack distortion and possible leakage during the cooling cycle. Under the higher temperatures of sterilisation some closures may also distort, vent, etc., hence if a good reseal is made after partial cooling, some degree of negative pressure may be created. Actual tests are therefore advised to establish the overall effectiveness of such closure systems.

However, positive and negative pressure tests must be advised if transport by air is to be regularly used (or in areas of the world where altitude differences may cause changes in pressure differentials). In these tests, temperature variations should also be borne in mind.

Transportation and warehousing

Having discussed how egress can be measured under 'normal' static conditions, 'closure efficiency' may still be influenced by conditions associated with transportation and warehousing (see above). Actual or simulated warehousing and transportation tests may be advised as part of a pack–closure evaluation.

The above more conventional procedures (newer procedures will be considered later) might be used to test product–pack efficiency in terms of its protective role against egress during the shelf life of a product. A similar series of tests can be considered where ingress may be the evaluation factor.

Ingress may refer to the following.

1 Moisture.
2 Gases of organic or inorganic origin.
3 General contamination which may be referred to as soilage, spoilage, etc. Contamination may be of a solid (particulates), liquid or gaseous form which may cause physical, chemical or organoleptic changes and can be a carrier of foreign substances (flavours, aromas, bioburden, etc.).
4 Microbiological contamination, included as part of 'spoilage', is totally undesirable when products are sterile. Pathogenic organisms should ideally be absent in products where the presence of such organisms would cause concern (e.g. *Listeria*, *Salmonella*, *Clostridium botulinum*).

The function of a closure to maintain a product in a pure and/or uncontaminated state, etc., has therefore an importance greater than product egress. Checking whether such ingress is controlled, limited or totally excluded by the 'closure' may follow the same or similar tests as those used to check product egress. However, some tests may be different, i.e. weight gain must replace weight loss checks. These tests therefore follow a similar order to those used previously, as follows.

Evaluation of drawings

The same comments apply, i.e. while imperfections in the closure/container system may be identified, the effectiveness of the 'seal' cannot be quantified from drawings. Excessive interference fits may actually cause container/closure distortion or, in severe cases, either breaking or cracking of either component. It is important that samples are compared with the drawing to ensure compliance. Any difference needs action on the drawing or samples (see previous notes on evaluation of drawings and checking samples with drawings).

Ingress to product

In common with egress, ingress can occur as:

1 total gain by pack
2 gain via (or through) the closure
3 gain via (through) the container.

Although (1) may equal (2) + (3), certain packs may absorb external constituents and others may migrate from the 'pack' to the product, e.g. certain plastics absorb moisture (e.g. Nylons), hence weight will vary according to the surrounding environment. Plastics which show absorption of moisture may have to be predried before they can be moulded.

Moisture gain can therefore occur as the reverse to leakage and seepage, permeation through the closure or the container, and moisture absorption from the atmosphere in which the pack is located. Since some packs have a series of closures, other than that used by the consumer, moisture gain (or loss) can occur via the secondary closures or seals, e.g. the folded and crimped seal in the case of a collapsible tube, the side and end seams in three-piece tinplate cans, the swaged-in valve cup with an aerosol.

Ingress, however, is not restricted to moisture and may, as indicated earlier, involve any solid, liquid or gaseous form of 'contamination'. Each of these may enter a pack via an ineffective seal and involve the 'breathing' of a pack. This may arise from changing pressures caused by atmospheric pressure variations (natural, changes in altitude), or changing levels of temperature (and RH), which cause the pack and pack contents to expand and contract.

Vacuum tests

Applying vacuum to an effectively sealed pack will mean that the internal atmosphere is under positive pressure. Under such conditions a flexible pack will possibly expand or inflate; a rigid pack may show no change. Applying a vacuum to a pack showing positive leakage will cause a similar vacuum inside the pack. Releasing the vacuum will allow the external atmosphere (or any external liquid) to enter the pack.

Pressure tests

Placing packs under a positive pressure external to the pack can provide a useful indication of possible ingress. The positive pressure atmosphere may use air, water under pressure, or a concentration of any gas (or liquid) which can be pressurised (see below for further details). For tests involving combined pressure and vacuum, comments apply as for egress.

Transportation and warehousing

Comments apply as for egress above.

Other tests and considerations

Since ingress may have more serious repercussions than egress, additional tests to those above are used to detect both moisture and possible microbiological contamination.

1   Desiccant tests. Dried desiccant tests (as defined in USP XXIII for tight and well-closed packs), provide a useful indication of moisture ingress. Possible desiccants are dried calcium chloride and dried silica gel, but although these usually provide a useful comparison between packs, relating this information to the product may prove difficult, particularly if moisture sensitivity equates with some form of chemical degradation.

2   Microbiological ingress. Bacteria, moulds and yeasts may 'grow back' through or via various closure systems. Normal leakage or closure efficiency tests may not establish whether organisms will penetrate through minute or small imperfections in the closure–pack systems. One check to ascertain whether microbiological contaminants will grow back is to contaminate the outside of the closure (or seal(s)) with a contaminated product, or growth media such as a broth, spiked with known organisms. For such tests a temperature of around 37°C (for incubation purposes) is likely to be preferable. Such tests are particularly relevant with sterile products and packs such as aerosols and pump systems, where product contamination would be unacceptable (e.g. wound care, eye care products). However, reproducibility of these as 'grow back' remains dubious.

3   Detection of foreign vapour ingress, e.g. leading to changes in organoleptic properties. Changes in flavour and aroma may occur because of foreign vapour entry via the closure. Since some undesirable contaminants (e.g. perfumes) may consist of a multiplicity of chemical substances, each ingredient may be absorbed into the material differently. The resulting off-flavours/aromas in the product may therefore be different to the original contaminant, as some separation of the constituents may have occurred as permeation or diffusion proceeded. Placing a pack in an enclosed concentrated atmosphere of possible contaminants is a useful way of establishing whether 'foreign vapour' transfer is likely.

4   Other gas permeation effects. It should be noted that all plastics are to some

degree permeable to gases. This means that even when the closure is highly effective, permeation into the pack can give rise to physical or chemical changes. Examples of these are as follows.

- LDPE bottle filled with an aqueous unbuffered product at pH 7.0 – after a period of storage a pH shift due to the inward permeation of carbon dioxide is most likely to occur (new pH approx. 4.5).
- LDPE bottle etc. as above, but product is buffered to pH 7.0. In such a case, carbon dioxide permeation will still occur but will not be detected by a pH change. If carbon dioxide reacts with the product (e.g. presence of carbonates could cause precipitation), this hidden ingress may not be considered as a possible cause of change or deterioration.

The above examples should tend to indicate that permeation ingress may occur by either the pack or the closure and give effects which are independent of general closure efficiency.

Discussion of egress and ingress should have highlighted the numerous ways in which a closure (or a seal) may need to be assessed or evaluated before a 'closure' can be pronounced as meeting 'fitness for purpose' (for egress/ingress only).

Before other functions, e.g. tamper-evidence/resistance, child-resistance, accuracy of delivery, can be discussed, general technical factors associated with ingress and egress need further consideration. Since these are common to 'seal' efficiency (i.e. ingress and egress) and may define seal quality, they were not covered under the headings used earlier. In the example used below a continuous screw threaded container–closure system has been employed as an indication of the typical variables involved. These are listed in Table 11.2 and then briefly discussed.

Table 11.2 applies to conventional continuous threaded preformed screw closures as applied to glass, plastic or metal containers, but is also relevant to multistart and lug type finishes. Certain features on the container have to be 'matched' against the closure.

Historically, screw closures have consisted of a threaded shell (originally metal) containing a wad or liner with a facing. The wad, which was made from cork agglomerate (gelatin or resin bonded), pulpboard, or feltboard, is gradually being replaced by alternative wadless systems. This provides for a resilient backing into which the seal is 'bedded'. The wad may be backed with Kraft paper and/or hot waxed if required. Although plain wadding may occasionally be used, most have a facing, which must be resistant to the product. Most facing systems are laminated to a sulphite or sulphate bleached paper. It may be one of many materials, as listed in Table 11.3.

In newer materials, such as polythene, plasticised PVC and EPE, it is possible to combine the wad/facing as one material, utilising the combined properties of resilience and resistance. Taking this one stage further, wadless caps can now be made from various plastics: LDPE, PP, HDPE, etc. In addition there are rubber compounds as discs, bungs or stoppers, i.e.:

1   natural rubber (ages, permeable, sensitive to excessive heat, but good on resealing, coring)
2   synthetics (butyl, chlorbutyl, bromobutyl, etc.)
3   silicone – inert, permeable and expensive (see Chapter 12, 'Sterile products and the role of rubber components').

Table 11.2 Typical variables for a container–closure system

Container	Factors common to both	Closure
	• Threads per cm or inch (pitch) • Thread type, i.e. interrupted or continuous • Thread form – semi-round, 60° (BS 1918), acme, buttressed (BS 5789 plastics), etc. • Thread length (turns), i.e. start to run-out • Thread height (above wall) • Thread base	
Thread OD (overall diameter)	Thread start – style of start (abrupt, tapered)	Thread ID (internal diameter)
Wall OD Sealing surface, width, shape and diameter Finish height Material: • Metal – type/style • Glass • Plastic	Thread helix angle	Wall ID Sealing feature (wadded or unwadded) Internal cap height • Metal • Plastic thermoset or thermoplastic • Preformed • Rolled on (metal)
Internal bore ID Parallel bore ID		Wadless – OD of bore Intrusion
Wall thickness		Thickness of wall, and head section • Style of wad retention, (glued-in, friction fit, flowed-in compound, etc.)
Presence of bead or transfer ring		
	With tolerances of all dimensions	• External shape, gripping areas (beading, knurling, ribbing, etc.)

Table 11.4 gives an elastomers selection chart.

Prethreaded screw caps

These can be fabricated from the following.

1 Metal – low carbon steel, tin coated, and aluminium, i.e. tinplate – corrosion protection can be improved by use of external enamels and internal lacquers.
2 Aluminium alloys – can also be enamelled, printed and lacquered.
3 Plastics (natural, coloured, metallised, etc.). May be either thermosetting or thermoplastic.

Table 11.3 Materials for facing systems

Material	Comments
Aluminium foil (soft)	0.025 mm or the same with a microcrystalline wax coating.
Tin foil	Very soft but expensive. Gives a good seal.
Polythene	Coated Kraft – usually 0.002 inches (50 μm)
Expanded polyethylene foam (EPE)	There are two grades of expanded polyethylene which in compression are similar to pulpboard (compression 10–20%) and compo cork (compression 45–55%)
Saran/PVdC film	Originally a 0.0075 inch DOW PVdC film, but this is inferior to dispersion coated PVdC in terms of moisture barrier.
PVdC coatings	An aqueous coated PVdC, varying in coating weight (an excellent barrier to moisture, gases and reasonably solvent resistant).
Polyester film (PET) i.e. Mylar and Melinex	50 or 100 gauge, rather hard (0.0005 or 0.001 inches).
Solid polythene	Occasionally used.
Solid PVC	Depends on plasticisers.
PTFE facing	0.002 inches very inert, hard and expensive, used with strong acids.
Flowed-in compounds	PVC plastisols, occasionally rubber latex, EVA variants.

Thermosetting, i.e. phenol formaldehyde (PF), Bakelite and urea formaldehyde (UF)

These may be wood, paper or flour filled, but be . !ert to possible release of ammonia, phenol, or formaldehyde residues from the moulding process. PF can be made by reacting phenol with hexamine (made from formaldehyde + ammonia).

In general (but not invariably) the unscrewing torque is 50–75% of the application torque. Examples of the torque instruments available are Torquemaster, Torquemeter and Kork a Torque. Unscrewing torques may, however, change according to storage conditions and length of time stored. Thermosetting caps, for instance, change dimensionally (moisture and coefficient of expansion) and metal/thermoplastic change mainly due to coefficient of expansion under changing conditions of storage. Phenol formaldehyde caps are slightly more dimensionally stable than urea formaldehyde caps. PF is available only in the darker colours, whereas UF is available in all colours. PF caps will withstand steam sterilisation, but urea will not.

Thermoplastic-based closures

See Table 11.5. The application of a prethreaded cap relies on a torque usually measured as N m, to make a good impression between two surfaces. Ideally one material should be hard, e.g. glass, so that it bites into a resilient (soft) material such as composition cork. The sealing surface of a glass finish may be radial or flat, or in certain circumstances stepped or tapered. Thermoplastic closures are generally less dimensionally stable than metal closures.

Table 11.4 Elastomer selection chart

Elastomer	Natural rubber	Butyl rubber	Chlorinated Butyl Rubber*	Nitrile rubber	Silicone rubber	Hypalon	Chloroprene	Viton	EPDM	EVA
Resistance against ageing	4	1	1	2	1	2	2	1	2	2
Sterilisable in saturated steam	3	1	1	2	2	1	2	1	2	2
Coring	1	4	4	4	5	4	3	5	2	3
Resistance against mineral oil	5	5	5	1	4	4	2	1	4	4
Resistance against vegetable oil	4	1	1	1	2	3	2	1	3	4
Resistance against aromatic solvents	4	3	3	2	4	3	3	1	4	4
Resistance against permeation of gas	4	1	1	3	5	1	2	1	3	3
Resistance against permeation of water vapour	4	1	1	3	5	2	3	1	4	4
Compression set	1	4	4	2	3	4	2	3	2	3
Flexibility	1	4	4	2	3	4	3	4	2	3
Resistance against heat up to	120°†	145°	155°	130°†	220°	160°	140°†	210°†	125°	120°

1 = excellent, 2 = good, 3 = average, 4 = poor, 5 = not recommended.   * Or bromobutyl.
† Only short time exposure (depends on cure system).
Reproduced by kind permission of West Pharmarubber Ltd.

Table 11.5 Thermoplastic-based closures

Material	Comments
Polystyrene (PS)	Hard, rigid, rather brittle: can be embrittled by chemical attack (isopropyl myristate), or crazed.
Polystyrene – medium or high impact modified grades (HIPS)	Reduced brittle factor.
Polythene LD (and LLDPE)	Rather soft, flexible – can be wadless, may stress crack.
Polythene: MD, HD	Less flexible and less soft; HDPE is now very popular.
Polypropylene (PP)	Fairly hard – can be wadless if special sealing 'ring' is incorporated. May be homopolymer (can crack at low temperatures) or copolymer.

Wadless closure systems

Wadless closure systems may be made from thermosetting or thermoplastic materials. The former were earlier used on plastic tubes, i.e. combining the hardness of the thermoset and the flexibility of the plastic tube.

Today wadless thermoplastic closures are used on glass, metal and plastic containers. The seal area may be achieved on the top, internal or external sides of the sealing surface of the container. The internal method of achieving a seal, known as a bore seal, is usually made with a tapered skirt or extending feature in the cap. When the top surface makes a seal this may be matched with a special flexible feature in the cap such as a crab's claw, a raised bead or a flat surface. The container sealing surface may also have raised areas such as ribs or beading. Finally, the outer wall of the container finish may be used as a seal area which matches with a taper or angle in the closure. Although some closure systems have claimed to make a triple seal by making contact within all three areas, the author believes that a single seal tends to be more effective, and bore seals are becoming increasingly popular.

Wadless systems are made from a range of thermoplastics, with polypropylene and high density polythene being widely used.

Plastic caps on plastic bottles

Loss of torque against time has been well documented with plastic caps on plastic bottles. This does not necessarily mean that the closure becomes ineffective, but there are occasions when a low torque only needs the vibration effects of transportation to become an unsatisfactory (loose/leaking) closure. Certain tamper-evident/resistant features such as sealed diaphragms and ratchet-type closure systems are likely to overcome such problems. Having the right combination of plastics may also eliminate or reduce this loss of torque. However, there is the converse where the use of the incorrect combination of plastics, or plastics with undesirable constituents such as lubricants, mould release agents, internal release agents, may actually exacerbate the loss of closure torque. This loss may be associated with thread forms, area of thread contacts, cold flow or creep of plastics involved, lubricants, etc.

Rolled-on pilfer-proof (ROPP) closures

Note that 'pilfer-proof' is early terminology, now replaced by TE (tamper-evident) or TR (tamper-resistant). This process usually applies only to metal shells made from aluminium alloy. But plastic caps with compound lining can also be formed on a container finish. The caps may contain either conventional wadding or a flowed-in gasket. In theory this type of closure provides a more consistent first seal than a prethreaded screw cap in that:

1   the operation of application applies a controlled top pressure which makes a seal between wad and container sealing surface
2   while still held by the top pressure, the thread is rolled into the metal, thus giving a finish which is tailor-made to the individual container
3   in the case of a pilfer-proof closure the skirt is rolled under the bottle retaining bead.

The ROPP closure has two torque measurements related to breaking the seal and the TE feature. Disadvantages can occur with the RO system where the glass finish is not up to standard, causing perforation of wad and difficulties in unscrewing. Reclosure is satisfactory provided the thread is fully formed, but shallow formed threads can be made to override due to the softer alloy metal.

The above in total represents over 100 variables which may exist within a conventional container/screw closure system. If one adds to this the variables associated with different grades of plastic and the constituents which may be contained therein, the torque range applied, the method of application, the temperature/RH of the environment at the time of application, etc., then the total variables can exceed 150 factors. Some examples of how these variables may interact are given below.

Torque

Screw closures 'lock' in position by the interlocking forces applied by the thread of the cap onto the threads of the container. The force applied is varied according to the diameter of the container, with the recommended force increasing as the diameter widens. This locking force is achieved through the contact area of the cap to container, hence the smaller the contact area, the greater the force per unit area of contact, and the greater the contact area, the lower the force per unit area of contact. Since the locking force applied by the thread contact is transferred to the area of seal, how 'effective' this force is in achieving a seal depends on a number of factors, i.e. whether seal involves:

- two 'hard' surfaces/materials
- two resilient surfaces/materials
- one resilient and one hard material.

Resilient materials will undergo a degree of impression or compression according to the nature of the material, the force involved and the area of contact taking the force.

The way the resilient material compresses will also depend on how it acts as a resilient or non-resilient 'cushion', i.e. at one end of the scale it may compress and have 100% recovery when the force is removed and at the other end collapse totally with no recovery. This in turn may be influenced by the applied force versus the contact area involved. Three examples are shown in Figure 11.1.

Figure 11.1 represents three sealing surfaces/walls on three different 28 mm necks of an HDPE bottle:

(a)   sealing surface is narrow with a width of 0.75 mm and an area of seal of 57 mm² (internal bore 23.5 mm)
(b)   sealing surface is 1.5 mm across, hence the internal bore is 22 mm and the area of seal is 110 mm²
(c)   sealing surface is 3 mm across, hence the internal bore is 19 mm and the area of seal 207 mm².

If a uniform torque is applied to each of the above, then the force to surface area ratio will reduce from (a) to (c). A situation therefore could occur where two of the three gave an ineffective seal, assuming the wadding system was, for example, a faced pulpboard on a liquid-based product, as follows.

(a)   The high force per area could cut through the facing and allow the liquid to penetrate the pulpboard, and slowly evaporate, giving rise to leakage and possible microbial growth on the wadding.
(c)   With a low force per area and minor imperfections in the sealing surface, there may be insufficient force (impression) to ensure a seal between the container surface and the faced wadding material.

In the above example an effective seal with (b) is assumed.

The transmission of the force applied between the container and closure threads has further implications which depend on both the wall section of the container and the wall sections of the cap (i.e. side walls and top section). In any of these instances the force applied may cause distortion or deflection of the container wall, the cap walls or the top section of the cap. Each in turn may reduce closure efficiency, which in instances

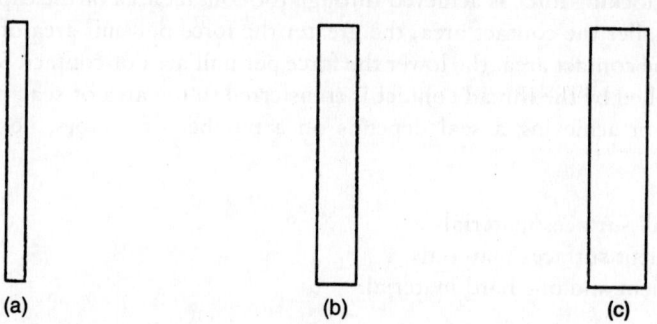

Figure 11.1 Examples of sealing surfaces/walls: (a) 0.75 mm; (b) 1.5 mm; (c) 3 mm (wall OD 25 mm)

may cause total loss of torque, hence a 'no seal' situation may be reached. Examples of this situation are sketched in Figure 11.2. Cap (a) is made from plastic with a very thin wall section, whereas (b) is a much thicker sectioned cap where distortion would be extremely unlikely.

When the situation in Figure 11.2(a) is applied to a fairly thin walled container, both the side walls may splay out (as shown in Figure 11.3) and the top wall section, which may initially dome, may ultimately crack open like a trap door.

The movement outwards of the side walls will depend on:

(a) the wall thickness
(b) the material employed (and constituents therein)
(c) the thread contours on pack and container
(d) the forces on each component and the cold flow–creep properties of each.

Table 11.6 gives some suggested torques for screw closures.

Thread engagement – turn to release

Thread engagement is normally checked by applying the cap onto the container at the recommended torque and then removing it with a slight lifting action until the cap loses thread contact. The degrees or parts of turn engagement are measured from position of tightness to where thread contact is lost (Figure 11.4).

A 180° or $\frac{1}{2}$ turn is usually unsatisfactory as pressure on one side tends to tilt the closure, hence compression is not even over the total surface. A 270° ($\frac{3}{4}$) to 540° ($1\frac{1}{2}$) turn is normally considered satisfactory. Although there may be reasons for $1\frac{1}{2}$–3 turns (to centralise a deep cap), this can be considered wasteful in application energy. This engagement will vary accordingly to:

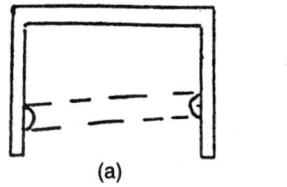

(a)

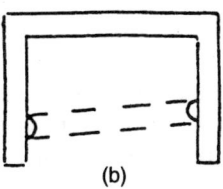

(b)

Figure 11.2 (a) Plastic cap with very thin wall section; (b) thicker sectioned cap

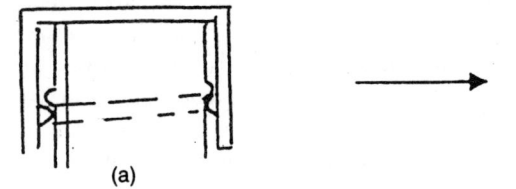

(a)

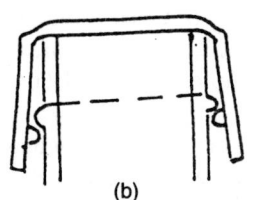

(b)

Figure 11.3 (a) Cap at recommended torque; (b) doming in cap head section – side wall distortion could reduce retention torque

Table 11.6 Suggested torques for conventional wadded screw closures (metal and plastic)

Closure diameter (mm)	Suggested application torque	
	(range in lb force inch)	range in N m
15	6–9	0.69–1.035
20	8–12	0.92–1.38
24	9–15	1.035–1.725
28	10–18	1.15–2.07
33	12–21	1.38–2.415
38	15–25	1.725–2.875
43	17–27	1.958–3.105
48	19–30	2.185–3.405
53	21–36	2.415–4.14
58	23–40	2.645–4.60
63	25–43	2.875–4.945
70	28–50	3.22–5.75

1 N m = 8.85 lb force inch = 10 kgf/cm. With double shell and shrouded type closure systems the torque should be related to the inner component diameter.

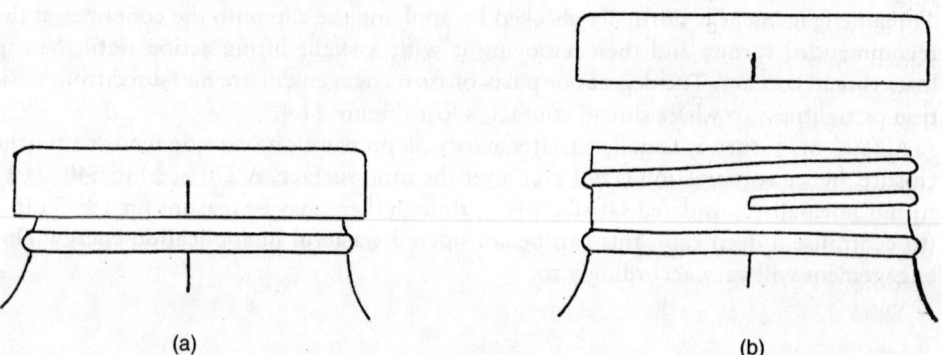

(a) (b)

Figure 11.4 (a) Cap and shoulder marked; (b) unscrew cap with lifting, i.e. one complete turn

1   wad thickness
2   container and thread starts
3   compression of any wad or wadless feature.

Multi-start versus single start threading

Multi-start threading, as usually found on lug systems and vacuum packs, generally provides more even pressure on the wadding or sealing media. Four start systems, for example, only need 90° or $\frac{1}{4}$ turn to remove and have threads or lugs of a steeper helix angle. Such systems rely on the vacuum for effective cap retention, as the steeper helix angle would make loss of torque (backing off) more likely, if only the interlock were involved. The vacuum is normally achieved by a hot fill or a steam headspace flush.

As mentioned previously, closures based on a single start thread may tilt or apply an uneven pressure if the turn of thread engagement is half a turn (180°) or less, except when such patented systems as Link-lok and Nek-lok are employed. The latter systems have a wedge-shaped bulge which is added to the container thread and/or closure thread at, say, 90° intervals under the container, or on top of the closure thread. These tend to centralise the cap on the container finish, thereby reducing or avoiding tilt. Such systems may also assist in closure retention and reduce loss of torque. There are other exceptions where a cap with half a turn engagement may be satisfactory, i.e. where used on solid products (thick ointments, solid paraffin-based products) which cannot suffer leakage and need virtually no special protection.

British Standard 1918 lays down the standard for the R3/2 (shallow), R4 (deep) and R4 (medium deep) threaded container finishes for glass or glass-like rigid containers. Standards for closures only exist by the fact that they are made to match a container finish. (For US equivalents, see Appendix 11.7).

British Standard 5789 1979 applies to plastic containers and closures requiring a buttress-type thread.

Thermosetting caps are compression moulded on either platen or rotary-type equipment. Pressure, dwell time and temperature are critical to the curing operation, otherwise brittle or soft caps may be produced.

Thermoplastic caps are invariably injection moulded. Extra decorative effects can be added by blocking, embossing in the mould, inserts and metal vacuumising. Plastic caps can also be printed by hot foil stamping or a process such as Tampoprint/Padflex. The cost of laying down injection moulds is usually high, probably £800–1,500 per single cavity, depending on the number of mould components. The cost per cavity reduces if multi-impression tooling is employed, as does the cost per closure. Unlike metal, plastics can be moulded into a wide range of shapes and colours, thus adding to the decorative appeal of the pack. Double shell metal caps are also available, which give a smooth finish similar to a plastic cap.

Note that compo cork is recommended as the wadding for wide mouthed closures as it takes up any unevenness (undulations) of the sealing surface, or one can use a suitable grade of expanded polyethylene, particularly where glass is involved.

Other metal closures for glass and/or plastics

The foremost metal closures in this category are the crown closure (beer bottle) and the foil heat seal used for yoghurt pots, or the induction sealed diaphragm. The crown cork closure is basically a tinplate shell which contains a wad/facing. This may be conventional, polythene or a flowed-in compound. Its application is similar to the RO in principle in that top pressure is applied first, followed by application of crimping action. It is designed as a one use closure. Foil (and plastic) seals involve a heat sealing operation (see also diaphragm seals for pharmaceuticals).

Metal lever cap (narrow neck mineral bottle)

Tinplate plus wadding. Can be resealed but is being rapidly replaced by Flavor-lok type closures.

Centre pressure cap

Tinplate plus wad. Press cap centre for cap removal. Press cap sides for retention. Used on glass jars but major use is on metal drums.

Metal vacuum seals

1   Top sealing disc plus rubber or plastic seal. This is held on by a safety band ring as used on jars of paste.
2   Light gauge aluminium cap incorporating a flowed-in gasket. The cap is crimped under the neck ring, i.e. jam, pickles, etc. Omnia (continuous beading) and Gerda (perforated beading).
3   More rigid closure usually made in tinplate applying a side seal on the neck by a rubber ring or flowed-in compound.

Note that certain flowed-in compounds can be used hot whereby threads or lugs can be moulded in from the heat of the container.

Other aspects of assessment

Although the effectiveness of a closure may relate primarily to the prevention of ingress and egress, many other aspects, as mentioned earlier, may be involved, such as the following.

1   Ingress and egress following use, i.e. can the closure be effectively reapplied and resealed (repeat earlier tests!) by all concerned? User assessment.
2   If closure system dispenses or assists in the administration of a product, does it do it effectively and reproducibly? (Query product contamination!)
3   Can closure be opened by the elderly, including those infirm, poor in sight, arthritic, etc. (and effectively reclosed)? Query age group.
4   Is the closure child-resistant, – i.e. has it passed BS 6652, 1989 or equivalent standard (US, ISO, etc.)?
5   Is the closure system tamper-evident, tamper-resistant? How can its effectiveness be established?
6   How can it be specified to give optimum on-line and off-line performance? What on-line performance is required? What quality standards need setting? How does it perform under compression and vibration (warehousing and transportation)?

Conclusions – reclosables

The total function of a pack relies on a successful marriage between the container and its closure. Over the years the role of closures has been extended and as a result the apparently simple act of putting a closure onto a pack has in certain instances become underestimated. Although the examples given in this chapter have in the main used screw-based systems, the principles offered for the assessment of closure efficiency can be applied to any design, i.e. push-in, push-over, etc. However, to achieve an effective seal, the design and the nature of the seal becomes dimensionally more critical. As in such systems at least one of the components (closure or pack) is likely to be plastic, the factors involved depend on the properties of both the container and the closure. In the case of plastics these variables include the moulding process, the type of plastic, the additives and processing aids included, moulding shrinkage, as well as the dimensional changes which occur according to climatic temperature and humidity variations. These all make the chance of 'getting it right first time' rather remote. The fact that many existing closure systems do have deficiencies, although unpalatable, has to be recognised. This should also make one aware that inventing any new concepts requires a series of trials and errors, evaluations and modifications, before the most effective compromise between container and closure can be achieved.

A final complication is the fact that closure systems (particularly those which assist in the dispensing or administration of a product) are becoming more complex and more sophisticated. The list which follows indicates many of the various closures and closure systems which are available for both primary and secondary packs: as seals or closures can be temporary or permanent, certain packs may have a series of closures created by the way in which they are converted or manufactured. A tinplate built-up aerosol container, for example, has four permanent seals, i.e. welded or soldered side seam, a cone and a dome held to the container body by double seams, a swaged-in valve cup, and an operational valve system (the in-use closure). Some of the systems will therefore be described in further detail.

1   Fold – overwrapping without sealing, fold over, fold down, grocer's fold, roll wrap, bread wrap, etc. Note dead fold characteristic of soft foil (see BS 1133) and over-wrapping, plus seal – i.e. heat, adhesive, etc.
2   Twist wrap – sweets, foil or special flexible cellophane or plastics where 'twist' does not unwind.
3   Bunch wraps – (also known as plunge wraps) where an item is pushed into a sheet and finishes with a pleated bunch, e.g. special soaps.
4   Ties – wire, paper–wire, plastic–wire, plastic for sacks, liners, bags. There are now a wide variety of locking plastic ties based on ratchets, loops, etc.
5   Adhesion with adhesives. Mechanical or specific adhesion to polar or non-polar surfaces (see below), e.g.

- self-adhesive or pressure sensitive (cold sealing)
- heat sensitive, or heat activated
- PVA (polyvinyl acetate)
- hot melt – 100% solids
- solder (lead and lead-free) and welding.

6   Heat seals and electrical sealing:

- direct and indirect heat sealing
- weld (melt)
- high frequency–radio frequency
- impulse, ultrasonic, laser, etc.
- induction etc. – see diaphragm seals.

7   Taping (plain and reinforced) – includes self-adhesive, water activated, heat activated:

- self-adhesive – usually plastic backed (PVC, polythene)
- cloths and laminated tapes – bitumen, foil, fibre, paper, etc.
- plastic tapes (polyester, HDPE, polypropylene).

8   Metal – nails, staples, screws, tacks for wood, fibreboard.
9   Strapping – wire, tensional steel, nylon, polypropylene, polyester.
10 String, thread and rope – stitching (sacks), tying using hemp, nylon, cotton, etc.
11 Taps (combined closure and tap) – tanks, drums, bag in box, etc.
12 Labels, tags and seals – destructible, non-destructible, water soluble, etc., may be used as tamper-evident features or a simple sealing aid, e.g. labels – paper + adhesive, pre- gummed, heat seal and pressure sensitive, plastic – self-adhesive.
13 Shrinkable sleeving and stretch sleeving, i.e. Viscose and PVC, PP, PET sleeving (items shrink by drying or heat). Stretch sleeving is usually based on polyethylene (LLDPE).
14 Foil – diaphragms, covers, lidding:

- heat seal – blister packs, moulded containers
- induction sealing – diaphragm and membrane seals.

15 Shrink and stretch wrapping – shrinkable films (PVC, polypropylene, polythene), sleeve or complete overwraps. Stretchable wraps, e.g. LLDPE, modified PEs.
16 Crimping – shaping, folding and crimping, e.g. collapsible tubes (metal). Aerosol valves for glass bottles. Overseals for injection vials.
17 Swaging – to shape with a swage (a die or grooved block for shaping). Aerosol valve in metal cans (1 inch orifice).
18 Tamper-evident and tamper-resistant closure systems. Tamper-evident closures, although seen as a specific group, offer a range of systems (see below).
19 Child-resistant closures – initially dating back to the Poisons Prevention Act introduced in the USA in 1970; cover both reclosable and non-reclosable systems – (see below).

Specific closures for containers (steel, tinplate, aluminium, plastic shipping containers)

1   Narrow neck (made in metal or plastic).
2   Press caps, screw caps, pourer taps, lever caps – orifices run from 28 mm upwards and may incorporate various pouring aids (e.g. spouts).
3   Full aperture – wide lug cover with sealing gasket, and ring locking system.
4   Fibreboard drums – slip lid/wide lug cover with sealing gasket.
5   Large aluminium containers – screw caps (plastic and metal)/bungs and plastic shives (antibiotics and perfumes)

Collapsible tubes (two closures) – nozzle and base fold and crimp

Metal

1   Operational aperture (see Figure 10.3):

- blind end nozzles or metal diaphragm
- screw caps – thermoplastic – no wad (wadless)
    – thermosetting – wadded.

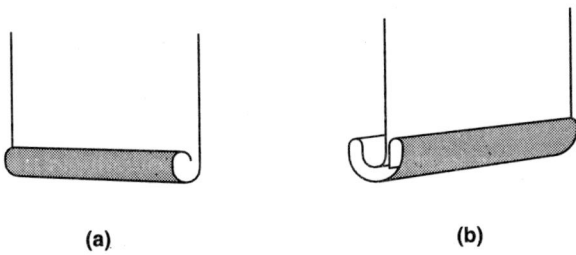

(a)   (b)

Figure 11.5 Metal closure

2 Filling aperture (see Figure 11.5), shaping, followed by double 1 or saddle fold 2 + crimp. The seals may be improved by incorporating a heat sealable or pressure sensitive band in the fold area.

Plastic

1 Operational end. If pliable material, rigid wadless caps thermosetting or HD polythene, polypropylene, polystyrene. If rigid material, wadded rigid cap, or wadless pliable (thermoplastic) cap.
2 Filling end. Heat seal, heat weld with cooling jaws usually essential (avoid presence of product). Also ultrasonic welding, hot air sealing, plus cooling jaws, etc.

Metal cans and composite containers

General line type containers

- Lever lid (paint).
- Lever lid + diaphragm – tablets.
- Vacuum lid with flowed-in compound – boiled medicated sweets.
- Hinged lid – pastilles.
- Screw cap – metal or plastic.
- Rotary (plastic) – talc.
- Jay-Cap (thermoplastic), flip-cap.

Open top cans

Open top cans are either three-piece built-up cans or two-piece cans. These may have a ring (pull) tab on double seamed aluminium lid (beer). Key opening (sardines) on double seamed food can (ham).

Most cans have double seamed ends (compound lined); these use five thicknesses of metal, e.g. most food type cans and some solid pharmaceutical products.

A double seam gives a good hermetic seal (Figure 11.6).

Note that the closure or sealing of other seams may be overlap or joint, plus solder, single seam (dry, soldered or cemented or doped), welded. Soudronic welding (butt welded) is now replacing soldered side seams. There is also a preference for two-piece rather than three-piece cans.

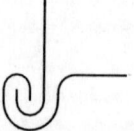

Figure 11.6 Double seam

Impact extruded aluminium cans

These were widely used in the UK for pharmaceutical tablets, powders, etc., but are now less popular in Europe and the USA due to cost compared with glass and plastic. Closures are plug (polythene), snap-on over bead (polythene), or metal screw cap fitted with conventional wadding or flowed-in compound lined. Extruded aluminium containers are still widely used for 10–30 ml monobloc aerosol cans.

Non-reclosables

Flexible packaging such as laminates, films, pouches and sachets relies on various styles of seal. These may be fin (inside to inside) from a single web, overlap (inside to outside) from a single web, inside to inside from two separate webs (four sided seal), or one web folded over by a centre fold (three or four sided seal).

The sealing may be achieved by heat involving temperature, dwell and pressure, together with removal of heat (while seal is under compression), with adhesives, or cold pressure sensitive sealing. Seals may be permanent, semi-permanent or peelable. Heat sealing may use direct (contact) heat, using a nitrocellulose, PVdC, heat seal coating, etc., or by indirect welding (hot air), using polythene (LDPE, LLDPE, ULDPE). The source of heat may also be created by ultrasonic, radio/HF welding, impulse, induction, laser, etc. Seals can also be achieved in certain cases between two different materials – i.e. melted or softened polythene will adhere to paper or board. In some circumstances two different heat sealants can create a peelable bond.

Note that although many films, laminates, etc. may have a 100% effective seal, the materials employed may be permeable to moisture, oxygen, carbon dioxide, etc. This property can be either a disadvantage or an advantage, e.g. plastic film overwrap can permit sufficient moisture permeability to cause a product to reach its critical (unacceptable) moisture level. Hence a laminate (without a foil ply) is not a hermetic pack.

The seal layers may be actual films, coatings or sealable lacquers quantified by caliper, i.e. micrometre or coating weight as g/m^2. The same base material may be used in a range of coating weights depending on the combination of the plies used, whether sealing mechanism is by platen or rotary sealing and the machine speed. Coating weight or caliper and the question, 'what is best?' are usually a trial and error exercise. What is best for one machine may not be ideal for another.

The sealing of non-reclosable materials, although predominantly reliant on heat sealing, involves other methods of sealing such as solvent, adhesive, cold sealing. These share a number of factors, including seal width, properties of the materials, cost, etc., with heat sealing remaining the most complex of the likely sealing processes. The following gives an indication of the other factors that may contribute or need consideration.

The properties of the materials of construction

Materials may be single or multiple layer. The latter may incorporate plies which provide strength (support plies such as paper, or tough, difficult-to-tear materials such as nylon or polyester), cushioning (paper), a barrier to gases, moisture, light, optimisation of cost (density, yield – basic cost, etc.), good printability, an ability to seal in the presence of contamination, etc.

The conversion process used to create material

Extrusion, lay flat tubing, calendering, casting, solvent or aqueous dispersion coating, etc. for single layer materials. Multilayer processes – wet or dry bonding (lamination), extrusion coating, coextrusion, etc.

Properties specific to heat sealing

Caliper, coating weight, softening, melting point, sealing range, viscosity, hot tack, ability to seal in the presence of contamination.

On-machine performance

Throughput, speed, possibly as metres per minute, how sealed by platen or rotary principles, how cooled and cut. Release following seal compression (jaw release) – depends on seal design, cleanliness of jaws, surface characteristics of materials, possible build-up from lacquers, varnishes, surface pick, pressure of inks, etc. External temperature applied and conductivity through to seal layer, cooling and cooling interfaces (air–metal, metal–metal and heat sinks), etc.

Reel factors (or sheet factors)

Width, diameter, core size, flagged joins (number permitted), maximum weight (handling by hand or mechanically), friction–slip characteristics (static build-up). Tightness of winding.

Storage factors

Type of storage position, i.e. normally flat, not on diameter, storage conditions, advised storage life – re-examination period, possibility of blocking.

Transportation factors

How handled, protected and packed. Position of travel.

Seal pattern

There is a diversity of seal patterns, i.e. flat smooth seal (no pattern), line pattern – all in same direction or at right angles, cross hatch or pyramid type patterns. Single (one-sided) or two-sided matching patterns. Seal pattern may encourage easy opening (tearing) or make opening difficult so that a propagation point is essential.

Width of seal

Seal width may be as low as 3 mm (small blisters), with 5 mm an advised minimum for sachets and strip packs. Width depends on web wander (a 10 mm width may be used where web wander may be ±5 mm, i.e. seal can be 5–15 mm.)

Design of pack

Pack design has to consider product volume, size/shape and weight and the seal width required to restrain/retain product. In certain processes, i.e. strip packs, flow packs, where the item actually extends the pack virtually at the time the heat (or cold seal) is being applied, the internal area must be large enough to prevent excessive pressure on the seals (thereby leading to stress, possible creases and capillary channels in the seals, or actual material perforation).

Material expansion and contraction during sealing

All materials expand or contract when heat is applied. If the web uses different constructions of materials each side, one is likely to expand more than the other, e.g. sachets using clear material one side and opaque the other. Whether this expansion and contraction lead to stress will partly depend on whether the full webs are subjected to heat or just the seal areas. Certain blister configurations suffer from tray curl, thereby making a cartoning operation more complex.

Heating methods and cooling

Heat may be applied by direct (e.g. contact heat) or indirect methods (e.g. hot air). Whatever the method of heating, the bonding materials must reach a specific minimum temperature for each combination of materials to weld together on cooling. This temperature is normally achieved by applying a much higher temperature to the surface. The transfer of the applied heat depends on the conductivity of the materials, the dwell time and the pressure. The strength of the seal made immediately after the heat is applied depends on the hot tack property of the heat sealing material(s). Although the seal can be improved (or achieved more rapidly) by cooling, hot tack is responsible for the initial weld or bond.

Hot tack varies between materials, increasing as follows:

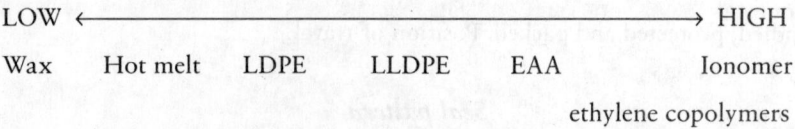

LOW ←——————————————————————————————→ HIGH

Wax   Hot melt   LDPE   LLDPE   EAA   Ionomer

ethylene copolymers

Cooling therefore is more critical to the materials showing low hot tack and may be achieved by air (cooled), water or chilled water.

The combination of temperature, dwell time, pressure (and cooling) will also depend on whether the sealing processes are platen or rotary, and whether the web is only heated at the point of seal or is preheated. As rotary invariably gives a tangential pressure between two cylinders, the dwell time is extremely short, thereby demanding a higher temperature than that used in a platen process for the same material, even when preheating is employed.

Temperatures at which heat sealing occurs generally range from around 75°C to 240°C. The list below goes from those sealing at a relatively low to high temperatures:

- (low) hot melts
- EVA
- ionomer
- lacquers
- LDPE
- LLDPE
- HDPE/PVdC
- (high) PP.

Heating or 'heat sealing' can also be achieved by impulse, ultrasonic (beware particle generation), induction, radio or high frequency, electromagnetic, vibration or laser methods.

Seal types

Seals may be permanent, semi-permanent, or peelable. Peelable systems usually consist of ethylene copolymers, possibly modified with polyethylene, or other films, lacquers or dispersions. Some are resealable, hence are not strictly tamper-resistant. Cold seals, typically based on a rubber latex, are usually non-resealable. These may employ the cold seal only in the area of the seal, hence avoiding any or limited product contact. Pattern systems are widely used for surgical materials and instruments.

Trimming and cutting (guillotine, die cut, scissors, shears, etc.) and perforating

As most heat sealing activities are based on reel-fed materials, cutting or trimming is an essential part of the overall process. Whether a material can be effectively cut depends on the cutting process, the material (metal) employed, how the web is held or restrained, the properties of the material(s) being cut and the temperature of the material when being cut, etc. Under certain conditions the cutting edges may blunt faster or give a poor cut. This also applies to perforation.

With die cutting this may be done by platen (intermittent process) whereby the web is stopped, or rotary (continuous motion). The latter process is considerably more expensive.

Ease of opening

Ease or difficulty of opening depends on the properties of the materials, the design and seal pattern. Polyester, Nylon and polypropylene may give rise to difficulties, hence it may be necessary to incorporate a propagation aid feature such as a V-shaped notch, a cut or slit. The other alternative is a peelable seal. The seal strengths of permanent and peelable seals are measured by a similar process.

Tamper-evidence, tamper-resistance and child-resistance

In general, heat sealable packs are not resealable once opened, hence they are inherently tamper-evident and tamper-resistant. Certain cold seal materials may be resealable, hence they do not comply with this parameter. Child-resistance properties are less easy to confirm, as the standard varies between countries. In the USA materials have to meet the test created via the PPA (Poisons Prevention Act 1970), in Germany DIN 55559, and the UK BSI 7236 1989.

Cost

Cost depends on the complexity of the material (especially multi-ply) and the yield. In terms of the heat seal ply cost, these are likely to increase as follows

$$LDPE/LLDPE \longrightarrow EVA \longrightarrow EAA \longrightarrow ionomer$$

and according to the caliper/coating weight, and the means by which they are applied (i.e. adhesive, extrusion, aqueous, or solvent coated).

Other factors

To the above can be added a few other rather obvious factors, i.e. non-blocking, non-exuding, non-tainting, with the correct slip/friction properties. State of the material surface, particularly with reference to oxidation, may also influence a heat sealing operation. This may be derived from a conversion process (e.g. pretreatment for printing). Other processes such as used to render a material sterile (e.g. gamma irradiation, steam sterilisation) and any surface active agents incorporated as additives or processing aids may also cause heat sealing problems.

The above still only covers some of the factors associated with a heat sealing operation. The primary factors remain: temperature, dwell, pressure and cooling.

Membrane or diaphragm seals

Although there are mixed views on membranes or diaphragms as a tamper-evident feature in that they are not visible until the closure is removed (i.e. not visible at point of sale), they do offer positive seal potentials. Diaphragms can be affixed to a container by adhesive, by a direct heat seal or by a pressure sensitive adhesive sealant. In the pharmaceutical industry the fourth method, induction sealing, has general preference. This involves a foil membrane coated with various plastics, which is retained in the closure and then subjected to induction (or eddy currents) after it has been applied to the container. At this stage, the induction head, which contains a water cooled copper coil, creates an electromagnetic field thereby inducing a current in the foil and producing an almost instantaneous heating effect. This heat seals the plastic facing attached to the foil onto the container neck and melts a layer of wax which retains the secondary liner in the cap when the foil seal is broken. Retightening of the cap is normally advised following induction sealing.

Various induction heat seal liners are available, such as the following.

1   On activating, the material separates to provide a foil seal with a pulpboard liner in the cap as a reseal.
2   Where pulpboard is inadequate (e.g. with liquids), a polyester faced liner on the pulpboard may be employed with a paper covered foil membrane.
3   This may involve a one-piece liner where the whole material forms a diaphragm-type seal. The diaphragm can be cut with a tab feature to aid removal.

Surlyn ionomer is the more widely used material. Seals can be achieved to LDPE, HDPE, PP, PET, PVC, PS and SAN.

With glass the contact ply depends on whether the glass is treated or untreated and whether the product is dry or wet. In certain circumstances special treatments may be necessary to give either a weld or peelable seals.

Membrane or diaphragm seals can provide very effective seals. This can be particularly important with plastic caps on plastic bottles which suffer loss of torque with the lapse of time. In these instances, the diaphragm provides an effective seal up to the point of use, after which the cap takes over the closure function.

Adhesive sealing

Adhesion is basically the joining or bonding of two materials by a third material. There are two primary methods of adhesion, physical or mechanical adhesion and chemical or specific adhesion.

Mechanical adhesion, as the title implies, is achieved by the open or porous nature of the substrate(s), whereby the adhesive penetrates into the cracks, crevices or gaps in the surface(s) involved. Specific or chemical adhesion involves the bonding of non-absorbent or non-porous surfaces such as found with glass, metals, including foil, and plastics. The bond achieved between these materials and the adhesive depends on molecular or electrical forces based on van der Waals' forces. Polar and non-polar materials need to bond with like adhesives.

Types of adhesive

There are three basic types of adhesive:

1   solution adhesives where the adhesive constituent is dissolved in a carrier (e.g. starch pastes, dextrines and contact cements such as polystyrene cement) or solvent
2   dispersion adhesives where the adhesive component may be as a dispersion, suspension or emulsion, e.g. polyvinyl acetate emulsion
3   hot melt adhesives which are made from 100% solids based on blending hot liquid thermoplastics which can be reactivated by heat.

Terminology associated with adhesion

Phrases that need to be understood include the following.

- Viscocity – resistance to flow.
- Wetting – the ability of an adhesive to flow and wet a surface by coming into close contact with it.
- Tack – the ability to form a bond of measurable strength immediately after the adhesive and adherent have been brought together.
- Setting time – the time needed to form an effective bond by mechanical or specific adhesion, e.g. a fibre tearing bond with paper-based materials.
- Open time – the elapsed time between the application of the adhesive to one or both substrates and the bringing together of the two surfaces to give an effective bond.
- Drying time – the time elapsed to form the final bond.

According to the circumstances, e.g. hand applied versus high-speed machine applied adhesive, the above factors will vary significantly. Hand applied operations normally need a longer open time, lower tack and longer setting time than machine applied, which requires a short open time, with high tack and a rapid setting time.

Classification of adhesives

Although there are many adhesives, there are only four main adhesive classifications, i.e. animal, vegetable, mineral and synthetic.

1. Animal glues are usually made from bones and hide. Casein from milk and fish glues are also of animal origin.
2. The main vegetable adhesives are based on starch and dextrine; the latter is a modified form of starch. Each has wide applications.
3. Mineral based adhesive systems involve materials such as sodium silicate but use of this, particularly for fibreboard, is reducing. Bitumens, asphalts and pitches could be put under this category.
4. Recently, synthetic adhesive systems have steadily increased based on synthetic rubber latices, polyvinyl acetate dispersions and hot melts, etc.

Factors influencing adhesion efficiency include the following.

1. Wetting out – the ability to create a continuous film (there are exceptions, see hot melts) which depends on both the adhesive and the substrate.
2. Viscocity – the resistance to flow. Adhesive must have good flow properties to achieve adequate coverage and uniformity of film thickness.
3. Polarity – like will bond only to like. Hence a polar surface needs a polar adhesive and a non-polar surface a non-polar adhesive. Both paper and wood are polar materials.
4. pH control, i.e. acidity/alkalinity extremes – unless controlled, the acid or alkalis could interact with material substrates, e.g. metal, causing corrosion or weakening of the bond.

5   Cleanliness – the presence of contaminants such as grease, dust, dirt can reduce adhesive–adherent contact, hence weaken the bond.

6   Microbial growth – certain adhesives (starches, dextrines) can support microbial growth, hence either preservatives will need to be incorporated or procedures used to minimise microbiological contamination.

7   Stress – adhesive film must be able to withstand stresses due to moisture (loss/gain), deformation from creep or cold flow, differential expansion and contraction, etc.

8   Adherent surface properties – ideally surface should be flat, smooth and not too porous.

9   Temperature – of adhesive and adherent at point of and immediately after a bond is made.

10   Water resistance or solubility – adhesives may be required to be water-resistant or water-soluble. This may influence bond quality and ultimate removal for material reuse, recycling, etc.

Methods of adhesive application

Adhesives may be applied in several ways, as follows.

1   Brush – a well-established method for hand application, but slow and variable consistency.

2   Dauber applicators – simple method of transferring an adhesive to a stationery area by a coated bar, finger or plate.

3   Wheel or rotary cylinder – the wheel or cylinder picks up adhesive from an open pot, tray or bath. This is thinned by a doctor blade or transfer roller system. The thinned layer is then transferred to the substrate. Viscocity properties are critical.

4   Low-pressure extrusion – via a nozzle head or die fitted with an on/off valve system.

5   High-pressure extrusion i.e. jetting – widely used for hot melt systems where a jet is 'fired' by a pressurised gun.

6   Spraying – similar to jetting except that adhesive is broken up into finer particles. Since this partially dries the adhesive, higher output speeds may be derived from this process.

Adhesive usage

Usage for adhesives is rather like horses for courses. Certain ones find very traditional applications. Animal glues are, for example, widely used for bookbinding, tube winding, including fibreboard, and for the production of so-called gummed tapes. Casein finds a specific application for bottle labelling where the product is chilled (e.g. beers and carbonated drinks) and there may be a film of moisture on the container. Casein has also been used in foil laminations. Mineral glues, and in particular sodium silicate, have been used for tube winding, corrugated board and the lamination of fibreboard. Sodium silicate's use is slowly reducing, partly due to the fact that it has high alkalinity. Bitumen is still used as a waterproofing layer in union Kraft type combinations. It can be applied as a hot melt or as emulsions or solutions in organic solvents. However, the use of solvents in any application is becoming less favoured. Vegetable adhesives still find extensive applications. Various types of starch are still used as a lap paste in wrap-around can and bottle labelling. Borated and unborated dextrines are used for envelopes, carton and case sealing, tube winding and bottle labelling. Vinyl-dextrines are used for remoistenable coatings.

In the synthetic category can be included dispersions and suspensions (but frequently called emulsions) which can be used on more difficult substrates where specific adhesion is essential (plastic, metal). They have a wide range of uses which include pressure and heat sensitive based materials. Various polymer systems are found based on both thermoplastic and thermosetting adhesive systems, e.g. vinyls, acrylics (increasing in use), polyamides, polyurethanes, ethylene vinyl acetate, vinyl acetate, ethylene acrylic acid (EAA).

Modern Plastics Encyclopedia lists the types of adhesive system which may be used to bond together similar and dissimilar plastics. These are usually coded under elastomeric, thermoplastic resins, thermosetting resins and miscellaneous systems.

In addition to adhesive, plastic components can be directly joined together or sealed by several techniques as described earlier.

Hot melts are 100% solids and can be formulated from a range of plastics to give various levels of tack with a range of setting times. Their benefit lies in cleanliness (no solvents or solutions to drive off), ease of application, short open time and fast setting times. They can also be used to seal virtually any substrate with the availability of good climatic properties from deep freeze to high tropical conditions. They are very resistant to water (waterproof and permeation).

Cold sealing

The use of cold seal adhesives, frequently laid out to a pattern (e.g. pattern lacquered), is becoming increasingly popular in the confectionery industry, particularly for flow wraps. Most cold seals are emulsion-based rubber latex systems applied by a gravure print roller. They have the advantage, as pressure sensitive systems, of achieving much faster sealing than conventional heat sealing. Some use is now being found for pharmaceutical application.

Closure evaluation – introducing new methodology

Methods for leakage detection are becoming increasingly complex in terms of instrumentation, with a trend, certainly for production packs, towards non-destructive testing. However, even so-called non-destructive tests may have conflicts with GMP.

Summary of leakage detection

Leakage (egress and ingress) can be related to liquids, solids, gases including bioburden and the methods associated with their detection. The list below includes those already mentioned together with others which have been or may be employed.

Observation of visual defects, e.g. pinholes, capillaries.

Vision systems could be included under this heading – see also 'Visual inspection systems' below.

Weight change

Loss or gain versus time under specifically defined conditions (and by chemical analysis).

Pressure–vacuum changes

By the application of pressure and/or vacuum under defined conditions (including fluctuating conditions), e.g. leakage by ingress/egress of external atmosphere or internal contents. This may involve the release of gases, e.g. air as bubble-type tests – limits of detection by visual inspection are usually around 1 cm^3 per minute with the 'possible' detection of pinholes down to 20–25 μm. Tests involving immersion in water may be carried out with or without wetting agents (to lower surface tension) and dyes.

Pressure decay systems normally operate to a specified pressure (usually within the pack) which is then monitored for pressure drop. Leaks down to $10^{-3} \text{ cm}^3/\text{s}$ can be detected. There is also a pressure increase method where leakage from a pack under vacuum can be detected as a positive pressure change (assuming an excellent vacuum chamber seal is achieved).

Certain flexible packs will extend or indent (i.e. undergo deflection) according to whether a pack is under vacuum or pressure when well sealed. A grossly leaking pack will show virtually no movement, and a slightly leaking pack less movement, than a well sealed pack. These movements or deflections can be quantified, e.g. by differential pressure, transducers (capacitive type) or spring loaded sensors. Typical instruments include the blister testers which sense deflection and, with larger packs (e.g. sachets), detect 'force' changes. Both these instruments are considered more sensitive than the older conventional vacuum with dye tests as pinholes down to 10 μm can be detected. These tests also have the advantage of being non-destructive.

In most instruments based on the above, the test period is kept to a short time (e.g. 0.5 to 1.0 s) so that temperature influences are minimised. It is also important to restrict creep, as certain materials will extend under unfavourable conditions.

Gaseous detection tests

These may use a specific gas associated with the product or a gas which can be specifically introduced for the leakage detection process, such as the following.

- Helium (sniffing) currently uses mass spectrometry which enables leakage to be detected down to $10–12 \text{ Pa m}^3 \text{ s}$ (this test can demand a high vacuum which may not be ideal for the component being tested). Certain halogens are also used for gas detection.
- Oxygen, i.e. Mocon Ox-tran – uses a stream of dry nitrogen whereby oxygen is detected coulometrically.

- Carbon dioxide, e.g. Mocon Permatran C detects carbon dioxide in another dry gas by infrared.
- Moisture vapour, e.g. Mocon Permatran W or Dynamic water vapour tester measures moisture by a photoelectric sensor.
- Radio isotope tracer gas, e.g. using krypton 85 where a high sensitivity is reported.

Burst tests

The strength of the seal on flexible packs (achieved by cold and heat seals) can be quantified by tensile tests as seal or peel tests or the air pressure required to create rupture of the pack. This can be carried out by a hypodermic needle arrangement followed by pressurising the pack at a specific rate until the pack bursts. Depending on the nature of the seal, the point of rupture may arise either in the body of the pack or the seals. An alternative method is to place the pack in a jig followed by a steady mechanical increase in compression.

Microbial integrity

Various procedures have been developed (under normal pressure and vacuum) to check whether highly contaminated liquid, gel or media based material will grow back or penetrate closure systems. Variable results suggest that alternative methods to detect leakage are preferable.

Crack, pinhole, capillary detection

Conventional dye/vacuum immersion tests were widely used to check the seal efficiency of ampoules. These have largely been replaced by electrical conductivity and capacitance type tests. Typical equipment includes the Nikka Densok ampoule inspection machine which employs a high frequency and high voltage. This distinguishes between good glass (which is a non-conductor) and areas of cracks or pinholes where current will flow between the inner and outer glass surfaces. Other machines use the principle of capacitance and dielectric constants, where a material with defects (penetrating cracks) will show a higher dielectric constant.

Thermal conductivity

These use a thermistor bridge which is balanced against air and is subsequently upset if another gas leaks into the air.

Chemical tracer tests

Used with materials which can be detected by interaction, i.e. ammonia on one side, hydrochloric acid gas on the other (formation of white cloud of ammonium chloride indicates transfer and leakage). This type of test has been used for pinhole detection.

Thermocouple gauges

Mainly used to detect a drop in temperature when solvent-type systems escape under vacuum. Could also be used to detect the presence of a warmer gas.

Physical or mechanical assessment procedures

These involve the widest variety of factors, e.g. screw caps are controlled by application torque and by removal torque. However, these change according to material, design, environmental factors, etc., some of which may never have been fully investigated. This equally applies to any closure system which relies on compression, interlocking, interference forces, etc. in order to make and maintain a 'seal'. Thus, although certain forces can readily be measured, e.g. torque, force to push in a plug, pull out a plug type system, force to apply or remove a press-over closure. The variables associated with most of these systems (see the appendices) tend to be quite horrific. Whether the measured forces equate with an effective seal will vary according to the quality of the materials employed and the perfection/imperfection of the surfaces involved between the two interfacing materials.

Some excellent work has been done in this area by Dr Dana K. Morton of Schering Plough, USA, who investigated the seal integrity of rubber capped vials using a range of techniques, types of vial (blown and tubular) and a range of coated and uncoated rubber components. This work concluded that control of (top) rubber compression, quantified as residual seal force measurement, could be correlated to seal integrity in terms of liquid, gas and microbial factors, measured in Pa m^3/s.

The West Company offers two pieces of equipment to check rubber–vial type closure systems, i.e. the Seal Force Tester, which quantifies residual compressive forces, and the Seal Force Monitor, which checks the forces applied during the capping and sealing operation.

Visual inspection systems

Visual (imaging) inspection methods are gradually replacing the previous human inspection where each unit was individually viewed (frequently under two times magnification) against a white or black background. Although not currently bearing a direct assessment of closure integrity, they can eliminate likely suspect packs.

Note that 'leak-tight', as defined by NASA (Aerospace), is when nitrogen at 300 psig leaks at a rate not greater than 1.4×10^{-3} cm^3/s. It should also be noted that the pressure exerted by a gas will change according to the temperature (Charles's law). This roughly means that a 1°C rise or fall will change the test pressure, up or down, by approximately 0.4%.

Special aspects of closures and their assessment

Closure systems are becoming more complex and sophisticated, incorporating features related to such aspects as tamper-evidence, tamper-resistance, child-resistance, special easy opening closures for the elderly, and product administration.

Tamper-evidence and tamper-resistance

The earlier use of the word 'tamper-proof' has been replaced by tamper-evidence and tamper-resistance. The Extra Strength Tylenol incidences between 29 September and 7 October 1982 in the USA, whereby seven people were killed by cyanide and the copy-cat poisonings which followed, provided a worldwide alertness to the issue. Although TE/TR cannot offer total security it does offer some assurance that the product has not been contaminated, some of the contents removed and possibly replaced (e.g. watered down), etc. Certain TE/TR features (sealed diaphragms, ratchet closures) also improve overall closure efficiency in that cap backing-off or loss of torque is likely to be less of a problem.

Definitions of TE/TR are as follows.

1   Tamper-evidence (TE) – 'if breached or opened, package will provide visible evidence that the said container or package has been tampered with'.
2   Tamper-resistance (TR) – 'that which creates a barrier to entry and has to be broken or removed before entry can be achieved and which is difficult to repair (if necessary) without leaving any evidence'.

In the UK the current types of pack which are considered to fall in the TE/TR categories are as follows (note the preference in the UK for the term 'security packaging').

1   Film wrappers – a transparent film wrapped securely around a product or product container. The film must be cut or torn to open the container and remove the product.
2   Bubble packs – the product and container are sealed within a mount or display card generally composed of card and/or plastic.
3   Shrink seals and bands – bands or wrappers shrunk by heat or drying to seal the union of the cap and container. The seal must be cut or torn to open the container and remove the product.
4   Bottle seals – paper or foil sealed to the mouth of a container under the cap. The seal must be torn or broken to open the container and remove the product.
5   Tape seals – paper and/or foil sealed over all carton flaps or a bottle cap. The seal must be torn or broken to open the container and remove the product.
6   Breakable caps – the container is sealed by a plastic or metal cap that either breaks away completely when removed from the container or leaves part of the cap attached to the container. The cap must be broken to open the container and remove the product.
7   Sealed tubes – the nozzle of a tube is sealed and the seal must be punctured to gain access to the product.
8   Sealed carton – all flaps of a carton are securely sealed and the carton must be visibly damaged when opened to remove the product.
9   Sealed units – dosage units individually sealed in foil, paper or plastic pouches, where the individual compartment must be torn or broken to gain access to the product (e.g. strip, blister and sachet packaging).

It should be noted that this follows the list approved by FDA regulations on

5 November 1982. However, since that time the USA has withdrawn the use of glued cartons, cellulose shrink bands and heat sealed (folded) overwraps based on the fact that some can be opened and resealed.

Child-resistance

The advent of the Poisons Prevention Act 1970 in the USA formally introduced child-resistant packaging. The Act required both reclosable and non-reclosable (blister, strip, sachet) packs to pass virtually the same test procedure if child-resistant properties were to be claimed.

BS 5321 1975 for reclosables basically followed the USA protocol. No equivalent standard for non-reclosables was introduced, as the Medicines Commission (1974) believed that blisters and strips were reasonably child-resistant and were concerned if large numbers of children were involved in testing procedures. BS 5321 has now been replaced by BS 6652 (see also ISO 28317) 1989 which permits a sequential sampling procedure of up to 200 children between the ages of 42 and 51 months, thereby allowing a closure to be passed or failed with the involvement of smaller numbers of children. UK approved reclosables include Poplok, Clic-lok, Tracer, Snapsafe, Squeeze-lok, Push-lok, Medi-Loc.

UK legislation currently covers aspirin-and paracetamol-based products and a series of household/chemical products introduced from 1 December 1987. For solid dose dispensed medicines there is a scheme which requires pharmacies to use child-resistant systems unless they are not required by the patient (i.e. elderly, arthritic, infirm, etc.). Child-resistant closures are also required on certain liquid products.

Child-resistance, tamper-evidence/resistance and OPD (original pack dispensing)

Blisters and strips by their design are inherently both tamper-evident and tamper-resistant. Although the Medicines Commission report of 1974 suggested that blisters and strips had child-resistant properties, positive evidence of this did not clearly emerge until Glyn Volans et al.'s reports appeared in Human Toxicology, July 1987. These reports indicated that both reclosables which had passed BS 5321 (now replaced by BS 6652 1989) and opaque blisters and strips had reduced poisonings when compared with non-approved or conventional reclosable systems. As a result of these reports the PAGB, with the support of the ABPI, produced 'Design Guidelines for Strip and Blister Packs (1987)', which basically eliminates any 'flimsy' blister or strip packs which may be questionably child-resistant. This document later became BS 7236 1989. As a result, blisters and strips which meet the guidelines were at one time termed to have 'child-safe' properties rather than being called child-resistant.

It should be noted that the Medicines Commission did not advise a test procedure (such as BS 5321) for blisters and strips since the variety of configurations and product sizes could have exposed a significant number of children to the challenge (and learning risk) of opening packs. Although the USA has always used the same test for reclosables and non-reclosables, this is questionable since an opening of a reclosable can expose a child to larger product quantities compared with the single opening of blisters and strips. Non-reclosables also offer another obstacle in being available in small quantities, and children may tire of repetitive activities. There is also a risk with a reclosable that the previous user may not have resealed the pack correctly. The Volans report therefore goes part of the way in challenging the use of the US protocol for blisters and strips. The BGA in Germany is, however, meeting the US protocol by a 'type test' which approves a material for any blister/strip configuration, product shape/size, etc. based on one test. The materials approved include perforations between blisters, a tissue/foil/heatseal lidding material and a range of other combinations. The children at the greatest risk fall into the $2-2\frac{1}{2}$ year age group which is not covered by the US protocol, hence using children of 42–51 months could be equated with an accelerated test. The ISO standard ISO 8317 has been approved for reclosables, but a standard for non-reclosables is still under debate. German standards for type approval are based on DIN 55559.

Packs for the elderly, including monitored dosage systems

The improved security and integrity achieved by certain closure systems make them more difficult to open (and reclose where relevant) for a growing elderly population. The fact that these people survive longer because of their medication will require increasing attention in the future. To assist in this, various compartmental-type packs (e.g. larger blister) have been developed so that all the medications required for a set time (e.g. 8.00 a.m., 12 noon, etc.) can be placed in special compartments. Although this placing of various products with each other was initially approved by the Royal Pharmaceutical Society for the short period involved (1 to 4 weeks' supply), pharmaceutical manufacturers would be concerned if interaction risks arose under the terms of 'product liability'. Whether the products need testing (a) for the short periods and (b) in contact with other likely products is now under debate as to whether any 'risks' need quantification. These new types of pack, classified under the heading, 'monitored dosage systems', tend to conflict with the concept of OPD, as bulk packs are required for economical transfer to the new packs. Other systems such as MEMS (medical event monitored systems) either record when medication is taken or alert the patient when to take the medication, and are also becoming more available.

Closure systems involving product delivery or administration

Historically some of the first closure systems to include dispensing features were those used for drops, those incorporating an applicator (e.g. corn solvent) or brush (paints), and atomiser sprays. These were followed by the more complex valve systems subsequently used for a wide range of aerosols. It was the era of thermoplastics that introduced the complexity of closure systems found today, starting with dropper plugs and spray systems invented and commercialised in the early to mid-1950s. Since that time closure systems involving product delivery have steadily increased. These now include such items as prefilled syringes, IV packs, a wide range of pump systems, and valves, etc.

Since most of the above have an additional role to play during the period of use, assessment of performance during use requires thorough evaluation. In the case of multiple dosage packs, this involves checks for uniformity of delivery, malfunction (sticking, blocking, microbial contamination, etc.), degradation/loss of potency during the whole period of use with and without extended periods of storage involving any likely misuse or abuse by the user. As product particle size has become more critical, particle size analysis is now essential to certain performance evaluations. Compliance associated with the instructions and the device also has to be assessed.

Since in many of the newer administration systems the pack and closure cannot be segregated it is perhaps useful to look at a likely total testing schedule. Defining the type of test which may be required will depend on the types of material involved, i.e. glass, metal, plastics, etc.

However, as packs become more complex and more innovative, plastic becomes the more favoured material for sound economic reasons (frequently associated with fewer components which provide simpler assembly procedures). Any testing schedule may be influenced in the final level of intensity by various additional factors, the route of administration and the risks associated with it. This normally places IV solutions and injections at the top of the 'risk' list, i.e. those at the top of the list demand the greatest intensity of evaluation. For more details see Chapter 8, Appendix 8.8.

Compliance and confidence – conclusion

It should be evident that if the user, patient, or professional administrator of the product has confidence in the product and its pack, the likelihood of 'success' and compliance can be enhanced. Evaluating this feature by market research, questionnaires during clinical evaluation and consultation with the professionals who handle the product–pack (doctors, dentists, nurses, pharmacists, etc.) will become more vital in the future. The user–patient, in being made more aware of packaging, frequently in a negative environmental cost-effective role, may also become more critical of pharmaceutical packaging. This will lead, in the long term, to more effective packaging and better instructions on how the product should be used.

Seal integrity has now reached a status of greater importance under the terms of GMP and the fact that recalls related to seal failure regularly occur. In addition to this the broader role of the pack places increasing demands on the closure, particularly at the point of use.

Appendix 11.1: Leakage detection in sterile products

It has been widely accepted that compendial tests for sterility do not give high confidence that sterility is both achieved and maintained. Starting with a low (controlled) bioburden, maintaining GMP which builds assurance into the processes, adequate validation, and effective closure systems are the essential prerequisites to satisfactory sterile products. These basic principles apply irrespective of whether sterility is achieved by an aseptic or a terminal sterilising process. Checking that the closure system is effective in preventing microbial contamination or recontamination is critical to both unit dose and multi-dose products. Many papers have investigated this subject related to ampoules, IV solutions, multi-dose vials, syringes, etc. Examples of some of these papers are listed in Appendix 11.2.

Ampoules

At one time, 'ampoules' was synonymous with glass as either single or double ended systems which were produced from tubular glass. Although glass ampoules are still widely used, plastic ampoules usually made by a form or blow fill seal process (Rommeleg or Automatic Liquid Packaging) have shown a steady growth. Although the principles of manufacture and sterilisation (predominantly terminal versus predominantly aseptic) are different, both are sealed by a welding/fusion process and tests are therefore required to check the integrity of each (see above).

Vials

Rubber-based closures have a good chance of flowing into minor imperfections and making an effective seal provided there is adequate compression of the rubber. Over-compression disc-type seals (e.g. combination seals) and relatively shallow stoppers may cause the material to distort, flow into the bore, ruck at the flange, etc., and thereby cause general loss of closure efficiency. Coated stoppers, especially when the coating is harder than the basic rubber to which it is attached, generally need higher compression forces to achieve an effective seal.

Seal efficiency may change under conditions of autoclaving (e.g. steam at 115 or 121°C) and with the passage of time/conditions of storage. As a result a closure may have to be evaluated for integrity during several stages of its shelf life.

Intravenous (IV) solutions

IV solutions were originally in heavy glass containers with screw closures. Although such systems suffered from several problems (possible contamination from cooling water etc.), they are still in use in various parts of the world. The introduction of the DIN standard with a rolled- or crimped-on overseal retaining a rubber stopper improved the seal efficiency. Plastic has gradually gained in popularity as either pre-formed or blow fill seal moulded containers. These have been available as single port or multiport versions, which may or may not involve rubber stoppers and/or welded extensions. Due to the nature of the product and its use, closure integrity is more critical with IV solutions. However, certain packs (which are not blow moulded) are manufactured by welding or heat sealing, hence these seals also need continual evaluation. (Ports may be sealed by a number of methods.)

Since many IV packs are overwrapped (some prior to autoclaving), usually to reduce gaseous or moisture permeation factors, this may also add to the overall pack integrity and needs evaluation before and after autoclaving.

Cartridge tubes and prefilled syringes

Cartridge tubes (which may be used in a cartridge holder, disposable or non-disposable syringe unit) and prefilled syringes both have two closure systems: a plunger-type seal which acts as an internal piston to expel the product and an end seal which may be pierced, ruptured, part removed, prior to expulsion of the contents. The plunger or piston internal seal must prevent leakage and microbial ingress while maintaining ease of movement during use. There is, therefore, a conflict between the degree of interference to retain a seal and the ease of movement, partly achieved by lubrication (e.g. silicones on the rubber).

The top seal (overseal) may be a small stopper, a modification of a stopper, a disc or a combination-type system. Each normally requires rubber under compression held in position by an aluminium crimped, rolled-on, etc. overseal. The second sealing surface may be glass or plastic. In the case of glass cartridge tubes, these are invariably produced from the tubular or cane glass process, hence suffer from imperfections associated with this 'shaping' process. Plastic cartridges have never proved popular but are available.

Prefilled syringes can also be made from tubular glass or by moulding in plastic (e.g. polypropylene). These units may consist of either a single or double (bi) compartmental type. The latter then involve three seals, as a seal must be achieved between the two compartments. Syringes are further complicated at the end seal by the presence of a fitment for a needle (e.g. Luer) or by having a needle already moulded or fitted. These protrusions may then demand a further cover or seal, e.g. to protect the needle and prevent microbial contamination.

Prefilled syringes are usually packed into individual (sterile or sterilised) sachets, hence this provides an additional barrier to gaseous/moisture exchange and microbial ingress. However, this does not eliminate the need for closure integrity control, and this must start with quality of design. Elimination of critical defects in glass and plastic components (cartridge tubes and syringes) is increasingly being carried out by inspection systems, e.g. visual and high-frequency, high-voltage units.

Cleanliness

Although low particulates put an ever-increasing demand on sterile products, their presence at a seal or closure interface adds to leakage seepage risks. Combination seals, which were renowned for the generation of aluminium particles (usually from movement during transportation), are therefore now less used. However, some seals can create particles during the closuring operation, particularly if rubbing or tearing occurs (e.g. against relatively minor imperfections).

Conclusions

To support their high standards, sterile products require the greatest attention to detail in the quality of design stage, the highest quality standards and most effective quality assurance and quality control procedures. The fact that the seal is usually based on rubber means that the effectiveness and integrity of the total closure system has to be evaluated at several phases of the product shelf life, i.e.

1 initially
2 after autoclaving or sterilisation of components and aseptic assembly
3 during several stages of the product shelf life
4 at the end of the shelf-life period.

Appendix 11.2: References – sterile products

1 Myers, J. A., Contaminated bottles of autoclaved fluid, *Lancet*, **1389**, 24 June 1972.
2 Myers, J. A., Microbial contamination of packaged fluids after sterilisation, *Pharm. J.* 308–310, 13 April 1974.

3 Allwood, M. C., Hambleton, R. H. and Beverley, S. Pressure change in bottles during sterilization by autoclaving, *J. Pharm. Sci.*, **64**, 333–334, 1975.

4 Hambleton and Allwood, Evaluation of a new design of bottle closure for non injectable water, *J. Appl. Bacteriol*, **41**, 109–118, 1976.

5 Felix, R. I., Bottles and closures for injection fluids, *Pharm. J.*, **51**, 17 July 1982.

6 Mitrono, F. P., Baptister, R. J., Newton, D. W. and Augustini, S. C. A. M., Microbial contamination potential of solutions in prefilled disposable syringes used with a syringe pump, *J. Pharm. Sci.*, **43**, 78–80 1986.

7 Sharpe, J., Validation of a new form fill seal installation, *Manuf. Chem.*, **59** 22, 23, 27, 55, 1988.

8 *Non Destructive Testing Handbook*, 2nd edn, Vol. 1, *Leak Testing*, USA.

9 Denyer, S. and Baird, R. *Guide to Microbiological Control in Pharmaceuticals*, Ellis Horwood, 1990.

Appendix 11.3: Aerosol seals

Aerosols differ from other packs partly because they are pressurised and partly because of the number of seals. For example, a tinplate can normally has about five seal areas.

Due to the complexities associated with the seals, most aerosols are pressure tested by passage through a water bath at 55°C. This test normally identifies the presence of serious leakage by the release of air bubbles. However, many aerosols can suffer from slow leakage which is frequently highest immediately after the filling and assembly of the can and valve system. This usually occurs because the rubber or synthetic gasket systems involved swell (thereby improving the seal) once in contact with the propellants which have solvent-type properties.

As this loss is far more serious with small aerosols (e.g. metered dose inhalation products), tests are carried out on a continuous basis to check that initial loss and subsequent steady loss (after the gaskets have swollen) are under control. This usually means that aerosols are trayed off for a period prior to final packing, i.e. labelling and cartonning, etc., and are then individually check weighed for higher losses. Sample aerosols are also kept under selected conditions with weight losses being checked over longer periods.

Where plastic packs are now used, additional weight losses may occur by permeation (through the plastic).

Appendix 11.4: Closure systems and stress cracking

As many closure systems rely on interference, impression, interlocking forces, etc. to achieve a seal, this applied stress provides potential for either physical stress cracking or environmental stress cracking. Which occurs may depend on the design of the moulding, whether any contact material (e.g. the product) acts as a stress cracking agent, or a combination of both. Examples of cracking include horizontal cracks which may follow the thread (screw caps), vertical cracks on push-on closure systems, flaps lifting from the top of the cap (frequently an extension of 'doming'), or vertical cracking in bore fitting systems. Each can usually be associated with flaws in the moulding operation, poor design or the presence of a true stress cracking agent. If the last of these is established, the choice of the wrong grade or type of plastic may lead to environmental stress cracking (ESC). This can initially be established by taking samples of plastic (in line with the Bell Telephone Test), putting in a notch or V shaped cut, and stressing them by bending in the product held at 50 or 60°C. The samples are then observed to check whether the notch extends into a crack after a relatively short testing period. Although this type of test may give an indication that the proposed material is suspect, running a parallel test with a known poor stress crack resistance grade may be useful, as this can indicate whether the formulation contains a stress cracking agent. Typical stress cracking agents are detergents, wetting agents, certain preservative systems (e.g. benzylkonium chloride and bromide) and volatile oils.

An additional test, however, is still advised on actual mouldings since processing aids (e.g. mould release agents) may add another dimension to the test. A typical test on screw caps is to apply them at a higher torque (probably double that which would normally be recommended) under the conditions of a Hedley test (pack filled or part filled with product) and then store at 60°C for 48 h (minimum period) to 2 weeks. Samples are regularly examined and the period leading to cracking recorded. If cracking does not occur with the product, but does in the presence of the standard Igepal, this normally reveals the long-term weakest point of the closure system. The removed neck test with overtight closures may be used as a QC test to check deliveries or as a test to compare different cap designs or similar designs from different manufacturers.

It should be noted that changes in mould dimensions (wear of moulds, changes in moulding conditions), even if these remain within acknowledged specifications, have to be assessed throughout the life of both closure and container mouldings. If regrind is allowed into the process, items produced from this will again have to be regularly checked.

Although environmental stress cracking was initially associated with low-density polyethylene, and one means of reducing this risk was the use of materials of a lower melt flow index (MFI), 'cracking' can occur with a range of plastics. The cause of this cracking may be associated with a strain which is in-built into the moulding or it may subsequently be created or increased by the wedding of the closure with a container finish. Tests such as those applied above may therefore indicate a weakness in the total system rather than specifically identifying the cause (e.g. if a component cracks on a circular object, i.e. a plug, 180° from the injection moulding point, cold welding work might be suspected). This, therefore, means that further work has frequently to be carried out before cause and corrective action can be identified.

In the case of a screw closure, it should be evident that a closure which has one turn or more of thread engagement will suffer less thread-to-thread stress than one of, say, $\frac{1}{2}-\frac{3}{4}$ turn (i.e. the same force (torque) is spread over less area with the latter, hence stress cracking could be more likely). This torque force is also conveyed to the sealing surface of the container and the contact surface of the closure, hence areas receive and convey a greater force (onto the cap). Studying how a stress occurs with the closure–container system is therefore a useful part of avoiding stress cracking problems.

Appendix 11.5: Upside-down, on-head, or on-cap stacked packs

Certain packs are designed for the container to be upside-down, i.e. sit on a wide flat cap. Typical examples are found in plastic tubes, and bottles which use wide diameter caps (i.e. shrouded caps). As the challenge to the closuring system in such instances may be greater than that found in right-way-up capped containers, leakage, or more likely seepage, tends to be more prevalent. This is because the inverted system has a product seal contact where any pressure change (dimensional or airspace, expansion/contraction) endeavours to force liquid out or air in. Some manufacturers recognise this risk by transporting upside-down packs closure upwards.

Appendix 11.6: Some references and standards

- BS 1918 Pt. 1 1984, Continuous thread finishes.
- BS 1918 Pt. 2 1981, Crown finishes.
- BS 6652 1982, Child-resistant reclosables.
- BS 3130 Pt. 3, Glass containers and closures.
- BS 3313 Pt. 1, Aluminium capping foil for glass containers.
- BS 3313 Pt. 2, Aluminium capping foil for skirted closures for plastic containers.
- BS 2006 1984, Specification for aluminium collapsible tubes.
- BS 4230 1977, Metal collapsible tubes for eye ointment.
- BS 4839, Blow moulded polyolefin containers.
- BS 5638, Blow moulded unplasticised PVC containers.
- BS 6499 1985, Specification for metal screw necks, caps and inner seals for metal containers.
- BS 5789, Specification for screw threads for plastic containers.

US methods

- Measuring torque, T3205.
- Thread application and removal torque, T3759, D3991.
- Screw cap liner compatibility, T3202.
- Screw cap MVT in lining, D3199, T3201.
- Heat seal strength, PIFA 2/74.

Pressure sensitive tapes

USA standards:

- Tensile strength, D3759.
- Unwind force, D3811.
- Peel adhesion 180°, D3330.

Holding power to:

- fibreboard, D3652
- caliper, D3652
- impact resistance, D3812
- water penetration rate, D3816.

Strapping:

- flat steel (and seals), D3853
- non metallic (and connections), D3950.

General references

1 *Code of Standards for Security Packaging*, PAGB.
2 Driscoll, D. J., New technologies enhance trend to fewer basic types of liner, *Packaging Technol.*, April 1982.
3 Aleff, H. P., A comparison of thermoplastic with thermoset closures, *Packaging Technol.*, April 1982.
4 Dickey, J. J., Individually tailor-to-fit seals with aluminium roll-on closures, *Packaging Technol.*, April 1982.
5 Pond, W., Aluminium foil/polymer laminates as hermetic seals on treated glass, *Packaging Technol.*, April 1982.
6 Keller, R. G. Control of factors relating torque to sealing force for C.T. closures, *Packaging Technol.*, April 1982.
7 Amini, M. A., Permeation and leakage in closures, *Packaging Technol.*, April 1986.
8 Amini, M. A., Methods of evaluating closure integrity, *Proceedings of the 3rd Wisconsin Extension Update Conference on Packaging*, October 1983.
9 Evans, T. G. *Fits and Misfits of Screw Closures on Containers*, Link Industrial Design.

Appendix 11.7: US finishes

US finishes are available through either the Glass Packaging Institute (GCMI finishes), Washington, DC, or glass manufacturers as special finishes e.g. OIG (Owens Illinois). Some of the more important finishes are as follows:

- GCMI 400 series, Shallow continuous thread (nearest UK equivalent BS 1918 R3/2).
- GCMI 405 series, As 400 but with depressed thread.
- GCMI 410 series, Medium continuous thread concealed bead finish.
- GCMI 415, Tall continuous thread concealed bead finish (UK BS 1918 R4).
- GCMI 425, Continuous thread for small diameters.
- GCMI 430, Continuous thread pour out glass finish.
- GCMI 450, CT thread finish – wide mouthed containers.
- GCMI 480, Pour out glass finish.
- GCMI 485, Combination CT and polyethylene sifter top snap cap glass finish.
- GCMI 490, Combination snap and screw cap finish.
- GCMI 500, 530, 550, 555, Threaded crown finishes.
- GCMI 600, 607, 609, etc. Crown finishes.
- GCMI/OIG 1600 series, Pilfer proof roll on.
- GCMI 2710, Biological finish.

12

STERILE PRODUCTS AND THE ROLE OF RUBBER COMPONENTS

N. Frampton and D. A. Dean

Introduction

The selection of the appropriate packaging materials and processes for sterile products presents a series of challenges of considerably greater complexity than for non-sterile products. A sterile product may be defined as a product which is totally devoid of all forms of life, both vegetative and sporing. Most important in this area is contamination by bacteria, fungi or moulds and yeasts. In all pharmaceutical products it is also becoming highly desirable to work towards much lower bioburdens. This involves the application of microbiological standards to both raw materials and finished products. These normally exclude certain pathogens such as *Salmonella typhi* and *Clostridium botulinum*, but it should be noted that even some non-pathogens can also cause problems.

In order to limit or exclude microbiological contamination in pharmaceutical products, a number of approaches are possible:

1 rigid (microbiological) specifications for all raw materials (especially water) and how they are 'packed and stored'
2 strict adherence to the code of good manufacturing practice (GMP) (facilities, personnel, procedures and documentation)
3 use of special processing techniques, e.g. control of air quality, dedicated positive pressure production areas
4 use of antimicrobial preservatives (where acceptable) which are essential to most multi-dose forms of product
5 use of a sterilisation process which may involve a terminal sterilisation or an aseptic process
6 the selection of the appropriate form of packaging, noting the advantages of certain (unpreserved sterile) forms of unit dose.

Various guidelines, including those on general or current GMP (CGMP), are available related to specific aspects of the above from both official organisations, such as the FDA, and specialised societies such as the UK-based Parenteral Society and the US-based PDA.

A terminal sterilisation process usually involves the filling and closing of product containers under conditions of a high-quality (low bioburden/particulate) environment

492

where the product, container and closure are usually also of high microbiological quality but not sterile. This is followed by a final complete sterilisation process. In an aseptic processing operation, the drug product, container and closure are subjected to separate sterilisation processes and then brought together. Since maintenance of sterility relies on the processing, compliance with high standards is critical to any aseptic operation. Each function therefore requires thorough validation and control at every stage of the process.

Antimicrobial preservatives can be added to many pharmaceutical products in order to give protection against microbial contamination. A wide range of preservatives is summarised in Table 12.1. It should be noted that preservatives should not be regarded as protection against poor processing techniques but as a means of minimising bioburden during poor storage and usage.

There are a number of official tests for preservative challenge, i.e. preservative efficacy challenge tests, which can be found in the British Pharmacopoeia (BP), United States Pharmacopeia (USP), and European Pharmacopoeia (EP). There also are 'in house' challenges which may be more rigorous than the compendial tests.

Since preservative efficacy may vary according to the product, analysis of preservative content often has to be supported by a preservative challenge test. This may also be relevant with certain emulsion systems where the preservative may partition between the different oil and water phases. For simple distribution phenomena, the partition or distribution law normally applies.

Because of problems which include toxic hazards and sensitisation, some preservatives are under suspicion, while others have been withdrawn from use. This has often encouraged the use of non-preserved sterile unit dose presentations. Preservatives have also suffered from absorption, adsorption and, where soluble and volatile, subsequent loss by evaporation. For example, preservatives suffering from adsorption include phenyl mercuric nitrate and acetate; benzalkonium chloride; thiomersal. Preservatives suffering from absorption include phenol; chlorocresol; cresol; and 2 phenyl ethanol.

These preservatives have a solubility in certain rubbers and plastics and will continuously diffuse through the polymeric matrix due to their volatile nature. These

Table 12.1 Antimicrobial preservatives

Substance	Approx. % used	Comments
Phenyl mercuric nitrate (PMN) and acetate (PMA)	0.002	Various usages but mercurials queried
Benzalkonium chloride	0.01	Oral, ophthalmic, topicals
Ethanol	15.0	Oral, topicals
Benzoic acid	0.1–0.5	Oral, topicals
Parabens	0.1–0.2	Creams, mixtures
Chlorhexidine	0.01	Eye products
2 Phenyl-ethanol	0.4	Eye products
Thiomersal	0.1–0.2	Eye/nasal products
Phenol	0.5	Certain multidose injections
Cresol	0.3	
Chlorocresol	0.1	
Benzyl Alcohol	1.0	
Bronopol	0.02–0.05	Creams

493

problems illustrate the view that sterile products generally put greater stress on all packaging materials. Thermal processing can cause physical changes to plastics, glass and multilayer materials, as well as the increased potential of interaction, exchange and extraction. Thermal defects may arise from differential expansion and contraction, as well as instant or delayed cracking of glass-based materials due to the effects of thermal shock.

Interaction between product and pack may involve:

- surface interactions
- leaching or migration of material from the pack into the product
- loss of constituents in the product into the pack, i.e. container or closure.

The history of injectables

Injectable products are sterile liquid drug preparations that are administered parenterally, i.e. introduced into the patient's body through the skin. Although injections are a relatively recent form of therapy, the history of the development of the technique can be traced back to the early seventeenth century. William Harvey described the circulation of blood in 1616, and later attributed death caused by snake bites to the distribution of the poison throughout the body via the blood.

The first recorded attempt to inject medication intentionally was in 1665 by Sir Christopher Wren, then Professor of Astronomy at Oxford and later to become a famous architect. Wren worked on animals, but later attempts by a Johann Taylor were with humans. Unfortunately the crude nature of the apparatus, the absence of pure drugs and ignorance caused the practice to fall into disrepute.

However, during the late eighteenth century and throughout the nineteenth century interest was spasmodically revived. Jenner used intradermal administration in the late eighteenth century for his smallpox vaccination and a Frenchman, Pravaz, introduced a plunger-type syringe in 1853 with leather components. Although the work of Pasteur and Lister pointed out the need for the development of aseptic techniques, it did not result in any immediate practical changes. Syringe materials were not suitable for heat sterilisation and the drugs were often heat sensitive, so by 1880 physicians were preparing their own injections at the time of use.

By the 1890s progress had been made in the use of bacteriological filters towards sterilisation, and at about the same time a French pharmacist called Simousin developed the first ampoule. These changes resulted in the manufacture of parenteral solutions passing from the hands of the individual pharmacist or physician to pharmaceutical companies.

Nevertheless, pyrogenic reactions continued to be associated with parenteral therapy. Florence Siebert demonstrated in 1923 that the pyrogenic inducing bodies came from the water used to prepare the solutions, and care in using a pyrogen-free water eliminated the fever problem. This lead to the official acceptance by the American Formulary in 1926 of injectable solutions, which is the true beginning of universal parenteral therapy.

Today parenteral products are divided into two types, namely large and small volume parenterals. Large volume solutions in containers of 100 ml or more are essentially for intravenous use, usually over an extended period of time. Such solutions are also for irrigation and dialysis. Small volume parenterals are for immediate injection by various routes, such as subcutaneous, intramuscular and intravenous.

Injections are often the most efficient way of administering a wide variety of essential drugs. There are of course both advantages and disadvantages associated with this method of drug administration over the oral form; these are detailed in Table 12.2.

Sterilisation of parenteral products

The basic pharmacopoeial accepted sterilisation processes include:

1 dry heat
2 moist heat
3 irradiation, including gamma irradiation and beta irradiation
4 gases
5 product and air filtration.

Dry heat

Dry heat sterilisation involves high temperatures such as 160°C for 3 h; 170°C for 2 h; 180°C for 1 h; 300–320°C for 3–4 min. Although glass and metal can withstand these temperatures, the use of dry heat sterilisation for rubber and plastics needs to be considered with care. There are relatively few 'engineering' type plastics and a limited number of rubbers that can meet these high dry temperatures and retain satisfactory physical properties.

Moist heat

Temperatures of above 100°C can be achieved by moist heat under pressure in an autoclave and, as with dry heat, there is a time–temperature relationship:

- 106–108°C (6–8 h)
- 115–118°C (30 min)
- 121–124°C (15 min)
- 134–138°C (3 min).

Moist heat sterilisation can be used to sterilise packaging components for aseptic filling or to terminally sterilise both the product and the pack. Because of this, various factors have to be noted.

Table 12.2 Parenteral products administration

Advantages	Disadvantages
Faster effect	More expensive
Maintenance of high drug levels	Professional administration
Little or no inactivation	Unpleasant for patient
Injected directly into target	

1   The product expands according to its coefficient of expansion as the temperature rises (note that alcohol expands more than water).
2   The air space or ullage above the product also expands according to its nature (air or nitrogen) and its pressure.
3   The combined expansion will depend on the product/ullage ratio and the pressure build-up will depend on whether the pack is rigid with limited expansion (e.g. glass) or flexible and extensible (e.g. various relatively thin-walled plastics).
4   Whether the packaging material is resistant to moisture (metal, glass) or absorbs and loses moisture according to the temperature and level of moisture present (e.g. certain plastic materials).

The above invariably means that closures may dimensionally change during the sterilisation process (especially screw-based systems). Also, certain materials may extend during the heating cycle (plastics) and hence become distorted when recooled. To minimise this distortion, an overpressure or balanced pressure autoclave is essential for some materials, i.e. bottles or bags. Control of this distortion depends on the plastic involved, the design of the pack, the nature of the product, the volume to ullage (air space) ratio, the time–temperature cycle involved, the overpressure and when and how it is applied. These have to be optimised by trial and error experimentation, as other factors (i.e. how the autoclave is loaded and the items spaced etc.) also play a part. This always assumes that the closure remains effective throughout the cycle and does not 'vent'. In this context this cannot happen with welded packs and, in general, closures made by effectively applying an aluminium overseal over a rubber stopper are superior to the older systems based on metal screw caps (older glass IV packs).

As indicated above, the properties of certain plastics may be temporarily modified by the combination effects of moisture and temperature during the autoclaving cycle. In general, the physical properties of rubber formulations are not affected by the moist heat sterilisation other than the fact that closure systems may absorb moisture (depending on the rubber formulation/materials employed) during the autoclave cycle. This can be an issue for lyophilised products or aseptically filled dry powders where long drying cycles for the rubber closures are sometimes employed to prevent desorption of moisture from the closure into the product.

Irradiation

Sterilisation by irradiation typically uses either gamma or beta radiation (electron beam). These two processes are significantly different in that gamma irradiation is a lengthy process involving penetrating rays, whereas beta irradiation is in comparison a short exposure process where the rays are much less penetrating, i.e. it tends to be a surface sterilising process. Typically gamma irradiation is achieved by a cobalt 60 source at a dose of 25 kGy. The items to be sterilised are slowly passed through the process, over a period of up to 24 h. These rays will penetrate most materials, including aluminium foil, paper, board, glass, rubber and plastics. Gamma irradiation has increased in popularity for the terminal sterilisation of medical devices and the sterilisation of packaging components for aseptic process.

Gaseous sterilisation

Although various gases can be employed, e.g. formaldehyde, ethylene oxide, most pharmaceutical processes relate to the latter. Since ethylene oxide (and its residues) are toxic and it forms explosive mixtures with air/oxygen, special precautions are essential to safe handling. Ethylene oxide is therefore mixed with an inert gas (usually CO_2) and needs a certain temperature (usually 55°C) and the presence of moisture to be effective, together with materials which are either porous (paper, Tyvek, board) or permeable to the gas (PVC, PS, PE, etc.). This means that there is a solubility or retention factor related to their use and a period must be allowed to reduce residues (by degassing).

Filtration

Finally, filtration should be mentioned as a means of producing sterile products or gases. In the case of aqueous-based liquids (of low viscosity), terminal filtration usually employs a special filter of 0.2 μm (or minimum 0.22 μm) pore size. Although a single filter can achieve effective sterility, there is a general trend towards a two filter process, i.e. 0.45 μm then 0.22 μm, where applicable. In the case of more viscous products, filtration may need an increase in temperature (which usually reduces the viscosity) and/or additional pressure. Filtration techniques generally assume that the product can be produced with low bioburden products.

Packaging materials

The efficacy, stability and safety of a parenteral drug on storage and administration depends largely on the nature and performance of the packaging components. In general the requirements of a modern parenteral product can be summarised as follows:

- the drug is medically effective
- the complete item is easy and quick to use
- the inside of the container and its contents must be sterile
- the drug and inside of the container must be free from pyrogens and toxic substances
- there must not be excessive contamination by particulates
- minimum interaction or exchange between product and pack.

All the above requirements must be maintained throughout the product shelf life.

Four main materials are used for the primary (direct contact with drug) or secondary packaging (part of the container or administration set but not in direct contact with the drug):

1 glass
2 plastics
3 aluminium
4 rubber.

The first three materials will only be touched on briefly since they are covered in full in earlier chapters.

Glass

Glass is available in four types, i.e. types I, II, III, NP (USA) or I, II, III, IV (Europe), the different grades relating mainly to their chemical 'neutrality'. Applications include:

- ampoules – single or double ended, open or closed (always single use containers)
- vials – normally produced from pregraded tubing and used as single dose or multidose containers, in sizes of 2.5 ml to 100 ml, with neck sizes of 13 mm to 20 mm
- bottles – various sizes and closure systems, produced by conventional glass moulding techniques.

Plastics

There are many different types of plastics and an even greater number of grades to meet virtually every product requirement. The main economical plastics used in pharmaceutical applications are the economical 'four' i.e. polyethylene, polypropylene, polystyrene and polyvinylchloride.

Plastics are used in virtually every pharmaceutical application (oral, topical, ophlthalmic, parenteral applications), either as a single material or in combination with other materials, as coatings or laminations.

Aluminium

Aluminium is used as an overseal to effect a seal between the rubber disc or plug and vial. An overseal must be rigid, yet sufficiently ductile and malleable to be clamped onto the vial. Since the overseal is a secondary closure, problems of drug compatibility do not occur. The aluminium itself is usually coated on the outer surface with an epoxy resin-based lacquer. This protects the aluminium from oxidisation, or from slight surface corrosion during autoclaving. Alternatively, the product may be coloured by using coloured anodised aluminium and a clear lacquer. The range of colours enable coding of products and further differentiation can be achieved using a D-I-D® overseal (decoration–identification–differentiation) which enables instructions, logos or product names to be printed on the overseal.

Rubber and elastomers

Rubber components are now used extensively for many parenteral packaging and administration applications including injection vials and prefilled syringes. Because of its varied chemical nature and risk of extractables, rubber is regarded by many as the most critical of the primary packaging materials, especially as a wide range of constituents can be involved (see below).

Up to the beginning of the twentieth century, closures were typically made from cork or glass stoppers. In the early 1900s solid rubber 'corks' or bungs, made using natural rubber as the base elastomer, replaced the cork and glass stoppers. The use of rubber bungs (a popular nomenclature used to describe rubber closures) provided a number of specific advantages summarised in Table 12.3.

Rubber formulations

In this chapter the word 'elastomer' is used to describe the base polymer and 'rubber' to describe the fully compounded finished component. A rubber formulation is a complex blend of ingredients, and a typical high extract sulphur cured natural rubber formulation is given in Table 12.4.

Elastomer

The choice of elastomer has the greatest effect on a formulation. The most common elastomers that can be used for closures for injectable products are given in Table 12.5. Of these elastomers, natural rubber, synthetic polyisoprene, butyl, chlorobutyl and bromobutyl rubber are typically used for the manufacture of rubber closures and stoppers used in the packaging and administration of parenterals.

Table 12.3 Special properties of rubber

Property	Advantage gained
Flexible	Conforms to shape of vial etc.
Resilient	Reseals after needle puncture
Non-thermoplastic	Tolerates most heat sterilising and other processes
Good compression set	Retains seal throughout product life
Can be varied by ingredient choice	Formulations can usually be developed compatible with most drugs

Table 12.4 Typical sulphur cured natural rubber formulation

Category	Ingredient	Mass % (w/w)
Elastomer	Natural rubber	60.00
Filler	Calcium carbonate	25.0
Pigment	Red iron oxide	4.0
Plasticiser	Paraffin oil	5.0
Processing aid/activator	Stearic acid	1.0
Activator	Zinc oxide	2.5
Vulcanisation system	Accelerator (e.g. sulphonamide, dithiocarbamate, thiuram)	1.5
	Elemental sulphur	1.0

Table 12.5 Elastomer characteristics

Polymer	Characteristic
Natural rubber	Good physical properties
Synthetic polyisoprene	Good physical properties
Butyl	Low permeability
Halobutyl	As butyl, but with lower water extractables
Nitrile	Mineral oil resistance
EDPM	Resistance to high pH solutions
Silicone rubber	High permeability
Neoprene	Lower oil resistance than nitrile

Natural rubber

This was the first type of polymer used in pharmaceutical applications, and was found to have desirable characteristics in that its resilience provided sealing properties and this resilience could be developed to allow the rubber to be pierced by a hypodermic needle, resealing after removal. This high level of resilience is partially due to its chemical structure, it being a straight chain elastomer (Figure 12.1).

During the curing or cross-linking process only 10–20% of the available double bonds react and this gives rise to the potential for breaking of the chemical chains upon exposure to factors such as heat, oxygen or ozone. This can result in surface tackiness, crazing and ultimately total degradation of the rubber.

Although natural rubber has been used for many years, there is an increasing awareness of an issue described as 'latex protein allergy' whereby naturally occurring proteins and natural rubber latex can cause allergic reactions and, in the most severe cases, anaphylactic shock. Items made from latex natural rubber typically include surgical and examination gloves, anaesthesia masks, and dental dams. During the period 1989–1993 the US Food and Drug Administration (FDA) received reports of over 1000 cases of injury and fifteen cases of death associated with latex allergy (Dillard and MacCollum, 1992). The cases of death related to a single supply of barium enema catheters which were believed to have been produced using poor manufacturing conditions. These were recalled and subsequently replaced by catheters made using synthetic rubber.

Rubber closures and components for the packaging and administration of parenterals are normally made from so-called dry rubber. Where such closures have been produced using dry natural rubber, the bioavailability of proteins has not been proved (Slater, 1993). It is postulated that the difference between latex and dry natural rubber is related to the processing of the base elastomer and rubber compound (Russell-Fell, 1993). The processing of dry natural rubber involves acid coagulation followed by a crumbling/creeping operation with extensive washing in water and drying at 100–130°C. During manufacture dry natural rubber compounds are typically compression moulded at high temperatures up to 160°C. A study of the extractable protein content of fourteen dry natural rubber samples and five dry natural rubber products found limits so low as to be at the limit of detection of the Lowry method (Yip *et al.*, 1995). There has been one reported case (Towse *et al.*, 1995) of an allergic reaction involving local erythema following an injection of insulin. The paper concluded that there was strong circumstantial evidence that the patient's allergic response was caused by latex antigens contained in the insulin vial and/or syringe. Reputable suppliers have been pursuing alternatives to dry natural rubber: one common approach is to introduce synthetic polyisoprene and to describe such materials as natural rubber latex free.

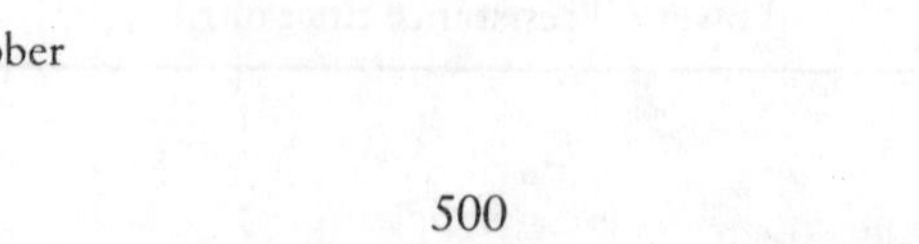

$$\left[\begin{array}{c} CH_3 \\ | \\ CH_2 - C = CH - CH_2 \end{array}\right]_n$$

Figure 12.1 Natural rubber

Butyl and halobutyl rubber (chlorobutyl/bromobutyl)

Butyl rubber shown in Figure 12.2, has been commercially available since 1942, and chlorobutyl and bromobutyl have been commercially available since 1960 and the 1970s respectively. All three polymers offer very low permeability to gases. The vulcanisation of butyl rubber requires a high level of curatives to effect cross-linking; the introduction of halogenated butyl rubber resulted in greater reactivity of the base polymer. As a direct result it was possible to use a lower level of curatives for halobutyl polymers and also to explore so-called unconventional vulcanisation systems that yielded a significantly lower level of extractables.

In certain cases it is desirable to combine the properties of the previously described natural rubber with those of the halobutyls. With straight butyl rubbers this was impossible due to the prolonged cure time of butyl which meant that the natural rubber would be overcured, resulting in an unusable 'non-homogeneous' mix.

Cure ingredients

During cure (or vulcanisation), the individual polymer chains become chemically linked together to form a three-dimensional structure. This minimises the tendency for permanent distortion under load at room temperature or for the rubber to 'melt' at high temperatures, such as at steam sterilisation. Certain additives are necessary as vulcanisation agents to provide the chemical cross-links, which are created at elevated temperatures, typically from 140°C to 200°C. Heat is applied to the rubber while it is being compressed in metal moulds, so that the forming and vulcanisation processes occur simultaneously. The most commonly used vulcanisation system in the general rubber industry is based on sulphur. Sulphur systems can be devised to fit most rubber processing conditions and can be applied to most polymers commonly used for pharmaceutical applications. Activators, usually zinc oxide and stearic acid, are necessary to activate the accelerators, but here the precise quantity is less critical. The detailed mechanism of the rubber curing process is complicated, but it is generally accepted that the sulphur combines with a zinc salt of the accelerator to produce a thio-intermediate which, in turn, reacts with the rubber. The inevitable residue of zinc–accelerator salts is slightly water soluble and can be extracted by aqueous solutions, if only at the level of a few parts per million. This tendency to contaminate is a significant disadvantage of a sulphur cure, although many sulphur cured rubbers have a long history of satisfactory use with aqueous injectables.

One such contaminant associated with sulphur-based vulcanisation systems is the organic accelerator 2-mercaptobenzothiazole (2-MCBT) and associated derivatives. In 1981 (Petersen et al., 1981) the presence of 2-(2-hydroxyethylmercapto) benzothiazole

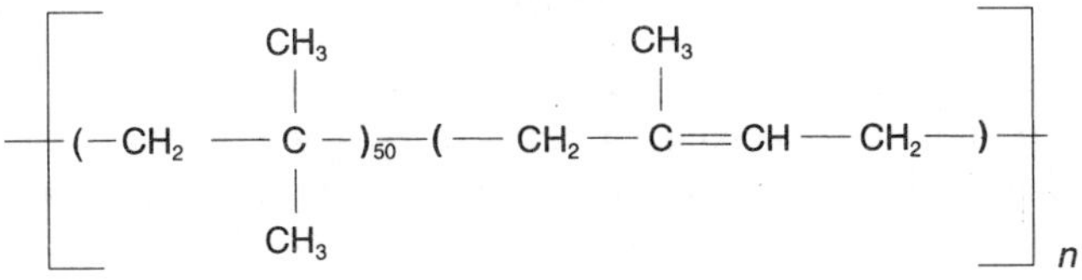

Figure 12.2 Butyl rubber

(HEB) was detected in the contents of a disposable hypodermic syringe. It was identified that the extractant was a reaction product formed between a 2-MCBT derivative and ethylene oxide used for sterilisation. Subsequently the oxidation product of HEB, 2-(carboxymethylthio)benzothiazole (CMB), was detected in the serum of premature babies receiving prolonged intravenous therapy (Meek and Pettit, 1985). So-called modem vulcanisation systems do not use sulphur as the cross-linking agent nor use 2-MCBT or derivatives, and are consequently free from this particular problem. These new vulcanisation systems show a considerable reduction in aqueous extractable matter and are often described as having low water extractables.

Fillers

Fillers are added to the elastomer in order to add bulk, lower cost and/or to improve physical properties such as hardness, strength and abrasion resistance. Typical fillers are materials such as carbon black, talc, china clay and whiting. Carbon black has been shown to contain polynuclear aromatics (PNAs) and there is concern regarding their carcinogenicity (Lee and Hites, 1976). However, despite extra controls there has been a move away from the use of carbon black as a filler in applications involving the primary packaging of parenterals. Its use continues as a pigment or colourant in rubber formulations but at substantially lower levels than that as a filler.

The use of calcined clay as a filler has shown to lead to the release of soluble aluminium from rubber closures into the parenteral solution (Milano et al., 1982). Various techniques for the determination of soluble aluminium in rubber closures have been proposed (Mondimore and Moore, 1983). There has been concern about aluminium since the 1970s, when a link was identified between high aluminium levels in tap water used for renal dialysis equipment and accumulation of the element in the brain. The injection of parenteral solutions into the body effectively 'bypasses' the normal defence mechanisms and under these circumstances may present a challenge to the normal metabolic processes (Massey and Taylor, 1989). In response to these challenges, suppliers have developed rubber formulations that are essentially free from materials containing aluminium compounds.

Protecting agents

These are added to reduce the ageing effects of the rubber and include paraffin wax added to form a protective bloom and antioxidants such as phenolic compounds. These protecting agents are required for natural rubber and are not necessary for modern synthetic rubber formulations.

Plasticisers

Petroleum oils (either naphthenic or paraffinic), are added to rubber to reduce the rubber hardness and improve processing characteristics. There are well-documented examples of other materials being used as softening agents in plastics and rubbers. The leaching of plasticisers from infusion bags such as di(2-ethylhexyl)phthalate (DEHP) are well documented. Another plasticiser, tris(2-butoxyethyl) phosphate (TBEP), was found to leach from a rubber stopper into a blood sample collected using an evacuated tube device (Shah *et al.*, 1982; Shang-Qiang *et al.*, 1983). The presence of TBEP was shown to cause displacement of certain drugs from plasma to erythrocytes and hence to distort the apparent concentration of drug in plasma.

Colourants

The main colourants used are inert inorganic materials such as iron oxide, titanium dioxide and, at small loadings, as previously noted, carbon black. With these materials, white, grey, black, brown, pink and red shades can be developed. Other colours are obtained by organic pigments, which can give bright vibrant colours but carry a cost premium.

The hypodermic syringe

The simple disposable syringe is well known and is supplied sterile by the manufacturer. These were introduced to overcome the problems of sterility within hospitals when multi-use non-disposable syringes were used. These syringes are supplied empty and are used in conjunction with vials or ampoules. The development of the disposable syringe has some interesting milestones in its history.

A metal and glass syringe was manufactured by Gemrig and Co. (Philadelphia) in 1857. Here the barrel was made of glass and the plunger rod from a metal, probably German silver. The piston or plunger had a frictional surface manufactured from leather. The 'Luer-Syringe' was invented in 1896 in Paris by Karl Schneider of H Walfing Luer and this was a major step towards the disposable syringe we know today. Obviously, the use of leather for the piston was one area in need of improvement and eventually the move to 'rubber' was made.

The disposable syringe comprises three main component parts, i.e. barrel, plunger rod, piston, and these are described below.

Barrel

The barrel of the disposable syringe is manufactured primarily from a sterilisable grade of polypropylene with an added nucleating agent to improve the clarity. Over the length of the barrel a scale is printed indicating the various dosage levels available from that particular size of syringe. At the open end of the barrel a feature known as the finger grip is incorporated which provides a firm platform for use when injecting into the patient. The administration end is fitted with either a needle or a standard medical luer which enables a wide variety of hypodermic needles to be attached.

Plunger rod and piston

The plunger rod is used to move the piston up and down the barrel. The piston is usually manufactured from a natural or synthetic rubber and is attached by either a simple latch or a screw thread to the plunger rod, and provides the effective seal required to withdraw drug from the vial/ampoule and administer into the patient. The seal is normally made via two, but occasionally three, circumferential ribs which, when inserted into the barrel and assembled on the plunger rod, exert radial interference and thus affect the seal. The seal integrity for such syringes can be evaluated using an aspiration test whereby the capability of holding a vacuum within the barrel is determined. It is this unique sealing characteristic of rubber that has resulted in its wide-ranging use.

In recent years a new challenge has emerged for large-volume disposable syringes in the form of syringe pumps. These are used to administer drugs automatically over periods of 24, 48 or even 72 h, and the break-loose force and sliding friction characteristics of the piston and plunger down the barrel are of paramount importance. The break-loose force is the measure of the force needed to start the piston travelling down the barrel, and the sliding friction is the force needed to maintain that movement, which should be constant with a smooth gliding action. The tendency for a piston to judder down the barrel ('stiction') makes a syringe unsuitable for use in modern syringe pumps. These syringe pumps are capable of delivering a variable amount of fluid and are equipped with overpressure alarms and an alarm to indicate an almost empty syringe. The latter alarm requires careful control of tolerances over the syringe itself to provide a constant final 'hard height' calculated from the plunger rod handle to syringe body fingergrip. These syringe pumps may be coupled to electronically controlled systems to provide controlled drug delivery.

Ampoules and vials

Technical details of the basic ampoule and vial have been given in earlier chapters. Here we detail the historical development of these packaging containers and also identify some recent design improvements which increasingly bridge the gap between a container and drug delivery device.

In 1886 Stanislaus Limousin devised a container for storing sterile solutions. This container was named an 'ampoule' and was manufactured with a long tapering neck at one end. After the ampoule had been filled the 'tip' of the glass was sealed using heat. Today the single dose ampoule has changed little from the original Limousin design.

The next major step was to introduce a rubber closure to seal a glass vial. This enabled multiple insertions through the rubber closure by a needle while retaining seal integrity, due to the flexible nature of rubber. The rubber stopper is held securely in place by an aluminium overseal which can be crimped onto the vial, thus making an effective seal between the rubber and glass. The aluminium itself is available in a number of designs depending on the application intended. These designs include the Flip-off® overseal (providing tamper-evidence) and fully removable overseals.

Advancements in vial/closure design have resulted in novel prefilled vial systems giving a range of benefits over the 'standard' package. One such system is the Becton Dickinson Pharmaceutical Systems Monovial® INF comprising a glass vial holding the drug in either a freeze dried or a liquid state and an integral transfer set. This system allows for the aseptic reconstitution of the drug and subsequent transfer into the infusion bag. The transfer set consists of a protective overcap manufactured from low density polythene, covering the main co-polyester needle guard capsule with an integral needle. The vial is filled and stoppered using one of two stopper designs, depending on whether the drug is lyophilised or in liquid form. The four-part transfer device is then assembled on the vial. In use the overcap is removed and the needle inserted into the infusion bag. Pressure is then applied to the transfer set which forces the rubber stopper down into the vial suspended by the transfer set. A seal is maintained by a secondary rubber 'O' ring on the transfer which moves down into the vial neck: subsequent mixing and transferring are then facilitated. This system reduces the number of basic steps performed by the nurse from sixteen with a traditional system to only seven for the Monovial system.

Abbott Laboratories also manufactures a novel vial reconstitution method, the ADD-vantage™ system. Here a purpose-made infusion bag has an integral 'vial port' which is accessed by removal of a protective cap via pulling an integral 'pull-ring'. This allows the unique drug vial to be screwed into the port. Activation of the system is achieved by pulling back the inner cap on the vial, inverting the bag and mixing.

Lyophilised products

Lyophilisation is the process whereby a pharmaceutical formulation containing the active ingredient dissolved in a solvent, usually water, is first frozen and then the water is removed under a reduced pressure by sublimation. The use of lyophilisation is increasing, partly because many of the new biopharmaceutical preparations are unstable when stored in solution. To provide a long shelf life, it is important that the stopper has low permeability to air and moisture. It is recognised that the main source of moisture into the lyophilised cake is through a process of desorption from the rubber stopper itself into the hygroscopic cake. Factors affecting the functional aspects of a stopper selection are:

1   partial insertion or half stop position (Figure 12.3)
2   component stability on the vial
3   insertion force
4   seal integrity
5   reconstitution and the withdrawal of active ingredient.

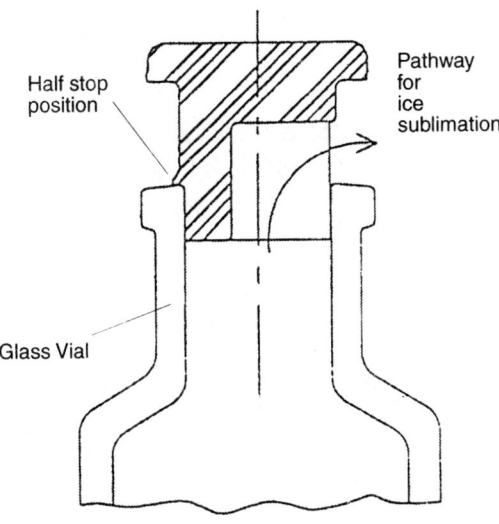

Figure 12.3 Half stop position

The half stop position, shown in Figure 12.3, is the fundamental role of the lyophilisation closure. The partially inserted closure must allow a sufficient pathway for ice sublimation to occur while being able to form an effective seal upon full insertion. Mechanical stability is provided by interference between the plug portion and the neck of the glass or plastic vial. Obviously a trade-off exists between mechanical stability and final insertion force. The seal formed between rubber and the glass container has two functions: initially it must provide a short-term seal prior to over-crimping and may require retention of a nitrogen headspace within the vial. After crimping, the seal must maintain integrity for normally 2 to 3 years. The first requirement is more a factor of geometry, whereas retention of seal integrity over time is more a function of correct rubber formulation selection to include suitable compression set characteristics and overcrimp procedure. In terms of seal integrity there are both primary and secondary seals formed between rubber and the glass container as shown in Figure 12.4.

The design of the lyophilisation closure significantly affects the reconstitution step. Certain stopper designs can retain part of the cake within the flutes of the plug section, resulting in only partial reconstitution. There are essentially three main designs of stopper with the variation occurring in plug portion, as shown in Figure 12.5:

1 two or three leg/peg
2 cruciform design
3 igloo or slot design.

The leg or peg design suffers from relatively poor stability in the half stop position. This results from the relative ease with which the rubber pegs can be forced inwards. The cruciform design has excellent stability in the half stop position because there is significant interference between the rubber and glass in that position. There are some concerns with this design because of cake retention in the flutes and central cone.

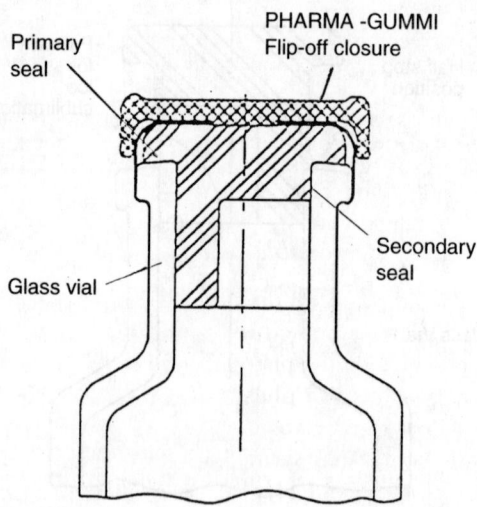

Figure 12.4 Stopper seal integrity

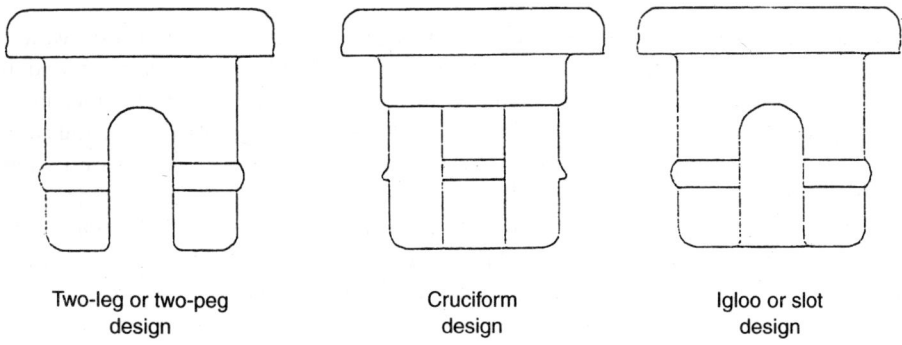

| Two-leg or two-peg design | Cruciform design | Igloo or slot design |

Figure 12.5 Lyophilised stopper designs

The igloo or slot design is widely regarded as being the optimum lyophilisation stopper design. Excellent half stop stability is achieved by rubber–glass container interference in this position. The slot prevents cake retention and thereby provides complete reconstitution.

Lyophilisation stoppers are predominantly made from butyl or halobutyl elastomer-based rubber formulations chosen because of their relatively low permeability to gases.

Prefilled syringes

A prefilled syringe combines the function of a primary container with that of a conventional syringe and prior to use contains the drug. The prefilled syringe has several advantages:

- immediate administration from one item
- can be used anywhere
- labour saving
- measured accurate dose
- low risk of errors in medication
- lower risk of contamination
- marketing advantage.

Removable seal system

This is ostensibly the most simple, with the design being very similar to the disposable syringe except that the barrel is manufactured from glass and is prefilled with the drug solution. This solution is sealed by the piston at one end and a rubber needle shield or plug at the other. In use, the shield or plug is discarded and the device is ready. Some examples of this prefilled syringe type are as follows. Becton Dickinson Pharmaceutical Systems offers the Hypak® prefilled syringe in two versions, the bulk, unsterilised Hypak® and the sterile, ready to fill Hypak® SCF (sterile, clean, fill). Bünder Glas GmbH offers a removable seal system called Variject.

Diaphragm puncture system

With the diaphragm puncture system there is a glass cartridge, one end of which is sealed with the rubber piston and the other with an aluminium overseal and rubber septum. The filled cartridge either is placed into a separate syringe body or forms the body of the syringe. When the piston is depressed the first action is to pierce the rubber septum with one end of a double ended needle. Further movement of the piston administers the drug.

Bünder Glas GmbH produces a range of systems of this type under the trade names Dipsoject, Diviject and Koniject. MIN-I-JET®, manufactured by International Medication Systems (IMS), patented in 1965, is also a diaphragm puncture system.

Single-component bypass chamber system

The glass tube is sealed at one end by a rubber plunger and at the other by a floating rubber piston. When the plunger is depressed, the pressure build-up moves the rubber piston from the glass tube into the plastic end cap. Bypass or flow-past grooves in the plastic end cap allow the parenteral product to be expelled. Duphar BV of Holland markets its prefilled syringe under the name of Dumpharject®, and this works on the bypass chamber principle.

Two-component drug system

Two-component drug systems are on offer from a number of suppliers with dual-chamber syringes for liquid–liquid and powder–liquid administration. The two compartments are separated by a 'floating' rubber piston and the design of the glass body includes bypass channels to allow liquid transfer.

There is a risk with the standard design that, if the nurse is a little careless, the rear piston will be pressed too quickly past the bypass slot. This could result in inadequate dissolution of the solid, possibly with leakage through the needle. To overcome this, the Vetter Lyoject® has a plunger rod that is partially threaded running through a mating thread at the top of the syringe. The rear piston is advanced slowly by screwing in the plunger. By the time the plunger reaches the end of the threaded portion, mixing is complete and the drug can be administered in the normal way by pressing the plunger.

BD Hypak® has addressed the problem of incomplete dissolution of the dry powder product by introducing a piston with a grooved front rib. This creates turbulence as the water flows past it, thus dissolving the solid more readily. Bünder Glas GmbH also offers a bypass syringe suitable for liquid–liquid or liquid–dry applications under the tradename Variject 2 system.

Auto-injectors

Single use

An auto-injection device for self-administration has been developed for military use by STI. A heavy spring fires the needle about 25 mm into the thigh muscle before drug injection takes place. This is designed to penetrate easily through four layers of battle dress clothing. Such systems are marketed by STI under the trade-names Mediject®, Astopen® and Combopen®, and by Duphar as MultiPen®. Two-component wet/dry systems can also be administered using the STI Binaject™ auto-injector. With this relatively new technology it is imperative that personnel are trained in the correct use.

Auto-injection devices have been developed for self-administration of sumatriptan for the treatment of migraine. Glaxo Wellcome has marketed such a device as Subject®

Multi-use

Diabetics have traditionally been forced to perform self-injection, so auto-injectors have been developed for use in this area and look like a modern felt-tip pen. Quantities of insulin can be pre-set by turning a knob on the pen which has features including an audible click, clear resistance prior to each dose and a visual indication on the scale thus helping to eliminate dosing errors. Quick and easy dosing is possible with such systems. Auto-injectors are marketed by a number of companies under the following tradenames: Novopen®, Novepen® II, NovoLet™, Optipen® II and D-Pen®. Pressurised needleless systems are also now available.

Selection of rubber formulation and component design

A large number of factors should be considered when selecting a rubber closure for the sealing of a new drug or package:

- active drug substance
- solvent used
- preservative
- pH and buffer system
- process of sterilisation and, if aseptic, fill or terminal sterilisation
- size of pack and fill volume
- single or multi-dose
- sensitivity to metal ions
- importance of gas or moisture vapour permeability or desorption
- the total manufacturing process of filling and capping the vials
- product shelf-life requirements
- route of administration
- disposal of the pack and toxicity of contents.

In the past the main focus was on compatibility, primarily because of the relatively high level of extractives present in rubber formulations. The focus has now moved to include aspects such as stopper cleanliness, processability and presentation to the filling line. These issues are of increasing importance with the industry interest in barrier or isola-tor technology. This technology is gaining importance within the pharmaceutical industry as a preferred method of manufacture for aseptic processing. The entire filling area is covered by a physical barrier and the vial washing depyrogenation tunnel and primary packing component lines can be integrated to provide a complete aseptic fill-ing system. Access to the filling line is provided by a series of specially designed ports

509

and intervention by the operator is provided via glove boxes. The flow of components such as stoppers and plungers has become critical since they must be supplied into the isolator in a sterile and clean condition. This requirement has refocused pharmaceutical companies on the potential to source such components in a ready-to-use or ready-to-sterilise format (see below).

Compatibility with the drug

The problems with interaction of a parenteral product and the rubber closure are well documented in the literature. So-called 'high extract' formulations are typified in the 1978 paper by Pikal and Lang where a haze was identified as being caused by paraffin wax and sulphur. The organic accelerators which are used in conjunction with sulphur have also been a source for contamination. Wells *et al.* (1986) identified amine impurities that originated from the decomposition of amine salts of dithiocarbamates. These impurities were detected in a water-soluble Vitamin E product intended for intravenous injection. The case of Merck Sharp and Dohme Research Laboratories' development of sodium cefoxitin is an excellent example (Portnoff *et al.*, 1983).

A haze was found to form on reconstitution of the stored lyophilised product. The haze was identified as containing paraffin, silicone oil and zinc. Despite screening of fifty different rubber formulations, the only viable solution at that time was to use the West Company's 'Teflon coated' injection stopper. With the development of so-called 'low extract' rubber formulations, MSD has been able to approve non-Teflon faced closures for this application. These 'low extract' rubber formulations are normally vulcanised using unconventional cross-linking systems and so avoid the problems of sulphur and organic accelerators.

The problem of haze reported by Pikal and Lang (1978), Wells *et al.* (1986) and Portnoff *et al.* (1983) has been studied further by Jahnke *et al.* (1990a, 1990b, 1991), who investigated volatiles from the rubber closures. Jahnke reported a complex mixture of volatile hydrocarbons from the butyl and halobutyl polymers routinely used to make vial closures. The oligomer identified from butyl rubber was 1-isopropenyl-2,2,4,4-tetramethylcyclohexane and that from chlorobutyl rubber was 1-(1-chloromethylethenyl)-2,2,4,4-tetramethylcyclohexane. Both are referred to as the C_{13} oligomer, and its contribution to haze formation on reconstitution of lyophilised powders has been confirmed.

Problems of closure-related compatibility can be resolved by the use of a stopper laminated with a fluoropolymer on the sealing face. Such products are commercially available as FluroTec® closures for injection, infusion and lyophilisation closures as well as plungers for prefilled syringes. To provide an integral seal, the upper part of the sealing area is not coated, as shown in Figure 12.6. The use of such closures has been proposed by Danielson (1992) as a means of 'reducing or eliminating much leaching of toxic compounds'. Franke *et al.* (1994) have been able to relate the haze formation in reconstituted solutions of parenteral antibiotic powders to volatile components from the closure adsorbed onto the powder surface during storage. To avoid this phenomenon, marketed products such as cefodizime-disodium are commercially packaged using fluoropolymer laminated closures.

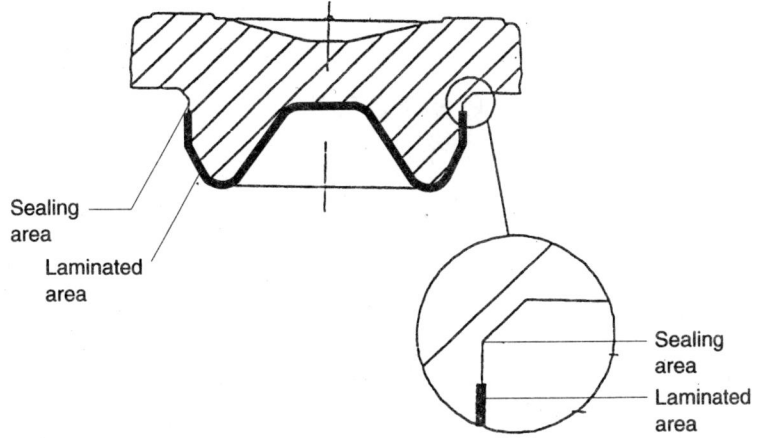

Sealing area

Laminated area

Sealing area

Laminated area

Figure 12.6 FluroTec® closure

Seal integrity

It has been highlighted earlier in the chapter that rubber, due to its chemical structure, has excellent resilience properties. This characteristic forms the basis for its widespread use for piston and closures. A review article by Morton (1987) highlighted that there is debate within the pharmaceutical industry as to where the 'true' seal is formed in a parenteral vial package. The true seal is defined as the primary seal and Morton confirmed the location of both primary and secondary seals as shown in Figure 12.7.

The primary seal is formed between the underside of the closure flange and top of the vial; the secondary seals are formed between the vial side wall and the plug portion of the closure (termed flange seal and bore seal). It has been postulated that correct selection and specification of the aluminium overseal is as important as the primary packaging materials, since it forms an integral part of the sealing mechanism.

Container/closure seal integrity has been reviewed by the Parenteral Drug Association (1983) and the Parenteral Society (1992). Variation in the overall height of the combined vial and closure will result in different closure-seal forces being applied at the crimping head. Quality control tests are proposed such as the dye intrusion challenge, liquid loss or bacterial challenge test. Methods for 100% on-line testing are also recommended to include high-voltage detection and seal force monitoring (Morton and Lordi, 1988).

The bore and flange seal interaction are used extensively during the filling of pharmaceutical products. Prior to over-capping with an aluminium overseal to effect the primary seal, the manufacturer must rely on the secondary bore seal to provide a short-term seal during processing.

Self-sealing and fragmentation

An important characteristic of rubber is its resilience, giving rise to so-called self-sealing properties. This property is the ability of the rubber to allow penetration by a hypodermic needle and 'snap' shut when the needle is removed, thus maintaining an

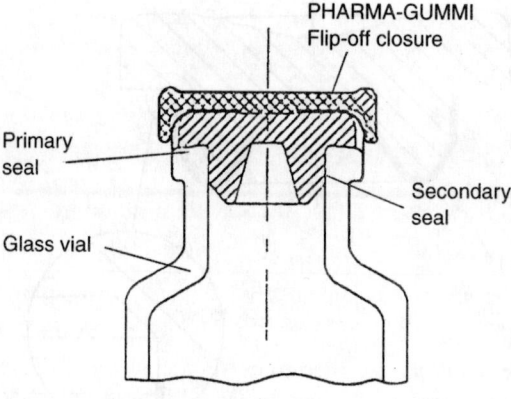

Figure 12.7 Primary and secondary seals in a parenteral vial

effective seal. This is an important consideration for a rubber stopper's coring or fragmentation performance. As the needle passes through a rubber stopper there is the potential for the frictional detachment of rubber particles and for larger fragments to be cut out by the 'heel' of the needle. Each of these in turn depends on the sharpness of the needle point (angle and use of side grinds) and the needle heel (angle and quality of cut). The quality of metal to construct the needle and absence of burrs also play an important role, as does the correct selection of rubber formulation. Determination of this self-sealing characteristic is covered in a number of applicable ISO standards together with the European Pharmacopoeia as follows:

- ISO 8362-2, Injection Containers for Injectables and Accessories [Closures for Injection Vials]
- ISO 8536-2, Infusion Equipment for Medical Use [Closures for Infusion Bottles].

Penetration force is a measure of the force required to insert a needle through the rubber septum. When a needle pierces a rubber closure it inherently generates a number of rubber particles and this phenomenon is termed fragmentation.

Another important authoritative standard is the European Pharmacopoeia: section VI. 2.3.1 relates specifically to rubber closures and is divided into chemical and physical sections. The chemical tests on autoclave extract determine the following properties:

- appearance of solution
- pH
- UV absorbance
- reducing substances
- heavy metals
- soluble zinc
- ammonium

- residue on evaporation
- volatile sulphides.

If the rubber closure or component is intended to be pierced by a hypodermic needle, then the physical test regime of the European Pharmacopoeia applies. This includes test method limits for penetrability, fragmentation and self-sealing categorisation (type I or type II closures), and methods for the determination of penetration force and fragmentation.

Cleanliness of rubber closures

Rubber closures by their very nature need to be subject to some degree of cleaning prior to use to remove particulates and to remove endotoxins from the stopper surface. Indeed, when aseptically packaging a 'sterile' product the closure must be 'sterile and pyrogen-free' itself, or it will contaminate the product.

Within the pharmaceutical and parenteral industry rubber closures can be supplied at differing degrees of cleanliness, with each level placing reduced requirements on the customer for further treatment. The various levels are shown in Figure 12.8.

Ready to wash closures

This level would represent the 'as manufactured' closure and as such was the accepted standard of presentation to the customer in the 1970s. It was accepted that in this state the closures required further processing, cleaning and lubrication with silicone oil by the pharmaceutical company before sterilisation. The closures in the as-supplied condition could be assumed to have moderate to high levels of microbial, pyrogen and particulate contamination.

Ready to rinse closures

Closures supplied ready to rinse have undergone a minimum hot water wash by the closure manufacturer to remove the potential hazards detailed above. For some

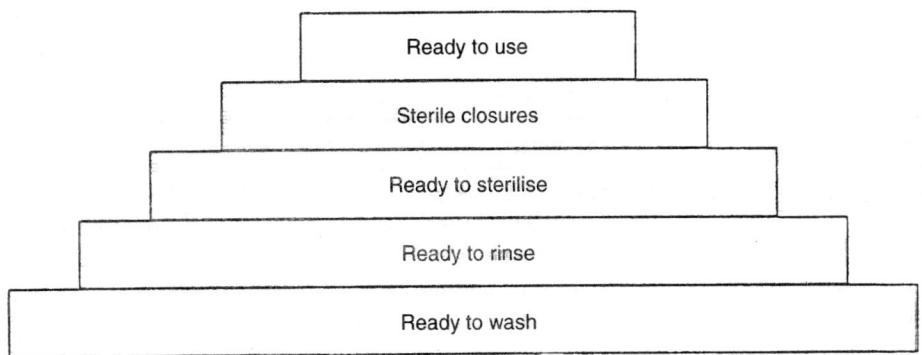

Figure 12.8 Stepwise approach to ready-to-use/sterile closures

applications this is considered sufficient and only the addition of surface lubricants is necessary as a post-treatment. However, if the closure is to be used in a 'sterile' package then depyrogenation must be carried out.

Ready to sterilise (RTS) closures

Ready to sterilise closures must as a prerequisite have been pre-lubricated, have a defined maximum particle burden and be pyrogen-free. Proved Clean® closures provide the required definable particle burden by objectively documenting the particulate cleanliness of the rubber closure for particles down to 25 µm in size. To achieve a low level of particulate contamination it is necessary to manufacture within a controlled environment and to complete the final washing stage and packing within a cleanroom environment. Experience has shown that each step of the manufacturing process should be optimised to provide the lowest particulate burden. For example, the polythene bags used to store cleaned stoppers have been identified as a major source of particulate contamination. This was one factor that led to the development by the West Company of a sterilisable bag manufactured using a combination of HDPE and Tyvek to facilitate steam penetration and drying. Rubber closures are routinely supplied in these sterilisable bags ready for steam sterilisation by the pharmaceutical company.

Particles found on the surface of rubber closures have been categorised as exogenous and normally originate from the environment associated with stopper processing. Endogenous particles released by the stopper are normally in the 2–5 µm range and typically include blooms, liquid migration and outgassed materials (Dölcher, 1990). The release of endogenous materials can be significantly reduced by the use of FluroTec® closures with the fluoropolymer laminate. To ensure that the closure is pyrogen-free it is subjected to a rinse in pyrogen-free water or water for injection (WFI). This water can be prepared by FIN-AQUA distillation.

Ready to use (RTU) closures

The 'ultimate' level of closure cleanliness encompasses all the requirements of RTS closures and also is subject to a sterilisation process. The sterilisation process for rubber closures can be achieved by a number of methods summarised below (Table 12.6).

The use of the RTU closures can offer a significant opportunity to reduce the total acquisition cost of a product.

Table 12.6 Methods of sterilisation for closures

Sterilisation method	Advantages	Disadvantages
Steam sterilisation (autoclave)	Preferred method, established effectiveness	Increased closure moisture level giving potential problems in lyophilised products
Ethylene oxide (ETO) sterilisation	No closure moisture level increase	Ethylene oxide sorbs into closures
Gamma irradiation	No closure moisture level increase	Not suitable for all rubber formulations

Lubrication

Most closures are lightly coated with silicone oil, such as a polydimethyl siloxane, as a means of reducing particulate formation as it acts as a lubricant between closures. It also reduces considerably the inherent tackiness in many rubber formulations. The main advantage of a silicone oil coat is that it facilitates the stoppering operation by lubricating the passage of the closures through assembly machines and insertion into the barrel or vial opening. The actual quantity of silicone can be adjusted to suit individual customer requirements. A vial closure silicone oil level of 0.005–0.020 mg silicone oil per cm^2 of rubber surface has been found to be optimum. Lower levels result in poor tracking and stoppering characteristics, while higher levels can result in 'pop-out' of the stopper from the vial. It has also been noted that silicone oil can contribute to particle counts as measured by a Coulter counter (Mannermaa *et al.*, 1992), and is a potential cause of haze formation, especially on reconstitution of stored lyophilised products (Wells *et al.*, 1986). A silicone resin coating can be applied to the surface of a closure followed by a cross-linking or baking step to adhere the resin. The coating provides the same advantages as silicone oil and is claimed to reduce significantly the level of endogenous particles released from the rubber.

Conclusions

Sterile products clearly place extra challenges on the pack in terms of the materials employed and the processes/procedures involved in the filling and packing operations. They also involve the greatest level of risk to the user/patient since the administration of sterile products involves direct injection, thus bypassing the body's natural defences. Because of this increased risk for the patient, the pharmaceutical company is exposed to a greater degree of responsibility and risk via 'product liability' claims.

The administration of these sterile products and ease of use have become a much more important criterion in recent times. This trend is expected to continue, as will the move towards drug delivery devices intended for easier application, with an increasing focus on self-application. These containers/drug delivery devices will inevitably use an increasing number of plastic components so that any complexity is involved in the assembly of the system rather than in the use of the delivery device. Rubber components have a significant role to play in the successful development of such devices, since there is no real substitute for rubber.

Advances by reputable manufacturers have removed some of the perceived disadvantages of rubber, in particular the refinement of rubber formulations to reduce the level of extractives. The development of a fluoropolymer-based laminate under the FluroTec® product range to provide real barrier properties has simplified the complex process of rubber closure selection and offered a level of security not available with a conventional closure. The use of such laminated closures is predicted to increase in the future, in particular these are likely to be specified as the closure system for biopharmaceutical applications.

The trend toward the use of isolator technology for sterile products to improve the quality level and reduce the manufacturing cost has placed a new emphasis on the importance of the primary packaging components. Existing systems for sterilisation and depyrogenisation of glassware fit readily with isolator technology, but there are recognised difficulties in the provision of sterile pyrogen-free rubber closures into the isolator. Solutions range from the supply of sterile rubber closures and metal crimps in disposable bags, each fitted with a special transfer port, to closures being supplied in specially designed recyclable containers. Alternatively, it is possible to gain access into an isolator using a special receptacle and a manual or automatic transfer port. The use of the latter system would not require any further advances by closure manufacturers, but such systems are likely to be suitable only for small volume production. The supply of closures into isolators would appear to suit ideally the use of gamma sterilisation, and although this method has been used to supply sterilise closures there are certain regulatory requirements that affect existing products. Changes in the sterilisation method will require a degree of evaluation by running stability batches and also validation of the sterilisation method, in particular the impact on the physical and visual properties of the closures.

References

Danielson, J. W., *J. Parenteral Sci. Technol.*, 1992, 46, 43.

Dillard, S. F. and MacCollum, M. A., Reports to FDA: allergic reactions to latex containing medical devices, *International Latex Conference: Sensitivity to Latex in Medical Devices*, 1992, 23 (abstract).

Dölcher, D., *PDA International Conference*, Arlington, February 1990.

Franke, H., Hencken, P., Ross, G. and Kreuter, J., *Eur. J. Pharm. Biopharm.*, 1994, 40, 379.

Jahnke, R. W. O., Kreuter, J. and Ross G., *J. Parenteral Sci. Technol.*, 1990a, 44, 282.

Jahnke, R. W. O., Kreuter, J. and Ross G., *Int. J. Pharm.*, 1991, 77, 47.

Jahnke, R. W. O., Linde, H., Mosand I. A. and Kreuter, J., *Acta Pharm Technol.*, 1990b, 36, 139.

Lee, M. L. and Hites, R. A., *Anal. Chem.*, 1976, 48, 1890.

Mannermaa, J. P., Muttonen, E., Yliruusi, J. and Juppo, A., *J. Parenteral Sci. Technol.*, 1992, 46, 73.

Massey, R. C. and Taylor, D. (eds), *Aluminium in Food and the Environment*, Royal Society of Chemistry, Cambridge, 1989.

Meek, J. H. and Pettit, B. R., *The Lancet*, 1985, 1090.

Milano, E. A., Waraszkiewicz, S. M. and Dirubio, R., *J. Parenteral Sci. Technol.*, 1982, 36, 116.

Mondimore, D. and Moore, C., *J. Parenteral Sci. Technol.*, 1983, 37, 79.

Morton, D. K., *J. Parenteral Sci. Technol.*, 1987, 41, 145.

Morton, D. K., Lordi, N. G., *J. Parenteral Sci. Technol.*, 1988, 42, 57.

Parenteral Drug Association Inc., *Aspects of Container/Closure Integrity*, Technical Information Bulletin No. 4, 1983.

Parenteral Society, *The Prevention and Detection of Leaks in Ampoules, Vials and Other Parenteral Containers*, Technical Monograph No. 3, 1992.

Petersen, M. C., Vine, J., Ashley, J. J. and Nation, R. L., *J. Pharm. Sci.*, 1981, 70, 1139.

Pikal, M. J. and Lang, J. E., *J. Parenteral Drug Assoc.*, 1978, 32, 162.

Portnoff, J. B., Henley, M. V. and Restaino, F. A., *J. Parenteral Sci. Technol.*, 1983, 37, 180.

Russell-Fell, R., *International Conference: Latex Protein Allergy*, 1993, 3.

Shah, P. V., Knapp, G., Kelly, J. P. and Cabana, B. E., *Clin. Chem.*, 1982, 28, 2327.

Shang-Qiang, J. and Evenson, M. A., *Clin. Chem.*, 1983, 29, 456.

Slater, J. E., *International Conference: Latex Protein Allergy*, 1993, 7.

Towse, A., O'Brien, M., Twarog, F. J., Braimon, J. and Moses, A.C., *Diabetes Care*, 1995, 18, 1194.

Wells, C. E., Juenge, E. C. and Wolnick, K., *J. Pharm. Sci.*, 1986, 75, 724.

Yip, E., Poon, N. K. and Lang, M. K., *International Conference: Latex Protein Allergy*, 1995, 33.

13

BLISTER, STRIP AND SACHET PACKAGING

D. A. Dean

Introduction

Although strip packs date from the late 1920s (starting with the single Aspro strip in waxed paper) and blister packs from the early 1960s, both are now well established forms of pharmaceutical 'unit dose' packaging. As unit dose packs offer individual protection until the dose therein is removed, personal dosage, tamper-evidence, child safety, no cross-contamination risks, no opening and reclosing problems, etc., their popularity has limited the growth of typical multipacks. Against these advantages, blisters and strips generally occupy larger volumes than their multipack equivalents. However, this increased pack external area, particularly when cartoned, may enhance the product display image and offer more label space.

Elderly patient compliance has been raised as a point for criticism. This has usually been a result of the question 'do you have difficulty in opening blister or strip type packs?' where 'have you tried opening them this way?' might have been more helpful.

Blister packs originally consisted of a thermoformed plastic tray with a lidding material made from plastic, paper, foil or a combination of these, with the product being removed either by pushing through the lid or via a peelable lidding. Today this definition has been extended by cold forming of plastic/foil combinations and the so-called tropical lidding over the blister.

Similarly, strip packs consists of one or two plies, made from regenerated cellulose, paper, plastics, foil or any combination of these, whereby an item is inserted into a pocket area against a recess in a heated platen or roller. However, some systems now involve the use of preformed pockets thereby making it increasingly difficult to differentiate between blister and strip packaging (Figures 13.1 and 13.2).

Blister packs

Blister machines utilise the fact that a plastic film can be softened by heat and then formed in a mould by:

1   mechanical forming between male and female moulds
2   vacuum or negative pressure – which draws the softened film over or into a mould
3   pressure – in which compressed air forces the film over or into a mould
4   combinations of the above.

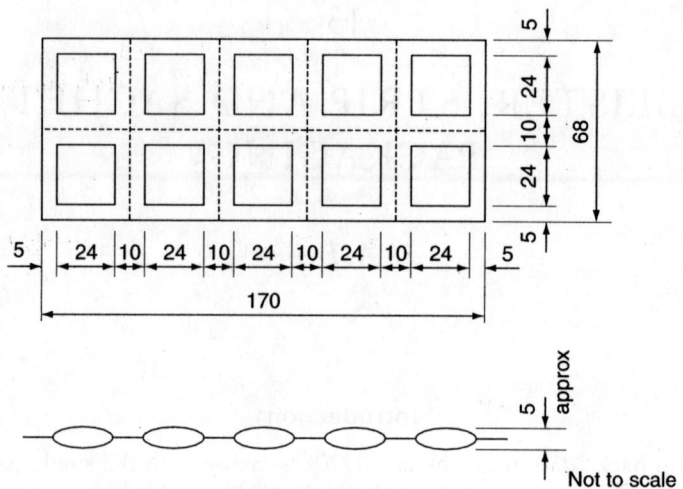

Figure 13.1 Strip pack (based on tablet 13 × 6 mm)

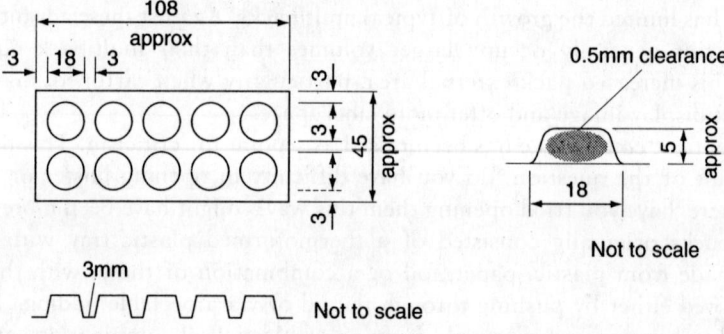

Figure 13.2 Blister pack (based on tablet 13 × 6 mm)

The trays thereby formed are subsequently filled, lidded and cut out into specific tray sizes and configurations.

The distribution of the wall thickness achieved by the moulding operation depends on the process: whether the material is formed into or over a mould, film thickness, depth of draw, softening temperature, type of plastic, etc. For an identical blister shape, pressure plus plug assistance generally gives the most uniform blister. Pressure forming usually gives a thicker top section and vacuum is thicker near the base of the web, thinning towards the top. In-built strain within the blister can be observed by viewing under polarised light (provided it is a clear or natural material).

Basic equipment principles

Fully automatic machines are based on either continuous or intermittent movement of the web through the unit, or a combination of the two. Until recently this motion depended on whether certain processes were carried out on platens or cylinders. It is now possible to use platens which have a reciprocating action whereby continuous motion can be maintained. The basic machine operations performed on a machine are:

1 heating + thermoforming or cold forming
2 filling
3 heat sealing of the lidding material
4 punching-out or guillotining the tray from the web.

Additional operations may be printing of the lidding web, registration reading units, batch marking, product check/rejection on not fully filled trays, perforating or scoring between blisters, code reading and disposal of trim (wind-up or shredding). Machines may also incorporate anticurl devices, stacking of the trays, cartoning, etc. (Figure 13.3).

Thermoforming

Heating of the reel-fed base (tray) web is usually achieved by either infrared heaters or contact heaters. Heat may be applied at the forming stage or at a preheat station with or without further heating. The preheat station may be either a cylinder or platens; in certain instances the platens may be differentially heated (top and bottom).

The moulds into which the plastic is formed can be cooled by air, water or chilled water.

The web may be held by grippers, rollers, etc. as it is passed through the machine. Platen machines usually impart less tension to the web but generally operate at lower speeds, i.e. 8–12 m/min whereas 12–16 m/min can be achieved by continuous motion or by reciprocating motion machine with platens.

In general only the simpler materials can be thermoformed on cylinders using vacuum (e.g. PVC, polystyrene, PVdC coated PVC). Platens using pressure forming, particularly with plug assistance, not only offer more uniform blisters but can utilise the more complex materials, e.g. Aclar/PVC, polypropylene, coextrusions (Figure 13.4).

Feeding and filling

The type of feeding mechanism largely depends on the product being fed, i.e. suppositories, ampoules, tablets, capsules, etc., size and the number of tracks across the web. Uncoated tablets and capsules are normally fed from a vibratory bowl via channels or tubes by gravity. Vacuum extraction is frequently applied to the bowl, tubes, etc. to minimise powder and tablet chips which may finish up in the seal or tray. Conventional flat-shaped uncoated tablets usually present no problems, but sugar-coated or bevelled tablets with little side edge thickness may cause difficulties due to dovetailing or shingling. In such cases a rotary table feed may be used. A flood and sweep fill may be employed for sugar-coated tablets when speeds in excess of 300 per track are possible.

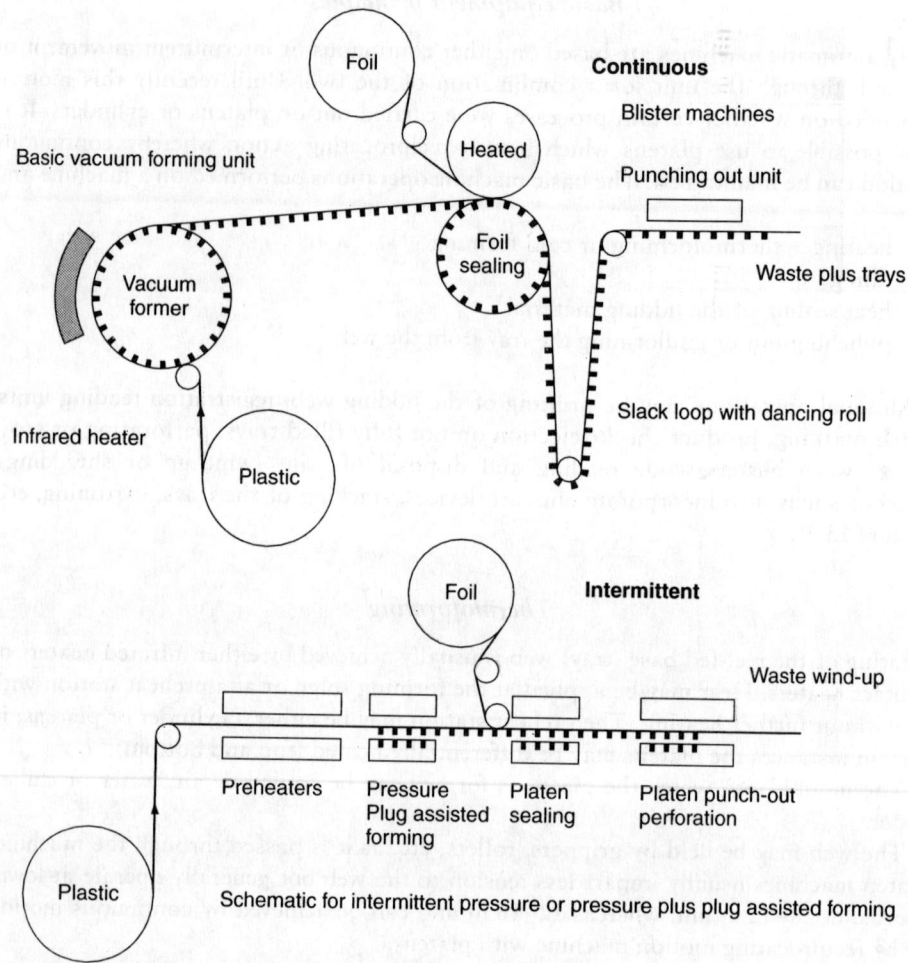

Figure 13.3 Blister machines

However, on most machines a fill speed of 250 items per minute per track is considered good. These speeds are related to the physical restrictions of feeding an item by gravity. Reciprocating tube fillers and chevron roller fillers are used on some machines where the close proximity of the tracks would cause restrictions to the filling speeds.

Lidding and heat sealing

As with the thermoforming process, heat sealing may be based on platens or cylinders or occasionally a combination of the two. Irrespective of the process the pocket must be sufficient to allow a clearance between the product and the lidding (normally around 0.5 mm), otherwise the product may adhere to the lid on heat sealing. The platen requires two uniformly flat surfaces with the base platen-shaped to accept the blisters. On certain machines one platen applies the heat via thermostatically or

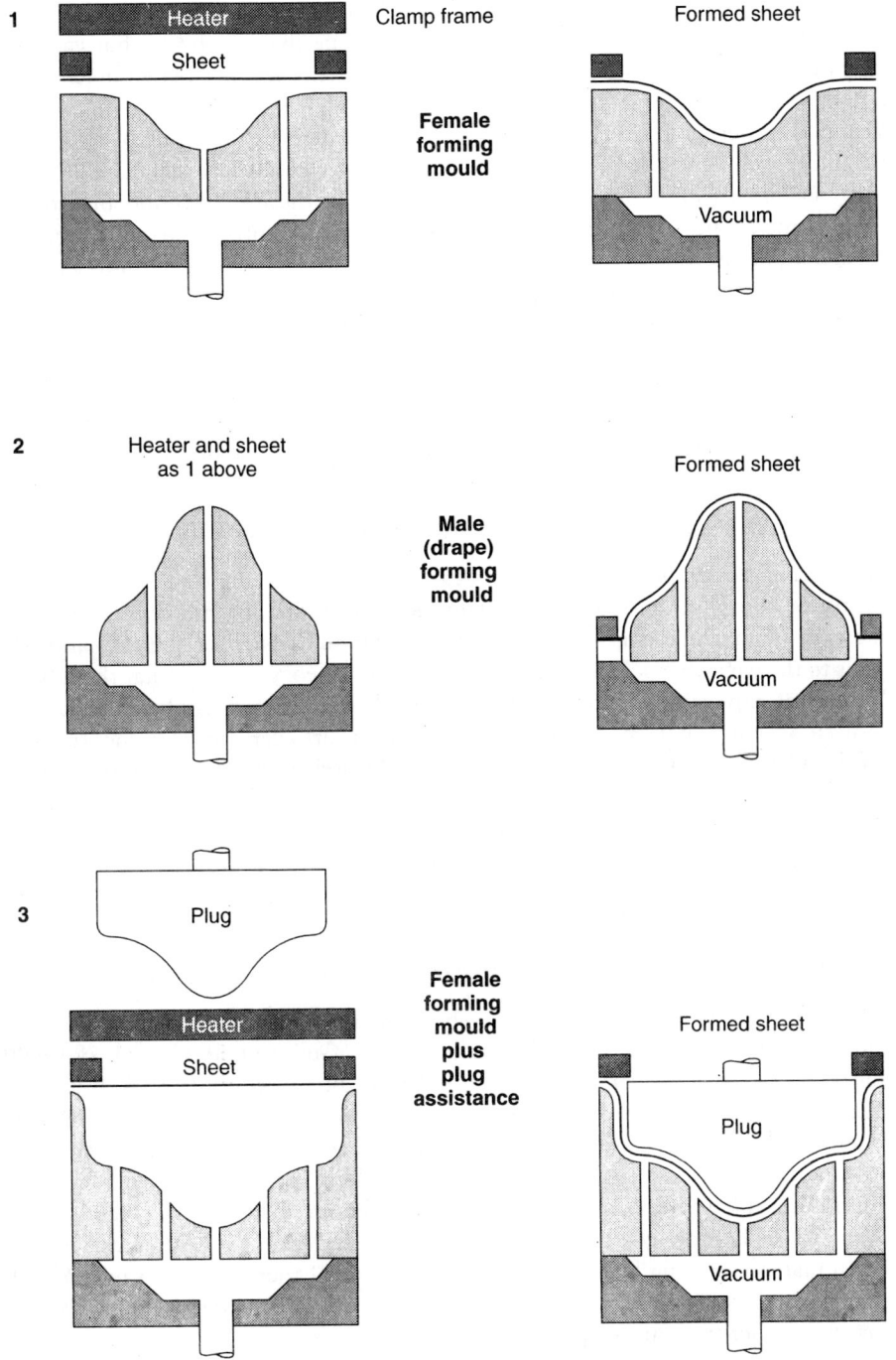

Figure 13.4 Thermoforming operations by vacuum

electronically controlled heaters and the other is cooled by air or water to facilitate rapid and effective sealing with minimum of web distortion. The platen process usually operates at a lower temperature and longer dwell time than cylinders, but can suffer from transferring more heat via the web to the product. On other platen machines the web passes through preheaters.

As stated earlier, uniformity of seal depends on the perfect matching of two platens which under well-controlled conditions undoubtedly gives a better seal. The pattern of seal may be line, pyramid or cross-hatch, but the last of these is invariably preferred. In the case of the cylinder type, the seal is achieved at the circumferential contact between two rollers, one of which is heated. As the process dwell time is very short, a higher temperature generally has to be employed.

It should be noted that the seal pattern is only on the heated platen or sealing roller, with the cooling platen or cylinder being smooth or flat (i.e. there is no impression or pattern on the plastic side of the web).

The effectiveness of either type of seal is checked by the uniformity of the seal impression, by vacuum tests or material deflection under vacuum/pressure.

Curl of trays (particularly relevant with hard foil)

The heat sealing operation can impart a degree of 'curl' into the tray, thereby creating problems for automatic enveloping or cartoning. The amount of curl depends partially on the type of machine employed, the type of web and design of the tray and what happens to the web when it leaves the sealing station. Theory suggests that the different coefficients of expansion for foil and film are partly the cause, plus film shrinkage due to molecular reorientation. Curl can be reduced or overcome by incorporating thermoformed ribs in the tray, or by reversing the web curvature by passing over a tension roller or through radiused guides. In the last of these the radius of the bend back has to be ascertained by trial and error experiments. Curl is less of a problem with soft foil as it stretches more readily. Between-pocket perforations or cuts can also reduce curl.

Removal from web (after perforating, where carried out)

Removal of the sealed trays from the web by punching-out or die cutting enables shaped trays without sharp corners to be produced. Guillotining, if used, invariably produces sharp corners which if not carefully handled may penetrate pockets of trays. Punching-out (unless a reciprocating or rotary unit is employed) is usually carried out as an intermittent action with platens. In the case of continuous motion machines the web is usually converted to intermittent by a 'slack loop' prior to either punching-out or guillotining. However, continuous motion can be retained by rotary die cutting, which is inevitably more costly in terms of dies and equipment. Wastage can be min-imised in platen punching by staggering the action, i.e. 2 then 1 in a 3 tray across the web configuration. Reciprocating cutting forms can also maintain a continuous motion, hence increase output speeds.

Product inspection and between-pocket perforation

Product inspection prior to lidding suffered problems when the web jerked or slowed down/accelerated whereby items could be thrown out of the previously filled pockets. Although this aspect has now been eliminated from most machines, the after-lidding option had further problems when clear materials were replaced with dark tinted or opaque or foil/foil blisters to improve either child-resistance or moisture, light, oxygen protection. Thus depending on the machine or/and web materials, the original before and after lidding options remain. Prior to lidding inspection now offers mechanical/electrical sensing or an imaging technique, while after lidding tends towards either infrared or X-ray methods.

Perforation or similar options offer a means by which pockets can be readily separated and/or the prevention of any opening method from exposing more than one product. In the US-type peelable packs, perforation or something similar is usually essential to control the peel. Perforation may be achieved by true perforation (a series of bridges and cut-through zones), a part cut through by sharp blades or knives, or the use of a form of laser technology. Such operations usually require a larger between-pocket distance (3 to 4 mm increases to 5 to 7 mm), adding to the overall size of the blister. The operation is normally carried out either prior to the punching out or within the punching, guillotine stage. It must be performed on well-cooled trays, as warm or flexible materials are less easy to penetrate and can blunt the knives more easily.

Machine summary

Although individual machines may be built for specific functions, standard machines generally offer fixed platen or cylinder sizes. The factors which may have to be considered in the choice of a machine are:

1   area available per stroke on machine (width and length)
2   size and configuration of trays
3   area of wastage or minimum wastage
4   size of product and physical–chemical characteristics
5   type of material used for lid and tray
6   type of feed, number of feed tracks
7   output required or strokes per minute
8   critical nature of blister wall distribution and seal effectiveness
9   type of blister (push-through, peelable)
10 number and frequency of change-overs
11 type of forming available or necessary, e.g. vacuum, pressure, mechanical plug assistance, and combinations of these
12 type of heating available – radiant, conducted, preheat, etc.
13 type of web transfer, i.e. continuous, intermittent, or a combination of these
14 type of removal from web, punch or guillotine, etc.
15 need for perforations, scores or slits between pockets
16 whether machine is integral with a cartoning unit or can be coupled to one.

On some machines printing of the lidding by gravure or flexography can be added. Batch marking can be achieved by printing, embossing or debossing. Various types of product detection systems are available.

Invariably any machine is a compromise between a number of the more important factors.

Tray and blister design

As indicated earlier, total efficiency will relate to the minimal wastage and the maximum throughput. Both imply that the layout of the trays allows the use of a full web and this therefore means that the theoretically ideal blister shape may rarely be possible. Blisters should avoid square or near right-angled corners or bases as this may make release from the mould difficult and lead to thinning in those areas. Similarly, undercuts should either be avoided or be well radiused. Generally blisters should have an adequate clearance with the product and have an adequate radius at both the top (dome) and where the blister emerges into the tray flange. As vacuum forming gives less uniform wall distribution, this can be partially compensated by changing the angle of the draw from say $6°$ to $12°-20°$, but this may add to cost if the tray size is increased to a point where output/tray per area is reduced.

Similarly, the draw angle is less critical with pressure and pressure plus plug assisted forming, where a draw angle of $3°-6°$ is usual.

Satisfactory seals can be achieved with a separation of 2–3 mm between blisters but there may be some danger of exposing the adjacent pocket when a product is pushed out. Thus 3–4 mm is more general for both between blisters and margin seals. With in-between pocket perforations or scores this distance becomes 5–7 mm. In the case of peelable blisters it is necessary to extend the peelable edge by at least 5 mm. Alternatively, a cut-away part of the blister tray either internal to the design or on an edge seal may be employed, to enable a good grip for the peel feature. Whether the edge seal remains uniform depends on such features as accuracy of registration, method by which web is held and drawn through the machine, method of tray removal from the web. If the tolerances of these is excessive then wider in-between blister and edges will be necessary. If a tray of the push-through type without perforations provides minimum wastage and maximum machine output, then any change to a larger tray (perforations, or perforations plus peel, etc.) will lead to fewer trays per stroke, more wastage and lower output. In the cost examples it has been assumed that the same output/wastage can be maintained with larger trays. This is based on the availability of machines with the best area per stroke. In practice this may not be possible.

Work in Germany by Professor Gadecke has shown that blister trays with properly designed perforations will meet the US protocol for child-resistant non-reclosable packs. In these tests children tended to be satisfied by tearing along the perforations rather than penetrating into the pack. Opaque or dark tinted plastics are essential to render the item contained therein less attractive. The advent of original pack dispensing (OPD) and the fact that the UK has not followed the European norm (European packs are based on 10s, 20s, 30s, etc., and UK on 7s, 14s, 28s, etc.) has led to various attempts to use common tooling for both. This has frequently meant that certain sizes have pockets blanked off, e.g. a 14 pack can be produced by incorporating a 'blank' in a 15 pack.

Protection and use

In order to obtain a full pack evaluation it is necessary to consider a number of requirements. For instance:

1   ingress from the atmosphere which may result in product deterioration, e.g. oxygen, moisture, carbon dioxide, microbiological hazards
2   migration of product ingredients from within the product to the outside atmosphere
3   migration from the pack into the product or reaction between the product and pack, e.g. discolouration, softening of the heatseal
4   mechanical damage to pack or product: note that on-edge stacking of blisters usually offers the best strength.
5   a convenient means for removing the product without exposing other units
6   the pack must satisfactorily retain the product for the declared 'shelf life'.

The above has to be established by laboratory testing prior to a formal stability programme. As with all pack selections, detailed knowledge of the product, the packaging materials and the process to be employed is an essential requirement. Blister packs are unlikely to give sufficient protection to products severely affected by moisture, oxygen, carbon dioxide, as all known plastic materials are to some degree permeable to these factors.

In such instances additional protection can be achieved by foil sachets, foil lined cartons or overwraps. If the last of these is used it is then necessary to establish that the 'shelf life' of a tray following its removal from its additional wrap is satisfactory for the 'in use' period.

Protection against moisture

The usual practice of making up a few blisters and placing them on test in a cabinet at 25°C 75% RH, 40°C 75% RH, etc., may produce very misleading results. In actual practice blisters may be enclosed in a carton (possibly overwrapped), placed x cartons per outer (overwrapped), y outers per pallet or with the pallet being shrink wrapped. All of these activities reduce the flow of moist air around the pack, and provide a possible series of moisture barriers. It therefore may not be surprising to find in 24–48 months' storage of a pallet that there is no actual moisture change in the product. Overwrapping of individual cartons or the outer can significantly increase the shelf life of the product. The predicted shelf life from a cabinet test may therefore carry an unnecessary safety factor or even indicate that a blister pack would not be suitable, when under actual conditions it could be acceptable.

Having established a pack/product by an adequate testing sequence, it is necessary to emerge with:

1   a fully and correctly specified product
2   fully and correctly specified packaging materials and finished pack
3   a recognised and defined means of bringing (1) and (2) together, i.e. SOPs.

The successful operation involves not only those who originated the pack and the product, but production and quality control. The latter will be involved in the inspection of incoming materials and the finished packed product.

Child-resistance, tamper-evidence/resistance and OPD (original pack dispensing, now called patient packs in the UK)

Blister and strips by their design are inherently both tamper-evident and tamper-resistant. In 1987 the PAGB, with the support of the ABPI, produced *Design Guidelines for Strip and Blister Packs*, which basically eliminates any 'flimsy' blister or strip packs that might be questionably child-resistant. The above design guidelines led to the issue of BS 7236 1989, *Non Reclosable Packaging for Solid Dose Units of Medicinal Products*. For further details see Chapter 11. An ISO standard based on ISO/EN 28317 has now been approved for reclosables but the standard for non-reclosables is still under debate. German standards for 'type approval' are based on DIN 55559 (more detail is given in Chapter 11).

OPD or patient packs

Although some people considered OPD as synonymous with blister and strip packs, any type of pack can be used. However, the advent of OPD will see a significant swing to blister and strip packs for a number of reasons, including the following.

1 Products are becoming more potent, hence tablets/capsules are smaller.
2 Sustained, delayed and controlled release products are reducing the 3 to 4 times a day dosage regime to 1 and 2, hence quantities and packs will become smaller.
3 Small packs are difficult to label and to accommodate the 70 × 40 mm or 70 × 35 mm community pharmacist's label.
4 Cartoned blister and strip packs give adequate label space and provide a means of collating a patient leaflet (i.e. flat rectangular cartons).
5 Cartoned blister and strip packs also provide adequate space for a bar code and a removable bar code if required for pricing bureau costings.

It should be noted that the volume resulting from the use of blister and strips will be more significant in the warehousing activities of the pharmaceutical supplier and the wholesaler. It will probably be less critical than the community pharmacist envisages, since lower stock levels of OPDs are likely to be kept compared with a bulk pack of 500, 1,000, etc., and the dispensing containers which have to be kept for their use. An actual reduction in space could occur as cartons stack better than bottles, particularly if the bottles are not contained in cartons.

Blister materials – trays and lids

The majority of the packs used in Europe are of the push-through variety. In these instances hard foil of 0.015 mm and above is used. This is adequate as the permeability of the plastic tray tends to be far higher than the foil.

Opaque or tinted materials are necessary if the pack is to meet the UK child-resistant requirements. Opaque films (usually incorporating titanium dioxide) tend to be slightly more permeable than clear materials. Permeation increases with the filler or modifier content of the plastic.

Note that impact modified grades of PVC usually soften at a lower temperature hence may improve machine throughput. Vinyl acetate is widely used as an impact modifier. Impact modified grades generally show higher moisture vapour figures than UPVC.

Lidding materials can also use soft (annealed) foil (0.025 mm) or laminations of soft foil and other substances (tissue paper, glassine, etc.). Soft and embossed soft foil extends in the push-through stage, hence may give added child safety provided it does not damage the item concerned.

Environmental concern with reference to PVC and the fact that burning (possibly as a distinction from controlled incineration) may generate obnoxious acid fumes has created pressure on the pharmaceutical industry to move away from PVC. The alternative materials which have been considered include PET (polyester) and PP (polypropylene). Both require higher softening temperatures than PVC and good heat control, which can be more readily achieved with modern equipment with an effective preheat system. However, this only applies to certain selected and special material grades. Although these materials can be coated with PVdC to improve the moisture barrier, there are pressures to ban PVdC as it also contains a chloride component. Suffice it to say that the replacement of PVdC and its associated barrier/heat seal features may not be easy to achieve. Current opinion is that PVC will not be replaced.

Currently specific grades of PP are being preferred to PET and most machine manufacturers are offering modified machines which will handle these materials. For cold forming, multilayer materials are now being offered with two thinner layers of soft foil which are separated by a plastic ply.

Blister materials (tray – plastics)

In the following list, 1 = moisture barrier provided by PVC; 2–10 = times improvement in WVP.

1 PVC or UPVC (1). Homopolymer – may be opaque or tinted.
2 PVC (0.7). Impact modified (usually with vinyl acetate), up to 50% higher permeability. Can be opaque or tinted. Note that impact modified grades show white in fold area when bent over.
3 PVdC coated PVC (3–5). Usually 36–100 g/m^2 PVdC on various calipers of PVC.
4 PVdC coated PP (3–5).
5 Aclar*/PVC (10–15).

- Copolymers (Aclar 22A/PVC, Aclar 33C/PVC, Aclar 88A/PVC)
- Homopolymers (Aclar R$_x$ 160/PVC, Aclar R$_x$ 160/PETG, Aclar UltR$_x$2000, 3000 SupR$_x$900).

6 Polystyrene PS (0.2). Rather more brittle than PVC – improved by the addition of modifiers (increases opacity).

---

* Aclar is the trade name of polymonochlorotrifluoroethylene supplied by Allied Signal. (Generally, UltR$_x$3000 offers the best moisture barrier.)

7   Polypropylene – copolymer (3–5). Good resistance to WVP but poorer gas barrier. Not easy to control when thermoforming due to higher temperature involved, but improving with specialist grades.

8   Polypropylene – talc filled (1–1.5). Better thermoforming, but WVP only slightly better than PVC. Chalk filled PP is also available.

9   PVdC–PE–PVC, sometimes called triplex.

10   PVC   PE   PVdC   PE   PVC
     100   30   180   30   100 μm

11   PET (polyester) selected grades (usually as a copolymer), e.g. PETG.

Blister lidding materials (push-through)

Foil hard 0.018–0.020 mm plus 6–8 g/m^2 wax, 4–12 g/m^2 vinyl type lacquer or PVdC coating of 10 g/m^2 and above. Lowest foil gauge in use is 15 μm. Note that special HS lacquers can be formulated to adhere to PVdC, Aclar, PP, etc.

Hard foil tends to be more expensive than soft foil if the former has to be subjected to the removal of lubricants by solvents before it can be washed, lacquered and/or printed. However, low-temperature heating (below the annealing temperature) has also been used to remove the oil-based lubricants.

Foil soft 0.025 mm and above plus wax, vinyl type, PVdC or HS coatings for heat seal – note that greater stretch risk with soft foil necessitates a thicker gauge. When soft foil is laminated with 35 g/m^2 glassine, improved child-resistance is achieved. Note that most foils have a primer coat applied on either side prior to coating, printing or laminating, etc.

Peelable

Paper-foil–heat seal lacquer of various combinations. Also cold seals.

Note that heat sealable lacquers have to be 'compatible' with the tray material. If PVC/PVdC is formed with the PVdC on the inside of the blister, a PVdC type compatible lacquer is necessary for the lidding material. All lacquers should be checked for peel strength both initially and at each shelf-life period (1, 3, 6 months, etc.) as ageing effects have been detected, e.g. push-through becoming peelable and peelable becoming permanent (Figures 13.5 and 13.6).

Cold forming (or mechanically formed blisters)

Laminations of plastic and foil, usually of 40 μm + foil, can be physically formed on modified blister packing equipment by a cold mechanical forming operation which is carried out between male and female dies. These laminations of plastic and foil enabled foil to flow without flex cracks during forming although limitations in draw angles and forming depth still remained. This limitation has been improved (but not totally overcome) by using a modified aluminium alloy, the selection of the lamination, the forming design and the best machine factors. The forming material currently consists of such combinations as a biaxially oriented plastic laminated to 40 to 60 μm, aluminium foil and an internal (third) layer of plastic (PE, PVC). Cold forming is also being achieved with multilayer materials containing two layers of soft foil separated by a polymer layer.

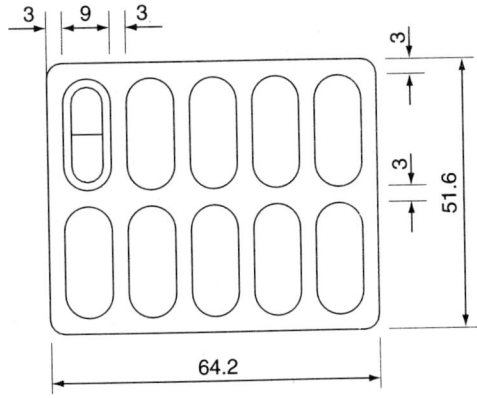

Figure 13.5 Conventional push-through pack

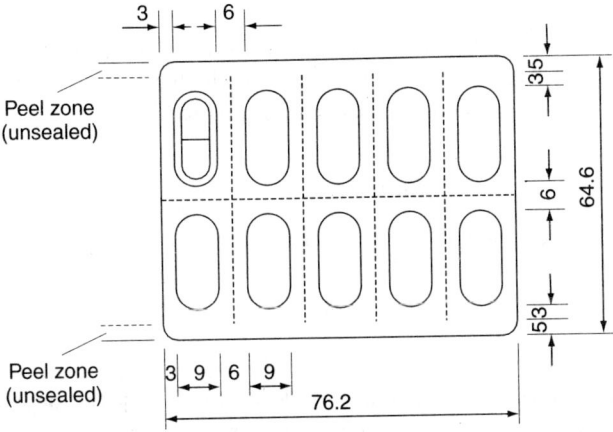

Figure 13.6 Same as Figure 13.5 but with peelable pocket perforations

Cold forming processes have been developed using a number of basic ideas, as follows.

1   Clamping the material and carrying out a true punch action where the non-held area is extended (stretch forming).
2   Taking a foil which has been embossed or finely creased; can be extended by air or mechanical pressure without showing flex cracks.
3   Taking a reel of material with regular cross-direction slits (as used on Servac suppository machine). A male/female mechanical forming operation is carried out between each slit. This mechanical operation forms the foil and the slit area moves (opens), thereby preventing any high degree of stress (uses 12.5 μm OPP/40 μm foil/HSL).
4   Latest innovations include a double forming operation which reduces the tray size to 20% (Advanced Forming Technology (AFT) process). These tend to use Teflon stretching dies.

Stretch or cold forming

Although foil is an excellent barrier material, gauges of 40 μm and less were difficult to form without fracture. This was partly due to the fact that metallic materials have a crystalline structure and commercially pure grades of aluminium foil had a grain size of around 40 μm (foil of 40 μm was likely to be a mono-grain layer). By the production of special foils of smaller grain size, new 40 to 60 μm foils consisting of multiple layers can more readily stretch without any fracture risk. Laminating this foil to biaxially oriented polypropylenes, polyamides and polyester films further added to the stretch forming possibilities.

It was also shown that the better the laminating bond between the foil and the plastic, the better is the forming operation. To date a typical forming ratio is approximately 1:2.5 (i.e. a cavity diameter of 20 mm would have a depth of 8 mm), using polyamide/aluminium 40 μm /polyamide/PVC film.

In the development of the above technological progress, two selected techniques have been employed:

1 the MAD unit developed by Bosch (a machine to measure multiaxial elongation)
2 Hoogoven screen – a specially printed screen from which stresses and deformation during forming can be quantified (also useful for plastic films).

Summary

Cold or stretch forming is growing as a commercial operation. The factors which influence the stretch forming operation include:

1 the gauge and type of foil used
2 the fineness of the crystalline structure of the foil
3 the design of the formed area including angle of draw and the depth of draw (width to depth currently does not exceed a ratio of 2:5)
4 the structure of the supporting or carrier lamination including the uniformity of the oriented plastic
5 positive lamination between foil and outer ply
6 the forming speed and the friction properties of the laminate
7 the quality of the die, especially the surface finish.

However, further improvements should not be overlooked. New laminations and configurations have recently become available to improve further the child-resistance features of both blisters and strips. In the USA these are typically peelable configurations.

Tropicalised lidding

While cold forming remains relatively expensive, alternative ways of obtaining excellent moisture protection will be sought. Putting a foil lid over the tray section and sealing it to the blister margins, known as the 'tropicalised' blister, is now available from several suppliers. This type of lidding may be achieved by a preforming operation, thereby allowing a seal with relatively narrow margins or by direct lidding (no stretch) with a more gradual 'draw' and wider margins. Both methods increase the pack size and add to costs.

Costs

Costs are related to material prices, output speeds, wastage, machine depreciation, downtimes, etc. (see below). Depending on the choice of material, blister packs of the push-through variety can be as economical as glass bottles in quantities up to around ninety items per pack. At quantities below twenty-five items, there are positive cost advantages in most cases. Both these comments must be accepted as rather general statements – the actual break-even point has to be calculated for each set of circumstances. The above indications assume that both a glass bottle and the blisters have to be packed into cartons, with a CRC fitted to the bottle pack.

Greater emphasis has been put on blister packaging systems in recent European developments. Most machines can be coupled with a leaflet/cartoning system. In many instances the cartoning operation is an integral part of the blister machine. Labour costs can change relatively rapidly, particularly at times of rapid technical development, allied to salary inflation, so it would be misleading to include details in this chapter. However, in general, labour costs on bottling/blister lines of a similar size will largely be comparable.

Continuing competition is expected between cold form and tropicalised blisters, which compared with straight PVC blisters, offer area ratios of 60×48 (PVC), 70×58 (tropicalised) to 112×66 (cold form) with cost ratios of approximately $100:170:285$.

Summary

Blister packaging equipment can extend from a fairly basic piece of machinery which covers a form fill seal, and removal from the web operation to a highly sophisticated unit covering a far more complex range of operations. Invariably complexity must be associated with higher prices, more highly trained operatives, less flexibility, etc. Plastic blister materials cannot offer full climatic protection, hence additional protection may have to be achieved by some form of overwrapping system.

A broad summary can be made of machines, materials, outputs, costs, etc. in comparison with glass and plastic bottles, metal cans, and strip packs as shown by the general costings. As the requirement for a unit dose or multiple unit dose increases, both blister and strip packs are ensured of a significant increase. Blisters may gain in space and cost saving but lose out in climatic protection, unless cold formed foil, a foil tropicalised blister, or an overwrapping system is used.

New machines, cold forming, a plastic/foil blister/pocket, which use areas of materials between those of blisters and strips are also likely to increase. Whether these are actually strips or blisters will depend on the forming process used.

In summary, any individual type of dosage form offers obvious advantages in product hygiene, personalisation and protection if the correct materials are selected. It also enables the patient to carry a daily dose readily.

Finally, in small quantities of items (say fewer than seventy-five) blister packs are likely to be both economical and competitive with other packs, showing in addition a weight saving with a volume increase.

Normally the lidding is printed (for transparent trays both sides can be printed) but not the tray. On-line or in-house printing of lidding materials is increasing.

Note that semi-automatic blister packaging employing large preformed trays which are filled by hand then lidded from reel or sheet, followed by punching-out or guillotining, can offer speeds of around 1,200 items per minute with two or three operators. Under such conditions prices can be reasonably competitive with more sophisticated automatic equipment, particularly if runs are relatively short and a variety of tray and product sizes are involved. This can be particularly useful for clinical trial supplies.

Controlled or monitored dosage systems for the elderly

Various blister tray systems using large blisters which will take several products are now being offered for elderly, infirm, arthritic patients, etc. These trays normally hold twenty-eight to forty-two blisters, which are filled with the patient's medication and then lidded. The nature of the medication can be marked in various ways, i.e. water tablets, heart capsules, etc., with clear indication when each is to be taken, e.g. morning, mid-day, bedtime. In some systems these times are colour coded.

Examples of these include:

- Manrex Controlled Dosage Medication Systems
- Nomad by SurgiChem
- PCI (Pharmacy Consultants Incorporated)
- Webster Systems (now taken over by the Boots Company)

and may be found in the USA, Canada, the UK, Holland and Australia.

It is forecast that these systems will increase in popularity, particularly as the elderly population is showing a steady increase, often residing in special homes.

The pharmacist normally purchases the blisters in reels, and has a special sealing machine for the lidding operation. The pockets can usually be individually labelled (on the lidding) using a computer-based system involving self-adhesive labels.

Since the monitored dosage systems conflict somewhat with the OPD concept (a pharmacist does not like transferring products from blisters and strips) there may still be a need for a bulk pack, particularly if the use of these dosage systems continues to expand.

Blisters – liquids and semi-liquids

Although conventional horizontal formed blisters can be used with semi-viscous to viscous products (or even smaller quantities of liquid), it is necessary to turn them to a vertical position if a higher fill volume per pack is to be achieved. Filling single or double sided formed blisters in the vertical position can be carried out in cut individuals, cut sticks or an intermittently or continuously reel-fed system. Initial attempts to utilise a double sided formed blister led to low operational speeds. The introduction of laminate or coated webs whereby the sides of each web can be heat sealed led to significant increases in output. For example, the Lamps san Prospero, Unifill machines (Elopak) can produce packs with liquid volume fills between 1 and 90 ml with output speeds of up to 20,000 an hour, Dott. Bonopace also offers machines, a development of its suppository packs, where preformed blisters are delivered in reels. In theory machines of these types should be capable of aseptic production and hence in the long term could compete with other machines which operate on aseptic systems.

In the food industry such equipment would use either a presterilised web exposed by a removable peelable layer, or UV or hydrogen peroxide as an on-line surface sterilising agent. Currently none of these would be acceptable for a pharmaceutical operation, although use for sterile oral liquids might bear consideration.

Strip packs

Strip packs present an alternative form of pack for a unit dosage. Strips can be produced from single or multi-ply materials, provided the two inner plies can be sealed by heat or pressure (e.g. cold 'self-adhesive' seal). Materials can range from relatively permeable plies to those which incorporate a foil ply of sufficient thickness (and effectiveness of seal) that an individual hermetic seal is produced for each dosage. To date strip packs are usually produced at lower speeds and also occupy greater volume than blisters. The break-even cost with glass containers largely depends on the material used, output speed, and item size.

Strip packaging process

Basically a strip pack can be formed by introducing an item which extends a pocket area during insertion or by a preforming operation prior to filling (see Figures 13.7 and 13.8). As the latter method gives less strain (or more controlled forming) to the pocket area and reduces the material needed by 20–35%, it is suggested that this type of strip pack may increase. Either one or both sides of the plies may be mechanically formed, but this process can only be applied to materials which will 'stretch' without tearing.

Strip packaging machines are far simpler and smaller than blister packaging units, usually simply consisting of a feed system, product insertion plus heat sealing, and a guillotining operation to size.

Feed is usually via a vibratory bowl with feeding tracks (usually up to a maximum of sixteen). Alternatives are a rotating table plus drop or sweep. Most machines employ a

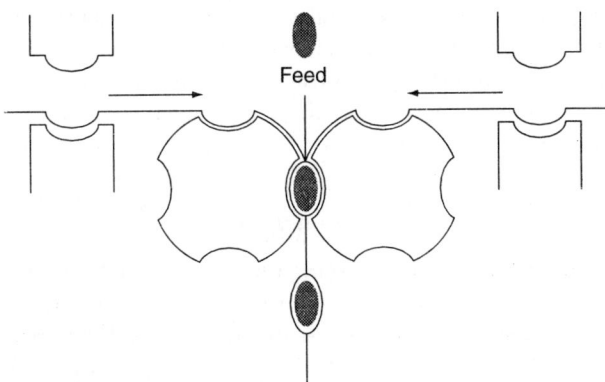

Figure 13.7 Strip pack preformed pocket

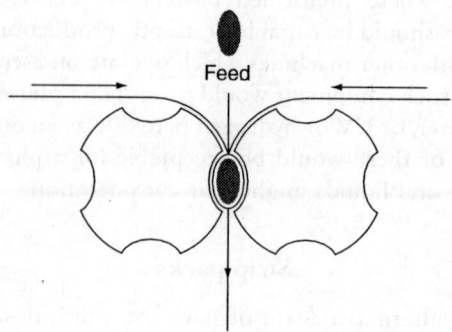

Feed

Figure 13.8 Strip packs in item formed pockets

vertical feed (gravity drop) but occasionally the web is run horizontally with a platen-type sweep. The pocket area is created by recesses either in a platen or more usually in a heat sealing cylinder, where a circumferential point seal is made between two inter-meshing cylinders.

As with blister packs, the maximum speed depends on the size of the item and grav-ity. A maximum speed of 250–300 per track is likely with a 325 mg (five grain) type of aspirin product. Removal of powder, chips, etc. is achieved by vacuum extraction.

Cutting of the emerging web is invariably done by either a scissors or guillotine motion or rotary die cutting. Additional stages which can be incorporated into the machine include printing, perforating, batch coding, magic eye registration, etc. As dis-tinct from blisters, perforation does not usually add to the seal width, as pocket seals are nominally 5 mm or more. Most machines use two separate webs but occasionally a single centrally folded web may be employed. Strip packaging is closely allied to sachet packing and in certain cases it is difficult to differentiate between the two. Two differ-ent plies can also be used (top and bottom) provided the sealants are compatible.

Machine speeds

A few eight-track machines exist (maximum output around 2,000 items per minute); four, two and single tracks are more usual with outputs of 1,000, 500 and 250 respec-tively. As a result of this speed limitation, few machines are coupled to a cartoning unit.

More recently sixteen- and thirty-two-track machines have achieved output of 4,000 and 8,000 items per minute. These are similarly priced to blister units and have an inte-gral cartoning option.

Strip designs

Strip designs are very basic, as the emerging units are invariably rectangular or square strips. The pocket portion can, however, be round, oval or square. The pocket area is critical to the diameter, shape and thickness of the product. If the pocket is too 'tight', tearing, perforation of the pocket periphery or wrinkling of the seal area may occur (Figure 13.9). The seal width may be as low as 4 mm, but usually 5 mm and above is employed. If the seal area is likely to wrinkle or crease then wider seals may be

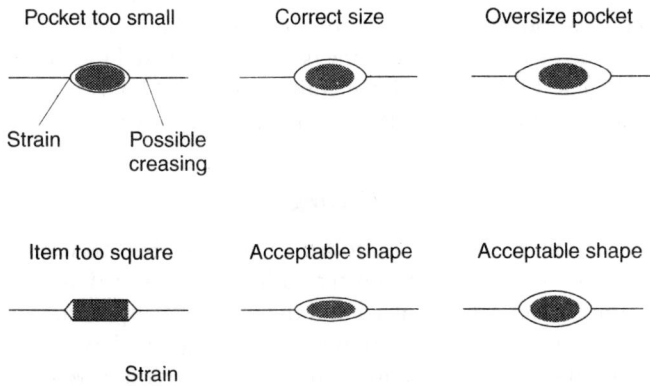

Figure 13.9 Strip packs in item formed pockets

necessary. It should also be recalled that the cylindrical-type sealing process does not usually have a distinct cooling cycle – hence any pull on the seal ply will tend to weaken the seal when the sealant is still pliable. This is particularly relevant with foil, where it may be necessary to have air cooling cylinders if a small seal margin is used. Warm materials are frequently more difficult to cut than cold materials. This may introduce a need for extra cooling or moving the cutting operation further away from the heat sealing area, as a 'soft seal' may string or prevent a clean cut. Use of cold seals (self-adhesive materials) is extending, particularly as such materials can be sealed at higher speeds than conventional heat seals.

Machine sizes and heat control

Most strip machines consist of two cylinders driven from a large one-sided control box. This inevitably creates possible heat control difficulties, particularly as the cylinders get either wider or of greater diameter (i.e. the drives act as a heat sink, whereas the ends furthest away from the drives are exposed to air). Based on this, the greatest heat is likely to be retained somewhere between the two ends of the cylinder, possibly causing overheating, metal expansion, leading to pressure increases, etc.), Latest machines therefore incorporate two-ended supports (or drives), thus allowing wider diameter and longer cylinders to be used.

Materials

Full details and examples of typical materials are given in earlier chapters, so they are not covered here.

Materials employing foil inevitably provide the best, indeed excellent, protection provided an effective seal is achieved and the foil is not unduly stretched to form perforations during the handling.

Vacuumised metal coatings are gradually improving. Tests indicate that these substantially increase the protection offered by plastic materials but do not equate with a ply of foil. Two plastic plies, each with a vacuumised foil, when laminated in direct contact with one another, can give excellent barrier properties. The barrier properties achieved by metallisation may reduce somewhat once the material becomes creased. Protection from some of these creasing effects can be improved by the incorporation of a more flexible ply (e.g. LDPE), i.e. PET metallised/LDPE. PET is very resistant to tear, hence needs a tear initiation feature. It also confers child-resistance.

Costings

Good protection means the incorporation of a foil ply, but such packs are usually greater in cost than either a blister or blister with an overwrap. This is due to the cost of the material, the greater area involved and the likely lower production rate.

Cheaper plies such as regenerated cellulose film provide the lowest cost form of unit pack coupled with restricted protection, but this can be improved by an overwrap. PVdC coated PP is the preferred substitute material today.

Volumes

The volume occupied by strip packs is invariably high. Some reduction can be achieved by preforming the pockets. Cartoning with the more flimsy materials may create difficulties. For single strips, envelope or catch covers are a useful alternative to cartons. They also make cartoning a much easier operation. Particularly useful for clinical trial supplies (Figure 13.10).

Identification

Strip plies are usually printed by gravure or flexographic processes either on or off the strip pack machine. Registration is usually carried out on one ply. Repetitive printing is frequently employed, i.e. three repeats to two pocket areas, so that one full print will appear on each unit.

Conclusions

Strip packs incorporating a suitable foil ply offer excellent protection and are superior to all reclosable packs (there are no risks associated with opening and reclosure) and conventional blister packs. In general strips are produced at lower speeds than blisters, occupy a greater volume, and are more expensive. Cellulose or OPP films (single ply)

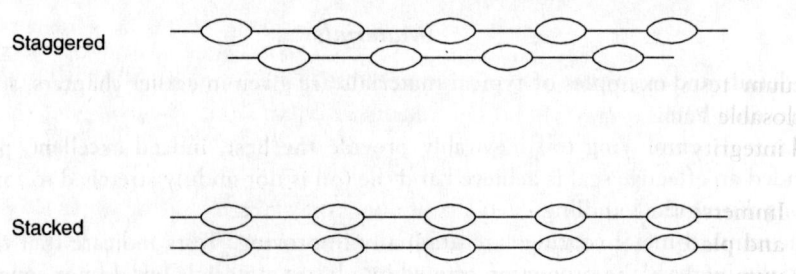

Figure 13.10 Staggered and stacked configurations

are likely to break even with bottles of 100 items, and a foil ply with 20–25 items. However, certain sophisticated machines handling 1 inch effervescent tablets offer high speeds of over 7,000 items per minute, hence are faster than most blister machines.

Strip packaging machines are generally more flexible than blister packers; change-over times are shorter and much lower in cost (except for the very widest machines). They are, therefore, more ideal for short runs. The largest machines with integral cartoning are similar in price to the fastest and largest blister units.

Machines can readily be coupled with catch covers (Wrapade and Siebler machines) and due to their smaller size have versatility in movement between packaging lines.

One of the most widely used materials with excellent moisture protection is paper, 40–45 g, extrusion coated LDPE, 12 g/m^2, 7–9 µm soft aluminium foil, 25 g/m^2 LDPE. The presence of two layers of plastic more than amply fills in any pinholes in the foil layer. The same laminate is also widely used for sachets and is technically preferred to a similar laminate with the foil on the outside.

Package integrity

The need to check pack integrity has increased in importance, both to guarantee product shelf life and to ensure that the product has not become 'contaminated' from some external source. Contamination may be related to organoleptic, physical, chemical or biological change, e.g. increase of bioburden, loss of sterility, which may be related to closure effectiveness.

Improving pack integrity can be related to on machine control (i.e. the quality assurance approach) or quality control (regular checks are made on the packs produced). Until recently the historical way of checking the integrity of blisters, strips, sachets, etc. involved the use of destructive-type testing, e.g. vacuum tests under water, burst tests. The more recent introduction of non-destructive tests should therefore not only improve output, but enable better on-line statistical evaluation to be carried out, thereby giving a better feedback on machine performance. This also means that where seal integrity is lost or is suspect more effective corrective actions can be undertaken, including improvements in on-line controls (i.e. more emphasis on quality assurance). Non-destructive testing equipment is usually based on a dry pressure vacuum procedure followed by detection of pack distortion (deflection) or non-distortion (non-deflection), i.e. packs with effective seals become concave then convex as positive pressure changes to negative pressure, while leaking packs either do not change or show less or limited distortion, depending on the scale of the leakage.

Vacuum tests

Vacuum tests under water vary from company to company. BS 7236 1989, Non-Reclosable Packaging for Solid Dose Units of Medicinal Products, gives the following seal integrity test.

Immerse the test package in a container containing coloured water (15–25°C) and place the container in the vacuum chamber. Apply the appropriate vacuum of 33 kPa (250 mm of mercury) for strip packages or 24 kPa (180 mm of mercury) for blister packages, for 30 s. Restore atmospheric pressure and remove the container from the vacuum chamber. Remove the test package from the container and blot off the excess water. Examine the package for ingress of water into the pockets.

Pinholes and foil (aluminium)

Pinholes normally refer to the minute holes which may be present in the foil after conversion. Foil of 0.017 mm caliper and above is generally recognised as commercially pinhole-free. 0.025 mm foil can normally be 'guaranteed' pinhole-free. Foil below 0.017 mm gradually shows an increasing number of pinholes. However, the WVP of foil of 0.006 mm is lower than any nominal gauge of plastic when used in a heat sealing lamination. When foil is laminated or coated the initial pinholes tend to be 'filled in', thus reducing any permeation risk still further. Permeation is then related to the plastic which covers the pinholes.

In the case of blister packs permeability via the foil side is extremely low, hence permeability relates mainly to the plastic of the tray and the wall distribution. With strip packs permeation may occur through edge seals, or more likely capillaries created by creases in the edge seal, as well as actual foil perforations. In general pinholes and perforations cannot be detected by vacuum dye tests as the plastic plies normally remain intact. Capillary leakage can be detected by this method – it may be assisted by adding a wetting agent to the solution.

Although the effect of pinholes may be minimal, the shelf life of the product can be reduced where the pack is exposed to high humidities for prolonged periods. Pinholes are likely to be irrelevant for short shelf life or rapid turnover products, where a certain degree of risk can be taken. See Chapter 10 for more details.

Sachets

Sachets achieved success when the first effective heat sealants were marketed. Their use, initially as a replacement for powders in folded paper, was extended into granules, moisture sensitive solid products and liquids (particularly shampoos).

Sachets can be fabricated from a single web with a centre fold, using a three or four sided seal or two webs using a four sided seal. The reels may be fed horizontally or vertically and be sealed by a series of heated platens or rollers (cylinders) or a combination of the two. In certain ways they are an enlarged version of a strip pack. The sachet seal can also be made peelable by a non-seal part on the web which may involve a pattern lacquer rather than a full heat seal coating. Difficult to tear plies, like PET, can also be used provided a cut or V-notch is added to initiate the tear.

Small sachets usually start with narrow seal margins of around 5 mm, but become wider as the weight of the contents increases. Like strip packs, an over-tight fill should be avoided, as this can lead to perforation on the inner side of the heat seal and capillary channels, resulting from seal creases. Although seal patterns can follow strip packs, line seals, either all parallel or across at the top and down at the sides, tend to predominate. A cross seal at the top tends to give a more secure seal whereas parallel downward lines make for an easier tear open feature. Although sachets can be received preformed for filling, reel-fed processes based on a form fill seal principle are preferred. Speeds of between sixty and ninety sachets per track can usually be achieved.

Sachets also have the advantage that they can be used for liquid and semi-liquid packaging. Flow wraps are a further extension of a sachet-type pack. Both have been widely used as a protective overwrap to extend the shelf life of blisters.

Recent developments in blister and strip packaging

Although this question could be answered in terms of material, machinery and their performance, where each may be influenced by the properties of the product, costs, change-over time, output, etc., there are broader issues today, i.e. what standards should be used for child-resistance, how does one improve moisture protection, etc.

Although cold formed materials started with 40 μm foil and utilised a relatively shallow well-radiused draw, perforation problems with the foil have arisen. As a result, 45–50 μm foil has been substituted with gauges available up to 60 μm.

Most machines, which are now based on pressure forming with plug assistance, can be adapted to cold forming. There has been a tendency for a machine to occupy less length by operating over two levels or by doubling back on itself. Although maximum speeds of over 6,000 items per minute are still relatively rare for conventional blisters, higher speeds are predicted.

Aclar copolymer based materials using 22A, 33C, 88A have more recently been challenged by the homopolymer R_x series with lower costs coupled to good moisture barrier properties. However, there are many alternative overwrapping systems which may be used to improve moisture barrier. In this context the Japanese have recently introduced silicon oxide coated PET overwraps. Use for thermoforming, a multilayer material, a coated material, or the lowest cost material with some form of overwrap remains an emotive issue as to which is most environmentally friendly. Multilayer materials are likely to be the most difficult to recycle, but recovery of energy may be possible by effective incineration. One newer material for cold forming uses two thinner layers of soft foil separated by a polymer layer, while another has involved a double forming process (AFT).

Machinery and machine improvements

Machine improvements include use of larger reels (frequently now without joins), various forms of preheat with variable temperature ranges either side of web, preference for pressure forming with plug assistance, improved cooling of moulds, possible preheat for foil sealing section, automatic splice facility, Geneva driven notched drum for accurate forward progress and accurate registration, on-line printing, e.g. flexo, accurate perforation or cutting, minimising of curl, improved GMP, faster changeovers, integrated cartoning, microprocessor–computer controls and fault diagnosis, etc. Removal of the blisters from the web with the minimum of wastage is now the rule rather than the exception. Machines have also become more compact, with a trend towards more versatile units. Modular machines and Servo technology driven systems are also being offered.

Deblistering units (on and off the machine) are more readily available.

Tamper-evidence, tamper-resistance and child-resistance

Emphasis on the above continues to grow, with the result that some companies do not know the current state of the art. Companies therefore continue to present attractive looking products to children in clear materials and design blisters where the products interact when the blister is bent into an arc, with the risk of the items literally 'popping out'. Fuller information on the subject can be found in Chapter 11. It is of interest to note that since the introduction of child-resistant packaging, commencing in the mid-1970s in the UK, there has been a significant reduction in the reported cases of child poisoning instances. This has involved those reclosable CRCs which have passed a test using children and non-reclosable packs which have not passed any test but have shown a significant growth in use over that same period. Although this implies that either many blisters, strips, sachets, etc. are inherently child-safe or children are less interested in a pack where the product is not visible or shows less rattle (compared with tablets in a container), there is still a need to improve the more 'flimsy' forms of pack. In addition, many child-resistant packs still present opening problems to the ever-increasing elderly population who rely on regular medication in order to survive. This can result in either inadequate replacement of the closure or the transfer to open containers, thereby exposing both the product and children at risk. The industry has still to address these concerns fully.

Costs

A summary of typical comparative costings based on glass, metal, strips and blisters is given in Table 13.1. Earlier published tables also gave comparisons in terms of volume and weight, related to both incoming materials and finished packs. It should be noted that costings can significantly vary according to individual circumstances.

It must be stressed that Table 13.1 gives examples based on specific circumstances where many of the factors can change between different companies, hence each organisation must do its own costing exercise for its own particular operation.

Table 13.1 Comparative costings (costs cover materials, labour, carton, outer pack, etc.)

Item	Pack	Cost ratio
Bottle glass	10s	1.15
Bottle glass	100s	1.9
Bottle plastic	10s	1.00*
Bottle plastic	100s	1.75
PVC push-through blister	10s	0.40
PVC push-through blister	100s	1.95
PVC blister, peelable, perforated	10s	0.55
PVC blister, peelable, perforated	100s	2.15
Can metal, aluminium	10s	1.70
Can metal, aluminium	100s	2.60
Strip (paper/foil/polyethylene)	10s	0.70
Strip (paper/foil/polyethylene)	100s	3.65

*Plastic pack taken as unity for ten items. Actual costs will vary according to the machine, output, labour, etc.

Semi-automatic blister packaging equipment

Other than being used to pack solid dose medication, blisters or bubble packs, as they are often known, may find further applications in pharmaceutical packaging. These may be as a protective overwrap against physical damage, to prevent ingress or egress, to aid display or to act as a tamper-evident/tamper-resistant feature (i.e. packs which are not involved with the solid dosage form).

Although the same principles apply to semi-automatic machines, sheets may be used instead of reels. The types of material and the process employed tend to be based on their economic and strength characteristics. Where a tray or container is not required for a direct form fill seal operation, the thermoformed item can be fabricated either in a female mould or over a male mould. The various combinations of vacuum, pressure and mechanical (plug assist) are indicated in drawings. With vacuum forming, and where a female die is used, the process is called straight vacuum forming. If a male die is used, the process is termed drape forming. In air pressure forming, greater pressures may be employed.

The majority of the individual type of blisters are made by vacuum forming either into or over (drape type) moulds, which are frequently made from metals such as aluminium. The choice between female and male moulds depends on a number of factors, as follows.

Female

Base (flange) is thickest, and uniform; top of mould is thinner. Formings can usually be put closer together therefore more mouldings per sheet. No webbing between moulds. Limitations in depth of draw. Good radiused corners required – not suitable for sharp corners. See Figure 13.11.

Male

Base (flange) is thin and non-uniform; top of mould is thickest. Capable of greater depth of draw for a given caliper. May tend to web if layout is not properly designed. Needs greater space between mouldings (rule of thumb 1.5 × draw height) therefore fewer mouldings per sheet. Capable of achieving relatively sharp corners. See Figure 13.11.

Plug assistance can be used, particularly where webbing is likely to occur, but this generally slows output. Air holes for venting vary between 0.50 mm and 1 mm for most small mouldings.

Mouldings can be 'ribbed' to improve strength or to enable a thinner material to be used, e.g. 300 µm reduced to 200 µm by ribbing. Improved wall distribution can also be achieved by extending the softened plastic sheet by vacuum or pressure prior to final forming (often known as balloon or bubble extension).

Materials

When clarity is required PVC, PS, PET, or cellulose acetate may be used. The last of these tends to cost more even though the moulding cycle is approximately 25% faster; this does not compensate for the higher material cost (+30%). Impact modified styrene or styrene is more widely used for coffret-type inserts which are invariably coloured or flock coated. Styrene offers a higher yield than PVC (note densities) and a faster forming time. PET is often the preferred material for surgical or medical device systems.

Male forming

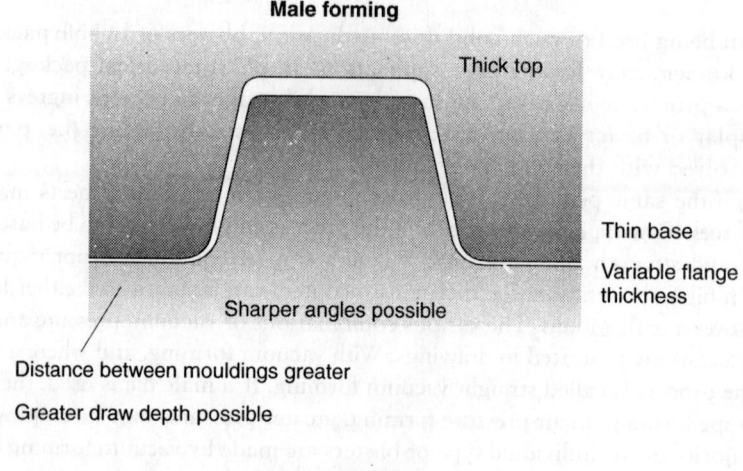

Female forming

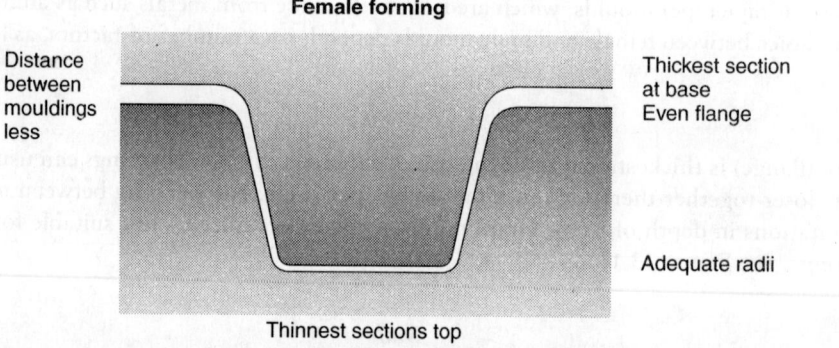

Figure 13.11 Male and female vacuum forming

Some relatively simple blister packaging equipment is produced on a rotary table principle whereby a blister can be formed, hand filled, lidded and the completed blister pack removed after four 90° movements. Others work on a reciprocating bed principle of forming and lidding. These are often used for optic lenses and opthalmic-type solutions for lens cleaning.

Some typical blister packs are shown in Figure 13.12. Various assembly and sealing methods can be used, e.g.:

- heat seal through lid (board, laminate or label)
- heat seal through plastic
- heat seal through plastic and lid
- blister locked between cards by adhesive or staples
- folded card – plus heat seal, adhesive or staples
- blister locked to card by label.

Blister packs offer good display advantage where clarity is essential. Punched hole systems provide for hanging cards.

Blister trays are particularly useful where several items are involved in the medication, i.e. lyophilised product plus water for injection.

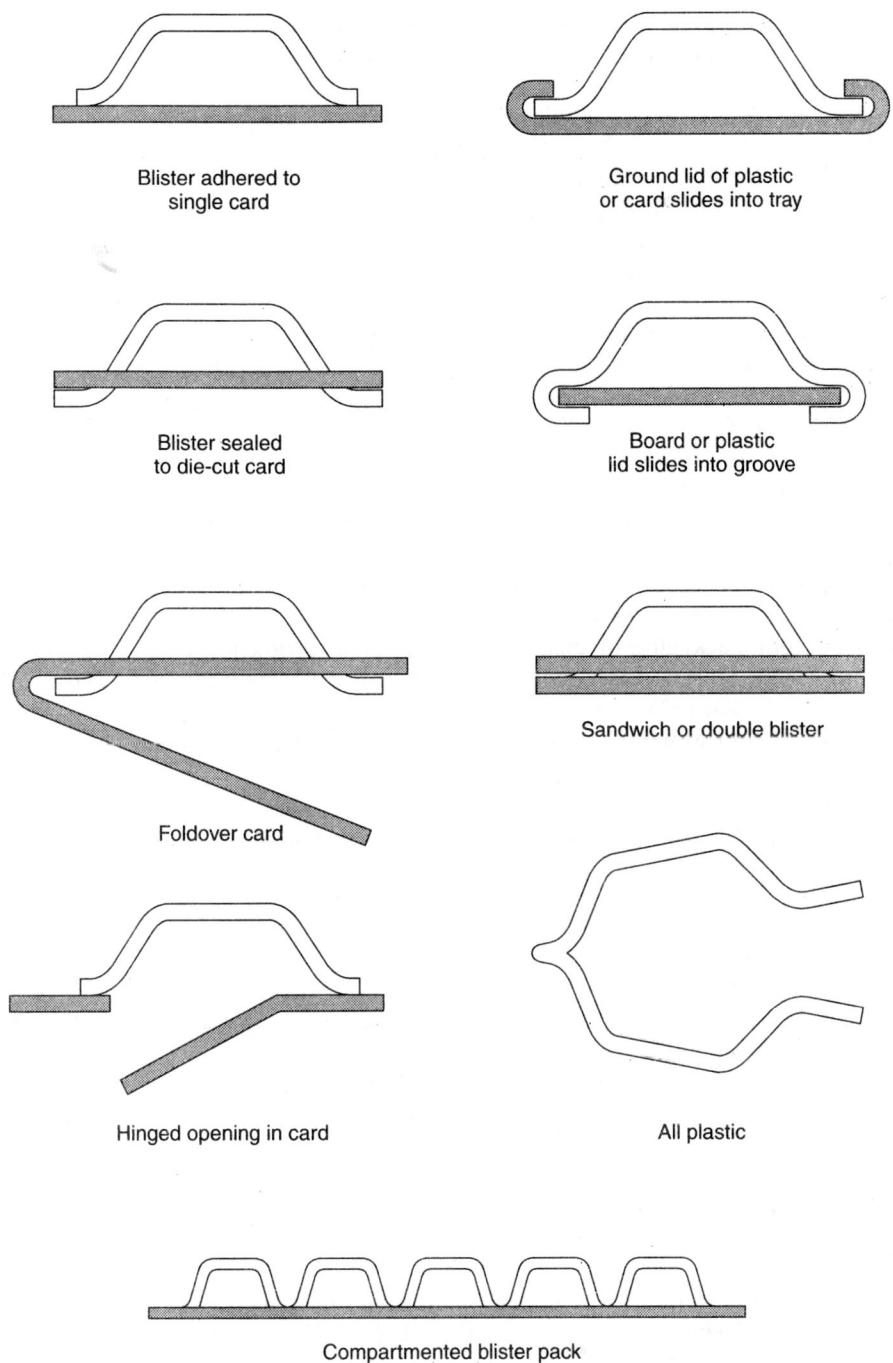

Blister adhered to
single card

Ground lid of plastic
or card slides into tray

Blister sealed
to die-cut card

Board or plastic
lid slides into groove

Foldover card

Sandwich or double blister

Hinged opening in card

All plastic

Compartmented blister pack

Figure 13.12 Thermoformed card pack constructions

References

Current blisters, strips and sachets technologies have a strong historical foundation through the developments reported over the past 30 years, as can be seen from the following references.

1 Dean, D. A., A review of blister and strip packaging of tablets and capsules, *Interphex 1974*.
2 Dean, D. A., Unit packaging of tablets and capsules, *Pharm. J.*, 9 September 1972.
3 Dean, D. A., The blister packaging of pharmaceuticals, *Pharma Int.*, 1972, 1, 5.
4 Dean, D. A., A review of development in the blister packaging of pharmaceuticals, *Pira Conference*, 27–29 March 1972.
5 Dean, D. A., Unit packaging pharmaceutical preparations, Institute of Packaging Conference, 27 September 1973, *Unit Packaging in Industry, Solid and Liquid Dosage Forms*.
6 Dean, D. A., Child resistance through unit packaging, *Institute of Packaging Symposium*, 9 January 1975.
7 BAFRA, *Barrier Properties of Aluminium Foil*, 1974.
8 DRG (UK), *Unit Dose Packaging of Pharmaceutical Tablets and Capsules*, 1974.
9 Medicines Commission, *Report on the Presentations of Medicines in Relation to Child Safety*, DHSS, August 1974.
10 Dean, D. A. *et al.*, Child resistant packaging, *Interphex*, 30 March 1976.
11 Mader, G., Blister packs and child safety, *Manuf. Chem. Aerosol*, April 1976.
12 Childproof packaging of medicines (from 'Child protection packs' compiled by Ciba Geigy, Hoffman la Roche, and Sandoz) *Die Pharmazeutische Industrie*, 37, No. 4, 279–283, 1975.
13 Kraus, W. and Maier, K., Coated foils and films for push through blister packs, *Drugs Made in Germany*, 18, 3 September 1975.
14 Gadecke, R., Campeao, D. and Muhlbacher, B., Studies of the protective value of press through packs of medicinal preparations in the preventions of poisoning in children, *Pharm. Ind.*, 37, No. 8, 632–635.
15 De Felice, W., Measures for the improvement of press through packs with reference to their child resistance, *Pharm. Ind.*, 37, No. 8, 635–640.
16 The ability of children to obtain tablets from different containers, *Med. J. Aust.*, 18 October 1969.
17 Dean, D.A., *A Review of the Current UK Situation and Basic Thoughts on Child Resistant Packaging in UK*, CPA Course, London, December 1974.
18 Dean, D.A., *UK Concepts in Child Resistant Packaging – New UK Trends, Samples, Economic Considerations to Convert to Child Resistant Packaging from Conventional Packaging*, CPA Course, London, December 1974.
19 Dean, D. A. Use of aluminium foil in pharmaceutical packaging, *Manuf. Chem. Aerosol News*, February 1978.
20 Thomas, R., Sr, *Flexible Film and Push Through Blisters*, CPA, 2 June 1981, Bristol Myers Co.
21 Mann, S., *An Improved Alternative PVC for Pill Packaging*, D and CI, March 1982.
22 *Tscheulin Information Materials Meeting*, DIN 55559, September 1983.
23 Dubouchet and Paisley, Blister materials options for packaging, *Packaging*, November 1984, 60–62.
24 The (multi) unit dose packaging of pharmaceuticals, *IOP Conference*, 8 October 1986.

25 Dean, D. A. *et al.*, Unit dose, *Manuf. Chem. Aerosol News*, January 1980.
26 Guise, W., Blister packaging today, *Manuf. Chem. Aerosol News*, November 1984.
27 Baumann, N., The adventures of PVC/PVDC, *Packaging Technol.*, June/July 1985.

Awareness of the advances in technology are often correlated through national and international conferences and the subsequential technical papers.

In 1998-9 a series of Blister-pack 2 day conferences were run in Cologne, Germany and Newark, USA to review and update blister packaging. Presentations were made by people well recognised within the industry and a list of papers, purchasable fron The Packaging Group Inc (US), 70 Valley Forge Drive, East Brunswick, New Jersey 08816, USA. is given below:-

September 23rd - 24th 1998

1. A global view of Blister Packaging for Pharmaceuticals
   Stephanie Batz
   Kalle Pentaplast Gmbh, Germany
2. Why use Blisters?
   Dieter Janek ®
   Managing Director, Horn and Noack, Division of Romaco Gmbh, Germany
3. Alfoil Polymer High Barrier Films (PVDC)
   Monique Roulin, Manager Technical Sales
   Aerni Leuch AG(AEL) Switzerland
4. ACI-AR High Barrier Films
   Mike Phillips
   Allied Signal Speciality Films (UK)
5. Cold Formed Aluminium Foil and lidding concepts.
   DR Erwin Pasbrig ®
   Development Technical Application – Pharma
   Lawson Marden Singen Gmbh, Germany
6. Replacing PVC – the alternatives
   Dieter Laube
   PCI Allpack Gmbh Germany
7. Evaluation and Shelf life testing with reference to the ICH Guidelines
   Mervyn Frederick, Head of Packaging Development,
   NV Organon, Akso Nobel (Holland)
8. Heat Sealing – rotary v platen ®
   Dieter Janek, Magaging Director
   Horn and Noack, Division of Romaco
   Gmbh, Germany
9. Non destructive leak testing of blisters.
   Paul Sharpe Business Manager
   AI Qualitek (UK)
10. Preventing recalls – on line inspection and printing
    John Mackenzie, Sales Manager
    Romaco (UK) Ltd
11. Machinery – future trends in blister packaging
    Marielli Criscuolo, Marketing Research Manager
    IMA, Pharmaceurical Division. Italy
12. Machinery – flexibility of blister lines,
    Markus Mazger, Product Manager, Pharmaceuticals
    Robert Bosch, Gmbh Germany
13. Machinery – Thermoforming Machine and Lines -Latest
    Technology. Advanced Forming Technology (AFT)
    Dirk Briskorn, Managing Director

Klockner Hansell, Gmbh, Germany
14. Machinery – ʃlister packs for Clinical Trial supplies –
Special equipment.
Matthew Vogelsanger, Managing Director,
Fleximation AG – Switzerland
15. Blister Packaging and Child Resistance – is there a future? Colin Scaife
CE Packaging Partnership
16. Strip – a substitute for blisters.
Paper by Siebler Verpackungstechnic
Presented by Dixie Dean (Consultant)
17. The role of the Contract Packer
Mr. G Russell, Sales & Marketing
PCI (Unipack) UK
18. Mobile Blister Machines, and deblistering – The neglected aspects!
A Ernest Parker, Managing Director
Sepa Products (Ireland) Ltd
19. Liquids and semi liquids in blisters ®
Werner Basler, Systems Manager
Unifil (International) Ltd
Krcuzlingen – Switzerland
20. The contract Packaging of Clinical Trial Supplies
Mike O'Donnell
Consultant acting on behalf of PCI – Unipack UK
21. Improving Barrier Properties by coating, coextrusion, lamination, metallisation and overwrapping
Dixie Dean (Consultant)
22. Future trends in Pharmaceutical Blister Packaging – an industry's point of view Mervyn Frederick –
Head of Pharmaceutical Development
NV. Organon, Akso Nobel (Holland)

A similar conference was run in the USA April 20th – 21st 1999. The speakers from the above event ® also presented the same papers. Different papers were produced by the following:
1) Evaluation and shelf-life testing – the influence of the ICH Guidelines
D A Dean (Consultant)
2) What's the Future for the Pharmaceutical
Blister Packager?
Dixie A Dean (Consultant)
3) Child Resitant Blister Packaging. US Regulations and Test Methods
Dr Suzanne Barone
Prof. Manager for Poison Prevention – US
Consumer Products Safety Commision
4) Aclar High Barrier Laminations – update and New Structure
Perry Fan General Manager
Rigid Films, Tech-Plex-Inc
5) Archieving longer term stability with PVC/PVDC
David Faghani, Marketing Sales Manager
Perlen Converting AG, US Region
6) Blisters and Clinical Trials: Recent developments
Mike O'Donnell – Consultant
7) Integrated Inspection on Packaging Lines
Geert Coudizer
CEO, Covan Vision Systems (Belgium)
8) Blisters and Contract Packaging – A Happy Marriage
Renard P Jackson, Exc V P Sales and Marketing
PCI USA
9) Blister Packaging – New Innovation in Child Resistance
Thomas Toren
Consulting Engineer, Australia

14

THE PACKAGING LINE

I. H. Hall

Introduction

In this chapter there is a discussion of the practical requirements of operating pharmaceutical packaging lines. This includes *all* the requirements of the packaging line including, where necessary, the staff required.

The objectives of any pharmaceutical packaging line can be simply described as filling, closing, identifying and protecting the product safely to a predetermined specification and at an economic cost. Unfortunately the design and operation is more complicated in reality.

Other requirements are:

- high consistent output
- zero downtime due to stoppages
- no rejects or wastage
- consistent quality
- low services, labour and maintenance costs
- high integrity, i.e. no risk of mix-ups
- high level of hygiene
- minimum depreciation
- minimum wear and tear
- regular and effective maintenance
- effective operator and maintenance staff training
- provision of safety for staff.

The typical pharmaceutical packaging line needs only:

1 materials – product and packaging materials supplied to agreed specifications
2 services – electricity, compressed air, etc. to agreed standards
3 personnel – effectively trained operators, engineering, QC and other support staff.

The activities of a typical packaging line may be broken down into the following broad steps, which form the backbone of this chapter:

- bringing the materials (both product and packaging) onto the line
- packaging line services required to make the line operate

- filling the product into the prime container
- closing the package, i.e. prime container
- labelling or identifying the prime container
- leaflet addition
- cartoning/display outers application, i.e. secondary packaging
- collation, casing and palletisation for warehousing and distribution
- on-line testing
- provision of motivated and trained production and support staff.

The filling and packaging operations may take place on one piece of machinery or be split across several machines, namely form fill and seal – e.g. blister packs where the product is filled, closed and identified on one machine – whereas a bottle of liquid medicine would need unscrambling, cleaning, filling, closing and labelling as separate linked operations to reach the same state of completion.

One of the most important considerations is that of the speed of the packaging line, which can be expressed as:

- design speed – the speed of the line running under no load and optimum conditions
- capacity – the upper sustainable limit of acceptable product passing a point on the line prior to warehousing
- running speed – the instantaneous operating rate
- output – the exact quantity of acceptable quality product which passes from the line, under load conditions, to the warehouse in a standard time.

There appears to be no pharmaceutical industry standard for measuring the efficiency of a packaging line. Line efficiency has been defined as the ratio of output to input, but a better measure is the ratio of the actual operating time (the actual time producing acceptable product) divided by the available time (when there is work available for the line) expressed as a percentage.

Looking at a typical complex packaging line, the most critical operation usually operates at around the required output speed. In most cases this is the filling operation. The other machines upstream and downstream should be designed so as to operate faster than the critical machine so that there is as little queueing of unfinished packaging as practical, for example as shown in Table 14.1.

There also may be a requirement to have accumulator tables upstream and downstream of the critical machine(s), each holding about one minute's worth of product. It should be noted here that the faster a packaging line goes, the greater is the need for higher quality packaging materials with lower, i.e. tighter, tolerances.

Bringing the materials to the packaging line

It is necessary to bring together the product and packaging materials at the head of the packaging line in order to pack them. It is sensible to discuss the various storage and cleanliness conditions first, so that the optimum conditions can be designed.

The major requirements of the proposed pack should be identified, e.g. is the line going to fill and close and pack the product in one or more operations?

Is the product particularly susceptible, e.g. sterile, moisture sensitive, oxygen sensi-

Table 14.1 Packaging line operations

Running speed (cpm)	Machine function	
113	Unload packaging materials ⎫	
110	Unscramble containers ⎬	upstream
105	Clean containers ⎭	
100	Filling the product into the prime container	
105	Closing the prime container ⎫	
108	Labelling the prime container ⎪	
110	Cartoning/leaflet addition (usually the same machine) ⎬	downstream
115	Collation of a standard quantity of prime containers ⎪	
117	Casing of a standard number of collations ⎪	
120	Palletisation to a preset stack pattern of cases ⎭	

cpm = containers per minute.

tive? Are special environments required and what level of cleanliness is required for the particular product, e.g. is the product dusty, or is the unscrambling of packaging materials a ready source of particulate contaminations?

There may only be need to fill, close and identify the primary container, e.g. many sterile filling operations store the filled prime containers for later packaging. This creates many problems, e.g. identification, storage of part finished packs (costs and specialist work in progress (WIP) stores etc). Having said this, the following general comments apply whether the pack is completed in one or more stages.

All the materials for a particular filling and packaging order should be brought together in a secure collation area, away from the filling and packaging line and fully checked against an authorised specification for identity and quantity, by a competent appointed person. It is essential that the co-operation of the planning, purchasing and stores departments is obtained in order to complete this detailed operation ahead of the scheduled packaging time.

The product should be closed as soon as practical after filling. The only major exception is freeze drying, where the container is filled with liquid, partially closed, freeze dried, then the closure operation is completed.

Sterile conditions produce their own problems where the primary packaging materials and closures are to be pre-sterilised and fed into a sterile area for aseptic filling and closing, or with filling and closing of the pack for terminal sterilisation e.g. sterile dressings with beta or gamma irradiation. In the first of these cases the secondary packaging would probably be done at a different time and in a different packaging area, whereas in the second case the pack could be completed to secondary packaging and only require separate tertiary packaging.

Note that *all* sterilisation procedures on packaging materials, e.g. heat, irradiation, do have an effect on the physical and sometimes chemical properties, e.g. plastics tend to go more brittle upon beta or gamma radiation. The sterilising of packaging materials is a specialised subject dealt with in Chapter 12.

The conditioning of containers or reel materials needs special attention, e.g. low temperature of storage containers brought into a warm moist atmosphere will induce condensation, thereby making the product damp and negating the adhesion of labels, due to the water film on the container. Storage of reels of material that are either stood on edge forming flats or in too moist or dry conditions giving 'dumb-bell' shaped reels should also be noted. Those packaging materials that are to be in direct contact with the product, e.g. containers, reels, wadding materials and closures, should be supplied in packaging that prevents contamination, is easy to clean, is easy to unload onto the packaging line, sheds as little contamination as possible, and is easy to store and recycle.

Open containers, e.g. securitainers or bottles, should always be inverted, blown with clean dry, oil-free compressed air injected by a dip tube from the base and vacuum sucked to remove as many particles as possible.

Unscrambling techniques have generally to be used for containers, closures, wads, etc., as they are of fixed shape and need to be manoeuvred into a queue and/or oriented for presentation to the filling/closing process. The ever-present problem is one of vibration and movement which attracts/sheds particles into the vibratory bowl or other moving parts of the unscrambler. No container should be allowed to be filled without going through some form of inspection for dirt or positive cleaning immediately prior to filling.

Reel-fed components are different in that they are usually fed through pre-set guides onto the machine main bed and the contact surface is usually on the 'inside' of the reel, thereby attracting less contamination.

Packaging line services

The packaging line cannot operate in isolation. It needs essential services, e.g. clean, dry, oil-free air, electricity, gases (nitrogen, oxygen), cooling water, vacuum, removal of waste material(s), removal of finished packs.

The services have been divided into three convenient headings, and should be considered before building the line:

1   atmosphere, sterility, level of cleanliness, environment, removal/disposal of waste
2   line layouts, operators, loading points
3   specifications, maintenance, planning, inventory control, testing off-line and QA/QC support.

The first consideration about general services is what atmosphere is to surround the line, is it to be clean or sterile, or are there requirements to isolate one section of the line, e.g. cartoning kept apart from filling as the cartons will shed fibres. This sort of requirement defines the level of cleanliness required in the packaging area. There should be, even in all non-sterile packaging areas, a good and efficient air-conditioning system with the ability to vacuum extract waste or contaminated air from the points of most contamination, e.g. container cleaning, unscrambling, cartons.

The solutions to the cleanliness problem may include the following.

1   Isolate the filling and closing operation in a GMP classified area (e.g. European class A or B; FDA class 100). In this case remember that *all* materials going into an aseptic area must be sterile. The output of the sterile area i.e. the closed sealed container, *must* be identified in some secure manner if it is going to be taken off the line and not labelled immediately.

2   For non-sterile situations build a floor to ceiling partition between the filling/closing equipment and the secondary packaging operations, and restrict the movement of fibre shedding materials.

3   Strip off all the fibre shedding incoming packaging materials in the collation area and send the materials to the line in internally recycled (plastic) containers and an aluminium pallet.

4   Keep the fibre shedding materials away from the immediate vicinity of the product contact materials.

5   Provide special closed container(s) for solid waste, e.g. cases, and cleaning cloths, plastic coverings, etc.

6   Special instructions for the recovery/reworking of reject packs produced on the line to minimise contamination.

The items in this section are contained in the later sections on 'On-line testing' and 'Operators and training'.

This section deals mainly with the external departments that have an influence on the line services and their operation, e.g. specifications, maintenance, planning, inventory control, testing off-line and QA/QC support. (Specifications of the packaging materials, product and final pack are essential, and are fully described in Chapter 4.)

Planning and inventory control have the task of ensuring that for any given order:

1   the services in the production building will all be available for the time needed for the order completion, e.g. heating, ventilation, air conditioning (HVAC), power

2   the requisite passed materials are available for the job

3   the requisite labour is available, including scheduling of line changeover; engineering, QC, etc. presence is available

4   there is internal transport, warehouse space, etc. available for the finished goods.

General principles of product filling

The following points are the major ones needing consideration when designing a packaging line.

1   How to unload the delivery of materials from the collation area, e.g. is there easy access to loading points on the line? All loading points, safety off switches, controls and warning panels should be on the operator side of the line. Operators should not be expected to crawl under, jump over or run around the line for routine topping-up of materials.

2   The physical state of the product will lead towards the design of the filling technique:

- gas – liquefied or pressurised
- liquid – sterile, viscosity, volatility, frothing
- semi-liquid – viscosity, separation, phasing into layers
- solid – powder, granule, tablet, capsule, regular or irregular shapes, free flowing or sticky or fragile.

3　The mechanism of filling may be achieved in one of several ways:

- volume – cups, pockets, auger filling, pump piston
- weight – one shot, dump and trickle
- level – vacuum, pressure, gravity
- arrangement – blister or column
- count – recessed cylinders, slats, regular objects queued then breaking a photocell beam.

The cleanliness of the chosen filling technique should be considered for potential contaminations, e.g. drips, product seepage, powder agglomeration. There therefore needs to be control of the following filling problems:

1　aeration of liquids, semi-liquids and powders, usually caused by excessive high-speed stirring
2　compaction, dusting, powder explosion risk
3　separation of liquids, semi-liquids and powders into phases
4　dusting and break-up of tablets and capsules due to being vibrated for too long in hoppers etc.

Common filling methods used for the various phases of product

Gas

This is usually used in the liquefied gas form as propellants for aerosols. Filling liquefied gas is usually by volume using a specialist high-pressure pump on a time or flow basis, usually filled backwards through the aerosol valve. Alternatively the aerosol container may be open in a highly refrigerated area, where the liquefied gas is dosed by a piston pump then the container is quickly closed.

Using gas as a flushing medium usually only requires a small volume of low-pressure gas, e.g. nitrogen or CO_2 to clear air out of the container, by means of a timed valve opening operation.

Liquid

With liquid filling the sterility, viscosity, volatility, and frothing characteristics of the product will eliminate some of the potential filling methods. Liquids may be filled by the following methods.

1　By volume, using a volumatic cup, a timed distribution from a pump, or by a piston in a sleeve dosing the correct amount. It is usual to use dip tubes which retract with the level of the fill to control the drips and reduce turbulence and frothing.
2　By level, where the liquid is pushed into the container and the excess liquid removed by vacuum, or pressure which forces excess liquid out through an overflow pipe or with gravity supplying the force required.

Semi-liquid

With semi-liquids the following physical criteria must be considered: viscosity, separation, phasing into layers. Sometimes too much stirring, or any stirring at all (in the case of creams), during filling can have adverse effects on the product.

Semi-liquids are usually dosed by volume using either an adjustable rotary pump or a piston and sleeve valve filler. Again the dip tubes which retract with the level of the fill help in controlling the amount of spillage.

Solid

Solids come in many forms, and the product form and speed of operation will determine the method of measurement.

There are probably more ways of controlling the various solids than any other pharmaceutical form.

1 By volume of powder using cups, pockets, and particularly by auger filling.
2 By weight of any solid form but most commonly using an auger fill either with one shot, or dumping the greater part of the product and trickle feeding the remainder. This latter is very accurate but usually needs an expensive feedback weighing system.
3 By level using either gravity or auger fill to a predetermined level in a transparent container.
4 By arrangement, e.g. in blisters, or columnar in the case of roll wrapped tablets etc.
5 By electronic count of regular shaped objects, e.g. tablets and capsules, using recessed cylinders, or slats, or regular objects queued on a rotating table then breaking a photoelectric cell beam to give a count.

Line fill checks include check-weighing, level of fill by light or X-ray or alpha radiation, pattern by artificial vision or feeler systems.

The two major forms of filling, i.e. with pre-made containers and with those that are form fill and sealed, will now be considered in more detail.

Container-based filling

The containers must first be unscrambled by various means depending on the shape, size and material of the container. Major risks are induced dirt from friction and static electricity from dry conditions and movement of plastics. Most containers used for sterile filling (ampoules, vials, bottles and collapsible tubes) are fed directly so that the operation of unscrambling should not be necessary. There are also certain types of pre-cleaned bottles which are supplied in clean layers, where the outer plastic protection may be removed and the above unscrambling operation may be excluded.

The non-sterile containers *must* in most cases be cleaned in line, e.g. invert; blow with clean, dry, oil-free, compressed air. The resulting dislodged particles are then sucked away from the container while withdrawing the air probe, but beware of induced static.

The objective is to have all the containers presented and fed to the orientation devices correctly, so the containers will next require queueing and orientation. Here the design and tolerances of the container are critical for high-speed filling.

Figure 14.1 shows containers that will queue well and therefore fill at high speed. Figure 14.2 shows containers that will have problems in orientation and presentation to the filling heads.

The containers may be presented to the filling apparatus in one of three ways:

1   gated – a preset number of containers are allowed through a feeding gate on a moving conveyor and stop by hitting a preset output gate positioned so that the container(s) are directly under the filling heads
2   scrolled, i.e. fed on a moving conveyer belt through a tapered screw so that the containers emerge evenly spaced on the conveyor infeed to the filler
3   placed, i.e. fed or placed into a 'puck' or bucket (usually used if the container is unstable, e.g. collapsible tubes).

The filling then takes place, usually by the methods mentioned above, prior to the container being closed.

Form fill and seal packaging systems

The types of pack that are sealed straight away on the filling line include blister packs, strip packs, pillow packs, ampoule filling and Rommelag/ALP form fill and seal systems.

Blister packs

Two basic types exist, i.e. hot formed and cold formed. The filling and closing operations are covered in detail in Chapter 13. Most blister packs will need to be collated and cartoned, with a leaflet, as they are not robust enough to survive the rigours of transport and distribution unprotected.

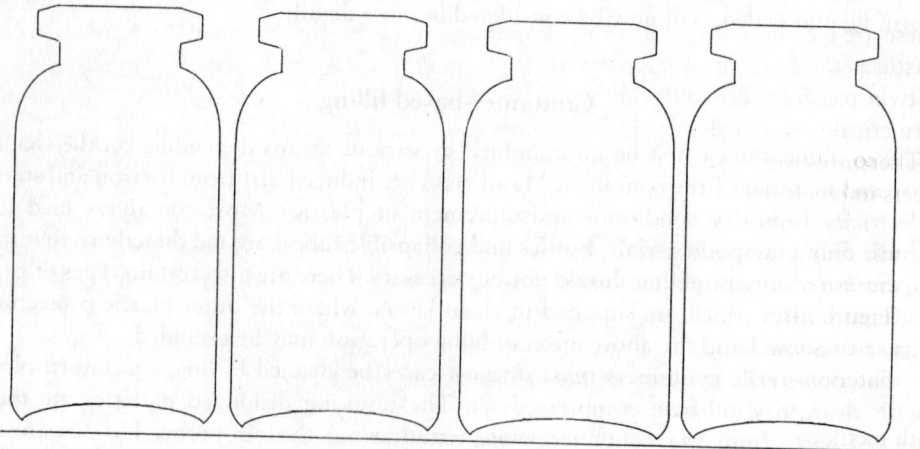

Figure 14.1 Good containers

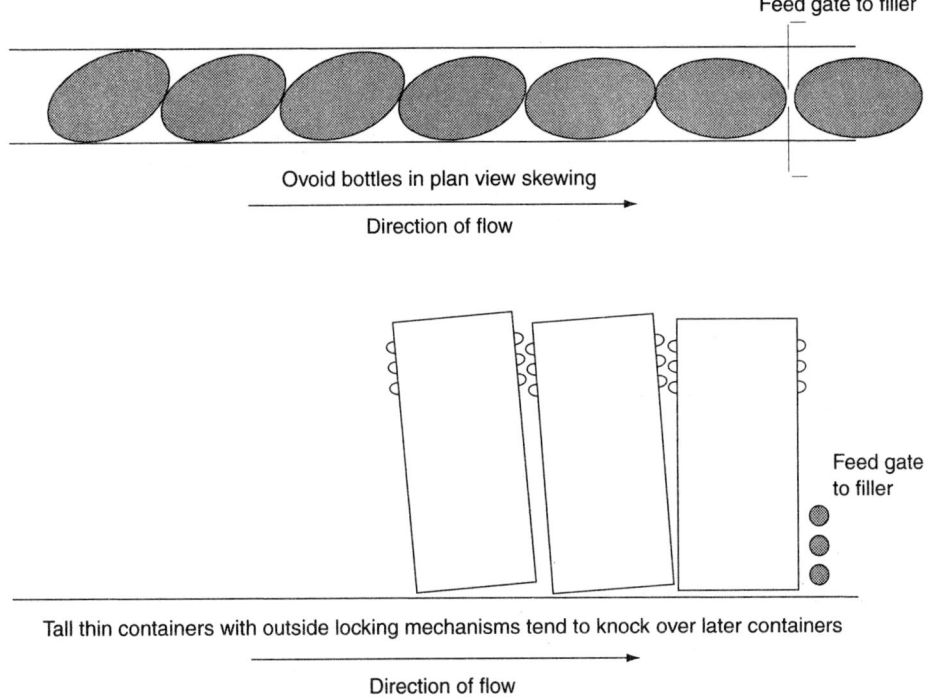

Figure 14.2 Problem containers

Strip packs

Usually two laminates of paper, soft temper aluminium foil and various plastics. Again the filling and sealing details are considered with the materials descriptions.

Sachets

These are usually a laminate with aluminium foil as the centre core and a heat sealable plastic as the product contact material. They can be made from either a single feed reel or twin reel feed. Firstly the carrying pouch is formed, then dosed with product, then hermetically heat sealed so that contamination is reduced to a minimum.

There are two basic ways of using the form fill seal process with laminates, films or sheets in reel form:

1   use only one stock reel of double the width but 'centrefold' it, the fold forming the base of the pouch (usually used in horizontal form fill seal operations) (Figure 14.3)
2   use two stock reels to form the two sides of the pouch; could have two different materials as the front and back of the sachet (Figure 14.4).

Both methods have been used for powders, granules, suppositories, liquids, pastes, and creams usually in the horizontal reel feeding mode. The control of the position of the print on the sachets is by the 'eye' mark and electronic registering method.

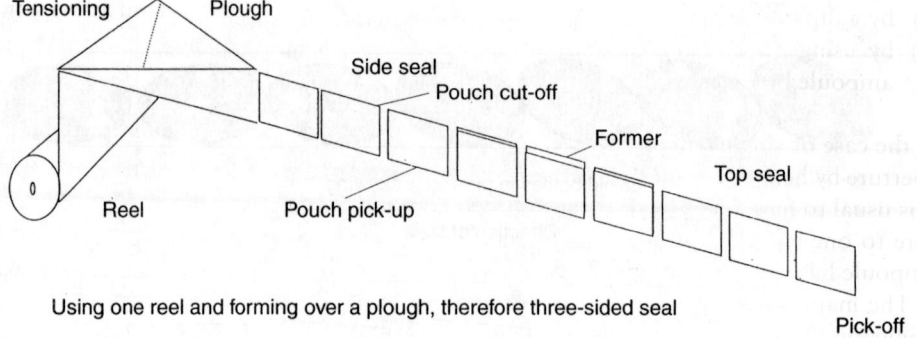

Using one reel and forming over a plough, therefore three-sided seal

Figure 14.3 Single web pouch operation

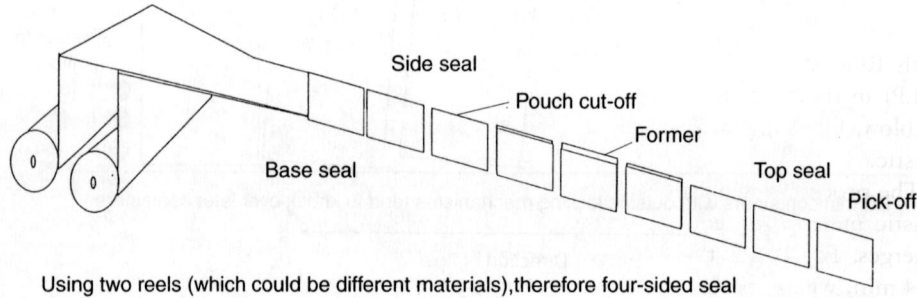

Using two reels (which could be different materials),therefore four-sided seal

Figure 14.4 Double web pouch operation

Pillow packs

These today are usually used for added protection as a secondary pack. In many respects they are similar to single reel sachet packs, but the product forms the outline of the pillow pack which is usually heat fin sealed up one edge and heat lap sealed/guillotined on each end.

Ampoules

These are in many shapes and sizes in glass, but have the common feature that they are always closed as soon as possible, by the use of gas/oxygen flames, after filling. Plastic ampoules are discussed under Rommelag/ALP systems below.

Glass (of whatever type) ampoules may be designed in different ways:

1 single ended
2 double ended
3 supplied with the end(s) open
4 supplied with the end(s) closed.

There are two ways to fill ampoules:

(a) by a dip needle dispensing the correct amount of fluid
(b) by using a tray and vacuum system, whereby the liquid is drawn into the open ampoule by vacuum.

In the case of single ended with end open and (a) above, there is just the closing of the aperture by heat to consider; in the case of double ended with ends open and (b) above, it is usual to have one end of the two-ended ampoule already closed, giving a heat closure to one end only; in the case of single ended with end closed and (a) above, the ampoule has to be first opened and then closed by heat.

The major problem with all glass ampoules is that when glass is cut there is a phenomenon of glass particle shedding. It is also difficult to fill any heat sensitive product when the temperatures might be >1000 °C locally in the neck area.

Rommelag/ALP systems

Both Rommelag AG (Germany and Switzerland) and Automatic Liquid Packaging (ALP) in the USA produce very specialised equipment, under the name 'bottlepack' or blow, fill seal. Each produces filled sterile products starting with dry granules of plastic.

The process which enables a sterile product to be produced operates as follows. The plastic material is fed into an extruder from which a round or oval tube (parison) emerges. For LDPE this typically involves heating to around 165–175 °C for about 3–4 min, where the bioburden is destroyed. The tube or a series of extruded tubes is fed into open single or multicavity cooled moulds which then close around the tube(s), sealing the base but leaving the top open and an extension which retains sufficient heat for welding. At this stage the 'bottles' are extended to the full mould size by either sterile compressed air (large containers) or vacuum (small containers), then filled with sterile, usually aqueous, liquid (achieved by double terminal filtration).

The top of the mould is then sealed using the residual heat in the above mentioned extension and is taken away from the machine to a final punch trim operation, to remove any waste. In the filling and closing stages the base of the mould remains cool, thereby adding little heat to the product. The forming and filling area is usually shrouded in a laminar flow cabinet. Prior to start-up the machines have all contact parts sterilised (automatically) by pressurised steam with a sterile wash through, i.e. SIP. The machine has to be regularly validated by microbial challenge.

Some regulatory authorities request that certain types of product, e.g. IV solutions, be subsequently subjected to terminal sterilisation. However, there is still an advantage in that a cleaner product is achieved, as the container is made, filled, sealed with the minimum of exposure and handling. Virtually all the risk is related to machine stoppage, clean-down after operating and the start-up period.

A range of machines are available with outputs from 800 units per hour (1 l + fills) up to 22,000 units per hour (0.2–2 ml fills). The latter are usually presented in 'sticks' of eight to sixteen units per stick. Certain machines have been designed to have the capability of inserting other sterile components, e.g. rubber stoppers, which are secured by the final top welding operation.

Materials used for the containers are LDPE, LLDPE, HDPE, PP, PVC, etc. The machines need a dedicated sterile area, so the capital costs for both machine and associated area vary from £1.5 million to £5.5 million. This would have to be justified, usually by 24 h operation.

Closing the package

Closing techniques are covered comprehensively in Chapter 11. All that needs to be said here is that the various methods of sealing listed below are critical to the whole of the integrity of the pack for three major reasons:

1 the closure is the weakest point in the pack design
2 the pack will have to be opened and may be reclosed
3 the closure may also have to act as a dispensing device.

There are two basic methods of closing the pack:

- integral sealing of the prime container, e.g. heat sealing of sachets, ampoules, etc., or by cold sealing techniques, e.g. pattern coating
- addition of individual closures, e.g. roll-on closures, screw closures.

Where vibratory bowl feeds are used for the separation and feeding of closures, it should be noted that the closures may pick up dirt and static electricity unless the feeding system is properly controlled. There is a case for ensuring that this type of feed has a vacuum extraction incorporated to remove as much of the induced contamination as possible.

Labelling or identifying the contents

Labelling techniques related to paper-based materials and the whole question of over-printing are covered comprehensively in Chapter 5. This leaves the need for a few comments on other forms of labelling, mainly involving plastics in the form of films.

Plastics are used in two ways as labels.

1 As a direct replacement for paper, i.e. used as sheet fed and applied adhesive (usually hot melt) or pre-coated with heat sensitive or pressure sensitive adhesive. The same application techniques are used for plastic labels as for paper, except that the presence of a clear plastic label can be difficult to detect on a labelling machine. This is overcome by either using 'eye marks' or adding a fluorescing material incorporated in the print or adhesive – reading with a UV sensitive reader. Another problem associated with 'plastic' labels is that, in general, they tend to be thinner than paper and have the property of picking up static electricity as they move in a dry atmosphere. Anti-static additives should be used in the plastic film as well as earthing the labelling machine.
2 Using the peculiar properties of plastic to be applied by either the shrinking or the stretching route (see below).

Stretch and shrink plastic labels

Most stretch and shrink labels are added to containers in a tubular form, generally relying on the stretch/shrink tightness of the material to retain label position for the life of the product. An additional feature is that the label may be extended over the closure to form a tamper-evident seal on suitable packs.

Stretch labels are unusual to date in pharmaceutical packaging but have the advantage of not requiring heat or specialised artwork to achieve a professional finish. However, they are difficult to use successfully on anything but regular shapes.

Shrink labels are used in the form of a full label or in the form of an additional label added for tamper-evidence, or both. A heat shrink tunnel is needed and, as the tube is fed loosely over the container and tightened, there is potential distortion of the print. This is catered for by distorting the artwork so that the finished shrunk sleeve copy is visually correct.

The materials used are generally LDPE, LLDPE, PP, OPP, or PVC in thickness ranging from about 30 to 100 μm.

A few additional general points on all labelling need to be stressed. Many form fill and seal styles of pack (e.g. blisters, sachets) use reel-fed preprinted materials which *must* conform to the same labelling/leafleting regulations as container labelled packs. Even though these reels may be thought of as labels, there is no independent action of labelling.

The shape of the container, its material and the closure type to be labelled all have a major influence on the choice of labelling machine. Cylindrical containers are the easiest to label, provided that they are clean and parallel sided with no protrusions anywhere on the plane to be labelled. Any other shape increases the difficulty of label placement and wipedown. If the closure of the container is of the dispensing type, e.g. aerosol valve, holding the container by means of top pressure during labelling will actuate the aerosol.

The particular labelling machine chosen for any particular job *must* be capable of easy cleaning so that full reconciliation of the label quantities can be achieved.

Other requirements

Leaflet addition

This is dealt with comprehensively in Chapter 5.

Cartoning/display outers

There are two basic types of equipment, loaded either horizontally (usually automatic) or vertically (which might require an operator).

1 Intermittent motion, achieved by a Geneva movement, works with lower speeds up to about 90 cartons per minute, but is more tolerant of poor cartons and robust.
2 Continuous motion – higher speeds up to 200+ cartons per minute, but requires tight toleranced cartons.

Collation, casing and palletisation

Overwrapping, stretch wrapping or shrink wrapping materials may be used on single items or bundles of 5, 6, 10, 12, 20, 24, 25, depending on the marketing preference. This is covered in more detail in Chapter 9.

Bundles may be cased and palletised: details are given in Chapter 15.

On-line testing

It is assumed that the incoming packaging materials have been supplied to an adequate authorised specification, quality controlled in an approved manner so that the materials arriving at the packaging line are known to be within the parameters of the specification. Therefore the testing that follows is that associated with putting the elements of the pack together.

There are some testing procedures that are essential to the correct functioning of the line, such as those that detect that the pack is incomplete:

- no container (or film) – no fill
- no container, no ullage filler – no closure
- no container – no label
- no container – no carton
- no leaflet – no carton.

This means that if any part of the total pack structure does not feed to the line, the feeding mechanisms for the subsequent materials will not be activated. It is also essential, as detailed earlier, to ensure that the correct fill of product has gone into the primary pack by whatever method is used.

Another essential area is the testing of the seal integrity of the closure:

- level/tilt position of applied closure
- inert gas 'sniffing' of form, fill and seal packs.

A fourth area considered essential for checking is ensuring that the correct identification is on the primary pack, i.e. bar code read or optical character verification (OCV) of the primary pack, label, leaflet, carton, outer casing or outer label. Bar codes and reading are dealt with in Chapter 5, but the techniques of optical character reading (OCR) or OCV are described below.

The OCR/OCV techniques have only become economically comparable with bar code reading in recent years. They are defined as follows.

1 OCR means that each individual character of text is compared with a preloaded series of type fonts, the results of the comparator output fed either to a display or to an accept/reject mechanism.
2 OCV means that a short series of printed characters is electronically compared with a short series of stored characters. It is therefore very much quicker in operation than OCR. Note that the same rules of loading the string of characters apply as are used for preloading bar codes, i.e. the information must be independent of the packaging material being delivered to the packaging line.

When one is contemplating the use of OCV, either OCR 'A' or OCR 'B' type fonts should be used, as they have been specially designed to minimise the problems of misidentifying characters. Some of the problem characters are:

2, Z; 1, I; S, 8, 9; 0, D, 8, 9; 5, 6, b

The comparator in the 'black box' is programmed to look very carefully at the problem characters, emphasising the differences between like characters by a high 'loading' of the scores of compatibility in the small differences area. Speeds in excess of 150 strings of 50 characters per minute have been achieved. The benefit of OCV over bar coding is that the already printed component item code, part number (or whatever it is called) may be used rather than the extra printing of a special security bar code.

Lastly, the product might need to be tested on line for the presence of unwanted metal objects, i.e. metal detection.

Operators and training

Packaging line operators should be encouraged to report any minor health hazards, e.g. cuts, minor skin infections, so that informed decisions can be made as to their suitability for working in controlled areas.

They should also have been formally trained on the particular machines that are in use on the packaging line, particularly in safety and observation, and have a thorough knowledge of how the marketable pack should look at all stages of its packaging. There should be SOPs for codes of dress, discipline, line processing, clean-down, etc. Training records should be archived.

The packaging line should be designed in such a way that the ergonomics gives the operator the least amount of time away from watching the line while loading additional components. Figure 14.5 shows a line designed to help the operator and the engineer; Figure 14.6 shows a badly designed line.

There must be planned routine maintenance, change-overs planning with the engineers, schedule planners and marketing in particular to maximise the economic order quantity (EOQ). The EOQ is defined as the point at which the cost of change-over equates to the cost of holding the extra inventory, by increasing production order quantities (Figure 14.7 shows a graph of EOQ).

All the time a packaging line is not producing finished packs it is consuming fixed overheads for no financial return. It is therefore essential that the downtime of the

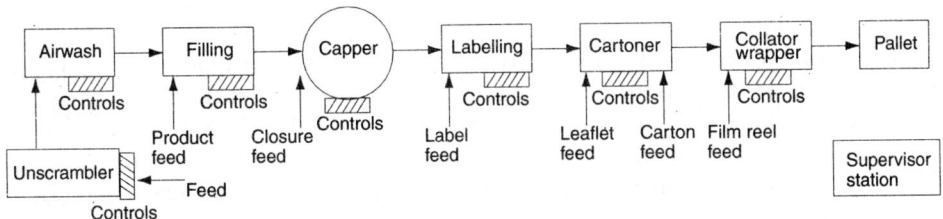

There is no need for the operators to leave the controls

Figure 14.5 A good compound line layout

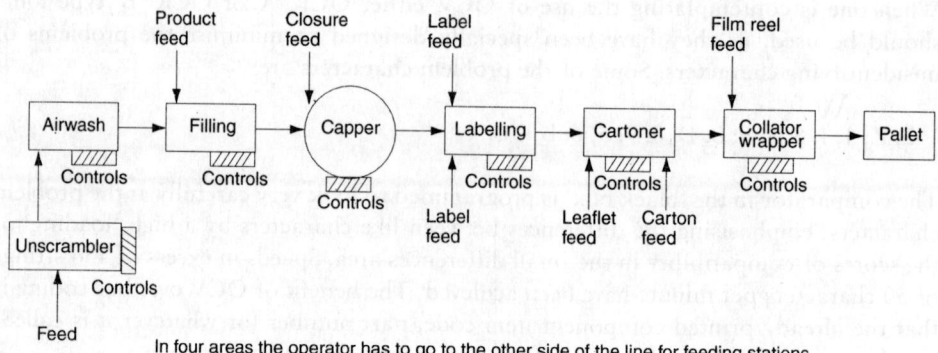

In four areas the operator has to go to the other side of the line for feeding stations

Figure 14.6 The same line as in Figure 14.5, thoughtlessly laid out

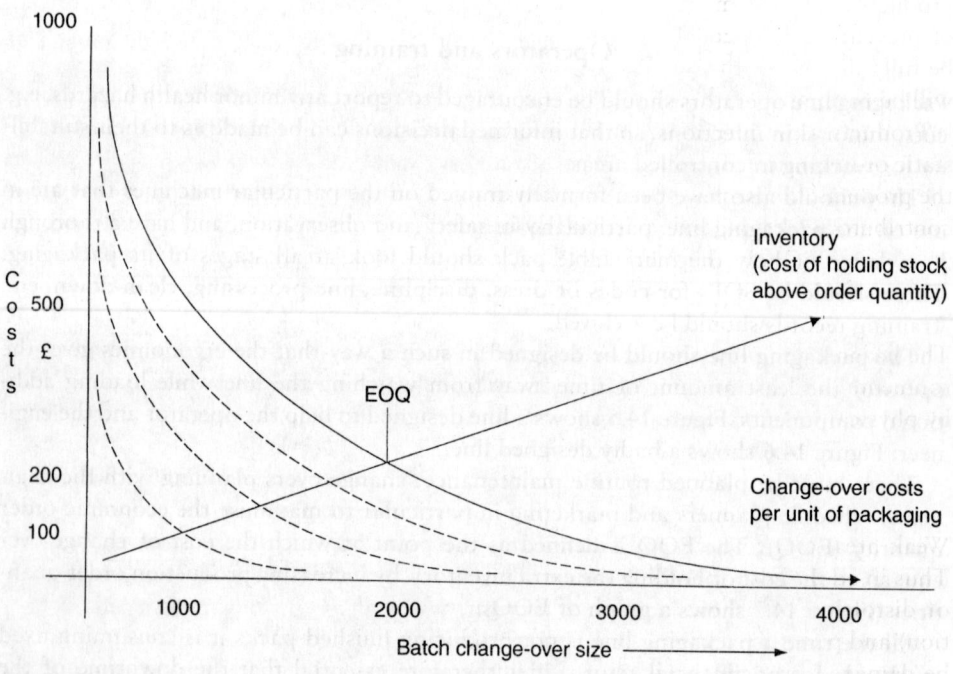

Figure 14.7 Economic order quantity (EOQ) graph

packaging line is minimised. This means that the EOQ becomes an important factor in the scheduling of work to the packaging line, as it has been calculated that a line with an output of about 100 pieces per minute, when materials and orders are available, costs about £20+ per minute to run. It therefore costs about £20+ per minute for the line to be standing still when it is scheduled to be operating. Companies cannot afford this, and must be aware of the need to programme and control all aspects of the process.

15

WAREHOUSING, HANDLING AND DISTRIBUTION

I. H. Hall

This chapter brings to the attention of the reader the general hazards suffered by all products and those most common to the full range of pharmaceutical packs. Methods of preventing damage in the warehousing, handling and distribution of products will be fully discussed. In addition, both internal UK packaging and packaging for export will be covered.

Products anywhere in the warehousing, handling and distribution chain are either static or in motion. This is an obvious statement, but both phases may involve 'risks' to the products. These risks can be broken down, identified and corrected by a number of contributory factors, as detailed in the following text.

Hazards in warehousing, handling and distribution

The hazards the product will be exposed to are physical (mechanical), climatic (environmental), biological, chemical, and some others. In practice the greatest risk is posed by physical or mechanical damage.

Physical or mechanical damage

Weak areas must be clearly identified and all physical forms of damage considered. Thus in addition to the effects of acceleration or deceleration (i.e. impact, drop, shock or distortion damage), compression, crush, vibration (including resonance and friction) and puncture during handling must always be checked. For example, an item can be damaged by top compression during warehousing or transit stacking, (with additional vibration effects).

It is important that the outer packaging:

1 does not collapse in warehousing or transit stacking
2 will withstand the total forces for the requisite storage and distribution time with adequate reserves in hand.

However, both these observations are dependent on other factors: e.g. type of pallet, how stacked on pallet, stacking of pallets, etc.

Impact, drop, shock, and to an extent distortion are caused generally by acceleration or deceleration of the pack itself or an object 'hitting' the pack, e.g. slips off a bench, kicked, dropped, slides about loose inside a container. Crush is the slow result of compression usually over a period of time and is covered under stacking.

Vibration is the term used where an object is oscillated back and forth in a direction at a certain speed (frequency) and by a distance (amplitude). The frequency of vibration (cycles of movement per second) will not in itself cause damage and is not really a concern except in the special case of resonance, which is the natural frequency of vibration at which a object will vibrate most freely. At the resonant frequency the amplitude increases quite dramatically and can lead to the pack/product being severely damaged.

It is very difficult to predict the resonant frequency of a pack, but a reasonable prediction of the transport frequencies that the pack is liable to meet can be made. This occurrence is not too common, but should be borne in mind if no other obvious solution to a breakage in transit problem occurs. Solutions to resonance can be:

1   cushion the goods from damage (see 'Cushioning' below)
2   isolate the vibration (use shock absorbers)
3   change the resonant frequency (alter weight or material)
4   change the driving frequency (lorry or conveyor speed etc.).

Vibration also leads to friction, causing abrasion and possible text damage. Certain surfaces (plastic, enamels, etc.) or decorated/printed items must avoid contact with abrasive materials (wood, fibreboard, paper and board, etc.) and be overwrapped in a less damaging material, e.g. PE/PP film, bags or an air cap.

Puncture is normally seen from some other external object which penetrates the pack, e.g. fork lift truck. However, sharp items may penetrate the pack from within, hence such sharp features may need some external protective cover or be restrained/contained in carefully designed packs.

Climatic (environmental) hazards

Temperature

Around the world the overall temperature can change from at least -50 to $+60°C$. Don't underestimate the heat and lack of heat attraction of the mode of transport, e.g. dark coloured containers can, during hot sunny days and cold clear nights, have a temperature difference of $60°C+$ at their skin.

Liquid water

Relative humidity (0–100%), humidity, moisture and condensation are terms for the intrusion of moisture into the packaging system which individually or in combination with other contaminants can lead to corrosion in metals or can soften papers and boards.

Humidity is the level of water vapour in the atmosphere. It is usually defined as the relative (RH) and absolute humidity. The effect of a temperature change is that in saturated air, if the temperature drops there is precipitation of water, e.g. rain or condensation onto exposed surfaces. Bear in mind the concept of equilibrium between atmosphere and water-absorbing products, e.g. cellulosic materials which may be considered as both moisture-absorbing and water-losing packaging.

Corrosion usually occurs on metals in the presence of water (or vapour), oxygen or acid on the product as well as the package. If the outer packaging is of cellulosic material and is wet, then the conditions for corrosion exist and the outer packaging has failed.

Radiation

The sun and artificial light, ultraviolet (UV) and infrared (IR) content of the source light can have serious effects on the printed text and identification, i.e. fading of inks, colours, etc. on the exposed surfaces of the outer packaging.

Air pressure

Either increased or decreased air pressure can create damaging forces on the pack and closure (e.g. changing altitudes).

Biological hazards

1   Microbial growth, bacteria, yeast, fungi and moulds can breed in favourable conditions, so specific precautions may have to be taken. Mould may grow on moist outer packaging.
2   Biological attack from rodents, birds, insects, termites, etc.

Chemical hazards

Seepage from nearby damaged product is obvious, but less so is contamination by stray by-products resulting from abrasion or mating surfaces (even though the primary cause is vibration).

Other hazards

Pilferages from criminal activities is not uncommon, so anti-theft devices and measures might be required as transportation has been a traditionally vulnerable point in the security system.

Hazards the product creates

Having dealt with the hazards to the product during warehousing and distribution, we now consider any hazards that the product or its packaging might hold for the community at large. At the pack design stage, the following checklist should be used.

1   Hazards of weight.
2   Hazards produced if there is a spillage.
3   Is the product toxic?

4   Is the product radioactive?
5   Is it an infectious substance?
6   Flammability of product?
7   Projections or protrusions which might catch on something.

All these questions about hazards must be asked at an early stage of the pack design so that the packaging may be designed to minimise any rejections in the storage and distribution stages.

Nature of the product

It is essential that the physical state of the product and its route of administration into the body are known, as the more facts that are known the easier it is to decide on the warehousing and distribution conditions and limitations, e.g. is the product an aqueous liquid needing to be kept cool but not frozen i.e. stored and transported between 2 and 8°C? The product itself will belong to one of the following categories:

1   solids, including tablets, capsules, powders, lozenges, suppositories, pessaries, pills, dressings and devices
2   liquids and semi-liquids, including oral liquids, emulsions, suspensions, solutions, lotions, creams, ointments, gels, aerosols and foams
3   vapours, vaporisers, propellants and gases, e.g. O_2, CO_2.

The routes of administration must also be taken into account in the assessment of firstly how to package the product and secondly how to protect it from all the hazards mentioned earlier. There might be special cases in compound packs where the fragility of an administration device has to be considered, as well as the risk to the product. These administration routes affect the overall design of the package and the protection necessary in warehousing or distribution.

Packaging materials and systems used

Several basic types of materials are used, all of which have been detailed in previous chapters, i.e. glass, metals, paper and board, plastics, wood and compound (comprising two or more of the above). Only those aspects of packaging design related to the warehousing and distribution modes will be addressed here.

1   Glass packaging today does not contribute anything to the discussion on warehousing and distribution packaging, save that it is fragile and needs good quality protection and as little handling as possible.
2   Metal packaging includes tins, cans, drums, pails, etc., which may be the primary, secondary and tertiary packaging in the case of transportation of bulk pharmaceuticals or pharmaceutical ingredients. Occasionally used for metal pallets and cage pallets. A common problem is that small containers can be easily dented.
3   Paper and board packaging is used mainly for secondary or tertiary packaging – labels, cartons, and corrugated cases – and is the main material used to protect the product in warehousing and distribution.

4   Plastics packaging is used in only a few minor roles in warehousing and distribution, namely shrink-wrap used as alternatives to metals (often has less to offer in terms of stacking strength).

5   Wood is used primarily for pallets and skillets, but is not considered as a 'clean' material, and can introduce physical or microbial contamination.

6   Compound materials are any two or more of the above five, e.g. foil-lined corrugated or plastic-lined fibreboard kegs may occasionally be used where an extra moisture barrier may be needed.

Nature of primary pack

The primary pack, i.e. that which immediately contains the product, is likely to be either rigid (securitainer or bottle, etc.) or flexible (blister pack, collapsible tube, etc.) and could be fragile, hence readily damaged in some way.

Although warehousing and distribution may be primarily associated with 'bulk' or the unit load packaging, they are also related to secondary packaging because sometimes these secondary packs are broken down (e.g. at the wholesaler) and sent out to their final destination as singles or twos. If this happens and the unit packaging is poor (e.g. poor quality carton), damage is likely to occur (rucking, creasing or crushing) thereby creating a substandard, unsightly or unsaleable pack, even though the contents may remain undamaged.

The interpretation of 'Bulk' may be as follows:

1   x cartoned products in a transit pack
2   x products in a divisional transit pack
3   one or more pallets of an item in its own transit outer (e.g. drums or sacks)
4   a pallet stacked in layers then stretch or shrink wrapped
5   any combination of the above.

In categories (1) and (2) above, removing single items from the transit pack for individual dispatch, or in the case of (3) and (4) removing single items from the pallet, may impose entirely new transit and stacking hazards on the product. This situation can be extended to complete transit loads, containerised loads, and systems involving specific palletised systems (e.g. cage pallets, box pallets, convertor pallets) where materials can be stacked to pre-controlled heights.

Handling – manual or mechanical

All goods will be handled many times from the end of the packaging line to the final consumer (the patient). An example is cartoned bottles to a UK retail pharmacy then dispensed to the patient.

The cartoned bottles will be collated into a dispatch amount, which will be either a tray and wrapping or a case. This will be handled probably manually and stacked to a predetermined pattern onto a pallet. The pallet will be moved off the packaging line when full to a holding area for QC passing, then to a warehouse and stacked (probably more than one high) awaiting dispatch. Upon dispatch either a pallet load or, more likely, a case or part case is moved from storage, stacked onto another pallet containing other products as a 'mixed load' (it will require additional protective packaging), moved onto a lorry and secured. From the lorry at the wholesaler's warehouse onto the ground, then into a stack, from which it will be placed in a 'picking' area where the outer case may be removed and picked into baskets/trays/Jiffy bags for van dispatch to the retail pharmacy. The retail pharmacist will give the bottle to the patient, probably in a paper bag.

This adds up to around fourteen handling/movements, and could include stacking, loading, unloading, repalletising, breaking down containers, breaking down secondary packs, etc. The warehouse handling of goods in recent years has become much more complex, starting with manual handling, passing through various mechanical transfer systems to fully automatic robotic systems.

Manual handling usually includes hands and feet (including kicking) and various non-motorised aids, e.g. wheel barrows, sack trucks, trolleys, mobile bins or cages. These involve the physical actions of lifting, lowering (dropping), pushing, pulling, throwing, catching. In each of the above, hazards to the handler (as well as the product/pack) must be considered, particularly in light of health and safety legislation.

Mechanical handling should present fewer hazards, provided that the goods are palletised and are properly stacked, stable and secure, and in good condition for their purpose.

Quantities involved

These will range over the industry from one or two ampoules or vials right up to shipping containers containing thousands of individual packages or even intermediate bulk containers (IBCs) for pharmaceutical chemicals.

It is difficult to quantify, but the classical pharmaceutical pack of filled containers will be of prime concern to the reader. The smaller the quantity, the more likely it is to become lost in a large warehouse and the more manual handling it will encounter.

Environmental changes during storage, handling and distribution

In the UK atmospheric changes are relatively mild, both naturally and due to changes in altitude above and below sea level. Severe changes in altitude can occur in air transport mode and within certain countries in the world. In air transport there are both pressurised and unpressurised aircraft. 'Pressurised' means that in flight the pressure is stabilised at 8,000 ft, equivalent, while non-pressurised means no control. If you are likely to export to Mexico City or Johannesburg, take note that their altitudes are 7,500 and 6,500 ft respectively. The pressure varies at about 0.475 lb/in^2 per 1000 ft of difference in altitude.

Other environmental changes could include:

1 temperature changes and their effect on dimensional stability, flexibility or rigidity of corrugated and cartonboard
2 static electricity pick-up is increased in warm dry conditions and excessive handling
3 condensation on the pack through bringing cold items into a warm, moist atmosphere

4   physical instability, e.g. 'dumb-bell' reels due to preferential moisture absorption at reel edges and the reverse.
5   RH changes as referred to earlier.

Corrugated boards and casing used for transit protection

Too little attention is usually paid to this important area of packaging. If the transit packaging is poorly designed, then the product will not reach the market in usable condition.

Structure of boards

Please refer to Chapter 5 for the construction of solid and corrugated boards.

Collation and casing of packs

In a packaging design there may or may not be a carton covering the prime container. If not, then a number of containers will have to be held together either in a tray or with some form of film wrap, e.g. deadfold wrapping, shrink wrap or stretch wrap. Product in a carton must be arranged so that the longest side of the carton is vertical, as this is the way to use the maximum strength of the carton. The cartons should then be collated into suitable numbers to suit the particular distribution system.

Structure of cases and design parameters

Cases should be designed to the FEFCO, sometimes called the International Fibreboard Case Code (IFFC), system. This is an international system which has codified the various designs of cases into a simple book of basic designs, to which the designer has only to add the dimensions and board specification (see Figure 15.1).

Moving and storage methods

Handling of goods was discussed earlier in the chapter, so that movement can be defined as either manual or mechanical. However at some point in the warehouse it is usual to store the goods, and this can be done in two ways.

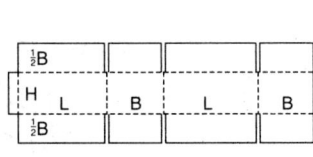
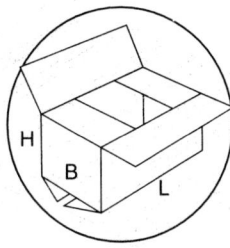

Figure 15.1 Example of FEFCO design

1 Random or floor storing, which is useful for single containers of bulk or single cases, but has the major disadvantage of the goods needing to be raised up from the floor to move them again. This imposes additional mechanical hazards, to say nothing of the problems of floor contact (cleanliness and moisture). Pallets or stillages may also be stored on the floor, but the space utilisation in a warehouse is limited.

2 Rack storing, which is preferable, may be on shelves, pallets on shelves, or moveable racking. The latter two usually require specialised lift trucks to operate the system successfully. This is discussed in detail later.

Palletised and non-palletised loads

Palletisation enables a unit load to be lifted, transported, loaded for distribution, unloaded, etc. with the minimum of manual handling. Pallets are designed to be stacked, and usually one onto another if the product/pack/pallet design permits. Pallets come in different sizes, styles and are designed to be handled by fork lift systems.

As stacks grow higher and weights increase, specialised and more costly high stacking trucks, cranes and robots could be employed. Manoeuvrability of these is vital as this relates to overall space utilisation (See 'Costs').

Using the non-palletised methods and depalletising to optimise transit vehicle space, warehouse space, etc. substantially increases manual handling. This can be reduced by the use of mechanical transfer systems (lifts, hoists, chutes, roller conveyors, etc.). Placing loads directly onto the floor in warehouses, vehicles, etc. is not recommended for pharmaceutical products. It is therefore advisable to try to raise the packaging 'off the floor' by the use of boards, duck boards, hardboard, slip pallets, slip sheets, etc., but these may cause other problems.

Pallet types

Pallets are usually divided between two-way and four-way entry styles. The two-way offers entry of lifting forks from two opposite sides of the pallet; the four-way from all four sides of the pallet. Various styles of pallet are shown in Figure 15.2. Please note in particular the variation in deck board gaps, which vary from a solid deck to gaps as wide as 6–7 inches. This will influence the choice of strength of secondary packaging material. Note also that the bases of the pallets are different, in that the number and types of cross-member in the base may differ from only two side bearers up to perime-

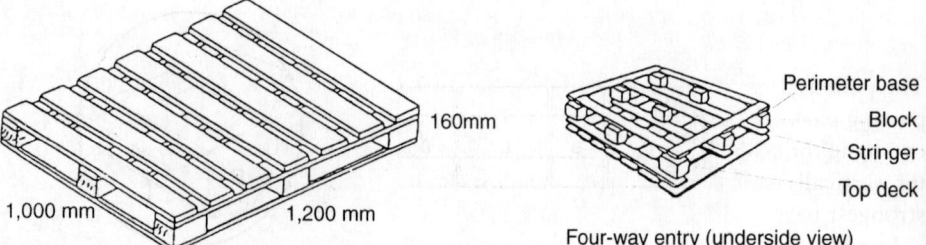

Figure 15.2 Types of pallet

ter base and centre cross bearer. This has a significant effect when pallets are stacked more than one high, e.g. in a lorry, trailer or container.

A pallet is a flat portable platform constructed to sustain a load, be stackable and permit handling by equipment. A stillage is a flat portable platform constructed to sustain a load and permit handling by equipment. Stillages are not designed to be stacked one upon the other.

A cage pallet is exactly what it says it is, usually a metal solid decked two-way entry pallet with demountable cage sides and lid. A box pallet is similar to the cage pallet but is usually of plywood sheet or heavy corrugated board construction (triwall).

Selection of pallet or stillage type requires consideration of the following factors.

1 Nature of goods being handled and whether the pallet is for one specific purpose or for general purpose use.
2 Distribution system(s) with particular attention to:

- number of directions that a fork lift truck needs to enter the pallet (two, four)
- handling by hand operated pallet trucks, as the base design may need to be different
- general handling and storage methods
- pallet 'footprint', i.e. the formation of the base of the pallet – this particularly applies when loading direct to aircraft floors and in stacking loads to greater than one pallet high
- gaps between the deck boards
- cleanliness and general pallet maintenance (to facilitate overall cleanliness and, in particular, use in 'controlled' areas, many companies are now specifying 'plastic' or aluminium pallets).

3 Cost in relation to goods carried and service life.
4 Destination, as there are several sizes of pallet in use. There are several 'standards' for pallet size, some of the more usual ones being:

- UK standard pallet size = 1000 × 1200 mm
- Europallet = 800 × 1200 mm
- US pallet = 1200 × 1200 mm approx.
- ISO pallet = 1200 × 1800 mm.

Note that pallets going to China, Australia and New Zealand must be 'treated' or tannalised to rid them of wood mites.

Fit to pallet

The palletisation of cases is probably the most frequently used safe method of transporting packaged product. There are certain factors that help, e.g. the load should not overhang the pallet perimeter, and must be stacked with the case edges on the perimeter vertically over each other to transmit the downward forces in the line of the strongest part of the case.

In addition there are several types of stack that can be designed, depending primarily on the case and pallet sizes chosen. Usually use a divided load which may be of interlocking or spiral stack types, but avoid columnar stacks as far as possible as they tend to fall off pallets when they are picked up by trucks, due to the pallet flexing under load, unless adequately stabilised.

To give an indication of pallet design, the following is a typical pallet specification.

1   Type: four-way entry, perimeter base 1,000 × 1,200 mm.
2   Materials: specify timber and blocks.
3   Timber components:

- top deck boards – 7 off 125 × 19 × 1,000 mm
- base boards – 2 off 100 × 19 × 1,000 mm
                       3 off 100 × 19 × 1,200 mm
- stringers – 3 off 100 × 22 × 1,200 mm
- blocks – 6 off 138 × 100 × 100 mm.
                  3 off 100 × 100 × 100 mm.

4   Construction: top deck boards will be evenly spaced so as to give 21 mm gaps. Annular ring nails are to be used for all joints, and each nail must be more than 20 mm from the wood edge.
5   Marking: brand 'user name' on two diagonally opposing blocks if required.

Load stability

The techniques of load stabilisation are designed to hold the load securely (whether just collated or cased) whatever type of pallet loading has been used. Load stabilisation facilitates handling and enhances the protection afforded to the contents by the package, while providing the means of effecting safe handling throughout the distribution chain.

Stablisation methods

Bonding

Drums, crates and trays are designed in such a way that when stacked in multi-tiered layers each interlocks with the one below. Trays, for example, can have plastic inserts or integral designs at each corner to support the tray above.

Interlocking stacking patterns

This is where rectangular packages are arranged in alternating stacking patterns to provide an overlapping bond on each layer. Although improving the stability, with corrugated cases it reduces the stacking strength.

Interleaving sheets

Otherwise known as tie layers. Low slip sheet material, normally paper or thin card, is placed between a set number of layers. This method is generally used for small packages or where the interlocking patterns cannot be achieved. The sheets can be applied automatically on the palletiser.

Incorporation of low slip materials

Used particularly for paper, plastic and composite sacks. With paper sacks use a creped Kraft paper on the outside ply. Even with dusty materials this increases the coefficient of friction of the contact areas, thereby reducing the chances of unwanted movement of one sack over another. Other treatments of paper use colloidal silica or compounds containing alumina.

Palletising adhesives

Used between the packaging to hold the load into one mass.

Strapping

In use today for the heavier end of the market, e.g. cases of filled vials. Care should be taken as strapping that is too tight on a load can cause severe crushing as it goes round right angles, unless edge/corner guards are used.

Stretch wrapping

One of the most popular forms of load stability in recent years. It consists of an anchored sheet of film being tightly wound around a load, manually or automatically. The control of tension is of great importance since if the wrap is too tight then crush damage occurs, particularly to the corners of the load.

Shrink wrapping

Can be used on either palletised or unpalletised loads. Properly applied it holds the load together well, forms a reasonable tamper-evident barrier and adds positive protection against vapour and water. If it is required the shrink or stretch wrap can be opaque, thereby obscuring the individual labels on cases.

Slings and sling bags

An alternative form of palletless loading, where the slings are arranged (may be with a shrink or stretch wrap) so that the load can be hoisted safely onto and off transport. Sling bags are a form of fabric IBC and can be used to utilise smaller loads, e.g. bags.

Height stacked and stack configuration

Round containers such as drums, pails and buckets have a poor space utilisation. Although a cube offers best utilisation of space it is not necessarily the best shape for stacking, as load interlocking by pattern arrangement is either difficult or wasteful of space. Rectangular or brick shaped outers which fit the pallet dimensions are preferable.

Computer software programs are available so that both stacking and transportation space can be optimised. In certain instances one might design 'backwards', i.e. select the optimum for the pallet and then produce a primary container size to fit this space.

This is significantly different to the classical design methods where the primary container was designed, then the outer pack size was calculated and these packs were then used to find the best arrangement for the pallet. This classical design method often does not fully utilise the area of the pallet, which can be important for warehousing costs.

The ideal height to which a single pallet should be loaded usually lies between 1 m and 1.25 m. However, the height to which a pallet or series of pallets can be stacked depends on a number of factors:

1   the compression strength of the transit outer
2   whether the primary pack will withstand compression, e.g. metal components, glass bottles (and note that compression and vibration may have an effect on the closure torque)
3   configuration of the stack
4   effects of environmental changes, particularly relative humidity (RH)
5   clearances between outer and contents, i.e. aiding or reducing compression, strength
6   base onto which the load is stacked, i.e. pallet deck footprint
7   type of pallet – feet or non-feet, pallet 'footprint'
8   security of loads for both stacking and movement can be improved by interlocking, corner stays, shrink wrap, stretch wrap, netting, or any combination of these.

The effects of the stacking height on the pack and product depend on whether loads are palletised or non-palletised. The height to which a product/pack can be safely stacked will depend on a series of factors. It should be noted that the word 'safely' can be interpreted in two ways:

1   the legal need for 'safety' conditions in the workplace, i.e. if the stack falls down and someone is injured the company could be legally liable
2   the protection of the product in terms of preventing physical damage by stack collapse or compression.

Any stacked product, even a static load, is still at risk from other elements, e.g. environment and movement of people, fork lift trucks, etc., which may be operating in the vicinity of the stack.

Modes of distribution and transport

Although UK distribution is today predominantly by road, distribution can take place worldwide using a number of different ways and modes, as follows.

1   Type of load.
  - Mixed load.
  - Bulk load.
  - Unit load (may be an intermediate bulk container (IBC)).
  - Container load.

2 Journey: distance, time, environmental conditions, stop-overs, etc. must be taken into account.

- Local.
- Internal UK short haul or long haul.
- Overseas to the continent.
- Overseas intercontinental.

3 Type of transportation used.

- If land transportation, this can involve road vehicles, end loading, side loading, with hydraulic tailboards or hoists, or on board cranes with varying degrees of protection. If the rail system, then container or package usually in a closed vehicle.
- Inland waterways face similar conditions to coastal shipping, while deep sea ships might be passenger or loose cargo or container and be coastal, cross-channel or intercontinental journeys. (Note that the time taken can be several weeks.)
- Air transport can use either passenger or custom-built cargo planes. Note that outside the 'Western world' there are many planes that are not pressurised.

Containerisation

This may be used for road, rail and water transportation, and is a useful method of ensuring that the goods are kept as much under the parent company's control as possible.

There are several sizes of container, but most are designed to be just over 2 m high, 2.5 m wide internally and of a suitable length to fit onto a 32 t lorry chassis. The container will probably be made of aluminium sheeting with reinforcing ribs internally, a solid steel/wood floor and, for shipping, steel reinforcing external ribs for stacking on docksides or onto ships. There are usually safety-locking doors only at one end.

The container can be loaded in one of two ways: by the pharmaceutical company itself, which has the advantage that once customs sealed it should not be interfered with; by an agent who will endeavour to fill the container to its maximum with a variety of goods, e.g. heavy loads on top of your goods.

It is generally accepted that the contents of containers will be stacked two pallets high, so it is essential that the goods are adequately attached to the pallet. The load will need to be stabilised as much as possible and this is done by systems of air bags blown up to take up the vacant load spaces, sacks of straw or plastic chips, or sometimes expanding plastic foams in specialised applications.

Each combination of transportation tends to produce different advantages and disadvantages, costs, etc. Each will also involve differing climatic, biological, drop, vibration, etc. hazards. Packaging designers must look all the way down the distribution chain before deciding on the final pack design.

Utilisation of warehouse space

Warehouse space is expensive, but it can be utilised most economically by the selective use of free stacking, shelving, bins, pallet racking, mobile racking, live racking (gravity feed systems), automatic (stacker cranes) or automatic flow-through using robotic systems.

There are several methods of optimising the space available. It is sensible to have the most popular product lines as close to the warehouse dispatch point as practical, thereby minimising the length of movement (and therefore time of operators, trucks, etc.) taken up in closing orders.

Several popular styles of warehouse space utilisation will now be described. Bear in mind that there is no theoretical 'right answer' to warehouse space utilisation problems without a thorough examination of all the operation and options of that warehousing system.

1   Free stacking of pallets is viable if the warehouse has a low roof and the goods do not occupy space for long periods of time, e.g. a QC quarantine area.
2   Shelving for small individual light items (which may have to be held for a short time) up to individual pallet loads. It is possible with proper design to have shelving designed to be as high as possible, with the operators using either mobile steps (for light items) or fork lift trucks (FLTs) for heavier items.
3   Bins would normally be used for small light items, particularly in wholesale warehouses, for individual pharmacy order picking. There could also be a gravity feed system of depalletised cases from a bulk stock area.
4   Pallet racking is fixed skeletal racking designed to fill from floor to ceiling.
5   Wide aisle is a term given to fixed pallet racking, where the aisle is wide enough for a standard FLT to turn and swing its forward projecting forks into the pallet picking-up apertures.
6   Narrow aisle is the term given to the configuration of fixed pallet racking where a specially designed side-lift FLT runs in a straight line between the racks, carrying a four-way entry pallet only in its short direction i.e. the 1 m dimension of the British pallet.
7   Mobile racking is a narrow aisle system with only one aisle per group of racks. The racks themselves are electrically driven so that the 'bin' is located by computer and the racks moved automatically so that the specific aisle is opened up to the lift FLT. There are of course safety features which prevent the racks from moving while picking operations are being undertaken.
8   Gravity feed systems (live racking) are a simple system of rollers where the product is fed on from the back and picked from the front, gravity providing the restocking force.

The decision whether to choose a simple or fully robotic warehouse rests with the inventory, type of pack involved, volume to be handled, destination, etc. Whatever is used, there is an increasing probability that computerised systems will be used for booking-in, stock location, booking-out, reconciliation, automatic label production, automatic routing, etc. Warehouses may be dedicated to only one function or several, i.e. a goods inward warehouse, production holding warehouse, QC quarantine warehouse, goods outward warehouse, which might be dispatching to either a wholesaler or to an individual.

It is essential in all cases to have quarantine areas, in which quarantine identified incoming goods and finished goods can be held pending QC release. The computer system must reflect the situation in the warehouse by 'locking out' any movement documentation until QC release is obtained.

Where warehouses are involved with the breaking down of outers (usually known as order picking), an analysis of orders should tell whether the ideal outer size is in use. This is particularly relevant where pick and place packaging is involved, as this is normally an expensive, labour-intensive, boring operation. Warehouse staff build up considerable knowledge on good and bad packaging, thus they have a valuable contribution to make to the consideration of the total pack design. It is advisable that consultation with the warehouse occurs, particularly in the field of minimising warehousing costs.

Storage and handling of packaging materials and components

Factors that need consideration in the storage and handling of packaging materials and components include:

1. the type of item, physical and chemical changes that might take place
2. the way the items are packed
3. the way the items are palletised and or stacked
4. the warehouse environment
5. whether the item is likely to change or deteriorate on storage, whether it needs a limited shelf life backed up by a re-test at intervals
6. facility for QC sampling, how the sample is taken, the pack resealed, inventory changes
7. the importance and level of cleanliness, hygiene, particulate contamination, bioburden, etc.
8. area segregation for quarantined goods
9. write-off procedures for out-of-date items – note that there are security aspects to this as well; goods should be destroyed if they are company-specific to prevent 'pass-offs'
10. control on pallets – all pallets should be the same, particularly where pallet exchange systems operate
11. contamination, e.g. spillage, roof leaking
12. physical or chemical changes of stock
13. avoiding the obvious hazards of overhead heaters, radiators, draughts, leaking roofs, light/heat/cold from windows, etc.
14. improper or inadequate packaging, overtensioned strapping, stretch wraps too tight.

Order picking

This may occur in the UK in either of two scenarios:

(A) the manufacturing company system catering for distribution to regional destinations
(B) the regional warehouse providing a service, usually twice per day, to every retail, community and hospital pharmacy and to dispensing doctors of any drug commercially available.

An order picking warehouse has different problems to the more conventional 'bulk' warehouse. Goods are picked from racking or bins, either by hand or lately by more sophisticated electronically controlled robotic systems for despatch. Depending on the warehouse type, the journey may be long distance by lorry with manual and/or mechanical handling in example 'A' above, or into a basket into the back of a van in example B.

The collation of picked retail packs for distribution from wholesale to retail is a very difficult area, as most of the individual items are of differing sizes and shapes, need protection during handling, packing, loading to transport, unloading, then movements within the retail environment. 'Mixed loads' are inevitable in this scenario and the packaging and protection of these loads is a skill acquired only with some thought:

1 put the heaviest, least crushable, items at the bottom of the load
2 ensure, as far as practical, that no part of the load overhangs the pallet
3 try to build up the mixed load with the most fragile materials inside gaining some protection from the surrounding packs
4 do not build up a mixed load too high, i.e. over about 1.2 m
5 ensure that the mixed load is secured by means of an anchored shrink or stretch wrap.

Remember that the retail unit, out of its secondary packaging, is very vulnerable to manual and mechanical handling – shock, vibration, drops, etc.

There may be occasions where there needs to be a system of distributing certain specialist products direct from the manufacturer to the individual patient, e.g. unlicensed drugs. This will involve sending probably only one container/course of treatment. This pack will be very small, i.e. too small for industrial distribution. The obvious method is by using the postal service. This service is usually very quick, economical and efficient, but carries a higher degree of risk of physical damage. It is essential that those products to be posted are carefully assessed for fragility and the secondary/tertiary packaging designed so that maximum protection is given for impact, low and medium vibration and crush.

Costs

Warehousing involves space, heating, lighting and labour. Typical 'space' costs (at 1994 figures) about £5–10 per year per ft^2, with overheads of £10–20. Based on this, pallets stacked three high (~4 m) on a 1000 × 1200 mm base area (~£315), plus handling space (2.5), would cost ~£790 per annum. If outers of 12 are assumed, 40/pallet, 3 pallets high = 1,440 units. Therefore one year's storage/item = about 55p per unit. Since keeping a unit in the warehouse for say 3.5 days will cost 0.53p or, if 4 weeks, 4.22p per pack, such costs need serious consideration. Involving stock in an order picking operation usually multiplies the costs by about 10 times.

Example:

- Load, unload and transport 1000 kg: assume 75p.
- Stack 1000 kg 1 pallet for 3.5 days, storage: assume £7.58
- Warehouse handling: assume £1.5
- To order pick 1000 kg, each item individually: £22.00 (expressed as a handling cost).

However, although considerable, distribution costs (or rather the proportion of product cost to distribution costs) are relatively small for pharmaceutical products (typically 2% of overall product sales revenue).

UN certification

There are various pharmaceutical products that fall into the UN dangerous goods category, e.g. aerosols. The UN dangerous goods regulations provide a structured method of assessing package performance and the requirements of performance of a package to carry dangerous goods safely, based on the defined degree of hazard.

The UN 'Orange Book' is the definitive guideline to the proper classification of products into one of nine classes, some with subdivisions (see Table 15.1). Each class and/or subdivision has three packaging groups: I, II, III. Each group defines a level of risk posed by the product, thereby defining the severity of the package testing required.

Group I contains the most dangerous goods of any classification and is likely to require that smaller amounts of the goods are carried, in addition to having much higher test specification. The limitations on the mass of product carried either per container or per load are usually applied to aircraft.

All substances to be carried by any means should be checked against the UN listings for dangerous substances (available from the Department of Transport). There are different limitations and definitions as to what is dangerous in each of the transport modes. ICAO, IATA, IMDG, ADR, RID are the abbreviations for the various bodies representing international air, sea, and European road and rail transport. Note that

Table 15.1 UN classification of products

Class	Material	Details
1	Explosives	Of no interest to pharmaceuticals.
2 with	Gases	2.1 Flammable gases, e.g., continuous spray aerosols butane propellant. 2.2 Non-flammable, non-toxic gases, e.g. continuous spray aerosols with CFC propellant. Division 2.3 Toxic gases, e.g. chlorine.
3	Flammable liquids	e.g. Liquids containing alcohol.

<table>
<tr><td></td><td></td><td></td><td>boiling point</td><td>flash point</td></tr>
<tr><td></td><td></td><td>(i)</td><td>$\leq 35\,^\circ C$</td><td>–</td></tr>
<tr><td></td><td></td><td>(ii)</td><td>$>35\,^\circ C$</td><td>$<23\,^\circ C$</td></tr>
<tr><td></td><td></td><td>(iii)</td><td>$>35\,^\circ C$</td><td>$>23\,^\circ C, \leq 60.5\,^\circ C$</td></tr>
</table>

Class	Material	Details
4	Flammable solids	Not likely to be of interest to pharmaceuticals.
5	Oxidising substances and organic peroxides	5.1 Oxidising substances which may contribute to combustion by producing oxygen. 5.2 Organic peroxides may be considered derivatives of hydrogen peroxide.
6	Poisonous (toxic) and infectious substances	6.1 Poisonous (toxic) substances, e.g. potassium cyanide. 6.2 Infectious substances, e.g. AIDS virus.
7	Radioactive materials	e.g. Medical isotopes.
8	Corrosive materials	e.g. Acetic acid.
9	Miscellaneous dangerous	Items not covered by the previous eight classes, e.g.

ICAO is the legal UN definition of what may and may not be carried. IATA covers the airlines and may not correspond to ICAO, but the classification and group testing specifications are the same.

All packaging must be tested by approved test methods by approved testing stations. All possible variations of packaging from all potential suppliers must be tested. The results are then scrutinised by PIRA (in the UK) and, if satisfactory, a certificate is issued. There are strict rules about the marking and labelling of UN approved packaging which must be followed to the letter, or the product which is classified as dangerous may be refused transport of any kind.

Cushioning of fragile packs

Cushioning is defined as the protection from physical damage afforded to an item by surrounding its outer surfaces with materials that have been designed to absorb the shocks or reactions caused by external forces. There are three major ways of achieving the prevention of damage using cushioning.

1   Spread the load caused by impact over a wider area, e.g. contrast a 50 kg package, size $250 \times 200 \times 200$ mm dropped from 1 m onto a corner and onto one flat base. The force to be dissipated is 50 kg m/s^2 (50 N). On the corner, only a few square centimetres take all the load, say 10 cm^2. Therefore load per unit area of contact is 5 kg m/s^2 (5 N). On the flat base the area is $25 \times 20 = 500$ cm^2; therefore the load per unit area is 0.1 kg m/s^2 (0.1 N).

2   Localise the forces, i.e. direct forces to the strongest parts of the package.

3   Absorb the energy in a resilient material by using a cushioning system, e.g.

- space fillers, e.g. powders and granules, shredded materials, wrapping materials
- crushing or non-resilience, e.g. foams, papers
- resilient cushioning devices, e.g. rubber, springs, steel or bulk materials.

When an object contained in a container falls, it accelerates. When it stops suddenly, the outside of the object stops before the inside of the object. This time is in milliseconds. The package must be designed so that the fragility of the prime container is taken into consideration and adequately protected.

Cushion packaging materials

Cushioning materials in widespread use include air bubble sheet, cellulose padding, cork-based granules/sheet, corrugated plastic corners, corrugated sleeves, embossed paper, expanded polystyrene, other expanded plastics, foam in place, free flow polystyrene, sawdust and shavings, straw, wood wool.

These materials have to be assessed on their cost, efficiency, versatility, compatibility, storage volume before use, fire risk, hygiene and disposability or reuse. There might also be an association with the product and sales image for marketing.

Conclusions

The objectives of warehousing and distribution can be summarised as:

- minimising total delivered cost
- storage for a minimum time period, involving the minimum quantity to meet all order demands while retaining an in-stock situation
- preventing damage or containing it to an economic minimum
- retaining customer goodwill
- minimising the cost of replacement/return and the need for repair/re-sorting.

16

PRINTING AND DECORATION

D. A. Dean

Introduction

Detail on printing and decoration as applied to planar surfaces such as paper and board can be found in many textbooks. However, the decoration and printing of packs, packaging materials and packaging components, many of which are non-planar surfaces, involves processes additional to the conventional ones. This chapter therefore briefly discusses these many processes, which continue to increase (comparatively recent additions include ink jet, laser and thermal printing).

Knowledge of the methods employed and the materials used, i.e. inks and the drying mechanisms, etc. are important to those in the pharmaceutical industry, as printing can be a source of contamination. This suggests that printing is best carried out either on presealed containers or after a container has been filled and closed. It also should be noted that it is somewhat difficult to achieve good colour matches using different printing processes on different materials, e.g. flat or radiused, glossy or matt.

Decoration or printing is the means of providing for a packaging material:

1   aesthetics or graphic design (to attract, enhance, stimulate sales of a product during display and use)
2   product identification
3   information related to 'labelling', e.g. product names, directions for use, warnings, shelf life, expiry date, use before, storage conditions, manufacturer and address, batch number, covering fixed and variable requirements.

Where the essential function is one of graphic appeal, effective overall design requires consideration to and understanding of a number of factors, such as:

1   knowledge of the product and the market (how, when, by whom used, etc.)
2   knowledge of the packaging materials to be employed (functional and structural detail, i.e. dimensions and tolerances of the item, area(s) to which decoration/printing may be applied, type of surface, etc.)
3   knowledge of the methods of distribution, marketing and sale
4   quantities of item to be supplied per year and quantity per order
5   knowledge of any legislative requirements (relating to general laws or specific products, e.g. foods, pharmaceuticals, dangerous chemicals)

6   knowledge of the various printing or decorative processes, including inks and drying methods

7   size, shape and colour of the background material (colour – clear/opaque, tinted/pigmented, opalescence, pearlescence, etc.).

Aesthetic design and decorative appeal which are covered by consideration of the above factors, may be improved/modified by both non-printing and printing processes.

Some processes are not strictly related to printing but can provide decoration, including:

- roller coating – kiss coating
- spraying
- vacuum deposition, e.g. metallising
- painting
- anodising
- plating
- colour-based material (natural colour)
- indentation, i.e. debossing and embossing
- labelling – by various methods
- decorative sleeving, i.e. shrink and stretchable sleeving
- flocking
- etching, e.g. acid etching of glass.

Decoration: features and terms

Decoration or printing must provide certain additional features associated with colour, illustration and typography, etc. These need consideration of the following.

Finish of surface to be printed

This covers surface reflectance, texture, smoothness, roughness, as well as gloss, semi-matt, matt, etc. Gloss may be achieved by the basic substrate, special inks, over-lacquers, varnishes, or a transparent laminated film.

Rub resistance (resistance to abrasion)

This is relevant to various stages of the handling of decorative or printed surfaces, i.e. on the production line, during transit (vibration), during stacking and handling, at the point of sale, or ultimately during use by the consumer. Many factors may contribute to rub, e.g. ink thickness, ink type, state of 'dryness'. Tests for rub resistance in the UK (dry or wet rub) are covered by BS 3110.

Note that the way a printed or decorated component moves, vibrates, rubs, etc. will relate both to the shape of the article and to the type and configuration of the packaging materials which surround it. For example, a cylindrical bottle in a carton or a divisioned outer will move from side to side, up and down and rotate in a clockwise or anticlockwise direction. A rectangular, square or oblong container is unlikely to rotate. Since the rotational movement with the round container is likely to be predominant and more damaging to the surface decoration, this may require a higher level of rub resistance.

Chemical resistance

This is related to:

1 product contact, i.e. product resistance over a range of temperatures, associated with the environment, point of usage
2 specialised processing or storage, e.g. sterilisation, storage in a deep freeze
3 contact with other substances, e.g. water, soap (particularly if used in a bathroom or kitchen)
4 human secretions, i.e. perspiration from hands may also cause marking or even reactions (particularly if these secretions are sulphurous, acid, etc.).

Temperature

This is associated with climatic, processing or with special storage recommendations. Packs may have to withstand severe cold, i.e. should resist cracking or flaking-off, or extremes of heat could cause softening or hardening (brittleness). Also shop windows, storage under bright lights, in the sun, or the boot of a car – especially if black.

If part of a decoration falls within a heat sealing zone, special heat-resistant inks/over-lacquers may be necessary. Alternatively, heat seal areas can be kept free from print.

Pick

Decoration should not lift, flake or crack under conditions of heat and/or pressure, e.g. heat sealing or the application of pressure sensitive tapes, i.e. substrate surface lifts. Heat seal jaws may be coated with PTFE to reduce ink 'pick'.

Key

A good key or bond between the printing inks and the substrate to which they are applied is essential if detachment or 'pick' is to be avoided. In certain instances surfaces need pretreatment (e.g. gas, or corona discharge) or a surface primer.

Odour and taint

Freedom from odour and taint is essential in the case of oral products where they may be detected by smell or taste, e.g. from residual solvents, from printing inks.

Toxicity and irritancy

Foodstuffs, pharmaceuticals, toiletries, cosmetics, etc. must avoid contaminants derived by direct contact or by migration from printing inks. Food grade inks can be specified. See also 'migration/contamination/reaction' below.

Light fastness and discolouration due to light

Light exposure may cause either fading or darkening of both materials and colours. (Note that temperature/humidity also influences change.) Ink fade is normally checked by Xenontest type equipment (main supplier Heraeus) and is measured against the British wool scale.

Note that other simulated tests include carbon arcs, fluorescent sunlamps, various xenon arcs, etc. Tests tend to be comparative once conditions have been standardised. North and south window tests are also used.

Slip

Surface slip (friction) characteristics may be important in certain packaging line operations, especially form fill seal equipment, and in stacking. Anti-set-off spray during printing can affect slip, where printed surfaces usually become 'gritty' to the touch, due to the excessive application of anti-set-off (to prevent print transfer to the underside of adjacent surfaces).

Colour control

Colour control is achieved by the setting of light and dark colour limits, and can now be accurately measured by colorimetry. Colour has hue, lightness and saturation and covers wavelengths of just below 400 nm to 760 nm.

Migration/contamination/reaction

Pigments/dyes or other constituents in inks, adhesives, varnishes, etc. may migrate through certain materials, i.e. plastics, and give rise to contamination/interaction, which under certain circumstances may either react with the ingredient in a product or cause toxicity, irritancy problems, or loss of potency. This risk may also occur with certain label adhesives.

Powdering

Powdering is usually associated with the detachment of small particles from a printed or coated surface. Powdering of surfaces can cause discolouration (e.g. change in surface reflectance, increasing rub, general particulate contamination, change in slip characteristics).

Grain direction

Machine or cross direction is a factor to consider in the case of cellulose-based materials, i.e. paper and board. Grain direction is important when these materials are wetted or heated, whereby various degrees of curl may be induced due to the swelling or drying-out of the fibres differentially according to the 'grain' direction. The cellulose fibres exhibit greater swell or expansion across the fibre, hence when wetted or dried the axis of curl will be parallel to the machine or grain direction. Dimensional changes can cause print registration problems.

Print terminology

Some explanation is required of the basic terminology used in printing and in artwork.

1   Line – areas of solid (continuous) colour with no variation in density, based on the original lino-cut type of plate.
2   Halftone (tone) – the image is broken down into a series of cells or dots by a screening process, using 40–300 per linear inch, giving a series from coarse to fine screen. (Look at the coarser process used in newsprint through an 8–10× magnification hand lens.)
3   Reversed out of – where areas of a solid colour are broken by shaped area (non-printed), which exposes the background surface or colour (see Figure 16.1).
4   Reverse printed or reverse side printed – applied on the underside of a transparent film which is then viewed via the top side. Eliminates external damage by abrasion or scuff.
5   Surface printed – direct printing onto a surface.
6   Sandwich printed – applies where printing is sandwiched between two materials, the upper layer being transparent.
7   Wet on wet – applies where a second ink is laid down on top of another while both are still wet. Not recommended but occasionally found (dry offset). Due to colour bleed and colour dilution, loss of clarity and general colour degradation may occur.
8   Print size – usually based on a point system, with 72 points per linear inch. Each type of printing process will have a minimum point size which will reproduce clearly. Most typefaces lie in the range of 6–14 point for main body text and 16–48 point for display text.
9   Print styles (typography) – found under various names, e.g. Modern Italic, Egyptian Bold, Modern Roman.
10 Contact printing – involves direct transfer of ink from plate to substrate or indirect transfer via an offset stage.
11 Non-contact printing – there is neither direct nor indirect contact (e.g. offset processes). Examples: ink jet and laser printing.
12 Origination and origination costs; originals. These phrases cover the photographic work and ancillary processes used to convert the original artwork (drawings, photos, transparencies, etc.) into film positives or negatives from which printing surfaces (plates, blocks, cylinders, etc.) can be produced, and the costs associated with them. These costs are usually recharged to the client.
13 Make ready time (printing machine). The make ready time is the time and labour required to set up a process ready for a print/decoration run. Since make ready times must be costed as part of a printing run, those costing the most to set up are usually associated with long runs and large quantities (e.g. gravure).
14 Stereos, forme, stereotype – various names related to the printing plate(s) and the machine location. A forme is usually flat whereas a stereo may be curved (around a cylinder).
15 Anilox roller. In the flexographic process ink is transferred from the ink fountain by a rubber transfer roller onto the anilox roller. The latter is usually an etched or patterned roller, giving cells of constant depth and size, from where it is trans-

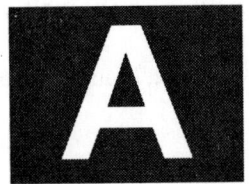

White reverse out of black

Relief process

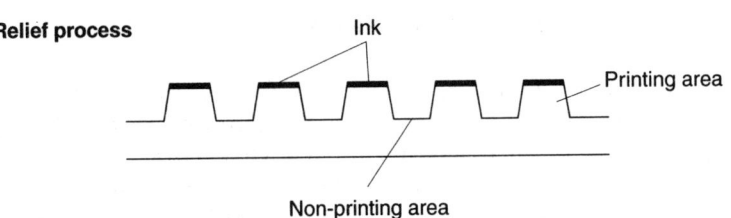

Planographic

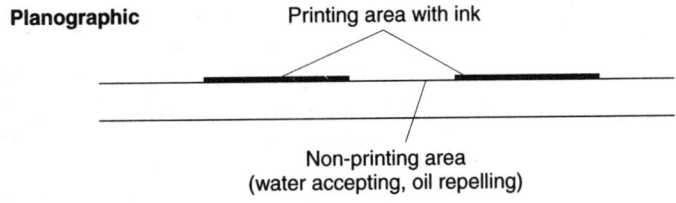

Intaglio

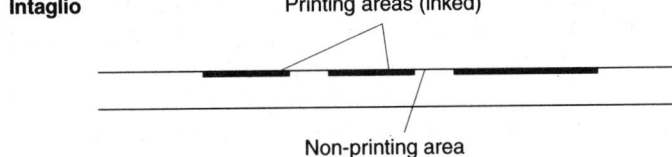

Stencil

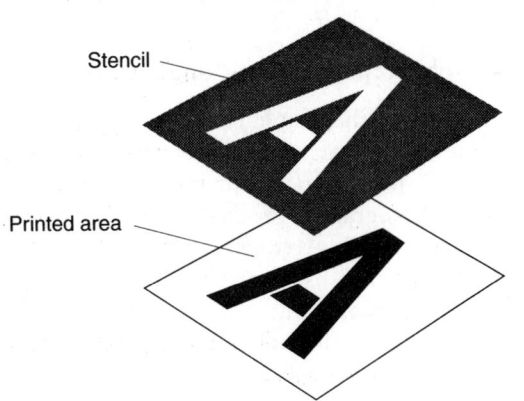

Figure 16.1 Printing processes

ferred to the relief plate (cylinder), without the ink being squashed over the sides of the relief characters.

16 Fountain – this is basically the box, trough, machine section in which the ink is held.

Decoration/printing – general processes

Decoration/printing may be carried out as follows.

1 In the flat as sheets or reels, e.g. paper, board, tinplate, films, foils and laminates. Materials in both sheet and reel forms may be further processed to give packs which may remain in the flat (e.g. collapsible cartons) until erected or are directly fabricated into a three-dimensional container (tinplate containers, composite drums, rigid boxes, etc.). Distortion printing also falls into this category.

2 After fabrication, e.g. two-piece metal cans, glass and plastic containers, collapsible metal tubes. Containers are manufactured and then printed or decorated by a secondary process. Since material and container shape impose certain restrictions, i.e. process used, design limitations, etc. some fabricated containers may use labels, printed sleeving, etc. rather than a direct decoration/printing process.

3 During fabrication – adding print during the fabrication process includes embossing, debossing and in mould transfer labelling.

Certain materials may need some form of pretreatment before they are printed. Examples include the following.

1 Applying a coating of enamel on flat metal sheets prior to fabrication into a container, or a round container after it has been fabricated. Both are carried out by a roller coating process followed by a curing/drying operation.

2 Applying a primer or key coating to aluminium foil.

3 Pretreatment of certain polymers such as the olefins to oxidise the surface by either flame or corona treatment.

A summary of the main decoration processes is given in Table 16.1.

Graphic reproduction ('origination')

Graphic reproduction may involve the simple action of typesetting, a combination of typesetting and artwork, pure artwork, or computer-based artwork. Typesetting may be carried out by hand (compositing), typesetting machine (linotype, monotype), via a special wordprocessor or a photographic process. Artwork may be based on monochrome (single colours) or multicolour. Artwork can be further divided into line (areas of solid colour with no variation in density) and half tone, where colour gradation is achieved via a series of dots per linear inch.

The conversion of original artwork through to a form (plates, blocks, cylinders) that can be reproduced can involve various stages, as follows.

Table 16.1 Main decoration processes

Process	In the flat	After fabrication
Printing process (contact)		
1 Letterpress	✓	
2 Flexography	✓	
3 Lithography	✓	
4 Gravure	✓	
5 Screen	✓	✓
6 Hot die transfer (gold blocking)	✓	✓
7 Dry offset letterpress		✓
8 Pad transfer (cliché)		✓
9 Thermal printing	✓	✓
Printing process (non-contact)		
1 Laser	✓	✓
2 Ink jet	✓	✓
Transfers		
1 Therimage		✓
2 Dinacal		✓
3 Letraset		✓
Miscellaneous		
1 Moulded in decorations (Transfer)	During fabrication	
2 Spraying	✓	✓
3 Roller coating (paint or enamel)	✓	✓
4 Anodising	✓	✓
5 Polishing and brushing	✓	✓
6 Dipping		✓
7 Vacuum metallising		✓
8 Bronzing	✓	
9 Flocking	✓	✓
10 Plating	✓	✓
11 Kiss coating	✓	✓
Preprinted items		
1 Labels (paper, plastic)		
2 Shrink/stretch sleeving		

Camera work and artwork

Camera work varies according to the type of artwork. It may involve photographic reduction or enlarging, colour separation, line and half tone reproduction, the production of negatives and positives, etc. These include the following.

Line artwork – single colour print

The artwork is photographed to produce a negative, usually on film.

Line artwork – multicolour print

The artwork may be pre-separated or composite.

1   Pre-separated: Each colour is drawn separately (in black on a white board) in registration, usually as a base artwork with overlays. Separate negatives are made for each colour by photographing the base artwork and each of the overlays.
2   Composite: The complete design is drawn in black on a white board with the required colour separation indicated. A set of identical negatives is made by photographing the artwork, with the negatives equating to the number of colours to be printed. From these are produced separate negatives for each colour, by painting out with an opaque lacquer the unwanted areas on each negative in turn.

Tone artwork – single colour print

The illusion of tonal gradation is produced by printing equi-spaced dots of varying size, the highlights (i.e. lighter areas) having small dots and the shadows large dots which may merge.

The artwork is photographed in the usual way to produce a negative, but the image on the artwork is broken up into varying sized dots on the negative by the introduction of a 'cross line screen' into the camera. This screen is a glass plate ruled with lines at right angles, varying from 50 to 300 lines (or more) per inch. Coarse screens are used for newspaper work, but for high-quality package printing screens of 150 lines per inch, or more, are used.

Tone artwork – multicolour print

The multi-coloured image is reproduced by printing, in close proximity, dots of varying size of three or more basic colours. The eye blends these coloured dots, giving the illusion of reproducing the original picture. This requires the production of separate printing plates for each basic colour and these are made from film negatives which are produced by 'colour separation' from the full colour artwork.

The artwork is photographed successively through coloured filters (together with the cross line screen which is always necessary for tone work) to produce negatives as follows.

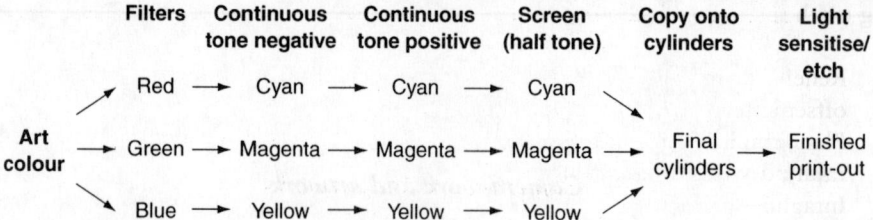

Note that continuous tone negatives and positives are black and white gradations of colour. The filters used are complementary to the final colours required, i.e. a blue filter will darken yellow but lighten green or blue (similarly red–blue (cyan) and green–magenta (red). Red, green and blue are the light or additive primary colours, whereas cyan, magenta and yellow (the complementary colours) are known as printer's or subtractive primaries.

For attraction, definition and sharpness it is usual to include an additional black printing plate. The black plate is produced by using a combination of filters. The three colours plus black are the minimum colours necessary for good reproduction of, say, a colour transparency photograph, being known as the process colours. This is the basis of four colour printing.

If there are large areas of a single predominant solid colour in a design, it is normal practice to use a special additional colour plate. For high-quality reproduction, fine screens and six to eight colour printing is frequently used (see gravure).

Printing down

The printing surface (plate, cylinder, screen, etc.) is coated with a light sensitive emulsion and light is passed through the negative (or positive) on to this emulsion. Multiple images may be produced and accurately positioned on the printing surface by the 'step and repeat' technique.

Developing and etching

The exposed image is developed and then processed in varying ways, depending on the type of printing surface being produced.

Desktop publishing (DTP) and digital artwork and reproduction (DAR), i.e. preprint to press (PTP) systems.

Modern wordprocessing and computer technology (electronic processing) can drastically speed up the preparation, proofing and correction of artwork. Reproduction of the design can be more rapidly followed up by the use of plateless (i.e. non-impact printing systems) or 'plate' printing systems. Such processes, initially used in their infancy for clinical trial supplies, are now being extended into production options.

Mechanical contact printing

The principles of the main printing techniques are based on mechanical contact printing (with reference to printing plate): see Figure 16.1.

1   Relief – print area is raised above the non-print area – letterpress, flexography, dry offset letterpress, hot die stamping.
2   Planographic – print area and non-print area are in the same plane – offset lithography, dry offset lithography.
3   Intaglio – print area lies below the non print area – rotagravure or photogravure.
4   Stencil – ink is forced through a stencil or screen, i.e. screen or silk screen.

Inks

The above printing processes (excluding hot die stamping) involve the use of inks which during the printing process are fed to the printing plate then transferred to the substrate being printed. These inks may be dried, fixed or hardened by:

- oxidation – chemical actions
- adsorption/absorption – penetration
- evaporation – loss of solvents
- precipitation
- curing
- heat setting.

The drying processes may be aided by:

- exposure to air (air drying)
- hot air – to aid air drying
- stoving – higher temperatures, i.e. a curing process
- direct heat – infrared
- UV drying (curing).

The ink involved may be oil-based (originally based on oxidisable oils), water-based, solvent-based (hydrocarbons, esters, alcohols, etc.), or heat-based (only mobile when heated).

Ink drying mechanisms

CHEMICAL ACTION, OXIDATION

Originally based on linseed oil; other oils have included tung, dehydrated castor oil and various resins. Drying action involves resinification by atmospheric oxidation. Drying can be accelerated by the addition of certain metals (lead, cobalt, manganese) as driers. Time to 'dryness' may be a few hours to a matter of seconds.

ADSORPTION/ABSORPTION – PENETRATION

Taken up initially on the surface and then absorbed into the media (can be very rapid, i.e. a fraction of a second with newspapers, where the pigments tend to remain on the surface, are powdery and therefore may rub easily).

EVAPORATION

Depends on volatile, solvent-type liquids such as alcohol, toluol, xylol, which evaporate very rapidly. With heat (hot air, infrared, etc.), setting takes only a few seconds. Water-based inks may also partially dry by evaporation.

PRECIPITATION

Caused by either moisture in the air or moisture already within the material being printed. This means that a solid (usually a resin) is made to precipitate out of a solution by moisture – hence the term 'moisture setting' inks.

POLYMERISED AND CATALYSED SYSTEMS

These are usually made from a two-component system which when mixed has a short life. Uses involve the screen printing of polythene containers, with either air drying or hot air drying.

The ideal ink system has to meet the requirements listed at the beginning of this chapter with instantaneous drying. The latter can already be achieved with a polymerised ink system used in conjunction with UV drying. Although UV systems are expensive to install, with an additional ink cost, their advantages usually outweigh any disadvantages.

ELECTROSTATIC PRINTING

This is increasing in use for variable wording. It relies on the attraction of dissimilarly charged surfaces, i.e. ink particles and surface to be printed of opposite charges (positive/negative). Design may be achieved by a screen or stencil. Note that modern photocopiers use an electrostatic principle coupled to a heat fixing process. See also 'Inkjet printing' below.

Main printing processes' specific drying methods

Letterpress – originally dried by oxidation but now a combination of penetration/oxidation. May also use quick-setting inks, moisture setting inks (mainly letterpress – low odour level), heat set, and oxidation on non-absorbent materials.

Offset lithography uses thinner inks than letterpress and originally oxidation (linseed oil), but now quick-setting inks are more widely used. On metal containers, oxidation was accelerated by heat but synthetic resins are now employed, thus giving a combination of polymerisation and oxidation. Heat also permits some evaporation, giving more rapid drying with a harder finish.

Photogravure – mainly evaporation (plus absorption with paper). With hydrocarbons the solvent is usually toluol or xylol. Alcohol is also used, particularly where a low odour is required. Nitrocellulose inks are thinned with esters, i.e. ethyl acetate. Use of UV inks plus UV drying is increasing.

Flexographic – evaporation. Inks may be alcohol-, solvent- or water-based, depending on material being printed. (With papers absorption is also involved.) UV inks and UV drying are available.

Screen – various combinations of evaporation, oxidation, penetration, polymerisation, etc.

Ceramic (glass) is a screen process employing powdered glass, pigments, plus carrier base. The pigmented glass is fused onto the surface by heat.

Colours may be achieved by dyes or pigments. Dyes are soluble; pigments are insoluble solids.

Thickness of ink film, dryness/drying time, ink rub are all interrelated, hence slow drying may lead to 'set off', i.e. the partial transfer of inked surface onto the underside of the surface above (sheet or reel). This may necessitate the use of an anti-set-off spray which in turn may change the surface film texture.

Printing ink thickness

The amount of ink which can be 'laid down' varies significantly between the processes. Average figures are:

- lithography, 2 μm
- letterpress, 3 μm
- gravure, 5 μm
- screen (thin ink), 10 μm
- screen (thick ink), 30 μm.

The choice of ink, printing process, etc. will depend on the form of the article to be printed and the substrate (material), i.e. the print drying process largely depends on the substrate, e.g. whether it is absorbent or non-absorbent, whether it will withstand the temperatures associated with the drying process. Printed plastic materials can be dried by air drying, hot air drying, UV curing, flame drying, infrared drying, again depending on the temperatures they will withstand. With air drying the inks may dry in stages, i.e. although they are sufficiently dry to be handled, drying may continue for a prolonged period before the ink is fully set. The more recent processes include flame drying (similar to flame pretreatment) and the use of special UV curing inks. The substrate material variables are paper, board, wood, plastic, metal, glass, fabric, etc.

Printing machine terminology

Before expanding the printing processes in detail, it is necessary to introduce some general printing machine terminology.

1   Feed – the input stage of the item being printed.
2   Printing plate – the area that carries the design or wording which receives the ink.
3   Plate cylinder – cylinder carrying the plate.
4   Impression cylinder – the cylinder which applies pressure to the item being printed, thus assisting the transfer of the print from either the plate cylinder or an offset cylinder.
5   Blanket or offset cylinder – cylinder onto which the cylinder image is transferred.
6   Ink rollers – those which take up the ink, provide for an even film thickness and then transfer the ink to the printing plate by direct contact.
7   Damping rollers – these apply water (similar to the ink rollers) to the non-print area of a lithographic plate.
8   Delivery cylinder – exit point from printing unit whereby item is delivered to winding-up or stacking point.
9   Fountain cylinder – cylinder in contact with ink reservoir.
10 Anilox roll – an engraved cylinder which transfers from inking rollers to the printing plate on a flexographic unit.

Printing machines and processes

Relief process

A printing plate can consist of two areas, one of which receives ink (printing area) and the other to which ink is not applied (non-printing area). In the relief process the printing area is raised above the non-print area. The main printing processes using this relief principle are now detailed.

Letterpress (either line or half tone)

Platen

This may be a V type hinged machine which may be fed by hand or automatically (see Figure 16.2). One arm of the V is stationary; this carries the printing plate which is inked when the machine is open. The hinged arm of the V opens and closes, carrying with it each time a paper for printing. The process is relatively slow.

Flat bed

The printing plate is laid on a flat bed or forme which passes backwards then forwards (reciprocating bed principle) (see Figure 16.3). At one end of its travel it is inked by rollers and then as it returns the printed item is passed between an upper impression cylinder and the plate. The impression cylinder then rises to allow the forme to return for inking. Due to the reciprocating action, speeds are relatively low, say 3,000 sheets per hour.

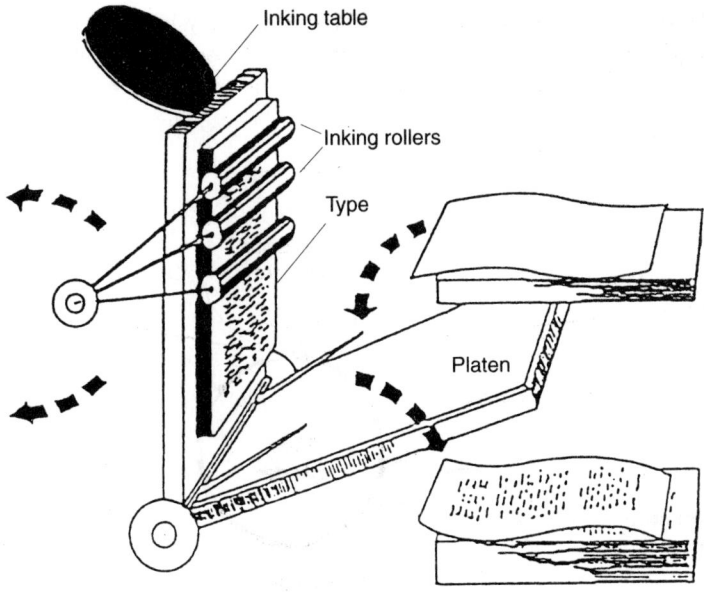

Figure 16.2 Letterpress platen

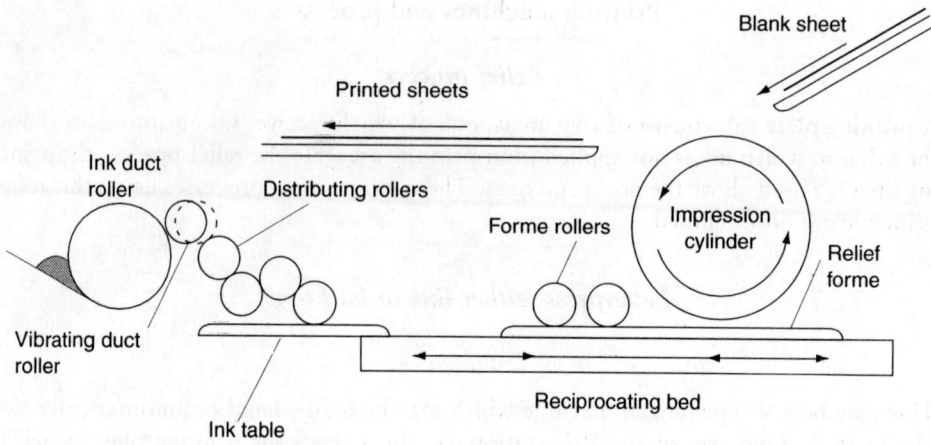

Figure 16.3 Letterpress flat bed

Rotary

Here the plate is on a curved cylinder and operates as in Figure 16.4. Speeds are high: 8,000 to 30,000 revolutions per hour. Feed is usually reel, but can be sheet. Plate cost varies – can be around £200–250 per colour (depending on size and screen). Main applications of letterpress are for the printing of paper and board.

Flexographic

Originally known as the aniline process, due to the use of water based aniline inks on paper (see Figures 16.5 and 16.6). Flexographic is a rotary letterpress process employing cylinder plates made from rubber, nitrile rubber, or special polymers. Excessive pressing may lead to squeeze-out, hence limitations to coarse half tones on certain equipment.

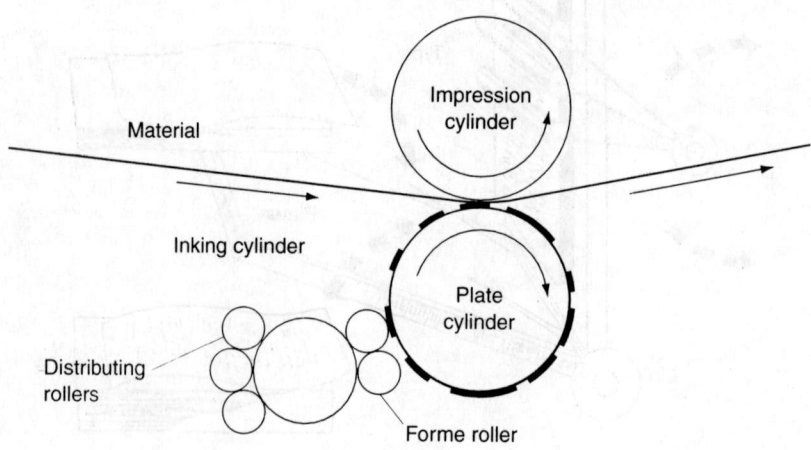

Figure 16.4 Letterpress rotary

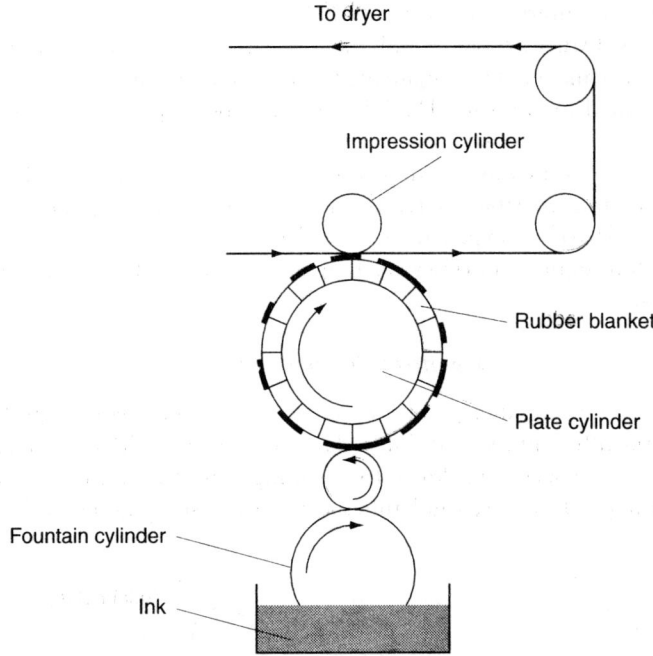

Figure 16.5 Flexographic, one impression

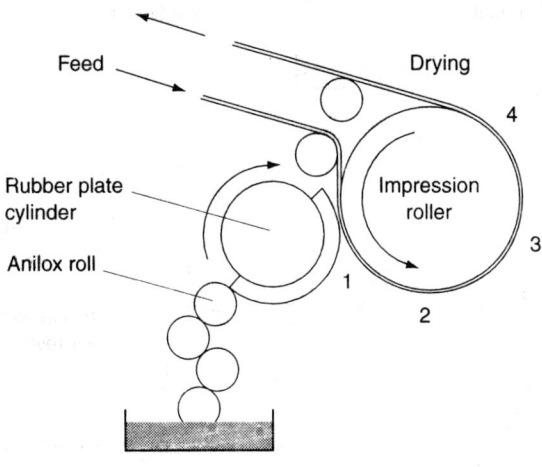

1, 2, 3, 4, Colour station

Figure 16.6 Flexographic process

Rubber blankets are suitable for spirit, aniline/glycol based inks. Special inks require ketones in PVC inks, hydrocarbons in polythene inks. (Nitrile rubbers are resistant to hydrocarbons.) Many inks now use pigmented polyamides (for plastics/foil) – silicones in waxes may be added to aid 'slip'. UV inks may also be employed, otherwise dry by evaporation.

Four colour process with common impression cylinder (4 in Figure 16.6) gives excellent registration with extensible materials. Now a relatively high-quality process. Printing plates are relatively inexpensive – around £175.

To be effective, foil requires a primer wash prior to printing (1–3 gm^2), e.g. nitrocellulose, vinyl resins.

Dry offset (letterpress)

The term has more than one interpretation, as some dry offset work is performed on conventional offset-litho presses (minus damping) using shallow relief plates. Alternatively, there are special machines for printing round or cylindrical items, i.e. plastic bottles, collapsible tubes, rigid tubes (seamless) (see Figures 16.7 and 16.8).

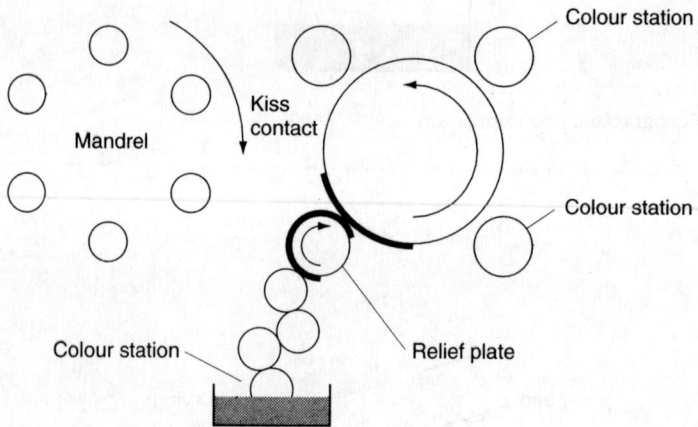

Figure 16.7 Dry offset, four colour

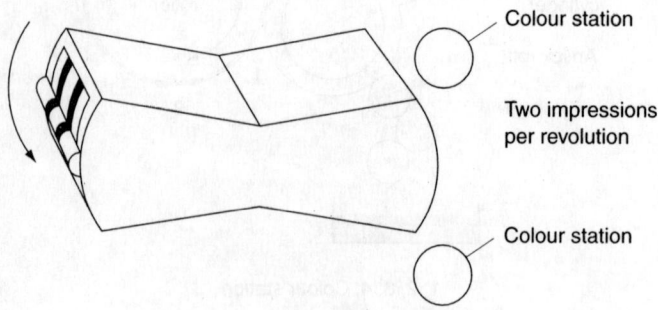

Figure 16.8 Dry offset, two colour

These are normally two or four colour machines, using letterpress plates. Some six colour units are also used.

Printing ink is transferred via a relief printing plate to an area on an offset rubber blanket. Kiss contact (the tube is held on a mandrel and, in the case of a plastic bottle, these are pressurised) is made with the item being printed which then makes one circumferential revolution. The print area is therefore slightly in excess of the circumference of the article (allows slight overlap in many instances). In the case of metal containers, printing is made on top of a roller coat of enamel. Drying is achieved by heat (hot air drying ovens).

Hot die stamping and gold blocking

In this process a carrier material is coated with a foil or pigment which under pressure and heat can be transferred to another surface (see Figure 16.9). It has certain advantages: no drying or surface preparation, quick for colour changes, no cleaning down. It can be printed on raised, on level or into recessed surfaces. Plates may be silicone rubber or metal. Soft plates provide for a kiss transfer whereas metal plates can be used to give a distinct impression into which the pigment or foil is deposited.

The carrier may be glassine, cellulose film, and polyester film. The choice of carrier relates to speed and transfer temperature. Polyester (i.e. Melinex) is the most common base. It is suitable for flat, cylindrical or radiused surfaces. The process is used for on-line printing. Metallic 'foil' consists of a carrier, release coating, lacquer metallised layer and a hot melt type adhesive specially formulated for the substrate.

Planographic

This process is usually the most difficult to understand. The printing area and the non-printing area lie on a common plane and are differentiated by the treatment of the printing plate. The print area accepts ink (oil) and the non-print area water, thus relying on the fact that water and oil do not mix. As seen in Figure 16.10, the plate is first wetted in the non-print area by damping rollers and then ink is applied by ink rollers to the print area. Only one printing process with variations uses this method, as explained below.

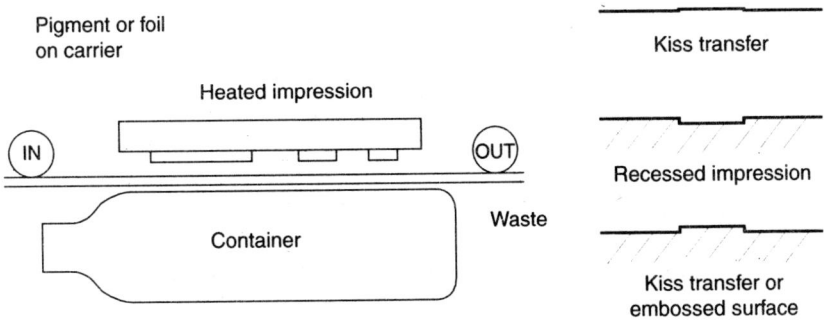

Figure 16.9 Hot die stamping or gold blocking

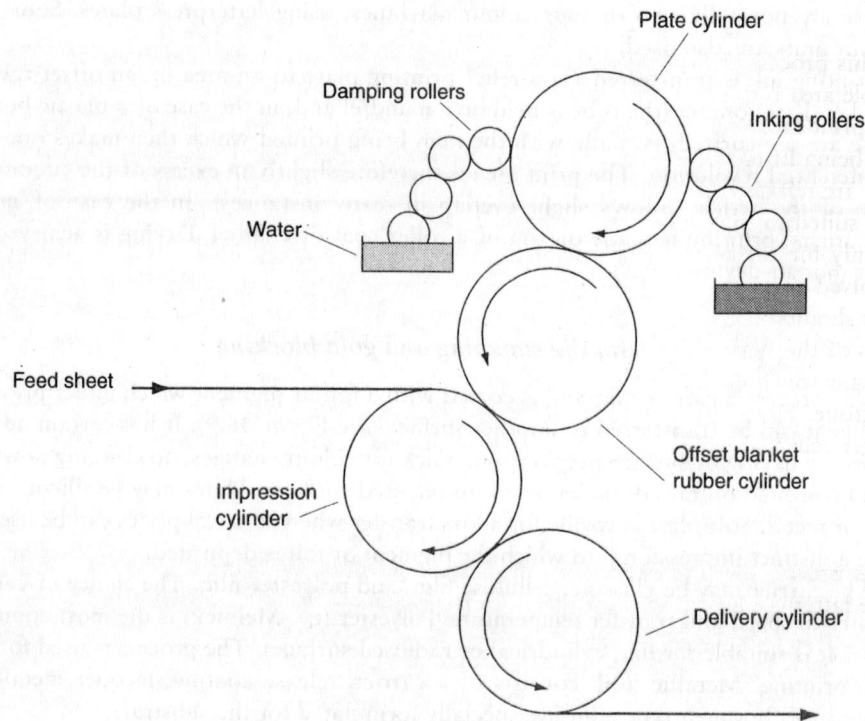

Figure 16.10 Offset lithography

Offset lithography

Plates may be either line or half tone. The inked image is offset onto a rubber blanket and then printed from this blanket onto the item being printed. It is used to print paper and board, metal in the flat sheet (tin plate) and occasionally plastic or foil. Offset lithography applies a relatively thin film of ink.

Dry offset lithography

Special plates are available where only the print area accepts ink without prior damping of the non-print area. These special plates are more expensive than conventional wet offset plates.

Web fed offset

This is now widely used for newspapers and uses heat to speed drying. This had disadvantages on paper and board (due to shrinkage), but has been used for certain carton board. It can produce over 40,000 sheets per hour.

Cost of lithographic plates is around £275 per colour.

Intaglio

In this process the printing area lies below the non-print area (see Figure 16.11). The whole area is flooded with ink, which is then scraped off the non-print area but left in the print area. The item being printed is pressed against the plate which results in the ink being lifted out of the ink cells. For example, gravure cylinders use a copper base and are relatively expensive to produce (£850–1,200 per colour/cylinder), but are ideally suited to long runs. Inks are usually solvent- (dried by heat) or water-based. Used mainly for the printing of board, paper, films and foil, usually where long runs are involved.

It should be noted that two types of gravure plates exist. Conventional gravure have cells of the same surface area which vary in depth. Areas of deep cells result in all ink flowing together to produce a solid area. Gravure also uses a process known as invert-halftone. Here the area of the cells vary so that small cells produce light tones and larger cells produce darker tones (i.e. variations in cell depth and size).

Stencil: screen

This process can use either solid stencils or screen (mesh) stencils (see Figure 16.12). The latter is called screen printing and was originally known as silkscreen, as silk-type

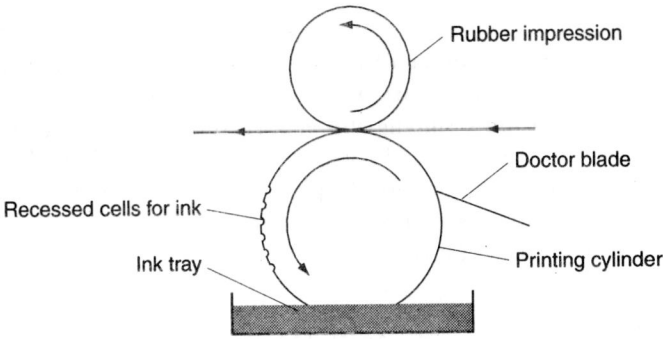

Figure 16.11 Photogravure or rotagravure

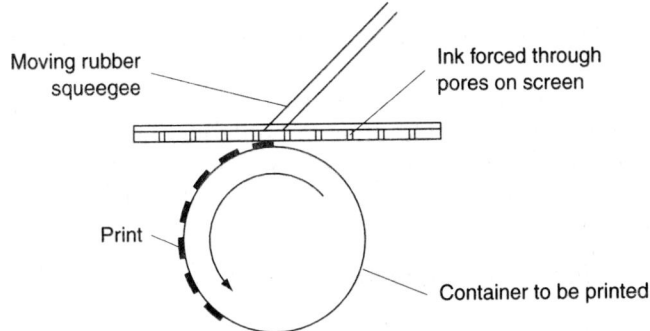

Figure 16.12 Screen printing

screens were employed. Present day screens are made of nylon, polyester or steel and are relatively low in cost, £45–75. Each screen may give 15,000 to 50,000 impressions. The ink is forced through the screen by a squeezer. Prior to this action the screen is separated from the item to be printed by a lift-off gap. This gap is reduced by the pressure of the squeezer whereby contact is made between the screen, ink and item. Screen inks are relatively thick, and are either air or hot air dried. The screen process can produce coarse half tones with thin inks.

Contact may be flat bed or cylinder, hand, semi-automatic or automatic fed. The speed of the process is limited by the drying. One to three colours can be printed in one pass by the use of split screens. The process is used to print paper, board, plastic or occasionally foil. Can be used for flat, cylindrical or radiused surfaces on preformed containers.

A costing of 1 p per pass is generally accepted. As more passes are employed the cost rises due to rejections, i.e. first pass 1 p, second pass +1.25 p, third pass +1.5 p, etc., giving total costs of 1 p, 2.25 p, 3.75 p respectively.

Due to the thickness of the ink, screen printing offers good body and a high gloss. Half tone type printing is achievable by the use of special thinner inks, particularly with UV inks and drying.

Other printing processes

Several named processes are based on transfer, i.e. Therimage, Letraset, Dinacal, etc.

Therimage is used for the printing of plastic containers. The basic image is printed by gravure onto a carrier material somewhat similar in construction to that described for pigmented foils under foil stamping above. Special turrets (costing around £3,000) are required to effect the transfer of the image under heat. When applied the printed image substrate has a greater affinity for the plastic being printed than the carrier base. Several types of heat sensitive bases are now available. Note that the image to be transferred is printed as a 'wrong reading'.

Letraset

This offers two basic transfer processes:

1   for in-mould decoration of plates
2   transfer printing of fabricated plastic containers.

Both employ a preprinted transfer (up to six colours). In the in-mould process the transfer is placed within the mould prior to bottle blowing or injection moulding. During the moulding cycle the printed transfer becomes 'fused' to the container. The printing can be produced by either screen or gravure and can be line or half tone.

Cliché or tampon transfer process, pad printing

Consists of either flat gravure plates (usually one to four colours) or solid line recessed plates which are flooded with ink, wiped with a doctor blade followed by a tampon descending onto a plate and lifting the ink from the recessed cells (see Figure 16.13). It then transfers it directly to the item being printed. With this process it is possible to print directly onto irregular or multicontoured surfaces (i.e. it is the only three-dimensional printing process: trade names Tampoprint, Padflex). The tampons usually consist of glycero-gelatin or silicone rubber.

Thermal printing

This involves two processes. In the first, a heat sensitive coating on a carrier changes colour on the application of heat, e.g. hot needles are used to give a dot matrix type of image. The material can be printed in up to four colours and can incorporate a barrier varnish. Dots are usually 6, 8, and 10.5 per mm. The second process transfers a thermally activated ink from a carrier ribbon. Various colours may be employed. The process is relatively slow, e.g. ribbon moves 5 inches per second. Now a popular process for on-line printing.

Non-contact printing processes

Ink jet printing

The ink is ultrasonically (or mechanically) broken up in to small particles, some of which are then charged, and deflected to the substrate being printed via a screen or stencil, while the remainder are condensed and circulated back to the ink reservoir. A speed of 600+m/min (based on a single line of dots) is possible. Up to six lines can be printed (see Figure 16.14).

Laser printing

A CO_2 laser beam is used to etch (burn in) or burn out (as used for batch coding and expiry dating). In the latter, a prior printed or enamelled surface has some of the ink removed by burning off, as used for batch coding etc. Note that other forms of laser printing processes can produce a high-quality conventional image.

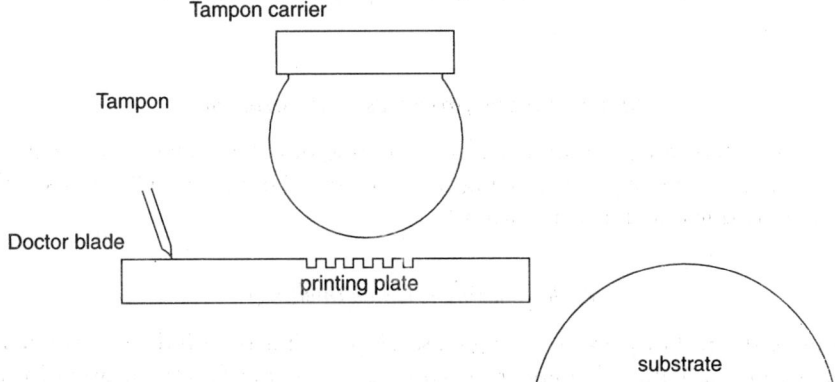

Figure 16.13 Tampon printing: transfer process

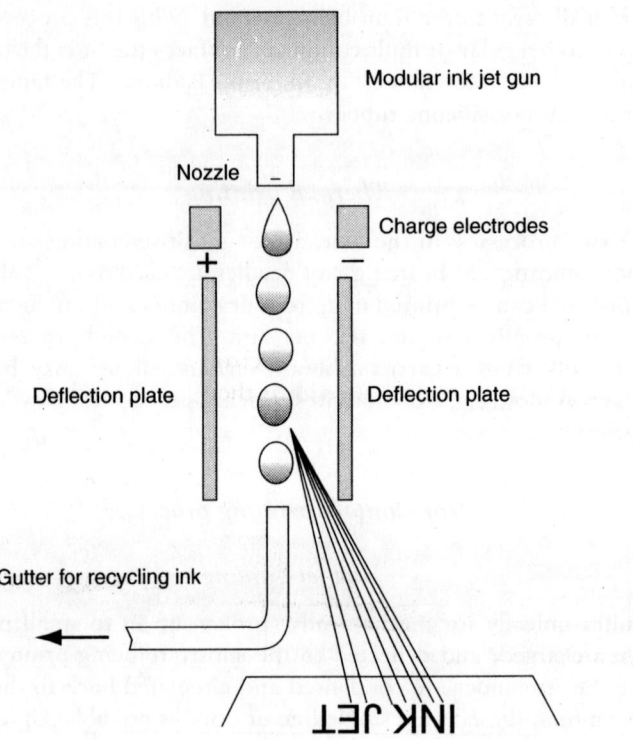

Figure 16.14 Ink jet printing

Embossing and debossing

'Embossing' means above the surface (raised). 'Debossing' means below the surface (recessed). Debossing or embossing may be achieved in a moulding operation by the use of male/female dies with or without heat. Embossing rollers or dies may also be used to produce surface designs/textures on foils, foil boards, papers and boards, metal containers and as a means of batch coding, expiry dating, etc., as part of an on-line production operation.

Miscellaneous processes of decoration

There are several ways of creating a surface coating or colour. These include painting (using a roller or a brush) and spraying (usually carried out in special booths with air extraction; used mainly for metal drums).

Roller coating (also enamelling)

A coating is thinned by passage through a series of cylinders with the lowest one being in contact with a 'bath'. The upper, or contact, roller transfers the coating from the roller to the item being decorated. The coating may be an enamel, lacquer, varnish, etc., which may vary in coating thickness. Metals (e.g. tinplate, aluminium) are enamelled in the flat sheet and metal collapsible tubes as a cylinder, both prior to final printing.

Dipping

Metal and glass may be immersion dipped to give either a coating or an etch (glass into hydrofluoric acid). Plastic coated glass bottles (as used for aerosols) are coated by dipping into a PVC plastisol.

Anodising

A coating of aluminium oxide is deposited electrolytically onto the surface of the aluminium component (pre-cleaned). The oxide is then dyed by immersion into a dye solution and colour set by steaming.

Vacuum metallising

Plastics can have a layer of metallic aluminium deposited on the surface by vacuum. Although aluminium is basically a bright silver, it may be lacquer tinted to give a wide range of metallic colours. Polyester, polystyrene, urea and phenol formaldehyde, and polypropylene are readily metallised. Other plastics need a pretreatment.

Plating

Tin coating of mild steel is basically a surface coating process. This may be achieved by a dipping process or an electroplating process (see Chapter 9).

Polishing and brushing

Small metal articles (usually aluminium) can be highly polished or wire brushed (scratched) to give various patterns which are either random or controlled. These may then be covered by a transparent over-lacquer to improve the effect.

Sand blasting

This was widely used to give glass a frosted appearance.

Moulded decorations

Surface texture or moulded-in configurations can be provided by many plastic moulding processes. Raised surfaces can additionally be 'kiss' blocked or coated.

Coloured base materials

Paper, board and plastic can all be produced as a coloured material. With plastic, colour can be introduced by dry or wet colourising or masterbatching.

Sleeving

Pre-printed sleeves are now available as heat shrink sleeves (based on oriented PVC, PP, PET, etc.) or stretch sleeves (based on LLDPE with a memory built in).

General

The above decoration/printing processes may be used singly or in combination. If a matching series is designed involving different materials and different decoration processes there are likely to be problems in achieving a good match. Other relevant parameters, i.e. print area, registration, colours involved, ink coverage required, shape of surface being decorated (particularly when round is compared with flat), may all need special consideration.

Where pharmaceutical packaging is involved, special attention must be given to food grade inks which are non-toxic and odour-free. Inks which are solvent-based need special monitoring.

Finishing

Labels, wrappers, etc., irrespective of whether they are printed as sheets or reels, are printed by multi-impression processes. For example, an individual label could be printed as a sheet (180 × 98 cm) carrying some forty labels (as a gang pull). These would be converted into 'cut singles' by a guillotine process.

Such printing is only allowed in the pharmaceutical industry if one common label is involved. Composite printing where different products or strengths are printed on a common sheet is not permissible due to admixture risks. Similarly, printing of reel-fed materials as 'jumbo' reels would be reduced to a number of smaller reels. Reel joins should be minimised and normally 'flagged'.

Security systems

Accountability, reconciliation, counting, etc., are all part of print security. These may be coupled with various coding options (bar coding, colour coding, edge coding, punched hole systems, metallic strips, etc.) so that print can be identified and checked against some form of 'code' reading system. In some processes (e.g. thermal, ink jet), items may be consecutively numbered.

Registration marks

Registration marks (e.g. thick colour bars read by a 'magic eye') and similar devices are necessary on form fill seal types of process where design registration is essential. Randomly printed designs, conversely, do not need registration.

Holography

This is now used as a decorative process to prevent counterfeiting. Currently showing a steady increase in use. For more detail see Chapter 5.

Other factors

Although the main printing processes and materials to be printed are covered, other minor processes do exist and newer ones are being investigated. Some materials and containers create design limitations due to the processes available, as detailed below.

State of surface – preparation of the surface

1   Impermeable surfaces (film, foil) – evaporation drying, gravure or flexographic.
2   Rigid containers (plastic) – dry offset, hot die stamping, screen, pad printing, ink jet, laser.
3   Smooth permeable surface for high quality printing – use letterpress, litho or gravure.
4   Rough permeable surface – litho best then perhaps gravure, but expensive.

Pretreatment

Certain surfaces require some form of pretreatment prior to printing. Foil usually requires primer wash, and polyethylenes and polypropylenes need to have the surface oxidised. The corona process is almost invariably used for films and flame treatment for bottles. Whether a surface has received treatment or not can be detected by immersing it in water and observing whether or not the water runs off. An oxidised surface has a lower wetting angle. If the surface is not printed soon after treatment another treatment may be necessary. Inks will not 'key' onto non-oxidised PE and PP and will be removed when a self-adhesive tape test is employed.

A more sophisticated peel test can be used to check the degree of surface treatment, and a suitable procedure is detailed in BS 2782 method 310. Another wetting test uses a dye in nitroethane which will remain as an intact film for up to 30 s with a treated material. A non-treated surface will show coalescence and form globules rapidly once the item is removed from the test solution.

Print adhesion

Print adhesion on plastics (and foil) is normally checked using a self-adhesive tape peel test. A few inches of a suitable standard tape is firmly pressed onto the print area then pulled off, slowly at first, then more rapidly. An assessment of print adhesion can be made from the quantity (ideally none) removed. Adhesion can vary according to the type and colour of the ink, the degree of pretreatment, the surface involved and the printing process, etc. In order to test print under likely use conditions, product immersion tests may be necessary: 60°C (140°F) is a frequently used condition, for 3 to 6 h. If product–pack may be used with soapy hands, a solution of soap can be employed. A print adhesion test, as above, can then be carried out, on the washed material, after it has been cooled to room temperature.

Application of ink and ink drying methods:

1   Absorption offers rapid drying but poor rub resistance.
2   Oxidation dries slowly – gives good rub resistance and good gloss if required.

3 Evaporation – rapid drying, possible solvent troubles (toxicity, fire risk, cost, safety).
4 Precipitation – poor rub resistance but almost odourless.

Note that UV inks can provide a high gloss.

Method of feed (i.e. reel-fed or cut sheet)

Reel – flexo, gravure, letterpress, litho. Note that a reel-fed machine using sheet form offers approximately 50% output of reel.

Rub resistance

If colour is very strong, litho in thin layers is not so rub-resistant as letterpress because of low varnish level. Note that rub resistance and brightness can usually be improved by the addition of over-lacquers or varnishes (based on shellac (spirit), nitrocellulose, Saran, vinyl, epoxy, water varnishes, etc.) or lamination (cellulose acetate, polypropylene, PVC, etc.). Coatings or laminations may also provide heat sealability.

Printing technology has made great advances over the past 15 years, with sheet speeds up to 15,000 per hour and reel-fed or cylinder models making up to 60,000 revolutions per hour. Computer controlled LED equipment has improved registration and colour control and reduced wastage, as well as increasing output and reducing make-ready times. Table 16.2 gives a comparison of the various processes.

Although decoration of paper and board is well covered by the literature, general understanding of the wider issues involved with 'other' materials has frequently been poor. This particularly applies when artwork is produced which although reproducible on paper or board, is unsatisfactory in terms of the printing/decoration processes available for another material.

It is also usual practice first to produce a design on paper or board then to endeavour to achieve a 'match' with other materials, when it would be somewhat easier to do the reverse. Matching of finished items is always difficult due to additional factors related to shape, surface finish, size, viewing/lighting conditions, etc.

Special considerations – pharmaceutical and cosmetics

Both pharmaceuticals and cosmetic packaging demand a high standard of decoration, with integrity, clarity and permanency. Colours in the form of dyes, pigments, inks, etc., must be non-toxic, non-irritant, fade- and/or discolouration-resistant, product-resistant and rub-resistant. In short, the highest quality standards are demanded in terms of visual appearance, functional usage, and safety. Although safety standards related to food substances may appear to be adequate, additional tests may be necessary as the 3–5 year shelf life required of a pharmaceutical pack may be considerably longer. Increased 'contact' time may therefore give rise to adverse effects associated with migration, interactions, absorption, adsorption, etc.

Although design and decoration are closely associated, wording requirements, particularly in pharmaceuticals, may be directly related to legislation. The gradual increase in the requirements related to the latter is leading to some concern, as the

Table 16.2 General comparisons (rough 1996 prices; IPH, items per hour)

	Letterpress	Litho	Flexo	Gravure	Screen
First costs including plates (per colour)	Low to medium £200–250	Medium £250–300	Medium £150–200	High £1,000	Low £60–100
Make ready	Medium	Low	Medium	High	Low
Production speed	1,500–2,000 IPH	500–2000 ft/min 1,500–45,000 IPH	500–2000 ft/min Up to 35,000 IPH	500–2600 ft/min Up to 35,000 IPH	Up to 6,000 IPH
Print quality (paper) Good material	High	High	Medium/high	High	High (design limitations)
Poor material	Low	Medium	Medium/low	Medium	High
Plate life	Medium to long	Long	Medium	Long	Short

The above provides only a very general comparison. For instance, costs/plate life will relate to the type of plate produced.

original concept that a pharmaceutical product should readily be identified is gradually being lost. Although colour has widely been used to differentiate products, or to provide association with a family series, it is generally not advised as a means of identifying different strengths of dosage form as in these circumstances there is no substitute for reading. The advent of coding systems, such as electronic bar codes and universal product codes (UPC/ANA/EAN etc.), must considerably improve product security, but again space to segregate these from the rest of the wording/design is not always easily found. Similarly, different printing processes have varying restrictions in terms of the amount of wording/colour which can be employed and the sharpness/clarity of print and the bar-type codings.

Decoration or aesthetic appeal obviously have different functions to perform between ethical and OTC pharmaceuticals. However, in the case of pharmaceuticals, functional and aesthetic appeal frequently become segregated, with the functional aspects receiving early attention, and the final aesthetic stages are not fully investigated and may be overlooked.

To conclude, thorough knowledge of all the decorative processes is essential for the packaging technologist who deals with both pharmaceuticals and cosmetics, as he or she must be capable of advising on all aspects related to aesthetic and functional design, plus safety. A day or so in the design/artwork and plate-making section of companies printing by the various processes will frequently convey more background knowledge than either a lecture or a textbook.

Finally, remember that printing has been recognised as a relatively 'dirty' process in the past. The industry is now attempting to 'clean it up'.

Recent trends

The introduction of computers has revolutionised print technology from origination, preparation of artwork, production of plates, on machine register and colour control, plate change-over, machine make ready, etc.

Desktop publishing (DTP) and digital art work and reproduction (DAR) are shortening publishing times, improving general quality and reducing origination times. Although this in many instances leads to some increased costs, subsequent downtime, wastage, etc. can be drastically reduced.

The new technology can be applied to both large-scale and small-scale production. In the latter case this is particularly relevant in the office and the production of special labels such as those used for clinical trial supplies.

Office printing

Earlier days saw limitations to office printing where stencils, typewriter (initially with a dampening pad, then a ribbon, a golf ball, etc.), and inked rubber pad were widely used. However, small-scale or office printing can now be achieved by a range of processes, i.e.

- photocopiers, based on an electrophotographic process
- laser printers (note: this is not burning out)
- LED (light emitting diode) printing

- ink jet printers
- colour copying
- dot matrix printers
- ion deposition
- direct thermal printing (usually as used on a fax)
- thermal transfer printing
- magnetography.

Virtually any of the above can be computer (or wordprocessor) led. Some of the above have been developed on a larger scale (magnetography) or find special usage (laser printing of proofs etc.). Other newer processes include the waterless version of offset lithography which uses special plates which accept ink on the print area without passing through a prior damping stage. These plates are more expensive than conventional wet/dry lithographic plates.

Printing inks may themselves be a source of contamination, particularly when based on solvents or oils. This risk usually lessens when water-based inks are employed (a current trend). As printing (and decoration) is a basic part of pharmaceutical packaging, knowledge of the processes and materials involved is essential if risks from these are to be avoided. As with the law, ignorance is not a viable excuse if problems arise.

Printing and printing inks

Printing inks vary in their composition and drying processes employed, according to the substrate and the printing process involved. Irrespective of the process, inks are usually at one stage 'wet' or mobile, even if at the later stage a 'dry' transfer (e.g. hot die stamping) is involved. Inks may vary in composition according to the process and the substrate, which may or may not be modified or pretreated in order to give a good ink key. Inks may be made to flow by the use of water, oils, or solvents. The last of these frequently falls under the UK Regulations, Control of Substances Hazardous to Health (COSHH) and prior to these The Health and Safely at Work Act (1974).

Solvent-based inks

Gravure acid flexographic inks have been conventionally based on solvents, particularly as the materials printed by these processes have typically been non-absorbent (i.e. foil, plastics). Solvents which are considered hazardous if inhaled include benzene, methanol, methyl and ethyl cellulose, hence these are no longer employed. A typical solvent based ink contains:

- 4–12% pigment or dye
- 0–8% extender
- 10–30% resin binder
- 2–10% additives
- 40–60% solvents.

This ink may be further diluted prior to use to give over 70% solvent. This solvent is lost via evaporation and drying. The solvents used include alcohols, esters, aliphatic hydrocarbons and glycol ethers, with a limited use of ketones and aromatic hydrocarbons. To prevent the venting of solvents direct into the atmosphere, solvent recovery or incineration systems may be used. Alternatively, water-based inks are being increasingly employed, possibly coupled to UV drying. However, even water-based inks may contain up to 15% of solvent, e.g. methylated spirit or isopropyl alcohol, and take more energy to dry (due to the high heat of evaporation of water).

Foils frequently use a wash coating of $0.5–2 \text{ g/m}^2$ as a print substrate. This may be a shellac, nitrocellulose or vinyl solution. Since many foil-based materials are heat sealed and foil is a good conductor of heat, most printing inks need to exclude light levels of wax and low melting point resins in order to avoid ink lift or pick.

Oil-based inks

As detailed earlier, offset lithographic printing operates on the principle that oil and water do not mix. With paper-based materials, conventional inks usually dry by oxidation and absorption. Early screen inks were also based on oil, drying by oxidation. These were used to achieve a thick film of 20–30 μm. Thinner inks were obtained by the use of non-nitrated cellulose derivatives, modified resins and white spirit. Ultra-thin film inks were subsequently introduced which gave films between 5 and 10 μm, thereby enabling the use of half-tone images.

Early oil-based inks were based on linseed and tung oils. Ink drying was speeded up by the use of cobalt driers (also manganese and lead), followed by high boiling hydrocarbons which allowed the introduction of quicker setting inks.

Heat setting inks

These were initially produced for higher speed rotary letterpress printing using inks based on synthetic resins in high boiling point hydrocarbon solvents which are rapidly dried with heated rollers. Heat set inks are still widely used for web printing and involve newer resin and solvent systems.

The growth in the use of synthetic resins and the variety and purity of solvents have allowed the use of many other drying processes: UV, IR, microwave, electron beam curing, etc.

UV curing inks frequently consist of 100% solids with no solvents (as used by screen processes). Since the use of UV creates some hazards (direct contact with UV and ozone residues), special equipment and precautionary procedures are essential.

Water-based inks

The risks associated with the use of solvents (toxicity, irritancy, flammability, etc.) and the costs of solvent control (e.g. extraction or incineration) have encouraged the development of water-based inks. Since water is a poor solvent for most synthetic resins, emulsions and dispersions have been developed. Water-based inks are used for gravure, flexography, screen and letterpress processes.

Conclusions

Inks, like rubber and plastic, need pigments or dyes as colouring agents, and several types of 'additive' to provide certain selected properties. The other main component is a carrier which may be based on oil, water or solvents, together with various synthetic resins.

The additives include slow or fast reducers, driers, retarders, varnishers, waxes, slip additives, stabilisers, etc., which may be specific to a particular printing process and the drying process associated with it.

17

PRESENT AND FUTURE TRENDS

D. A. Dean

Introduction

Before looking at present and future developments in the packaging of pharmaceuticals, some historical background in terms of products and packs may prove useful. Although certain product forms have existed for centuries, to some it may be difficult to envisage even 50 years ago when the majority of OTC and dispensed products were liquids, usually of a none too pleasant taste, and presented in glass bottles closed with corks. Today solid dosages are the major product form, coupled to a more scientific approach to medication where consideration is given to compliance, bioavailability, dissolution, disintegration, bioburden, mode of delivery, impurities from process residues and degradation, purity, etc. Having been brought up initially on the BP 1932, where purities of 90–100% seemed quite acceptable, it is amazing that one failed 50 years ago to ask the obvious question: what is this other, up to 10%? Today, although we place no less emphasis on purity, we concentrate on identifying the impurities or degradation products to establish that they are both acceptable and safe. In parallel with this change in attitude towards products, there have been significant changes in pharmaceutical packaging. Now there is a highly intense form of investigation where marketing, medical and technical knowledge are brought together to establish the best pack. This 'best pack' is inevitably a compromise of many factors, i.e. how does one balance the need for child-resistance, tamper-resistance, etc. with an increasingly elderly population who survive by their regular medication?

Having set a base line for some 50 years ago, what was the state of packaging art up to yesteryear? Glass and corks were supported by metal cans and tins, metal screw caps, thermoset caps, paperboard boxes and cartons, glassine and waxed papers, composite paper board containers, glass ampoules and cartridge tubes, collapsible metal tubes and the Aspro waxed paper strip.

Real awareness of packaging did not start until after the Second World War, and this intensified somewhat when thermoplastics entered the scene around about 1953. About the same time foil strip packs appeared, followed by pharmaceutical aerosols and squeezepacks, blisters in the early 1960s, pumps in the 1970s, child-resistance in the mid-1970s, elderly patient packs in the early 1980s, to mention a few packaging highlights.

The revolution that has taken place in the allegedly conservative pharmaceutical industry has resulted in greater attention to detail, with high spending on R&D functions in order that product safety aspects are fully covered. Lead times from drug discovery in research to product launch have therefore substantially increased. More sophisticated synthetic products (there were very few in 1938 when most drugs were of vegetable, plant or animal origin) have demanded more and more attention to packaging detail. Thus, although packaging can be described under a definition which equally applies to other packaged products, the emphasis on certain selected pharmaceutical aspects is continuously changing. This initial definition required that packaging should economically provide protection, presentation, identification, information, containment, convenience, compliance and confidence for a product during storage, distribution, display and ultimate use.

The shelf life is the period during which the product remains acceptable in terms of safety, efficacy, conformity and uniformity of content, reproducibility and product liability, with pharmaceutical elegance and acceptable quality.

Since 'standards' associated with the above rarely stand still, upgrading rather than downgrading is an inevitable trend. Under the broad heading of safety, tighter control and/or standards are continually being considered for:

- product–pack security and integrity
- Interaction or migratory exchanges between product and pack
- tamper-evidence, tamper-resistance, child-resistance, child safety, etc.
- dosage delivery etc.

All packs are a compromise, and finding the right compromise is increasingly difficult as the factors which need consideration steadily increase. This is accompanied by expanding facets of control, i.e. by GMP (good manufacturing practice), which start at product inception, through development, scale-up, manufacturing, packing, warehousing, distribution, sale/dispensing, use, to final disposal of the product and pack.

To meet these demands requires both improved knowledge and a more critical approach to all activities and operations, including packaging.

Present and future trends

These include improving required standards by both the pharmaceutical industry and those companies supplying the industry. This will be reflected in more sophisticated specifications, tighter specifications and the overall stricter control of packaging materials, manufacturing processes and the containers, components, materials which are produced.

Compared with other products, i.e. food, confectionery, beverages, etc., pharmaceuticals are a relatively small user of packaging materials, hence the industry is low in purchasing power. In response to the demand for higher standards, specialist and dedicated suppliers are emerging which give the required quality and security at a premium price. In the case of machinery, specialist machines are built, but often new technology for the food or beverage industry is modified after it has been established, to suit the needs of the pharmaceutical industry.

Changing process trends and changing technology, therefore, tend to follow other established practices but the level of expertise ultimately required by the pharmaceutical packaging technologist is second to none.

Broad policies established via the government, trade associations and the

Pharmaceutical Society can have a significant influence on industry. Recent UK policies include the OPD (patient packs) revolution, and the introduction of an ethicals blacklist which has moved certain products into a successful OTC category, and which has also been encouraged by the 'See your pharmacist first' campaign. In terms of product trends, there has been a significant growth in packs which aid product administration, packs which act as devices and can be used in devices.

Packaging of pharmaceuticals has been slowly moving away from glass to plastic and is likely, in the long term, to use more combinations of materials. One must, however, remain aware of the environmentalists who see packaging as waste in the dustbin, with criticism of the poor total use of materials and energy. Reuse, recycling, conservation of energy with minimal pollution risks, are becoming well recognised phrases. The professional packaging technologist must therefore be aware of these issues and keep up to date on the activities and responses of the big packaging material users to these ever increasing environmentalist pressures.

Finally, among these broad trends there is the confusing picture caused by cheaper parallel imports. Preventing such imports conflicts with the Treaty of Rome, but it does seem reasonable that a pack should use English text, particularly now that OPD advises the inclusion of user friendly leaflets to better inform the patients.

In the UK, pharmaceutical exports contribute over £5,000 million (1997) to the country's revenue, and there is still an expanding demand on a worldwide basis. However, this is currently being offset by a steady increase in imports. This growth industry, although expanding in total, could reduce in the UK in the next 5–15 years as many countries are now well advanced in setting up local pharmaceutical manufacture, using expert support from the UK, the rest of Europe, Japan and the USA. The expertise created in the so-called developed countries is an essential factor for the success of less developed ones setting up new industries. One difficulty is to decide the standards to which they should operate, since in many instances one is facing not just a 50 year technology gap but one of 100 years.

Some of the major influences will therefore be discussed under a number of headings, i.e.

- product trends influencing pack trends
- changes and trends in packaging materials
- changes in packaging processes
- other special considerations.

Product trends influencing pack trends

As previously identified, the swing from liquid or semi-liquid dosage forms to the solid dosage form is ongoing. This does not mean that liquid products will disappear, as they are still essential for young children and the increasing elderly population, who either cannot swallow a tablet or capsule or are concerned that it may have a 'choking' risk. Paediatric products are, however, changing as emphasis is placed on sugar free (for the prevention of dental caries), freedom from synthetic colourings, which allegedly cause allergies, freedom from synthetic flavourings, the elimination of alcohol, and the avoidance of preservatives which may also give rise to adverse sensitising effects. This trend may slow down at some time, since materials of natural origin are not always free from adverse reactions.

Liquid products are still very popular with many OTC products, so perhaps the apparent inconvenience of measuring it out actually helps to remind the user that a dose should be taken.

Liquids are still an essential form for injectable products both as multidose and unit dose presentations. Unit dose injections which can eliminate the need for a preservative are increasingly preferred. One can therefore predict a steady trend in growth with cartridge tubes, disposable syringes and prefilled syringes. Prefilled syringes include both the single compartmental and the bicompartmental type of syringe, which is useful where the mixing of components, immediately prior to injection, has certain distinct advantages (e.g. due to shelf-life restrictions). In the area of IV solutions there has already been a significant trend away from glass, coupled with a need for administering an increasing number of additives. Prepacked additives with a means of transferring them to IV solutions by injection or via IV pack ports will therefore increase.

Although glass has been holding its own in terms of vials, ampoules, cartridges, tubes, one can predict increasing competition to the tubular glass industry which to date has not suffered in the same way as blown glass containers. Plastic ampoules produced on blow fill seal equipment are gaining in popularity, as are vials which resist breakage, especially for expensive biotechnology products.

Plastic is currently having considerable success with unit dose liquid products, i.e. ear, eye, nasal products, as an addition to the multidose products market which it captured from glass some 25–35 years ago. The unit dose products are usually presented in sticks as either preformed units which are filled and sealed aseptically, or as a form fill seal process such as the Rommelag (Bottlepack) or ALP (USA) blow, fill, seal system. Increasing competition between preformed units and form fill sealed units can obviously be predicted, with emphasis on cleanliness (freedom from particulates), high sterility, confidence/credibility and cost. Unit dose systems without preservatives appear to offer advantages over preserved systems (in fact some consider that 'unit dose' should be synonymous with the absence of a preservative system), but have to be balanced against disadvantages involving higher costs per dose plus greater storage volumes.

Although a few oral products are also emerging in unit dose packs, particularly where the absence of any preservative offers advantages (food allergy conditions), expansion in this area is likely to be limited. For multidose liquid products (oral liquids, emulsions, suspensions, local applications, etc.), plastic continues to make inroads on glass. Whereas it has been relatively easy to find suitable plastics using opaque containers (HDPE, PP, etc.), the clarity and sparkle of glass has been difficult to match economically. Although it has been accepted that no one plastic can offer the inertness of glass, particularly with reference to retention of certain preservatives, flavours and active ingredients, it is relatively easy to find a plastic which is suitable for a specific product – albeit occasionally with a slightly reduced shelf life. Under this category various grades of PETP and PETG (polyester variants) are steadily growing in use. Since under normal handling polyester is much less prone to breakage and is lighter than glass, any cost premium can be readily offset. Polyesters generally show good retention of such volatile substances as menthol, camphor, esters of salicylic acid. Coated and multi-layer plastic containers offer further potential usage for liquid products. Silicon dioxide ('glass') coated plastics are also of interest (SiO_x coatings). These are being closely followed by carbon 'diamond-like' coatings.

Solid dose medication

The past 20 years has seen continuous growth of the hard gelatin capsule. However, the 1982 Tylenol incidents in the USA identified the ease with which capsules could be tampered with, and caused a severe setback for capsule usage in the USA. The discovery of more potent synthetic drugs has also meant that tablets (and capsules) have become smaller. Film coating has partly replaced the use of thicker sugar coatings. Controlled, delayed and sustained release forms have further reduced the occupancy volume for many new products and the frequency of administration. If one adds to this the growing influence of OPD (original pack dispensing), then there is a trend and a need for smaller packs for solid dose forms both now and in the future.

Other medicinal products which influence packaging trends

Although 'targeting of drugs' is a popular phrase, certain newer drug forms are clearly targeted to or via specific areas. These include a whole group of drugs that use the lung and are presented in a fine particle liquid or powder. In these instances the pack may act as a device (e.g. a metered dose powder aerosol), or a separate device may be used, e.g. Spinhaler (Intal), Rotahaler (Ventolin), Diskhaler (Ventodisk), etc.

Dermal patches are another new trend that challenges ingenuity in terms of the material used for the patch and the packaging. In fact it is interesting to note that the theory adopted by the dermal patch, i.e. a drug is incorporated in a polymer matrix from which it diffuses out at a steady rate to penetrate (permeate) the skin, is the converse of that which is normally required for a plastic pack, where no exchange between product and pack is desired.

Growth in biologicals and diagnostic agents are also putting new demands on the pack, especially where $-70°C$ is used.

Changes and trends in packaging materials

As changes to packaging materials occur relatively slowly, the materials which might be considered of historical value are still in wide usage. This particularly applies to the use of glass and metal, which extends back over several centuries.

A slight reduction in the use of glass has occurred in recent years, and it is likely that this will continue as a slow downward trend. However, glass is generally seen as environmentally friendly, hence this trend could reverse.

Metal containers are showing a much more serious usage drop in terms of containers for tablets and capsules, ointments, granules, powders, etc., and even survival as collapsible metal tubes is doubtful with the advent of laminated tubes. Rigid aluminium containers, other than aerosol containers, showed a rapid drop in usage some 8–10 years ago, when costs, compared with glass and plastic, became unfavourable. The conversion of bauxite to aluminium involves high energy levels. This means that aluminium is top of the recovery list in terms of the widely used packaging materials with a value of £600 to £700 per tonne when recycled (cf. glass £45–55 per tonne).

Composite containers involving laminations to board with metal or plastic ends are surviving to a degree, but use will undoubtedly be limited to a few mainly OTC types of product and possibly a growing healthcare/healthfood market. Lined carton systems incorporating foil compete with composites for similar markets.

The basic materials cited above being on the decline, the reverse can be expected for the remaining basic materials, i.e. plastic, paper and board, and films, foils and laminates.

Paper and board are likely to increase due to an expanding label market (greater quantities of smaller pack sizes) and their associated need for cartons (to give sufficient label area) for OPD products. The latter point is a contentious issue and the debate on where the community pharmacist should place the label will continue. However, if a bar code is essential (and possible) with smaller pack sizes, a carton may be the only way to combine an adequate surface area and a means of collating a patient leaflet.

Films, foils and laminates, including coextrusions and metallisation

Although OPD is not synonymous with the use of blisters and strip packs, and products will be found in small glass and plastic containers, the unit type of pack offers possible advantages, especially when the item and quantity, occupies a relatively small volume. Films and combinations of films, foils and paper as laminations, together with metallised substrates, coatings and coextrudates, etc., will all be part of an overall growth. This growth will not be related solely to thermoformed and cold formed blisters, but also to strips, sachets, overwraps, etc. and growth of shrink and stretch materials in the form of secondary packaging for warehousing and transportation. Again this may conflict with some environmental factors where composite or compound materials are difficult to recycle or reuse.

Metallisation (coatings of aluminium/oxide), which is more effective as a barrier when two materials are metallised and then laminated with the two metallised surfaces in contact, is likely to provide a better barrier than most plastic combinations (even Aclar–PVC). However, for an excellent barrier, foil of 0.025 mm and above will continue to be a popular choice as, provided the heat sealing is effective, a hermetic pack can be achieved. Lower gauges of foil down to 0.006 mm when part of a lamination incorporating a plastic ply or plastic plies also provide a high degree of protection against moisture, oxygen, carbon dioxide, etc. Although such a construction inevitably contains small pinholes, permeation through these is extremely low provided the foil layer is not stretched and/or perforated during machine handling and sealing.

Coextrusion, e.g. a process incorporating two or more plies of a plastic, will undoubtedly find more use in flexible pharmaceutical packs. Coextrudates can also be moulded into rigid containers, bottles, tubes, tubs, etc. subject to the quantities justifying the costs.

It is with some regret that in discussing plastics, one has to again admit that the glass–metal era is now in decline. In fact it can be positively stated that in the introduction of any new product, plastic now receives first consideration. Glass is frequently still used as a control in any test procedure, perhaps as a mark of respect for a material which has served the pharmaceutical industry with honour.

The history of plastics dates back to the mid nineteenth century when celluloid and Bakelite were discovered. Bakelite (phenol formaldehyde) and urea formaldehyde, both thermosetting plastics, found wide use in the pharmaceutical industry in the form of screw closures and are still used today. Although recognised as plastics, the thermosets play only a minor role as a packaging material and it was not until around 1953 onwards, when the first thermoplastics were used as low density polythene squeezee packs, that the real plastic revolution began. In 1996 five, in fact the most economical five, were the ones most widely used. These include the:

- polyethylenes (PE) – LDPE, MDPE, HDPE, LLDPE, ULDPE, VLDPE
- polypropylenes (PP) – homopolymers and copolymers of polypropylene
- polystyrenes (PS) – crystal and to some extent impact modified polystyrene
- polyvinylchlorides – unplasticised PVC and plasticised PVC
- polyesters – PETP and PETG.

These materials cover a wide range of properties, e.g. a range of densities 0.9–1.45, are clear to very hazy, hard, brittle to flexible, some virtually unbreakable; from highly permeable to ones of low permeability (with reference to moisture, gases, solvents, etc.), relatively inert to only fair inertness, etc., and all cost in the region of £700–800 per metric tonne (except PET at around £1,100 per tonne).

Changes in packaging processes

In the past 25 years there have many progressive changes in packaging processes, and several significant improvements are detailed below.

Form fill seal processes for liquids and semi-liquids

The Bottlepack system (Rommelag, Germany) and a similar process by Automatic Liquid Packaging (USA) – blow fill seal – continue to be successfully used for pharmaceutical products. These processes are now found throughout the world and container manufacturing details are covered in previous chapters.

In use they usually operate in a clean area but also with a laminar flow type hood over the moulding–filling stations. With these precautions the unit can produce sterile non-preserved products. Output largely depends on the pack size, but with a 10×2 ml stick the Rommelag 3012, 305 and 4010 M machines have outputs of approx. 4,000, 8,000 and 20,000 singles per hour. The machines also offer the advantages of very low particulate levels. ALP has a 301 and a 303–624 with six parisons coming from a single extruder giving 24 moulds. Special machines can also insert sterile components, e.g. rubber stoppers. Machines can handle PE, PP, PVC, PET, etc.

Container cleanliness

Many years ago it was common practice to store glass containers in crates out in the open. Washing was an essential prerequisite prior to use, but today producing containers and components clean in terms of both bioburden and particulates and then keeping them clean by effective handling is rapidly becoming the norm. This is now common practice in both the glass and plastic industries and, with a few exceptions (sterile and aseptic packaging operations), washing is now rarely used. (Note that rubber stoppers are normally washed (and siliconised) at the supply source.)

Faster strip and blister packaging

Filling via slat counters into bulk packs brought speed capabilities in excess of 20,000 items (tablets and capsules) per minute, thus making small OPD type products both comparatively slow and relatively costly.

Unit dose packaging in the early years suffered from speed limitations where a maximum of 250 items per row per minute represented the best that could be achieved, i.e. the faster 4 and 8 row strip packers achieved 1,000 and 2,000 per minute (maximum) and blister packs of 8 and 12 rows, 2,000 and 3,000 per minute (maximum). Today wider webs (more rows) and higher feed speeds per row have brought about outputs of up to 7,200 in strip packs (Siebler) and over 6,000 on blister pack machines.

In addition to catering for conventional thermoformed blisters using a plastic tray and a foil-based lid, most blister machine manufacturers now offer facilities to increase moisture protection, by use of either a tropicalised blister (by an additional foil over cover) or a cold formed, foil-based tray. Considerable competition is expected between these and similar options, where a high level of climatic protection is required. The other options include blisters in sachets and overwraps to cartons. Output speeds, climatic protections achieved, overall cost and patient/marketing preference, will influence the final pack choice.

Machine efficiency has also been improved by faster change-over times (15–30 min) and trim waste has been significantly reduced.

To improve child-resistance (see BS 7236), opaque or dark tinted packs and between-pocket perforations can be employed.

Faster lines, pregauging on-line or pregauged components and tighter specifications

Years ago the pharmaceutical industry was handicapped on output speeds, cost and security by the short runs, maximum line flexibility syndrome. This has gradually changed, particularly where companies have become international or streamlining of inventories has provided larger quantities for a few companies. Small runs, however, still frequently apply to generics.

As a result of this and generally expanding sales, many companies now have dedicated lines which have moved away from 60 packs per minute to 200 to 300 packs, with better flexibility (e.g. on-line changes). High speeds have inevitably required better material control, and tighter specifications. New techniques have been introduced to negate faulty containers, components and materials either interrupting production line flow or resulting in a substandard or faulty pack emerging from the production line. These new techniques frequently involve video technology with such processes as imaging, where individual components can be matched against a standard in dimensions and the identification of imperfections. SPC is now widely applied to achieve quality improvements.

Line segregation, dedicated machines and areas, cubiclisation, cleaner areas and clean air classifications

The need for cleanliness and the trend towards producing materials clean was identified above. The onus is then on the pharmaceutical manufacturer to maintain this cleanliness throughout the packaging process. There is also a need for improvements in product security with ideally a nil risk of admixtures, incorrect labelling, etc. All these aims can be optimised by clear segregation of operations, dedicated areas, the use of cubicles, operating under positive air pressure using filtered air, with properly clothed and trained operators, etc. These factors, which are all embraced by GMP, need to be supplemented by validation procedures and total accountability, reconciliation of materials delivered to and taken away from the production area. These latter security activities may be further improved by prior label scanning/ reading with a possible repeat operation on a production line using such processes as 'imaging'. However, sophisticated equipment of this nature not only is expensive but requires more frequent validation. End of line inspections are therefore receiving increased attention, as are 'isolation' units for sterile/aseptic packs.

Packs and devices

In introducing product trends which could influence the pack, drug targeting was identified as an important factor. In this targeting activity, packs can be identified with an administration role or packs may be tailored to more readily fit an actual device (see Appendix 17.1).

Examples of this include metered dose pump systems, which to some extent are replacing the well-established nasal squeezee pack.

Powder inhalation devices are currently proving very popular, in spite of the fact that patients generally prefer metered dose aerosols. However, this preference is counterbalanced by the fact that compliance is much more difficult to achieve with aerosols. There is also a third category where the pack and the device are totally independent, e.g. a unit dose of nebuliser solution which is subsequently transferred to a pressurised or an ultrasonic nebuliser unit for delivery to the patient.

Other special considerations

There are occasions when demands or considerations related to a pack conflict. This applies to some of the general observations listed below, and in certain instances an acceptable compromise may be difficult to achieve.

Tamper-evidence

The 1982 Extra Strength Tylenol incidents have had worldwide repercussions. Demands for a totally tamper-proof pack are difficult to achieve, certainly economically. Even so it is reasonable for a patient or user to expect that none of the product has been removed, substituted, diluted, contaminated, etc. Tamper-evidence is therefore both advisable and justifiable for pharmaceutical products provided the recipients do not expect it to safeguard them against the ingenious adulterator out to do mischief against 'life and limb'. However, the pharmaceutical company should not be liable provided reasonable steps have been taken to safeguard the patient under normal conditions. Freak conditions, as created by the maniac, are virtually impossible to safeguard against and prevent. The use of the word 'tamper-proof' is therefore not advised, but 'tamper-evident' and 'tamper-resistant' are accepted expressions.

Child-resistance

Child-resistance as such must receive everyone's support. However, child-resistance can frustrate the elderly, infirm, poor of sight, aged, arthritic, to a point where the product is transferred to an alternative (unsuitable!) pack, or the closure is never adequately replaced. There is therefore a need to recognise these problems in a growing elderly community and to find an acceptable solution. Effective answers to this, have to date, been complex and expensive.

It should be noted that the guidelines issued by the (UK) Pharmaceutical Society and the Association of British Pharmaceutical Industries (ABPI) on OPD indicate that packs should be both tamper-evident and child-resistant.

Security coding

There are many ways in which packed products can be security coded: edge slits, coloured edges, printed edges, punched hole codes, bar codes, colour bar codes, ink jet codes, laser codes, just to mention a few. Most manufacturers operate to some coding system which frequently adds to the total 'wording' complexities. Although bar codes plus scanning or imaging appears the simplest long-term answer, on-costs will play a significant part in any ultimate decision or solution.

Labelling – self-adhesive labels

Although 10 years ago the US pharmaceutical industry predominantly used heat seal labels, the UK was rapidly moving to the more expensive self-adhesive labelling systems. Since Europe is now predominantly using self-adhesive, there appears to be an international trend even though it is a more expensive label process. It has the advantage, with the correct choice of materials, that it will adhere to most substrates.

Lower microbial limits and lower particulates

The need for higher standards of cleanliness and hygiene has already been mentioned. Since the safety factors for aseptic processes and terminal sterilisation processes rely on a low initial bioburden, attempts will continue to minimise contamination. Packaging manufacturers of materials, components and containers will therefore slowly adopt GMP procedures currently found as part of the 'Orange Guide' in order to lower both bioburden and particulates. Cleanliness and improved hygiene are an order of the day, in terms of facilities, procedures and training.

Sterilisation methods

Although sterilisation methods may initially appear to be well documented, there is a need to review how each may change both the physical and chemical properties of packaging materials, containers and components.

This entails residues related to ethylene oxide sterilisation, and physical and chemical changes when gamma irradiation or accelerated electrons are employed, particularly when plastics are involved. It should be noted that plastics include lacquers, enamels, certain adhesives, etc. Surface analysis is emerging as a critical evaluation for any 'treatment' process. The need to establish the purity/impurity of packaging materials will also become necessary for most sterile products.

The need for cartoning, leaflets and packaging inserts

The USA, which is not OPD-oriented, has during the past 10–15 years moved away from the use of cartons, and leaflets have been attached to the primary pack by banding or adhesives. Although these means of attaching leaflets are available in the UK and the rest of Europe, the greater use of blister and strip pack and reluctance to change tradition should retain the carton for at least the next 5–10 years. If the move to OPD is accelerated, then a substantial growth in the use of cartons and patient (information) leaflets can be predicted. This will mean extra business for specialised printing industries, which have the security/GMP aspects of pharmaceuticals well covered.

Batch and expiry dating

Batch coding is not new, but expiry dating is essential for virtually all forms of pharmaceutical packs. However, when and where this is printed will be an interesting topic, with ink jet printing and possibly laser printing being some of the main contenders for an on-line production operation. Laser printing, which burns off colour/printing/decoration, should be coupled to vacuum extraction for safety reasons. The legibility/clarity of debossing and embossing codes is constantly being criticised.

In-house printing

It has already been mentioned that many pharmaceutical companies serve an international industry, thereby contributing to the balance of import/export payments. Since exports frequently demand different print layouts, and one or more languages in the text, there have always been problems associated with small print runs. In-house printing is expected to increase either as a separate printing operation away from the production line or as an on-production line process. Although several printing processes can be employed, hot die stamping and thermal printing, which gives good quality print, quick drying and reasonable freedom from rub and smudging, is currently leading the field. Letterpress, direct and offset, and flexographic printing are also employed. The advent of DAR (digital artwork and reproduction) is making a major contribution to faster origination.

Bar coding

Bar coding, coupled to scanning and the use of computerised data/record keeping, can serve several purposes from security aspects, stock keeping and accountancy to data retrieval (i.e. product information etc). With products which are sold via various outlets (community pharmacies etc.), the EAN or ANA code is an obvious choice. This is, however, frequently used in addition to the PIP code which was introduced by the National Pharmaceutical Association (NPA) some 20 years ago. The EAN code suffers certain weaknesses if it is to form part of a security code, and this problem may be resolved by better reading equipment or the introduction of a more user friendly code system. Coding therefore remains a highly debatable topic, with little chance of standardisation immediately in sight.

Computer dispensing and costing

The OPD guidelines have requested the use of the EAN code for stock control (hospitals and retail) and as a simplification for the UK Pricing Bureau where a peelable code is transferred to the prescription (form FP 10) for pricing and reimbursement to the dispensing pharmacist. The fact that other European countries have used a similar system (e.g. the Vignette, France) which was introduced many years ago does not necessarily mean that it is ideal for tomorrow's technology. Rapidly expanding computer technology could therefore bridge the gap and benefit the doctor and community pharmacist, by use of electronic transfer systems.

Original pack dispensing (OPD) (now termed 'patient packs')

In any attempt to discuss future trends there must be at least a few comments on this subject. Guidelines have been agreed between the Pharmaceutical Society and the ABPI, but the most contentious issue still derives from the 7 versus 10 common denominator for solid dosage forms. Argument has been put forward for the preference of multiples of 7 (7 day week), 4 week (28 day/month etc.) whereas other parts of Europe are based on 10s. Since multiples of 10 appear more prevalent in Europe, why do we have such an insistence that UK OPD can only relate to a unit of 7? Having a pack size suitable to take a label measuring 70 × 35 mm also causes problems, particularly as tablet/capsule sizes get smaller and fewer doses are needed per day with delayed and sustained release products. Of course there are ways of achieving an area of 70 × 35 mm, i.e. use blisters or strips in cartons or prohibit the use of container sizes below, say, a 40 or 50 ml capacity. Australia achieved this through a minimum pack size of 35 ml. This could, on some occasions, find seven tablets of small dimensions occupying only, say, 5–10% of the container volume. This raises questions as to whether it be filled with cotton wool, and whether the high space to volume changes product stability aspects, etc.

Although there are other, less contentious issues, the proposed changes inevitably introduce on-costs to the pharmaceutical industry, the wholesaler (initial costs have been given) and possibly the community pharmacist.

Controlled dosage systems (also called monitored dosage systems)

Controlled dosage systems are basically aimed at use by the elderly, infirm, or partly infirm, poor of sight, arthritic, as an aid to improving medication compliance. Doses or dosages of medication are enclosed in individual sealed compartments on a card, or in multiple blister packs, usually with a medication identity code (heart tablets, water tablets, etc.) together with clearly written instructions as to when each medication should be taken (day 1, 2, 3, etc. plus times, e.g. morning, afternoon, evening). These systems, of which there are now many, are already operating in the USA, Canada, Australia, Holland, and other places. However, they somewhat cut across OPD philosphies, particularly if a country is 100% OPD, since the quantities prescribed have to be transferred from bulk to the system which is then labelled or printed with the directions, solid medication codes, patient's name, etc.

The recent successes with these systems indicate that they should increase in use, subject to costs being acceptable.

Conclusions

It is evident that no pack is perfect or ideal (some are undoubtedly better than others), hence all packs are a compromise involving consideration of many factors – some of which are conflicting. The number of factors which need this consideration constantly increases.

Packaging has now come of age and packaging expertise, combined with packaging technology, should receive the highest respect. This is essential if the most effective compromise is to be reached between those involved with such decisions, e.g. marketing, medical, production, regulatory. For this purpose a packaging co-ordinator who provides an overview is becoming increasingly essential.

GMP is not simply the 'Orange Guide' and the interpretation of it, but ongoing improvements in pharmaceutical quality. This means more control over the total packaging function and a greater use of computerised data, records and information.

The packaging technologist must remain aware of the environmental issues, not because pharmaceuticals are a large user compared with food, beverages, household items, etc. but because it is known to be a caring and responsible industry – hence it could be prone to attack. This risk is increased by the fact that many companies use 'care' titles, e.g. healthcare, skin care.

Pharmaceutical packaging is very intense and the clearance of the primary pack (the packaging components in contact with the product) involves in-depth knowledge of product and packaging materials, including highly sophisticated testing procedures. Changes to the primary pack are therefore expensive. As the industry often over-packs in terms of the secondary packaging which covers warehousing and distribution, this is one area where cost savings can be achieved, without re-submission of data. Materials, space utilisation and handling methods, when studied together with computerised records, should therefore warrant investigation as this has until recently been a neglected area in the packaging chain.

Thus if we repeat the initial definition of packaging – 'Packaging is the means of economically providing protection, presentation, information, identification, convenience, containment, and compliance for a product during storage, distribution, display and use' – the complexities of what this simple statement entails will now be better appreciated. In the hands of an expert, everything looks simple. Packaging is now an advanced technology where training is achieved through experience as there are few books on the topic, and even where there are they rapidly become, at least in part, out of date.

The writer would like to stress that making predictions is becoming increasingly difficult, because of general consumer pressures (i.e. a more aware and critical general public) and the environmental/ecological issues.

The USA and Japan are using more and more coextrusions and what might be termed composite materials, consisting of layers of various materials. Such materials are increasingly being criticised by the environmentalists in Europe as they are difficult to reuse or recycle (except as the scrap for the conversion process). Several years ago one would have predicted an enormous future for these composite materials, but whether they will have a future is now becoming a serious question.

There is a call for the use of single effective materials. Predictions were made for plastic coated glass and silica (glass!) coated plastics. Does this mean that the future for glass and/or plastic will change? If plastic coated glass becomes widely used, does this mean that special equipment is required to eliminate the plastic from the cullet or are expensive 'scrubbers' to be added to all glass furnaces so that the plastic can be 'burnt off' without the emission of suspect gases into the atmosphere? Does this also mean that the material used in the sophisticated versus Third World countries will become significantly different, i.e. could one predominantly use glass while the others predominantly use plastic?

Consumer pressure (other than environmental issues) are highlighting needs for higher quality, convenience in use, restriction in so-called overpackaging, the need for special packs (which are easy to open and reclose) for an increasing elderly population, etc. The last of these may conflict with child-resistance, tamper-resistance, tamper-evidence, etc. and provide even greater conflict if coupled with environmental concerns. What is the future?

Ten years ago or so the USA led the world in the removal of 'cartons', with labelling systems combining leaflets or shrink/stretch sleeving in which a leaflet could be retained. It was predicted that the rest of the world would follow the USA. Today there is a move back to cartons for a number of reasons: improved stacking, space reduction, all-around recognition, better presentation coupled to good graphics, and as a means of retaining/collating a packaging insert/leaflet.

Trends therefore tend to follow cycles, emotive issues and consumer demands, which may be logical or totally illogical.

Packaging, which was earlier company-oriented, is gradually moving through national and international trends. These trends are divided according to what can be afforded in the developed and developing worlds. At one extreme packaging can be costly, complex, and sophisticated, while at the other the key phrase is minimum cost.

The effectiveness of the treatment is now being judged by the total cost of a disease/symptom and its treatment. This involves not just the cost of the packed medication but the cost of the GP, improved (specialist) diagnosis, reduced hospitalisation, etc. A pack involving an improved mode of delivery at a higher cost may therefore be the most effective form of treatment. This is found under the broad heading of 'disease management'.

While some trends come and go, others, related to GMP/CGMP, security and integrity, intensify. This also applies to legal issues which extend as law, directives and guidelines (FDA, ICH, EU, etc.). Counterfeiting or 'pass-offs' are one of the current concerns, and no doubt this trend will result in increased technology and improved practices.

ICH guidelines which define climate conditions for formal stability tests give a greater challenge to the pack and make the assumption that prior to formal stability the pack has been thoroughly challenged. Both these put a greater responsibility on the packaging technologist in terms of the test used and the conclusions reached. Packs must therefore be better challenged using both the ICH and other conditions. The latter should include those aspects which are not effectively covered by the ICH guidelines, as packaging people were only 'indirectly' consulted when the guidelines were devised. Some of this information can be learnt from directives, and guidelines related to devices (see Appendix 17.1).

Appendix 17.1: Packaging and medical devices

In some companies packaging and medical–pharmaceutical devices share areas of development and evaluation. For example, most devices are made in plastics using injection moulded components, which have factors common to closures and certain types of container. However, directives on medical devices tend to be ahead of those on packaging, hence packaging technologists should be conversant with the directives, if only to consider whether they can or cannot be applied to packaging. The device related directives are as follows:

- Medical device directive (MDD) 93/42/EC
- Active implantable medical device directive (AIMD) 90/385/EC
- In vitro diagnostics directive (IVD).

The MDD covers four classes of device:

- Class: I Low risk devices
- Class: IIa Selected medium risk devices
- Class: IIb Selected medium risk devices
- Class: III High risk devices.

Typical Class I devices include powder delivery systems to the lungs such as the Spinhaler, Rotahaler, Diskhaler, spacers which are used in conjunction with a drug and are part of a drug submission. Typical Class IIa devices include power operated nebuliser systems which are usually sold separate to the drug.

The amount of detail for approval of the device increases from Class I to Class III. In the UK submission of data and subsequent approval is through the Medical Device Agency (MDA). Devices have to be independently assessed by MDA Notified Bodies, which on approval can issue the authorised CE mark; this allows unrestrained distribution across Europe.

INDEX